Reproductive Medicine: Role of Follicle Stimulating Hormone

Reproductive Medicine: Role of Follicle Stimulating Hormone

Editor: Jasper McIntosh

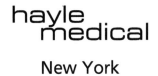

New York

Hayle Medical,
750 Third Avenue, 9th Floor,
New York, NY 10017, USA

Visit us on the World Wide Web at:
www.haylemedical.com

ISBN 978-1-64647-590-2 (Hardback)

Trademark Notice: Registered trademark of products or corporate names are used only for explanation and identification without intent to infringe.

Cataloging-in-Publication Data

Reproductive medicine : role of follicle stimulating hormone / edited by Jasper McIntosh.
    p. cm.
Includes bibliographical references and index.
ISBN 978-1-64647-590-2
1. Reproductive health. 2. Follicle-stimulating hormone. 3. Human reproduction.
4. Fertility, Human. 5. Embryology, Human. 6. Birth control. I. McIntosh, Jasper.
RG133 .R473 2023
613.9--dc23

Contents

Preface

Over the recent decade, advancements and applications have progressed exponentially. This has led to the increased interest in this field and projects are being conducted to enhance knowledge. The main objective of this book is to present some of the critical challenges and provide insights into possible solutions. This book will answer the varied questions that arise in the field and also provide an increased scope for furthering studies.

Follicle-stimulating hormone (FSH) is a glycoprotein polypeptide hormone. It stimulates the gonads i.e., testes in males and ovaries in females. It is synthesized and secreted by the anterior pituitary gland's gonadotropic cells and regulates the body's development, growth, pubertal maturation, and reproductive functions. FSH and Luteinizing hormone (LH) operate together in the reproductive system. FSH is a glycoprotein heterodimer consisting of two polypeptide units, alpha and beta. The alpha subunits of Luteinizing hormone (LH), thyroid-stimulating hormone (TSH), and human chorionic gonadotropin (hCG) are identical but their beta subunits vary. High FSH levels and low FSH levels both are diseased states. Premature menopause, poor ovarian reserve, gonadal dysgenesis, Turner syndrome, Klinefelter syndrome, castration and Swyer syndrome are some of the conditions associated with high levels of FSH. Polycystic ovarian syndrome, obesity, hirsutism, infertility, Kallmann syndrome, hypothalamic suppression and hypopituitarism are some conditions related to low levels of FSH. This book unfolds various researches related to the function and use of FSH. These studies can prove to be crucial to the research in the field of reproductive medicine. It will provide comprehensive knowledge on role of follicle stimulating hormone to the readers.

I hope that this book, with its visionary approach, will be a valuable addition and will promote interest among readers. Each of the authors has provided their extraordinary competence in their specific fields by providing different perspectives as they come from diverse nations and regions. I thank them for their contributions.

Editor

Clinical Use of FSH in Male Infertility

*Hermann M. Behre**

Center for Reproductive Medicine and Andrology, University Hospital Halle, Martin Luther University Halle-Wittenberg, Halle, Germany

Correspondence:
Hermann M. Behre
Hermann.Behre@medizin.uni-halle.de

The established clinical indication for FSH use in male infertility is the treatment of patients with hypogonadotropic hypogonadism for stimulation of spermatogenesis that allows the induction of a clinical pregnancy in the female partner and finally the birth of a healthy child. Several clinical studies with urinary, purified, and recombinant FSH preparations in combination with hCG have demonstrated the high treatment efficacy regarding these clinical endpoints. Shortcomings of this hormone therapy are the long duration of treatment, sometimes longer than 2 years, and the inconvenience of injections every second or third day. However, improvements of therapy might be expected with new hormonal treatment options already available for infertility treatment in the female. FSH use for treatment of patients with normogonadotropic idiopathic infertility and oligozoospermia is still considered experimental in most countries. Recent meta-analyses have shown that FSH can significantly increase pregnancy rates in the female partners of these patients, but the effect-size is relatively low. Therefore, predictive factors for treatment success have to be identified, including FSH pharmacogenetics, to select the right normogonadotropic patients with idiopathic infertility for FSH therapy.

Keywords: FSH, hMG, hCG, male infertiltiy, hypogonadotropic hypogonadism, idiopathic male infertility

INTRODUCTION

In male infertility, the indication for treatment with follicle stimulating hormone (FSH) is the induction and maintenance of spermatogenesis in patients with hypogonadotropic hypogonadism (1). As these patients are normally azoospermic without gonadotropin stimulation and during testosterone therapy, the presence of sufficiently high numbers of progressively motile and normally formed sperm in the ejaculate during exogenous gonadotropin therapy might result in the desired clinical pregnancy for many infertile couples. On an experimental basis, and in some places already in clinical routine, FSH preparations are also used for treatment of normogonadotropic infertile men with idiopathic impairment of spermatogenesis (2, 3).

The primary goal of FSH therapy in the hypogonadotropic or normogonadotropic patients is not the stimulation of testicular growth or spermatogenesis *per se*, but the induction of a pregnancy in the female partner of the infertile couple, and finally the live birth of a healthy child. This review summarizes the effects of FSH treatment on this primary clinical outcome in these two patient groups with male infertility. The administration of FSH to children or during adolescence is not the topic of this review.

FSH THERAPY FOR MALE INFERTILITY IN PATIENTS WITH HYPOGONADOTROPIC HYPOGONADISM

In patients with hypogonadotropic hypogonadism, male infertility is due to the lack of stimulation of spermatogenesis by the gonadotropins FSH and luteinizing hormone (LH). In so-called idiopathic/isolated/congenital hypogonadotropic hypogonadism (IHH or CHH) and Kallmann syndrome, the core pathophysiological feature is the disturbed hypothalamic synthesis or secretion of gonadotropin-releasing hormone (GnRH) (4). This leads to diminished or absent LH and FSH synthesis or secretion by the unstimulated pituitary gland and finally to endocrine hypogonadism with low testosterone serum levels and infertility with azoospermia or severe oligozoospermia as the respective laboratory markers. Various other diseases including secondary GnRH deficiency lead to the same pathophysiology (4).

Other causes for hypogonadotropic hypogonadism are pituitary insufficiency due to tumors (especially makro-prolactinomas), metastases of the pituitary and the hypophyseal stalk, post-operative states, radiotherapy of the pituitary region, traumata, infections, hemochromatosis, vascular disorders, and others (4). Hypogonadotropic hypogonadism is caused by the insufficiency of the pituitary gland to secret significant levels of LH and FSH. The clinical picture in these patients is additionally influenced by possible disturbances of the other pituitary hormones.

The therapy of choice in patients with hypogonadotropic hypogonadism due to various pathophysiologic causes as mentioned above is—for most of the time of the life-span—the exogenous substitution of testosterone to maintain all androgen-dependent functions. This therapy is well established over decades, relatively convenient for the male patients and comparably inexpensive (5).

In case the patients develop the wish to have children with their female partner, the testosterone substitution therapy is no longer sufficient and has to be interrupted. The patients should then be treated with FSH preparations and in addition with a pharmacological preparation to stimulate intratesticular testosterone production by the Leydig cells. As no LH preparation is currently approved for male hypogonadotropic hypogonadism, patients are usually treated with human chorionic gonadotropin (hCG) preparations with similar, but not identical bioactivity (6). hCG has a longer elimination half-life than LH and patients can be treated effectively by two injections per week (4).

In patients with hypogonadotropic hypogonadism caused by hypothalamic disorders, exogenous pulsatile GnRH can also be used for treatment, as this will stimulate the FSH and LH secretion from the pituitary gland (4, 7). Because of the complex and time-consuming pulsatile therapy, today only few patients with hypogonadotropic hypogonadism are treated with pulsatile GnRH. Pulsatile GnRH therapy seems to have no proven advantage over FSH plus hCG therapy in patients with hypothalamic hypogonadotropic hypogonadism. However, the lack of sufficient well-designed, randomized prospective studies does not allow firm conclusions on the best therapy for infertility in these patients (8, 9).

Early Experience With hMG in Combination With hCG Therapy

FSH has been used successfully for infertility treatment of patients with hypogonadotropic hypogonadism for more than 50 years, initially with urinary menopausal gonadotropins having FSH activity. It is worth reading the initial reports of FSH therapy in hypogonadotropic patients. MacLeod and coworkers reported on the successful therapy with urinary menopausal gonadotropins of a 37-year-old patient who underwent complete hypophysectomy in 1963 (10, 11). The patient had provided a semen sample 1 day before the hypophysectomy that showed 576 million sperm per ejaculate and quite good sperm motility and morphology. After surgery, the ejaculate quality decreased significantly and, following several weeks after hypophysectomy, the patient was unable to provide semen samples any more. Approximately 14 weeks after hypophysectomy, a bilateral testicular biopsy was performed which showed involution of spermatogenesis to the level of spermatogonia and only few areas with primary spermatocytes. One day after the first testicular biopsy, treatment with hMG (human menopausal gonadotropin originating from human urine with mainly FSH and some LH activity) was initiated in the patient, at a dose of approximately 206 I.U. per day.

After 64 days of menopausal gonadotropin treatment, another testicular biopsy only of the right testis revealed stimulated spermatogenesis, showing all stages of spermatogenesis including late elongated testicular spermatids. However, the restoration of spermatogenesis appeared only qualitatively normal, not quantitatively. As a patient was still unable to produce an ejaculate probably due to the insufficient low LH activity in the hMG preparation and therefore low testosterone serum levels, hCG therapy with 4000 I.U. on alternate days was added to stimulate testosterone production by the Leydig cells. At the same time the hMG dose of 206 I.U. was given no longer daily, but only every second day (alternating with hCG injections). With the combined therapy of hMG and hCG the patient regained the ability to produce an ejaculate that showed a total sperm count of several million with progressive sperm motility and normal sperm morphology, that were still decreased compared to the levels analyzed before hypophysectomy (11). Later the patient decided not to continue with hMG therapy and, unfortunately, no fertility data are available. However, this early comprehensive case report demonstrated clearly the principle of FSH therapy in combination with hCG for stimulation of spermatogenesis in patients with hypogonadotropic hypogonadism.

Clinical Studies With hMG in Combination With hCG Therapy

Since then, several patients with hypogonadotropic hypogonadism were treated successfully with hMG plus hCG, for stimulation of spermatogenesis and achieving the desired pregnancy in the female partner. One of the most comprehensive studies on the treatment efficacy in patients with different etiologies for hypogonadotropic hypogonadism was published by Büchter et al. more than 20 years ago (8). This study might be regarded as one reference study for hMG treatment of these patients, as at that time hMG has been replaced more and more by highly purified or recombinant FSH preparations in the andrology clinic (12, 13). In this study by Büchter and colleagues, 21 patients with hypogonadotropic hypogonadism due to pituitary disorders were treated with hMG plus hCG. As in some of these patients more than one treatment course was performed, 30 treatment courses could be included in the study analysis. Another 18 patients with hypogonadotropic hypogonadism due to hypothalamic disorders such as Kallmann syndrome or congenital hypogonadotropic hypogonadism were treated with hMG plus hCG (18 cases, 20 treatment courses). Altogether, 31 of the 50 treatment courses with hMG plus hCG were initiated for the induction of pregnancy in the female partner and 19 of 50 courses only for the induction of spermatogenesis.

In all of the 30 treatment courses (100%) in patients with a pituitary disorder, spermatogenesis was stimulated from azoospermia to the presence of sperm in the ejaculate. In patients with a hypothalamic disorder, gonadotropin therapy induced spermatogenesis in 18 of 20 treatment courses (90%). The duration of therapy until the first detection of sperm in the ejaculate was quite variable. In the patients with a pituitary disorder, the average treatment time was 4 months (range 2–16 months). In the patients with a hypothalamic disorder, the average treatment duration was 6 months (1–18 months). The duration of time until induction of pregnancy of the female partner in patients with pituitary disorders was 10 months (2–46 months), and 8 months (1–15 months) in the patients with hypothalamic disorders. For this review article, the information on pregnancies was included that was added in proof of the publication by Büchter et al. (8). An additional pregnancy in the female partner occurred after gonadotropin treatment of one patient with pituitary disorder for 42 months as well as one patient with hypothalamic disorder treated for 48 months. Including these data, hMG plus hCG therapy in patients with a pituitary disorder resulted in 18 pregnancies in 21 treatment courses (86%) and 6 pregnancies in 10 treatment courses (60%) in patients with a hypothalamic disorder (8). Compared to other current treatments of infertility including application of assisted reproductive techniques (ART), this "causal" therapy of male infertility in patients with hypogonadotropic hypogonadism proved to be highly effective (14).

Factors Influencing the Efficacy of Treatment

While hMG plus hCG therapy of infertile patients with hypogonadotropic hypogonadism appears to be quite successful regarding stimulation of spermatogenesis and finally clinical pregnancy induction in the female partner, the treatment might last quite long. Patients have to be informed that hormone therapy might last for several months and even years before the desired pregnancy can be achieved. Therefore, it is relevant to identify predictive factors influencing treatment efficacy (**Box 1**).

In an recent study on 51 adult patients with hypogonadotropic hypogonadism who had undergone one treatment cycle with FSH (urinary or recombinant FSH) plus hCG, those patients who had hypogonadotropic hypogonadism acquired after puberty or had a pubertal arrest showed significantly better treatment outcome (15). These patients achieved higher final bilateral testicular volume and higher final sperm concentrations compared to patients with hypogonadotropic hypogonadism manifesting before the normal onset of puberty. Most relevant, the pregnancy rate of 62% was higher in patients with post-pubertally acquired hypogonadotropic hypogonadism compared with those patients with pre-pubertally acquired hypogonadism (42%). In addition, a conception in the female partners of patients with post-pubertally acquired hypogonadotropic hypogonadism occurred significantly earlier (20.3 ± 11.5 months) than in the female partners of patients with pre-pubertally acquired hypogonadism (43.1 ± 43.8 months).

The therapeutic success was also higher in patients without previously undescended testes, in patients with higher baseline testicular volume and in patients with higher baseline inhibin B serum concentrations (15). The identification of these predictive factors is in line with various clinical studies by other study groups (16–21).

Clinical Studies With Recombinant or Urinary FSH in Combination With hCG Therapy

No adequate large, randomized controlled trials (RCTs) have been performed to compare efficacy of recombinant or highly purified FSH with the urinary hMG preparations in males—quite in contrast to the application of FSH preparations in females for ART. From the available information, it seems that the efficacy of the various FSH preparations in male patients with hypogonadotropic hypogonadism is quite comparable, regarding stimulation of spermatogenesis and inducing the desired pregnancy in the female partner (13, 18, 20–25). Today, in Germany only recombinant FSH and no longer urinary FSH preparations are approved for this therapy in male patients.

Common Dosing Schemes

One of the most common dosing schemes of gonadotropins in male hypogonadotropic hypogonadism is the administration of 150-225 I.U. FSH two or three times a week in combination with 1000-2500 I.U. of hCG two times per week (4). Several

---

Box 1 | Predictive factors for treatment success.

Clinical factors at initiation of FSH plus hCG therapy of adult male patients with hypogonadotropic hypogonadism predicting successful infertility treatment (15)

- History of normal puberty or pubertal arrest
- No history of cryptorchidism
- Higher baseline testicular volume
- Higher baseline serum levels of inhibin B

physicians start treatment with hCG alone for e.g., 3 months, as some patients—maybe those with some residual FSH activity—achieve stimulation of spermatogenesis by hCG alone (13, 20, 25, 26). However, the sperm concentrations seen after hCG therapy alone appear to be lower than those with the combined treatment with FSH plus hCG (27). Therefore, FSH should also be added in these hCG-treated patients at some time-point to achieve best treatment outcome. In addition, it has been shown that induction of spermatogenesis achieved by FSH plus hCG treatment in hypogonadotropic hypogonadism can be maintained qualitatively, but not quantitatively in most of the patients with hCG alone (28). On this line, a sequential therapy with 3 months treatment with FSH plus hCG alternated by hCG therapy alone for another 3 months has been proposed to reduce the relatively high costs of gonadotropin therapy (29). However, it is not known if this dosing regimen has the same high efficacy on the primary outcome clinical pregnancy rate.

The dose and injection interval of FSH might be adapted in individual hypogonadotropic patients to achieve optimal treatment outcome. The efficacy can be monitored by the increase of testicular volume, the stimulation of spermatogenesis, the serum levels of FSH achieved, the serum levels of testosterone achieved, and other factors. Unfortunately, large randomized comparative studies with different FSH preparations, different doses and different injection intervals are missing (13, 24). A retrospective study suggested that lower weekly FSH doses are sufficient to stimulate spermatogenesis and allow induction of the desired pregnancy in the female partner (24). Others have argued that the hCG dose in combination with FSH might be too high for optimal treatment effects (30). As the current FSH plus hCG dosing schemes have still the drawback of a quite long treatment duration before the desired pregnancy is achieved, it still seems rewarding to test different FSH and hCG preparations and dosing regimens by proper designed randomized controlled clinical trials to improve treatment outcome of gonadotropin therapy in male hypogonadotropic hypogonadism.

FSH in Combination With Recombinant hCG or LH

In Germany, recombinant hCG and LH preparation are approved for reproductive hormone therapy in women. In men, so far no adequate studies have been published comparing these preparations with urinary hCG. A combination of recombinant FSH with recombinant LH or hCG in one injection pen would allow easier self-administration, more fine tuning of individual therapy, higher compliance and maybe higher treatment efficacy. In addition, it could be speculated that LH instead of hCG therapy in combination with FSH could lead to much better clinical efficacy regarding stimulation of spermatogenesis and pregnancy rate in male hypogonadotropic hypogonadism (6, 30). So far injection pens with recombinant LH are only approved for treatment of females and it is about time to provide these options also to male hypogonadotropic patients. The pharmaceutical

companies should be encouraged to initiate the respective clinical studies.

Long-Acting FSH Preparations

Another option for treatment improvement would be to use long-acting FSH analogs that are already used successfully in the fertility care of women. In a recent phase III multicenter clinical trial of corifollitropin alfa in azoospermic men with hypogonadotropic hypogonadism, it was demonstrated that administration of 150 µg of a long-acting FSH preparation given every second week leads to significant increase of testicular volume and induction of spermatogenesis, comparable to the effects seen with short-acting recombinant FSH preparations (25).

FSH THERAPY IN NORMOGONADOTROPIC MEN WITH IDIOPATHIC INFERTILITY

Early Non-randomized Studies

As FSH therapy proved to be quite successful regarding stimulation of spermatogenesis of patients with hypogonadotropic hypogonadism and pregnancy rate in their female partners, it was tested whether this therapy can also be applied successfully in male patients with normogonadotropic idiopathic infertility. Early uncontrolled studies in these patients with hMG plus hCG therapy over a treatment period of 3 months demonstrated an increase of total sperm number in the ejaculate and also pregnancy rate in the female partners (31). The increase in pregnancy rate was especially evident in the so-called responders who were defined by an increase of sperm output of at least 25 million per ejaculate (31).

Placebo-Controlled Randomized Studies

However, it could not be excluded that the positive FSH effects in the normogonadotropic patients in uncontrolled trials were due to the well-known regression-to-the-mean phenomenon. The efficacy of hMG plus hCG treatment for 13 weeks in normogonadotropic patients with oligozoospermia was consequently revisited in a randomized, placebo-controlled, double-blind clinical study. The positive effects seen in the uncontrolled trials could not be confirmed by this randomized study. The effects on the classical variables of ejaculate analysis according to WHO were similar in the verum and placebo group (32). However, two of 19 patients treated with hMG plus hCG achieved a pregnancy in the female partner within 2 months after cessation of treatment while no pregnancy was induced by the 20 patients treated with placebo.

Because of the low number of patients included, this randomized controlled study did not have enough power to allow conclusions about pregnancy rates. In addition, the conventional ejaculate analysis might not detect all positive effects that are relevant for fertility. FSH therapy has clear positive effects on sperm DNA condensation and fragmentation that seems to be quite relevant for fertility (2, 33–37). These aspects might be overlooked by the standard procedures for semen analysis currently recommended by WHO (38).

TABLE 1 | Main results of two recent meta-analyses on pregnancy rates after FSH treatment of men with idiopathic infertility.

Inclusion criterion	Number of patients treated with FSH*	Number of patients treated with placebo or untreated	Odds ratio [95% confidence interval] for spontaneous pregnancy rate[#]	Reference of the meta-analysis
Randomized controlled clinical trials	201	211	4.94 [2.13–11.44]	(39)
Controlled clinical trials	384	308	4.50 [2.17–9.33]	(40)

*In one clinical trial included in each meta-analysis (n = 19 patients in verum and n = 20 patients in control group) hMG + hCG injections were given instead of purified or recombinant FSH. [#]Test for overall effect: Z = 3.72 (P = 0.00020) (39) and Z = 4.04 (P < 0.0001) (40).

Meta-Analysis of Controlled Studies

As there are no published controlled studies with sufficiently high numbers of participants yet, the effects on the pregnancy rate can only be assessed by meta-analysis. In 2013, an updated Cochrane review summarized the scientific evidence on efficacy of gonadotropin therapy in idiopathic male factor infertility to increase clinical pregnancy rate in the female partner (**Table 1**) (39). In this review, only RCTs with FSH/hMG alone or in combination with hCG for patients with idiopathic male factor infertility were considered that had a control group with placebo or no treatment. Finally, six RCTs were included in the analysis. The spontaneous pregnancy rate resulting from natural intercourse of 16% in the female partners of patients receiving gonadotropin treatment turned out to be significantly higher than the spontaneous pregnancy rate of 7% in the partners of men receiving placebo or no treatment (Peto odds ratio [OR] 4.94, 95% CI 2.13–11.44; 5 clinical studies; 412 participants; moderate-quality evidence). No difference was seen for pregnancy rates between the verum and control groups after additional treatment with intracytoplasmic sperm injection (ICSI) or intrauterine insemination, but the number of included patients was too low to allow final conclusions.

Recently, another comprehensive meta-analysis (**Table 1**) on clinical pregnancy rate as the main outcome variable was performed by Santi et al. including all controlled clinical trials on FSH administration (including one small study with hMG plus hCG) to male partners with idiopathic infertility (40). Randomization was not an inclusion criterion for this analysis. Altogether, 15 controlled clinical trials were included with 614 men treated with FSH and 661 patients with placebo or untreated patients. Nine of the 15 studies reported on spontaneous pregnancy rate (384 FSH-treated patients, 308 control patients). The spontaneous pregnancy rate in these nine studies was significantly higher in patients treated with FSH compared to controls (OR 4.50, 95% CI 2.17–9.33). Eight studies evaluated pregnancy rate after FSH therapy and application of additional ART (322 FSH-treated patients, 275 controls). The ART pregnancy rate in this meta-analysis turned out to be significantly higher in the female partners of male patients with FSH treatment compared to controls (OR 1.60, 95% CI 1.08–2.37).

Effect Size of FSH Therapy on Pregnancy Rate

Although these meta-analyses have demonstrated that FSH therapy in idiopathic normogonadotropic male infertility can increase clinical pregnancies in the female partners, the effect size is still relatively low. It has been calculated that 10 patients have to be treated with FSH to achieve one spontaneous pregnancy (40). Eighteen patients have to be treated with FSH to achieve one additional pregnancy after ART (40). As FSH preparations are quite expensive and many physicians involved in infertility treatment consider this effect not high enough, FSH treatment in idiopathic male infertility is so far not part of the routine treatment regime and not covered by insurance companies in many countries (3).

Selecting the Right Normogonadotropic Patient for FSH Therapy

To overcome these shortcomings, it is mandatory to select the right patients for FSH therapy. The evidence on FSH therapy in normogonadotropic patients is so far restricted to idiopathic infertility, which means that no identifiable, generally accepted cause for male infertility could be detected. Therefore, all male patients have to have a proper diagnostic andrological work-up before initiating any FSH therapy, and also the female partner needs to have a proper diagnostic gynecological work-up! Normogonadotropic male patients with identifiable and possibly treatable causes for male infertility (e.g., obstruction) should not be treated with FSH. Obviously, male patients with elevated bioactive FSH serum levels should not receive FSH therapy. It has been suggested not to provide FSH treatment to infertile patients with hypospermatogenesis associated with maturational disturbances at the spermatid level (2).

In addition to these factors, FSH therapy in normozoospermic infertile patients might be improved by optimizing the FSH dose, injection interval and especially treatment duration (1). In a recent prospective, double-blind, placebo-controlled clinical study in China including 354 patients with idiopathic oligozoospermia, the best results were seen in patients treated with the highest FSH dose of 300 I.U. every second day and for the longest treatment duration (maximal treatment duration in this study was 5 months) (41). Using the knowledge from the gonadotropin therapy in hypogonadotropic patients, it could be speculated that longer treatment of normogonadotropic patients would also improve pregnancy rates in the female partner (8).

One other promising approach to improve treatment outcome might be the application of FSH pharmacogenetics. Single nucleic polymorphism (SNP) p.N680S in exon 10 of the FSH receptor gene (FSHR) has been shown to influence the ovarian response during controlled ovarian stimulation (42). Therefore, it was logical to test the effect of p.N680S also regarding FSH therapy for normogonadotropic patients with idiopathic infertility (34). In this study, the primary outcome variable was DNA fragmentation index (DFI) of sperm in the ejaculate (36, 37). It could be shown that total DFI decreased significantly from baseline to the end of the study—a surrogate effect indicating improved fertility—in male patients with the p.N680S homozygous N polymorphism, but not in the patients with p.N680S homozygous S polymorphism of the FSH receptor. These findings indicate that a selection of the right normogonadotropic patients for FSH therapy might be possible, and probably different treatment regimens could be used for different patients groups.

Several pharmacogenetic studies have been performed in normogonadotropic men over the last years that tested SNPs of the FSH beta subunit gene (*FSHB*), SNPs of the *FSHR*, or combinations thereof (34, 35, 43, 44). These trials have been reviewed comprehensibly by Schubert and co-workers in this Research Topic of Frontiers in Endocrinology (45). Unfortunately, these clinical trials come to quite divergent study results, probably due to study design, inclusion criteria, and as one of the main factors FSH doses and injection intervals. However, only large, placebo-controlled, randomized multicentre studies with pregnancy rate—and not any surrogate marker—as the primary outcome variable will finally allow a conclusion on the value of FSH pharmacogenetics to select the right normogonadotropic patients with idiopathic infertility for FSH therapy.

FSH Therapy in Patients With Failed TESE

FSH therapy is currently suggested by different clinicians for patients with idiopathic azoospermia after failed testicular sperm extraction (TESE) (46–48). So far, these studies are case reports or have low patient numbers and do not include a randomized

control group. Therefore, no firm conclusion on the efficacy of FSH therapy in these patients with idiopathic azoospermia is possible, yet.

PERSPECTIVES

Although ART treatment is quite effective for infertile couples regarding the desired clinical pregnancy and the birth of a healthy child, there is a growing demand from patients and health authorities to apply effective causal therapies for the infertile male whenever possible and meaningful. Therefore, a systematic andrological examination of the male partner of the infertile couple should always be performed, even when some gynecological reasons for infertility have already been identified. In Germany, the thorough andrological work-up is now mandatory before any ART therapy can be initiated (49).

Hypogonadotropic hypogonadism is a good example how causal hormone therapy of male infertility can be applied with high clinical efficacy regarding induction of pregnancy in the female partner. It remains to be seen if FSH therapy will also be useful and generally accepted for treatment of male infertility in normogonadotropic patients with idiopathic impairment of spermatogenesis.

Without question, more well-designed, prospective randomized studies are needed to identify the best FSH treatment for the infertile male patient. All relevant players in the healthcare system should be stimulated to provide the respective resources for optimizing treatment outcome of male infertility—in the male!

AUTHOR CONTRIBUTIONS

All work for this article was done by HB.

REFERENCES

1. Oduwole OO, Peltoketo H, Huhtaniemi IT. Role of follicle-stimulating hormone in spermatogenesis. *Front Endocrinol.* (2018) 9:763. doi: 10.3389/fendo.2018.00763
2. Barbonetti A, Calogero AE, Balercia G, Garolla A, Krausz C, La Vignera S, et al. The use of follicle stimulating hormone (FSH) for the treatment of the infertile man: position statement from the Italian Society of Andrology and Sexual Medicine (SIAMS). *J Endocrinol Invest.* (2018) 41:1107–22. doi: 10.1007/s40618-018-0843-y
3. Colpi GM, Francavilla S, Haidl G, Link K, Behre HM, Goulis DG, et al. European academy of andrology guideline management of oligo-astheno-teratozoospermia. *Andrology.* (2018) 6:513–24. doi: 10.1111/andr.12502
4. Behre HM, Nieschlag E, Partsch C-J, Wieacker P, Simoni M. Diseases of the hypothalamus and the pituitary gland. In: Nieschlag E, Behre HM, Nieschlag S, editors. *Andrology. Male Reproductive Health and Dysfunction.* 3rd ed. Berlin: Springer (2010). p. 169–92.
5. Nieschlag E, Behre HM. Testosterone therapy. In: Nieschlag E, Behre HM, Nieschlag S, editors. *Andrology. Male Reproductive Health and Dysfunction.* 3rd ed. Berlin: Springer (2010). p. 437–55.
6. Casarini L, Lispi M, Longobardi S, Milosa F, La Marca A, Tagliasacchi D, et al. LH and hCG action on the same receptor results in quantitatively and qualitatively different intracellular signalling. *PLoS ONE.* (2012) 7:e46682. doi: 10.1371/journal.pone.0046682

7. Young J, Xu C, Papadakis GE, Acierno JS, Maione L, Hietamaki J, et al. Clinical management of congenital hypogonadotropic hypogonadism. *Endocr Rev.* (2019) 40:669–710. doi: 10.1210/er.2018-00116
8. Büchter D, Behre HM, Kliesch S, Nieschlag E. Pulsatile GnRH or human chorionic gonadotropin/human menopausal gonadotropin as effective treatment for men with hypogonadotropic hypogonadism: a review of 42 cases. *Eur J Endocrinol.* (1998) 139:298–303. doi: 10.1530/eje.0.1390298
9. Mao JF, Liu ZX, Nie M, Wang X, Xu HL, Huang BK, et al. Pulsatile gonadotropin-releasing hormone therapy is associated with earlier spermatogenesis compared to combined gonadotropin therapy in patients with congenital hypogonadotropic hypogonadism. *Asian J Androl.* (2017) 19:680–5. doi: 10.4103/1008-682X.193568
10. Macleod J, Pazianos A, Ray BS. Restoration of human spermatogenesis by menopausal gonadotrophins. *Lancet.* (1964) 1:1196–7. doi: 10.1016/S0140-6736(64)91212-7
11. MacLeod J, Pazianos A, Ray B. The restoration of human spermatogenesis and of the reproductive tract with urinary gonadotropins following hypophysectomy. *Fertil Steril.* (1966) 17:7–23. doi: 10.1016/S0015-0282(16)35821-6
12. Kliesch S, Behre HM, Nieschlag E. Recombinant human follicle-stimulating hormone and human chorionic gonadotropin for induction of spermatogenesis in a hypogonadotropic male. *Fertil Steril.* (1995) 63:1326–8. doi: 10.1016/S0015-0282(16)57619-5

13. Bouloux PM, Nieschlag E, Burger HG, Skakkebaek NE, Wu FC, Handelsman DJ, et al. Induction of spermatogenesis by recombinant follicle-stimulating hormone (puregon) in hypogonadotropic azoospermic men who failed to respond to human chorionic gonadotropin alone. *J Androl.* (2003) 24:604–11. doi: 10.1002/j.1939-4640.2003.tb02712.x

14. Blumenauer V, Czeromin U, Fehr D, Fiedler K, Gnoth C, Krüssel JS, et al. D·I·R annual 2017 – the German IVF-registry. *J Reproduktionsmed Endrokrinol.* (2018) 15:217–50.

15. Rohayem J, Sinthofen N, Nieschlag E, Kliesch S, Zitzmann M. Causes of hypogonadotropic hypogonadism predict response to gonadotropin substitution in adults. *Andrology.* (2016) 4:87–94. doi: 10.1111/andr.12128

16. Burris AS, Rodbard HW, Winters SJ, Sherins RJ. Gonadotropin therapy in men with isolated hypogonadotropic hypogonadism: the response to human chorionic gonadotropin is predicted by initial testicular size. *J Clin Endocrinol Metab.* (1988) 66:1144–51. doi: 10.1210/jcem-66-6-1144

17. Miyagawa Y, Tsujimura A, Matsumiya K, Takao T, Tohda A, Koga M, et al. Outcome of gonadotropin therapy for male hypogonadotropic hypogonadism at university affiliated male infertility centers: a 30-year retrospective study. *J Urol.* (2005) 173:2072–5. doi: 10.1097/01.ju.0000158133.09197.f4

18. Liu PY, Baker HW, Jayadev V, Zacharin M, Conway AJ, Handelsman DJ. Induction of spermatogenesis and fertility during gonadotropin treatment of gonadotropin-deficient infertile men: predictors of fertility outcome. *J Clin Endocrinol Metab.* (2009) 94:801–8. doi: 10.1210/jc.2008-1648

19. Warne DW, Decosterd G, Okada H, Yano Y, Koide N, Howles CM. A combined analysis of data to identify predictive factors for spermatogenesis in men with hypogonadotropic hypogonadism treated with recombinant human follicle-stimulating hormone and human chorionic gonadotropin. *Fertil Steril.* (2009) 92:594–604. doi: 10.1016/j.fertnstert.2008.07.1720

20. Dwyer AA, Raivio T, Pitteloud N. Gonadotrophin replacement for induction of fertility in hypogonadal men. *Best Pract Res Clin Endocrinol Metab.* (2015) 29:91–103. doi: 10.1016/j.beem.2014.10.005

21. Liu Z, Mao J, Wu X, Xu H, Wang X, Huang B, et al. Efficacy and outcome predictors of gonadotropin treatment for male congenital hypogonadotropic hypogonadism: a retrospective study of 223 patients. *Medicine.* (2016) 95:e2867. doi: 10.1097/MD.0000000000002867

22. Anonymous. Efficacy and safety of highly purified urinary follicle-stimulating hormone with human chorionic gonadotropin for treating men with isolated hypogonadotropic hypogonadism. European Metrodin HP Study Group. *Fertil Steril.* (1998) 70:256–62. doi: 10.1016/S0015-0282(98)00156-3

23. Bouloux P, Warne DW, Loumaye E, FSH Study Group in Men's Infertility. Efficacy and safety of recombinant human follicle-stimulating hormone in men with isolated hypogonadotropic hypogonadism. *Fertil Steril.* (2002) 77:270–3. doi: 10.1016/S0015-0282(01)02973-9

24. Sinisi AA, Esposito D, Bellastella G, Maione L, Palumbo V, Gandini L, et al. Efficacy of recombinant human follicle stimulating hormone at low doses in inducing spermatogenesis and fertility in hypogonadotropic hypogonadism. *J Endocrinol Invest.* (2010) 33:618–23. doi: 10.1007/BF03346659

25. Nieschlag E, Bouloux PG, Stegmann BJ, Shankar RR, Guan Y, Tzontcheva A, et al. An open-label clinical trial to investigate the efficacy and safety of corifollitropin alfa combined with hCG in adult men with hypogonadotropic hypogonadism. *Reprod Biol Endocrinol.* (2017) 15:17. doi: 10.1186/s12958-017-0232-y

26. Fraietta R, Zylberstejn DS, Esteves SC. Hypogonadotropic hypogonadism revisited. *Clinics.* (2013) 68 (Suppl 1):81–8. doi: 10.6061/clinics/2013(Sup01)09

27. Yang L, Zhang SX, Dong Q, Xiong ZB, Li X. Application of hormonal treatment in hypogonadotropic hypogonadism: more than ten years experience. *Int Urol Nephrol.* (2012) 44:393–9. doi: 10.1007/s11255-011-0065-0

28. Depenbusch M, von Eckardstein S, Simoni M, Nieschlag E. Maintenance of spermatogenesis in hypogonadotropic hypogonadal men with human chorionic gonadotropin alone. *Eur J Endocrinol.* (2002) 147:617–24. doi: 10.1530/eje.0.1470617

29. Zhang M, Tong G, Liu Y, Mu Y, Weng J, Xue Y, et al. Sequential versus continual purified urinary FSH/hCG in men with idiopathic hypogonadotropic hypogonadism. *J Clin Endocrinol Metab.* (2015) 100:2449–55. doi: 10.1210/jc.2014-3802

30. Casarini L, Santi D, Brigante G, Simoni M. Two hormones for one receptor: evolution, biochemistry, actions, and pathophysiology of LH and hCG. *Endocr Rev.* (2018) 39:549–92. doi: 10.1210/er.2018-00065

31. Schill WB, Jungst D, Unterburger P, Braun S. Combined hMG/hCG treatment in subfertile men with idiopathic normogonadotrophic oligozoospermia. *Int J Androl.* (1982) 5:467–77. doi: 10.1111/j.1365-2605.1982.tb00278.x

32. Knuth UA, Honigl W, Bals-Pratsch M, Schleicher G, Nieschlag E. Treatment of severe oligospermia with human chorionic gonadotropin/human menopausal gonadotropin: a placebo-controlled, double blind trial. *J Clin Endocrinol Metab.* (1987) 65:1081–7. doi: 10.1210/jcem-65-6-1081

33. Kamischke A, Behre HM, Bergmann M, Simoni M, Schafer T, Nieschlag E. Recombinant human follicle stimulating hormone for treatment of male idiopathic infertility: a randomized, double-blind, placebo-controlled, clinical trial. *Hum Reprod.* (1998) 13:596–603. doi: 10.1093/humrep/13.3.596

34. Simoni M, Santi D, Negri L, Hoffmann I, Muratori M, Baldi E, et al. Treatment with human, recombinant FSH improves sperm DNA fragmentation in idiopathic infertile men depending on the FSH receptor polymorphism p.N680S: a pharmacogenetic study. *Hum Reprod.* (2016) 31:1960–9. doi: 10.1093/humrep/dew167

35. Casamonti E, Vinci S, Serra E, Fino MG, Brilli S, Lotti F, et al. Short-term FSH treatment and sperm maturation: a prospective study in idiopathic infertile men. *Andrology.* (2017) 5:414–22. doi: 10.1111/andr.12333

36. Muratori M, Baldi E. Effects of FSH on sperm DNA fragmentation: review of clinical studies and possible mechanisms of action. *Front Endocrinol.* (2018) 9:734. doi: 10.3389/fendo.2018.00734

37. Santi D, Spaggiari G, Simoni M. Sperm DNA fragmentation index as a promising predictive tool for male infertility diagnosis and treatment management - meta-analyses. *Reprod Biomed Online.* (2018) 37:315–26. doi: 10.1016/j.rbmo.2018.06.023

38. WHO. *WHO Laboratory Manual for the Examination and Processing of Human Semen.* Geneva: WHO Press (2010).

39. Attia AM, Abou-Setta AM, Al-Inany HG. Gonadotrophins for idiopathic male factor subfertility. *Cochrane Database Syst Rev.* (2013) CD005071. doi: 10.1002/14651858.CD005071.pub4

40. Santi D, Granata AR, Simoni M. FSH treatment of male idiopathic infertility improves pregnancy rate: a meta-analysis. *Endocr Connect.* (2015) 4:R46–58. doi: 10.1530/EC-15-0050

41. Ding YM, Zhang XJ, Li JP, Chen SS, Zhang RT, Tan WL, et al. Treatment of idiopathic oligozoospermia with recombinant human follicle-stimulating hormone: a prospective, randomized, double-blind, placebo-controlled clinical study in Chinese population. *Clin Endocrinol.* (2015) 83:866–71. doi: 10.1111/cen.12770

42. Behre HM, Greb RR, Mempel A, Sonntag B, Kiesel L, Kaltwasser P, et al. Significance of a common single nucleotide polymorphism in exon 10 of the follicle-stimulating hormone (FSH) receptor gene for the ovarian response to FSH: a pharmacogenetic approach to controlled ovarian hyperstimulation. *Pharmacogenet Genomics.* (2005) 15:451–6. doi: 10.1097/01.fpc.0000167330.92786.5e

43. Ferlin A, Vinanzi C, Selice R, Garolla A, Frigo AC, Foresta C. Toward a pharmacogenetic approach to male infertility: polymorphism of follicle-stimulating hormone beta-subunit promoter. *Fertil Steril.* (2011) 96:1344–1349.e1342. doi: 10.1016/j.fertnstert.2011.09.034

44. Selice R, Ferlin A, Garolla A, Caretta N, Foresta C. Effects of endogenous FSH on normal human spermatogenesis in adults. *Int J Androl.* (2011) 34(6 Pt 2):e511–7. doi: 10.1111/j.1365-2605.2010.01134.x

45. Schubert M, Pérez Lanuza L, Gromoll J. Pharmacogenetics of FSH action in the male. *Front Endocrinol.* (2019) 10:47. doi: 10.3389/fendo.2019.00047

46. Barbotin AL, Ballot C, Sigala J, Leroy M, Rigot JM, Dewailly D, et al. Pregnancy after intracytoplasmic sperm injection following extended sperm preparation and hormone therapy in an azoospermic man with maturation arrest and microlithiasis: a case report and literature review. *Andrologia.* (2017) 49:e12665. doi: 10.1111/and.12665

47. Cocci A, Cito G, Russo GI, Falcone M, Capece M, Timpano M, et al. Effectiveness of highly purified urofollitropin treatment in patients with

idiopathic azoospermia before testicular sperm extraction. *Urologia.* (2018) 85:19–21. doi: 10.5301/uj.5000253

48. Laursen RJ, Elbaek HO, Povlsen BB, Lykkegaard J, Jensen KBS, Esteves SC, et al. Hormonal stimulation of spermatogenesis: a new way to treat the infertile male with non-obstructive azoospermia? *Int Urol Nephrol.* (2019) 51:453–6. doi: 10.1007/s11255-019-02091-8

49. Bundesärztekammer. Richtlinie zur Entnahme und Übertragung von menschlichen Keimzellen im Rahmen der assistierten Reproduktion. *Deutsches Ärzteblatt.* (2018) A1–A22. doi: 10.3238/arztebl.2018.Rili_assReproduktion_2018

2

Modulation of Gonadotropins Activity by Antibodies

Elodie Kara [1]*, Laurence Dupuy [1], Céline Bouillon [1,2,3,4,5,6], Sophie Casteret [1] and Marie-Christine Maurel [1]

[1] Igyxos SA, Nouzilly, France, [2] Service de Médecine et Biologie de la Reproduction, CHRU de Tours, Tours, France, [3] Biologie Intégrative de l'Ovaire, INRA, UMR85, Physiologie de la Reproduction et des Comportements, Nouzilly, France, [4] CNRS, UMR7247, Nouzilly, France, [5] Université François Rabelais, Tours, France, [6] IFCE, Nouzilly, France

*Correspondence:
Elodie Kara
elodie.kara@igyxos.com

Gonadotropins are essential for reproduction control in humans as well as in animals. They are widely used all over the world for ovarian stimulation in women, spermatogenesis stimulation in men, and ovulation induction and superovulation in animals. Despite the availability of many different preparations, all are made of the native hormones. Having different ligands with a wide activity range for a given receptor helps better understand its molecular and cellular signaling mechanisms as well as its physiological functions, and thus helps the development of more specific and adapted medicines. One way to control the gonadotropins' activity could be the use of modulating antibodies. Antibodies are powerful tools that were largely used to decipher gonadotropins' actions and they have shown their utility as therapeutics in several other indications such as cancer. In this review, we summarize the inhibitory and potentiating antibodies to gonadotropins, and their potential therapeutic applications.

Keywords: potentiating antibodies, inhibitory antibodies, follicle-stimulating hormone, luteinizing hormone, chorionic gonadotropin, signaling

INTRODUCTION

Gonadotropins, namely follicle-stimulating hormone (FSH), luteinizing hormone (LH), and chorionic gonadotropin (CG) are heterodimeric glycoproteins, constituted by an alpha- and a beta- subunit. The alpha subunit is common to all glycoprotein hormones, including thyroid stimulating hormone (TSH) (1). FSH and LH/CG receptors are G-protein coupled receptors (GPCR), mainly expressed in granulosa cells in female ovaries and in Sertoli cells in male testis for FSH receptor (FSH-R) (2), and in granulosa and theca cells in female and Leydig cells in male for LH receptor (LH-R) (3).

Because of their role in reproduction, gonadotropins are routinely used in fertility treatments in men and women for assisted reproductive technologies (ART) (4, 5). In women, it consists on daily injections of FSH or a mixture of FSH/LH, for 8–12 days, to grow and mature follicles. The final maturation is then completed with an injection of human CG (hCG) 36 h after the last injection of FSH. In men, FSH and hCG injections 2–3 times a week for several months are used to treat hypogonadotropic hypogonadism and induce spermatogenesis (6–9). Currently, the preparations used are either endogenous FSH extracted from post-menopausal women urine (human menopausal gonadotropins, hMG), highly purified urinary FSH, or recombinant FSH. The first recombinant versions of FSH (follitropin alpha and beta, corifollitropin) and all their biosimilars were produced in Chinese hamster ovary (CHO) cells. The follitropin delta approved in Europe in 2015 (Rekovelle™) and follitropin epsilon still under development are produced in human cell lines: PER.C6 for follitropin delta (10) and GlycoExpress for follitropin epsilon (11). For LH and hCG, recombinant versions produced in CHO cells are also available. In animals, equine CG (eCG), formerly named pregnant-mare serum gonadotropin (PMSG), is widely used to induce ovulation in small ruminants (12). Porcine pituitary extracts are used for current superovulation treatments in cattle (13), whereas ovulation in swine herds is induced with a mixture of hCG and eCG (14).

Despite all the preparations that are on the market, the only ligands available for gonadotropin receptors as therapeutics are native hormones. New biased ligands or ligands with different potencies and efficacies on gonadotropin receptors can help better understand receptor signaling, decipher the implication of the different signaling pathways in physiological and pathophysiological mechanisms, and finally bring to the market new molecules to improve ART treatments. In 2015 in USA, 182,111 ART procedures were performed leading to 59,334 live-birth deliveries (15). Among other strategies like small molecule ligands, one way to modulate the gonadotropins' activity could be the use of antibodies, targeting either directly the receptor itself, or its ligand to modulate hormone's activity.

Antibodies are useful tools that help to better understand gonadotropins' structure by epitope mapping (16–18) and their function by neutralizing the effect of endogenous gonadotropins (19–22). They also allow their quantification by the development of radioimmunoassays (RIA) and enzyme-linked immunosorbent assays (ELISA) (23–27). Finally, antibodies permitted the development of specific purification methods for gonadotropins, making them safer to use as therapeutic agents (28–30).

The effect of antibodies, if any, is expected to be inhibitory on antigen activity by impairing its interaction with its receptor. Surprisingly, some of them were described as being able to increase the activity of their antigenic protein. Potentiating polyclonal antibodies directed against epidermal growth factor (EGF) and insulin were first described by Shechter et al. in 1979 (31, 32). A few years later, potentiating monoclonal antibodies (mAbs) were described for ovine (o) and human (h) growth hormones (GH) (33–35). When hypopituitary Snell dwarf mice were treated with hGH in complex with a mAb, the actions of hGH on growth and body composition were enhanced compared to animals treated with GH alone (34, 35). The same kind of antibodies were described for TSH: mAbs directed against TSH were able to enhance its biological activity in vivo in Snell dwarf mice (36), suggesting that glycoprotein hormones' activity may be modulated by mAbs. Anti-receptor antibodies with stimulating activities were also described for TSH receptor (37, 38).

In this review, we give a brief overview of antibodies modulating gonadotropins' activity, either positively or negatively.

STRUCTURE AND FUNCTION OF GONADOTROPINS

Alpha- and beta-subunits of gonadotropins are non-covalently linked. The alpha-subunit is common to all glycoprotein hormones in a given species, and presents two major sites of N-glycosylation (1). The specificity of each hormone is conferred by the beta-subunit, that contains 2 N-glycosylation sites. hCG, eLH and eCG present a longer beta-subunit with an additional carboxy-terminal peptide (CTP) that is ~30 amino-acids long and contains multiple O-glycosylation sites.

eCG originates from uterine endometrial cups and is extracted from pregnant mare serum (39, 40). eLH and eCG beta-subunits are encoded by a single gene (41) but they differ in glycosylation. They both exhibit N-glycans on alpha- and beta-subunits, and O-glycans on the carboxy-terminal peptide (CTP) constituted of the last 29 amino-acids of the beta-subunit (beta 121–149) (42). With a carbohydrate content higher than 40% (43) and N-glycan chains terminated by sialic acids, eCG is the most heavily glycosylated glycoprotein hormone and has a longer in vivo half-life than other gonadotropins (~60 h) (44, 45). eCG binds to LH receptors in equine, but exerts FSH and LH actions in non-equine species by stimulating FSH and LH receptors respectively (46–51). Its dual FSH/LH activity and its longer half-life were the reasons why eCG was widely used since decades to induce ovulation in breeding animals, especially in goats and ewes for out-of-season breeding to allow artificial insemination.

hCG is mainly produced during pregnancy, by syncytiotrophoblast cells and a hyperglycosylated isoform is produced by cytotrophoblast cells. These two isoforms are implicated in implantation and early embryo development. Regular hCG for example promotes progesterone secretion by corpus lutea, angiogenesis of uterine vasculature, or growth, and differentiation of fetal organs, whereas hyperglycosylated hCG stimulates implantation by invasion of cytotrophoblast cells or stimulates growth of placenta (52). However, hCG can also be produced in non-pregnant women: it is produced at low levels by gonadotrope cells of the anterior pituitary, and seems to have an LH-like activity during menstrual cycle. Free beta-subunit of hCG is produced by multiple non-trophoblastic cancers. It is elevated in most cancers such as bladder, renal, prostate, gastrointestinal, lung, breast, neuroendocrine, gynecological, head and neck, and hematological cancers (53) and promotes their growth and malignancy by blocking apoptosis in cancer cells (52). hCG beta-subunit is thus used as a tumor biomarker usually associated with poor prognosis (53).

hCG, unlike eCG, has an LH like activity only and does not bind FSH-R (1, 54). CG and LH exert their effects via the same receptor, LH/CG receptor (LHCGR), that is coupled to Gs and Gq in granulosa cells and theca cells (55). However, the receptor is able to differentiate the binding and activity of these two hormones (56), and hLH and hCG differentially regulate signaling pathways (57, 58).

FSH plays an important role in reproduction. In females, it is implicated in follicular growth. FSH-R is expressed in granulosa cells and it is mainly coupled to Gs, which activates adenylyl cyclase and induces the secretion of cyclic adenosine monophosphate (cAMP), but it is also known to be coupled to Gq. In males, FSH regulates spermatogenesis. FSH-R is expressed in Sertoli cells and signals *via* Gs and Gi (59). In HEK 293 cells expressing FSH-R, FSH stimulates Gs/cAMP/PKA signaling pathway as in granulosa or Sertoli cells, but also signals *via* a beta-arrestin-dependent pathway, leading in both case to extracellular signal-regulated kinases (ERK) 1/2 phosphorylation but with different kinetics (60).

FSH-R is also expressed in other tissues than reproductive organs, such as osteoclasts (61) or adipose tissue (62), suggesting that FSH may play other physiological roles. In adipose tissue, FSH-R is coupled to Gi. An increase in Ca2+ influx induces the phosphorylation of cAMP-response-element-binding protein, which in turn activates an array of genes involved in fatty acids and triglycerides biosynthesis (63). FSH is thus implicated in lipid biosynthesis and its storage in adipocytes, which may contribute to age-related obesity and diseases due to high FSH levels in aging populations (62, 63). The first paper mentioning the role of FSH in bone mass regulation was published in 2006 (61). The authors proposed a mechanism where FSH was able to increase osteoclasts formation and function via a Gi2a-coupled FSH-R expressed in these cells and their precursors (64), suggesting that high circulating FSH levels were responsible for post-menopausal osteoporosis.

ANTIBODIES MODULATING THE ACTIVITY OF CHORIONIC GONADOTROPINS

Antibodies Modulating the Activity of eCG

Most of the antibodies against eCG were developed for structural analysis purposes. Maurel et al. identified an antibody able to inhibit eCG binding to LH and FSH receptors (65). Chopineau et al. analyzed the affinity and the specificity of 14 mAbs directed against eCG (66). The aim of this study was to analyze the epitopic sites of eCG and permitted to draw a topographic map of antigenic and functional sites of this hormone. The affinity of antibodies for eCG was ranging between 10^{-7} and 10^{-11} M. Ten of them were alpha-subunit specific because they recognized both native eCG and free alpha-subunit, but not free beta-subunit. One antibody exhibited a higher affinity for alpha-subunit than for the native eCG, and 13 mAbs exhibited a better affinity for the dimer than for the free subunits. The effect of these mAbs was then tested on FSH and LH bioactivities of eCG in *in vitro* bioassays. One beta-subunit specific, one alpha-subunit specific and one native alpha/beta dimer specific antibodies did not show any effect on FSH and LH bioactivities. Nine alpha-subunit specific antibodies either weakly or strongly inhibited both bioactivities. Finally, two mAbs were potentiating FSH bioactivity of eCG: one was beta-subunit specific and the other was native dimeric eCG specific. They did not inhibit eCG binding to LH-R. The degree of inhibition of inhibitory antibodies was correlated with their affinity for eCG, but it wasn't for the two antibodies potentiating FSH bioactivity of eCG.

These data suggest that the inhibitory or potentiating effects of mAbs on eCG bioactivities neither depend on their specificity nor their affinity. Moreover, the two antibodies potentiating the FSH bioactivity of eCG were either not affecting or inhibiting weakly the LH bioactivity of eCG, demonstrating that the effect on both bioactivities can be opposite (inhibitory or potentiating), with different degrees of activity (none or weak) on hormone bioactivities, highlighting the potential multiple mode of action of antibodies.

The high carbohydrate content makes also eCG highly immunogenic. Repeated injections of eCG for ovulation induction decrease the fertility of goats from 60 to 40% (12, 67). Roy et al. detected an immune response in animals treated with eCG for ovulation induction (68, 69), and demonstrated that the secreted antibodies from a previous treatment were inhibiting the action of eCG injected for the following treatment. The goats with high antibody levels at the time of eCG administration did have a much lower kidding rate (41%) than the other females (66%). This immune response was thus altering the fertility of these animals by delaying both the onset of estrus and the preovulatory LH surge. However, a deeper analysis revealed that some of the goats secreting high levels of anti-eCG antibodies did have a fertility beyond expected, ovulating and getting pregnant after each treatment, even after four treatments. The antibodies from the plasma of hypo-fertile or hyper-fertile goats secreting high levels of antibodies were purified and the IgG fractions were analyzed for their effect on FSH bioactivity in Y1 cell line derived from a mouse adrenal cortex tumor stably expressing human FSH-R, and for their effect on LH bioactivity in rat Leydig cells. The plasmas and the corresponding IgG fractions from different eCG treated goats exhibited either inhibitory, enhancing or no effects on FSH activity of eCG by modulating progesterone secretion by Y1 cells, and on LH activity of eCG by modulating testosterone secretion in Leydig cells (70). As expected, antibodies were mainly recognizing carbohydrate chains of eCG. Twenty-one either inhibitory, potentiating or neutral antibodies for LH and/or FSH bioactivities of eCG were analyzed. None of the antibodies cross-reacted with totally deglycosylated eCG or alpha-subunit of eCG. Interestingly, the inhibitory or stimulatory effects of these antibodies were not correlated with the affinity of the tested antibody for eCG (70). All together, these data demonstrated that gonadotropins' *in vivo* bioactivity and animals' fertility can be modulated with antibodies, especially since these antibodies are naturally occurring.

Later, Wehbi et al. (71) analyzed the effect of eCG in complex with three of these antibodies on FSH receptor signaling pathways. The eCG/antibody complexes effect was tested on HEK 293 cells expressing mouse FSH receptor and on granulosa cells punctured from slaughterhouse cows for their effect on cAMP production. The tested antibodies were differently modulating cAMP production: two of them were potentiating and one was slightly inhibiting eCG effect. In contrast, all three antibodies were enhancing ERK1/2 phosphorylation in HEK 293 cells expressing mouse FSH-R. Deeper analysis revealed that the antibodies were potentiating eCG signaling preferentially *via* beta-arrestin pathway, *via* cAMP/PKA pathway or *via* both. An antibody complexed to eCG was thus able to change the full agonist effect of eCG into a biased agonist effect, modulating differentially the balance between the signaling pathways induced by this hormone. This paper was also the demonstration that these antibodies were achieving the same *in vivo* effect in goat (i.e., high prolificity) *via* different signaling pathways. That was the first report of biased agonism at FSH-R and the authors suggested that such antibodies could help optimize glycoprotein hormones' bioactivities and thus the development of new therapies.

At the very beginning of infertility treatments, eCG was also used to treat women. The first successful treatment with eCG was described in 1945. Although its use lasted more than 30 years, scientists realized very early that women treated with eCG extracts, like animals, did produce "antigonadotrophic substances" which neutralize hormone's effect over time and after repeated injections. The immune response induced by eCG and the arrival of less immunogenic pituitary gonadotropin extracts led to the market withdrawal of eCG [reviewed in (4)].

Antibodies Modulating the Activity of Human Chorionic Gonadotropin (hCG)

As for other gonadotropins, anti-hCG antibodies were essentially developed for epitope mapping and variant specific mAbs permitted the development of immunoassays, leading *in fine* to pregnancy tests (72–74).

Naturally occurring endogenous antibodies were also reported: patients treated with exogenous gonadotropins can develop anti-hCG antibodies that impair fertility. They were detected in young men with hypogonadotropic hypogonadism treated with hCG (75, 76). These antibodies, detected in a 15 year-old patient following a secondary resistance during a third treatment to hCG, were low affinity but high binding capacity antibodies (76). A few years later, seven additional young men with hypogonadotropic hypogonadism, aged between 11 and 18 years, and resistant to classical hCG regimen were tested for the presence of anti-hCG antibodies. Four of them showed antibodies, but the neutralizing effect of hCG could be counter passed by increasing the doses of hCG used (75). The same kind of antibodies were described in women (77, 78). Immune response against hCG impairs fertility of women and induces pregnancy loss within the first trimester of pregnancy. To thwart this negative effect, Muller and collaborators described a treatment that was successful in three women positive for hCG antibodies. This treatment combined membrane plasmapheresis, prednisolone, and intravenous immunoglobulin therapy (78).

Anti-hCG auto-antibodies were also detected in sera of men and women that never received any injection of exogenous hormone (79). These antibodies were low affinity and did not interfere with hormone activity. However, few years later, antibodies with high affinity and the capacity to neutralize hCG and LH activities were detected in a patient with a history of spontaneous abortion, that was never exposed to exogenous hormone therapy (80).

ANTIBODIES MODULATING THE ACTIVITY OF FSH OR LH

FSH and/or LH Neutralization With Antibodies

Several inhibiting antibodies were described for FSH and most of them were used to better understand its physiological functions *in vivo*. Antibodies permit to block reversibly the action of one or several hormones, at a precise time of the lifespan of the studied model, rather than suppressing a whole organ like in hypophysectomy or a gene like in transgenic animals. For example, for female studies, in 1969, Goldman and Mahesh used an anti-sera obtained by rabbit immunization with ovine LH, that neutralized FSH as well as LH, to study the role of these hormones in ovulation (81). In 1970, the same group published data on the effect of the same anti-sera on neonatal rats (82). In 1971, Eshkol and Lunenfeld used the strategy of neutralization with antibodies to demonstrate the crucial role of FSH and LH in ovarian development during the first 2 weeks of life in rodents. FSH was found to be responsible for the stimulation of granulosa cell proliferation, organization and structure. FSH plus LH initiated secretory activity of granulosa cells, increased intrafollicular spaces, antrum formation, enrichment and maintenance of the theca layer, and development of the vascular system (19). At the same time, it was shown that LH anti-sera could block ovulation in rat, but not FSH anti-sera (83–86). Schwartz et al. suggested that FSH neutralization during estrus cycle could have a deleterious effect on follicles destined to grow and ovulate in following cycles (86). Several other studies have confirmed the role of LH as the indispensable trigger of ovulation, whereas FSH was required for the recruitment of antral follicles at the start of a new cycle in rat and hamster (87–91). The neutralization of FSH or LH with antibodies also permitted to study the role of these hormones in the synthesis of estrogen (92), on ornithine decarboxylase activity (93) and on gonadotropin surge-inhibiting factor/attenuating factor bioactivity (20) in rat and/or hamster. In monkey, the antibody neutralization of FSH highlighted the importance of FSH during follicular growth and showed that the mature follicle becomes less sensitive to FSH about 48 h before ovulation (94).

For male studies, Wickings and Nieschlag actively immunized *Macaca mulatta* against ovine FSH and observed a spermatogenesis suppression over a period of 2 years, confirming the importance of FSH for spermatogenesis (21). The importance of FSH in spermatogenesis was further confirmed by active immunization of *Macaca radiata* (95). In rat, even if the first studies obtained with immunoneutralization of FSH were controversial on the role of FSH in spermatogenesis (96, 97), later works with either passive (98) or active (22) immunization against FSH confirmed its crucial role in the maintenance of spermatogenesis. For active immunization, peptides from region 19–36 of rat FSH beta-subunit were used

(22). Altogether, these results suggest that immunoneutralization of FSH could be used as a contraception in men by suppressing spermatogenesis. However, Nieschlag recommended to abandon the approach of immunization as a contraception because a complete suppression of spermatogenesis was not achieved even after 4.5 years of immunization (99). Nevertheless, Moudgal and collaborators carried out a pilot study in 1997 where five male volunteers were immunized with ovine FSH isolated from sheep pituitaries (100). The subjects only responded to the first two immunizations (day 1 and 20), and did not respond to the boosters given at day 40 and 70. Ovine FSH vaccination generated antibodies against human FSH, but only 25–45% of the antibodies generated against ovine FSH were able to bind human FSH and the sperm count reduction was around 30–64%, which is not enough to consider this method as a contraception.

Anti-FSH antibodies were also detected in women. Two types of antibodies have been identified: naturally occurring anti-FSH antibodies (101, 102) and anti-FSH antibodies resulting from exogenous gonadotropins (103–106). First, Haller et al. found naturally occurring anti-FSH antibodies in patients with endometriosis or polycystic ovary syndrome (PCOS) and none of these patients had undergone ovarian stimulation for IVF. They also detected anti-FSH antibodies in healthy non-pregnant women but at lower rates than for patients with endometriosis or PCOS (101). Likewise, Shatavi et al. found spontaneous anti-gonadotropin antibodies in 27% of patients with unexplained infertility and never treated with gonadotropins, but only in 8% of women in the general population (102). To explain the presence of such spontaneous antibodies, it was supposed that an alteration of the immune system might be necessary and that the antigen responsible for their production could be either the circulating FSH from the female organism or the FSH in seminal fluid that may upregulate the anti-FSH immune response in females (101). In in vitro fertilization (IVF) patients, Haller et al. demonstrated that anti-FSH antibodies increase in infertile women with common autoantibodies (against nuclear antigens, smooth muscle, gastric parietal cells, b2-glycoprotein I, cardiolipin, and thyroid peroxidase) and with a history of IVF stimulation (103, 104). Shatavi et al. also found that anti-FSH antibodies were more recurrent in infertile patients with history of gonadotropin treatment than in infertile patients never treated with exogenous FSH or in women in the general population (102). Anti-FSH antibodies could also be associated with anti-ovarian antibodies (AOA) in patients with history of gonadotropin treatment (102, 107). The association of anti-FSH antibodies and AOA was also detected in infertile patients never treated by FSH and in women in the general population but at a lower frequency (102). Other studies have investigated the consequences of the presence of anti-FSH antibodies on the results of controlled ovarian stimulation (COS). Some studies found that anti-FSH antibodies were associated with poor ovarian response to IVF stimulation (104, 105). Thus, anti-FSH antibodies might have an inhibitory effect on FSH by preventing the binding of the hormone to its receptor or by trapping FSH in immune complexes (101, 107). On the contrary, Reznik et al. identified a higher proportion of anti-FSH antibodies in patients with a good response to COS compared to patients with a poor response (106). Antibodies produced in patients with a good response might have either no effect or a potentiating effect on the action of FSH. However, in humans, no in vitro study of the inhibitory or potentiating action of anti-FSH antibodies on FSH receptor signaling has been published yet. In human FSH, one of the major epitopes seems to be the 78–93 amino acid sequence of the β-chain (101, 107). This region contains a loop called cysteine noose which plays a role in the specificity of FSH receptor binding (101). Therefore, it was supposed that the binding of the hormone to its receptor could be modulated by antibodies directed against this region (101). To explain why some infertile patients develop anti-gonadotropin antibodies, some studies focused on the Major Histocompatibility Complex (MHC) Class II (103). The role of the MHC Class II is to present exogenous proteins to immune cells, which leads to a humoral immune response. In IVF patients, only anti-FSH IgA were associated with HLA-DQB1*03 (103). However, the development of anti-FSH antibody response to exogenous FSH treatment remains controversial. Indeed, a recent study conducted in healthy oocyte donors and infertile women has concluded that repeated gonadotropin treatments for IVF do not induce an immune response to FSH (108).

Antibodies Potentiating the Activity of FSH

The first anti-FSH mAbs described were directed against human FSH (16). Their binding specificities were well-characterized, but their effect on FSH activity was not investigated. The second anti-FSH mAb described in the literature was directed against bovine FSH (29) and was beta-subunit specific. It did not cross react with ovine or porcine FSH, indicating that it recognizes an area of bovine FSH not homologous to ovine or porcine hormones (29). Glencross et al. tested this antibody later on for its effect on bovine FSH bioactivity in hypopituitary Snell dwarf mice (109). The mAb injected in complex with FSH increased uterine weight whereas FSH alone or the mAb alone at the same concentrations did not have any effect, showing for the first time a potentiating effect with an anti-FSH mAb.

Holder's group described anti-sera directed against peptides derived from the beta-subunit of bovine FSH (110). When injected to hypopituitary Snell dwarf mice concomitantly with ovine FSH, these anti-sera produced by sheep immunized with peptides corresponding to 31–45 and 38–49 amino-acid regions of bovine FSH beta-subunit were able to enhance FSH activity, as measured by an increase in uterine and ovarian weight, and an increase in the percentage of keratinized cells in vaginal smears. The authors hypothesized that the administration of anti-peptide anti-sera precomplexed with FSH or active immunization of breeding animals with these peptides should result in a superovulatory response, and that the potentiating anti-sera strategy, in the case of FSH, could be used for several clinical situations, such as treatment of ovarian disorders related to low FSH secretion, induction of estrus and treatment leading to increase spermatogenesis.

ANTI-GONADOTROPIN ANTIBODIES AS THERAPEUTIC AGENTS

Therapeutic Antibodies in General

MAbs, initially developed for scientific purposes, now take part of the human therapeutic arsenal. Over the last three decades, they have grown to become more than 55% of the overall biotherapeutic market of the drug industry sales (111).

The regulatory story of therapeutic mAbs started in 1986 with the first FDA-approved therapeutic mAb, the murine mAb Orthoclone OKT3® (Muromonab CD3) indicated for the prevention of kidney transplant rejection. Unfortunately, the development of murine mAbs has been hindered because of the risk of immunogenicity in humans due to their murine elements. Replacing the constant region of murine mAb by human sequences resulted in the generation of the chimeric antibodies (∼30% murine content). The first-approved one, Rituxan® (Rituximab) in 1997, was used for the treatment of low grade B cell lymphoma. To overcome immunogenicity risk even further, new technologies for the generation of predominately or entirely human origin mAbs were developed. The humanized mAbs (5–10% murine content) are tailored by replacing all sequences by human except antigen binding complementary determining regions, which were derived from the mouse. The humanization technology developed by Sir Winter lead to the first humanized therapeutic antibody CAMPATH-1H® (Alemtuzumab, approved in 2001). Sir Winter was awarded the 2018 Nobel Prize in Chemistry along with George Smith for this technology and the fully humanization using phage display. Fully human mAbs (last generation) were developed by replacing the whole of the rodent sequences by human sequences. Humira® (Adalimumab) is the first fully human antibody approved in 2004, for the treatment of rheumatoid arthritis. Thanks to these new technologies, the rate of approval and mAbs available on the market for the treatment of various diseases has increased dramatically. In 2017, the FDA and the European Medicines Agency broke the record and approved 10 new therapeutic antibodies (112). Currently, more than 70 mAb products are available on the market, most of them being humanized (32%) or fully human (54%) (113).

To date, approved mAbs are from different isotypes, but the preferred mAbs in clinical use are of the IgG1 isotype (80%) (114). Additionally, there are five monovalent antibody-fragments on the market, four antigen-binding fragments (Fab) and 1 single chain variable fragments (scFv) (114). More sophisticated forms have been engineered, such as Fc-modification, IgG2/IgG4 hybrid Fc, glyco-engineered mAbs, bispecifics, or antibody-drug conjugates. These types of sophisticated mAbs reach more and more clinical trial studies (114, 115). According to Zhou and Mark (116), common mechanism of action proposed for mAb drugs include: (i) disruption of ligand–receptor interaction; (ii) target cell elimination via antibody-dependent cellular cytotoxicity (ADCC), complement-dependent cytotoxicity (CDC), and antibody-dependent cellular phagocytosis (ADCP); (iii) engagement of cytotoxic T cell by bispecific Abs; (iv) receptor downregulation by enhanced internalization and degradation; and (v) targeted drug delivery.

The indication of treatment for ∼80% of the therapeutic mAb drugs could be classified into oncology and immune diseases. The last ∼20% are used for the treatment of infection and cardiovascular diseases, orthopedic, eye and rare diseases (113). Despite the high treatment cost, the success of therapeutic mAb has recently reached the veterinary health with the launch in the European Union, in 2017, of Cytopoint® (Lokivetmab), a treatment for atopic dermatitis in dogs. Notwithstanding all the therapeutic mAbs developed to date, so far, none of them have succeeded in the field of fertility, and none of them are potentiating antibodies.

Therapeutics Involving Anti-gonadotropin Antibodies

Neutra-PMSG®, an Antibody Against eCG/PMSG

The unique antibody commercialized until now in the field of animal fertility is Neutra-PMSG®. This anti-eCG mAb is alpha-subunit specific and inhibits both LH bioactivity on small bovine luteal cells and FSH bioactivity on granulosa cells of bovine follicles (66). It was developed and marketed for cattle to limit the adverse effects of PMSG to improve the embryo production after superovulation treatment (117, 118). Due to a long half-life, PMSG had the disadvantage to cause a prolonged stimulation of follicular growth after preovulatory LH peak, inducing a poor response to superovulation treatment for cattle (117, 119, 120), sheep (121), and goat (122). Neutra-PMSG® injected 1–2 days after PMSG in superovulation treatment neutralized the adverse effects of PMSG by reducing its half-life in systemic circulation, improving embryo production. This mAb did not recognize endogenous gonadotropins in treated animals. Therefore, Neutra-PMSG® was highly specific for PMSG (117). Currently, most cows are superovulated using pituitary extracts containing FSH and LH (13), mainly because the pharmaceutical company (Intervet, The Netherlands) that developed the Neutra-PMSG® mAb stopped production in the 1990s.

Active Immunization Against hCG

A vaccination against hCG was also considered in the 1970s as a contraception method to avoid pregnancy in women (123, 124). The aim is to induce the secretion of antibodies that will bind hCG and block its activity, thus impeding pregnancy. Because an immunization with the whole dimeric hCG (alpha+beta-subunits) was raising antibodies not only against hCG but also against human LH (125), a special preparation of beta-hCG was made by processing it against heterologous anti-LH immunosorbents (124) and conjugating it to purified tetanus toxoid as an immunogenic carrier (123). This processed molecule was able to induce an immune response with antibodies specific to hCG. The antibodies produced were able to abrogate the binding of hCG to its receptor and its biological effects in *in vivo* bioassays. Moreover, the antibody titer declines over time, indicating that the vaccination is reversible (126). This vaccination system went through phase 1 clinical trials in several countries (India, Finland, Sweden, Chile and Brazil) under the International Committee on Contraception Research of Population Council. A slightly different preparation consisting of a dimer of hCG beta-subunit non-covalently associated with ovine LH alpha-subunit conjugated to tetanus and diphtheria toxoids (127) underwent phase 1 and phase 2 clinical trials in several centers in India. Eighty percent of treated patients generated sufficient antibody titer (>50 ng/ml) to be protected against pregnancy, and only one pregnancy was recorded over 1,124 cycles in fertile and sexually active women with an antibody titer higher than 50 ng/ml. After 12 years of inactivity on this project, Talwar and his collaborators are now working on a genetically engineered recombinant vaccine that is expected to go through clinical development in the next few years (128).

A similar approach was also tested for colorectal and pancreatic cancer treatments. In 2000, AVI BioPharma collaborated with SuperGen for the clinical development and marketing of Avicine, a synthetic vaccine constituted of the C-terminal peptide of hCG (CTP-37) conjugated to diphtheria toxoid. The vaccine went through several clinical trials until phase 3 pivotal study. In phase 2 efficacy study for colorectal cancer, 73% of treated patients developed an immune response against hCG and this response was associated with an improved median survival time (129, 130). As far as we know, the product has not reached the market yet. Recently, another group proposed another vaccine, where one residue in the amino-acid sequence of hCG beta-subunit is substituted (hCGβR68E) to eliminate cross reactivity with LH and conjugated to heat shock protein (Hsp70) as carrier to increase its immunogenicity (131). This vaccine has not been tested in humans yet.

Other Potential Therapeutic Antibodies
Antibodies Targeting FSH
To consolidate the assumption that high circulating FSH levels were responsible for post-menopausal osteoporosis, Zhu et al. showed that blocking FSH action attenuates bone loss in ovariectomized mice via two mechanisms: by inhibiting bone resorption and by stimulating bone formation (132). To do so, they used a mouse polyclonal antibody targeting a 13-amino acid sequence (LVYKDPARPNTQK) of mouse FSH beta-subunit that is a receptor-binding domain.

Liu et al. hypothesized that a pharmacological blockade of FSH action could also reduce body fat mass. In fact, they have shown that the same polyclonal antibody targeting the receptor-binding domain of FSH beta-subunit, injected daily for 8 weeks in mice, prevented the gain of body fat induced by the diet in male and female mice (133). This decrease of body fat was associated with an increase of fat thermogenesis (133, 134). For the purpose of potential therapeutic application in human, this team has developed a mAb targeting the same epitope in human FSH beta-subunit (LVYKDPARPKIQK) that had the same effects on body fat and thermogenesis on the mouse as the mouse polyclonal antibody directed against a sequence that is 2 amino-acids different (LVYKDPARPNTQK) (135, 136). The modulation of FSH activity by anti-FSH antibodies may be considered as therapeutic means to reduce the risk of obesity in elderly people with high levels of FSH (133). It was thus proposed that the same antibody could both inhibit bone loss and body fat gain (133, 136). However, while some of the other studies published on the subject supported the role of FSH in bone mass regulation (137–141), some others were contradictory (142, 143).

Moreover, clinical studies on human subjects reported that FSH suppression with GnRH agonist had no effect on bone resorption in women (144). In men, this suppression either increased bone loss (145), or had no effect when a testosterone supplementation was given (146). Furthermore, body fat mass is also increased in men treated with GnRH analog (147). Altogether, these data suggest that further investigations are needed to better understand the mechanisms underlying the role of FSH in bone mass and body fat regulation before a therapeutic approach can be envisaged (148). A therapeutic antibody to prevent osteoporosis is on the market since 2010. Receptor activator of nuclear factor-kB (RANK) ligand (RANKL) is a cytokine necessary for the development and the activity of osteoclasts. A fully human antibody, denosumab (Prolia®, Amgen) prevents RANKL binding to its receptor RANK. Denosumab, when given subcutaneously twice yearly for 36 months, reduces the risk of vertebral, non-vertebral, and hip fractures in women with osteoporosis (149), demonstrating that the strategy of therapeutic antibody can be used in this indication.

Antibodies Targeting hCG
Antibodies able to inhibit hCG activity were first described in 1980 (150). They were specific of the beta-subunit of hCG and did not cross react at all with other gonadotropins. Recently, one of these antibodies (mAb PIPP) was expressed recombinantly in tobacco leaves in different formats (scFv, diabody and entire antibody) and tested, after their extraction and purification, for their efficacy to neutralize hCG. The three formats of the same antibody were able to inhibit in vitro testosterone production induced by hCG in Leydig cells. In vivo, the entire mAb was able to block uterine weight gain in mouse model (151). These antibodies were envisaged as a contraception method by passive immunization in women, and were considered as a better method than active immunization where the response may be variable between patients, and a sufficient titer determined as the protective level of antibody was observed in 80% of the patients only. These anti-hCG antibodies have not entered a clinical development so far.

The same antibody was used for the development of an immunotoxin targeting hCG-expressing cancer cells (152). The VH and VL domains of the full antibody were linked together to form the scFv fragment (scFv PIPP). This scFv's gene was then fused with a gene expressing Pseudomonas exotoxin (PE38) and expressed in Escherichia coli as a recombinant protein (scPiPP-PE38). Once purified and tested on cancer cells, the immunotoxin showed 90% killing of hCG beta expressing histiocytic lymphoma, T-lymphoblastic leukemia, and lung carcinoma cells in vitro. However, further studies are needed to evaluate the potential of scPiPP-PE38 as a therapeutic agent for management of cancer cells expressing hCG or its subunits.

CONCLUSION

Many different antibodies against gonadotropins were developed and have proven to be very useful tools for many applications. They can also be naturally secreted due to a humoral immune response to endogenous or exogenous gonadotropins. With the same structure, immunoglobulins can have inhibitory or potentiating effects depending on their paratope defined by CDRs and their epitope (binding site) on the antigen. In the case of eCG, its naturally occurring potentiating antibodies have demonstrated that a differential activation of signaling pathways of FSH-R could lead to the same *in vivo* effect, i.e., high prolificity in goats (71). The development of antibodies with a range of modulating effects on the potency and the efficacy of FSH on its signaling pathways could help deciphering the importance of each pathway for FSH roles in reproduction, bone mass and body fat regulation. Moreover, these antibodies can represent potential therapeutics, targeting one pathophysiological or physiological condition in particular. Several applications for anti-gonadotropin antibodies have already been proposed and are under exploration, like osteoporosis, obesity, contraception, or cancer. All of these indications require inhibition of gonadotropins' action. On the other hand, in small ruminants, the naturally occurring anti-eCG potentiating antibodies induced a better fertility and prolificity demonstrating that it is possible to improve fertility by potentiating gonadotropins' activity during several estrus cycles, without any side effects. All these studies demonstrated that it is possible to target each gonadotropin very specifically despite their similarities.

To conclude, the development of antibodies modulating gonadotropins' activity could not only provide new tools to better understand their roles in different physiological processes, but could also bring to the market innovative drugs. Taking into account the state of the art and the clinical development time, there is a long way to go until a therapeutic antibody targeting a gonadotropin can reach the market.

AUTHOR CONTRIBUTIONS

All authors listed have made a substantial, direct and intellectual contribution to the work, and approved it for publication.

REFERENCES

1. Pierce JG, Parsons TF. Glycoprotein hormones: structure and function. *Annu Rev Biochem.* (1981) 50:465–95. doi: 10.1146/annurev.bi.50.070181.002341
2. Simoni M, Gromoll J, Nieschlag E. The follicle-stimulating hormone receptor: biochemistry, molecular biology, physiology, and pathophysiology. *Endocr Rev.* (1997) 18:739–73. doi: 10.1210/er.18.6.739
3. Huhtaniemi I, Zhang FP, Kero J, Hamalainen T, Poutanen M. Transgenic and knockout mouse models for the study of luteinizing hormone and luteinizing hormone receptor function. *Mol Cell Endocrinol.* (2002) 187:49–56. doi: 10.1016/S0303-7207(01)00698-0
4. Lunenfeld B. Development of gonadotrophins for clinical use. *Reprod Biomed Online* (2002) 4 (Suppl. 1):11–7. doi: 10.1016/S1472-6483(12)60006-6
5. Lunenfeld B. Gonadotropin stimulation: past, present and future. *Reprod Med Biol.* (2012) 11:11–25. doi: 10.1007/s12522-011-0097-2
6. Boehm U, Bouloux PM, Dattani MT, de Roux N, Dode C, Dunkel L, et al. Expert consensus document: European Consensus Statement on congenital hypogonadotropic hypogonadism–pathogenesis, diagnosis and treatment. *Nat Rev Endocrinol.* (2015) 11:547–64. doi: 10.1038/nrendo.2015.112
7. Dwyer AA, Raivio T, Pitteloud N. Gonadotrophin replacement for induction of fertility in hypogonadal men. *Best Pract Res Clin Endocrinol Metab.* (2015) 29:91–103. doi: 10.1016/j.beem.2014.10.005
8. Han TS, Bouloux PM. What is the optimal therapy for young males with hypogonadotropic hypogonadism? *Clin Endocrinol (Oxf).* (2010) 72:731–7. doi: 10.1111/j.1365-2265.2009.03746.x
9. Zitzmann M, Nieschlag E. Hormone substitution in male hypogonadism. *Mol Cell Endocrinol.* (2000) 161:73–88. doi: 10.1016/S0303-7207(99)00227-0
10. Koechling W, Plaksin D, Croston GE, Jeppesen JV, Macklon KT, Andersen CY. Comparative pharmacology of a new recombinant FSH expressed by a human cell line. *Endocr Connect.* (2017) 6:297–305. doi: 10.1530/EC-17-0067
11. Abd-Elaziz K, Duijkers I, Stockl L, Dietrich B, Klipping C, Eckert K, et al. A new fully human recombinant FSH (follitropin epsilon): two phase I randomized placebo and comparator-controlled pharmacokinetic and pharmacodynamic trials. *Hum Reprod.* (2017) 32:1639–47. doi: 10.1093/humrep/dex220
12. Baril G, Remy B, Vallet JC, Beckers JF. Effect of repeated use of progestagen-PMSG treatment for estrus control in dairy goats out of breeding season. *Reprod Dom Anim.* (1992) 27:161–8. doi: 10.1111/j.1439-0531.1992.tb01135.x
13. Bo GA, Mapletoft RJ. Historical perspectives and recent research on superovulation in cattle. *Theriogenology* (2014) 81:38–48. doi: 10.1016/j.theriogenology.2013.09.020
14. De Rensis F, Kirkwood RN. Control of estrus and ovulation: Fertility to timed insemination of gilts and sows. *Theriogenology* (2016) 86:1460–6. doi: 10.1016/j.theriogenology.2016.04.089
15. Sunderam S, Kissin DM, Crawford SB, Folger SG, Boulet SL, Warner L, et al. Assisted reproductive technology surveillance - United States, 2015. *MMWR Surveill Summ.* (2018) 67:1–28. doi: 10.15585/mmwr.ss6703a1
16. Hojo H, Ryan RJ. Monoclonal antibodies against human follicle-stimulating hormone. *Endocrinology* (1985) 117:2428–34. doi: 10.1210/endo-117-6-2428
17. Lunenfeld B, Isersky C, Shelesnyakmc. Immunologic studies on gonadotropins. I. Immunogenic properties and immunologic characterization of human chorionic gonadotropin preparations (HCG) and their homologous antisera. *J Clin Endocrinol Metab.* (1962) 22:555–63. doi: 10.1210/jcem-22-6-555
18. Weiner RS, Dias JA, Andersen TT. Epitope mapping of human follicle stimulating hormone-alpha using monoclonal antibody 3A identifies a potential receptor binding sequence. *Endocrinology* (1991) 128:1485–95. doi: 10.1210/endo-128-3-1485
19. Eshkol A, Lunenfeld B. Biological effects of antibodies to gonadotropins. *Gynecol Invest.* (1971) 2:23–56. doi: 10.1159/000301850
20. Tio S, van Dieten JA, de Koning J. Immunoneutralization of follicle stimulating hormone does not affect gonadotrophin surge-inhibiting factor/attenuating factor bioactivity during the rat ovarian cycle. *Hum Reprod.* (1998) 13:2731–7. doi: 10.1093/humrep/13.10.2731
21. Wickings EJ, Nieschlag E. Suppression of spermatogenesis over two years in rhesus monkeys actively immunized with follicle-stimulating hormone. *Fertil Steril.* (1980) 34:269–74. doi: 10.1016/S0015-0282(16)44961-7
22. Yao B, Yi N, Zhou S, OuYang W, Xu H, Ge Y, et al. The effect of induced anti-follicle-stimulating hormone autoantibody on serum hormone level and apoptosis in rat testis. *Life Sci.* (2012) 91:83–8. doi: 10.1016/j.lfs.2012.04.026
23. Aono T, Taymor ML. Radioimmunoassay for follicle-stimulating hormone (FSH) with 125-I-labeled FSH. *Am J Obstet Gynecol.* (1968) 100:110–7. doi: 10.1016/S0002-9378(15)33647-4
24. Check JH, Nazari A, Kuhn R, Lauer C. Relationship of early follicular phase sera follicle stimulating hormone and luteinizing hormone levels as measured by a radioimmunoassay and an enzyme-linked immunosorbent assay to number of oocytes retrieved. *Clin Exp Obstet Gynecol.* (1996) 23:83–6.
25. L'Hermite M, Niswender GD, Reichert LE Jr, Midgley AR Jr. Serum follicle-stimulating hormone in sheep as measured by radioimmunoassay. *Biol Reprod.* (1972) 6:325–32. doi: 10.1093/biolreprod/6.2.325
26. Midgley AR. Radioimmunoassay for human follicle-stimulating hormone. *J Clin Endocrinol Metab.* (1967) 27:295–9. doi: 10.1210/jcem-27-2-295

27. Odell WD, Parlow AF, Cargille CM, Ross GT. Radioimmunoassay for human follicle-stimulating hormone: physiological studies. *J Clin Invest.* (1968) 47:2551–62. doi: 10.1172/JCI105937

28. Donini P, Puzzuoli D, D'Alessio I, Lunenfeld B, Eshkol A, Parlow AF. Purification and separation of follicle stimulating hormone (FSH) and luteinizing hormone (LH) from human postmenopausal gonadotrophin (HMG). II. Preparation of biological apparently pure FSH by selective binding of the LH with an anti-HGG serum and subsequent chromatography. *Acta Endocrinol (Copenh).* (1966) 52:186–98. doi: 10.1530/acta.0.0520186

29. Miller KF, Goldsby RA, Bolt DJ. Immunoaffinity chromatography of bovine FSH using monoclonal antibodies. *J Endocrinol.* (1987) 115:283–8. doi: 10.1677/joe.0.1150283

30. Zandian M, Jungbauer A. An immunoaffinity column with a monoclonal antibody as ligand for human follicle stimulating hormone. *J Sep Sci.* (2009) 32:1585–91. doi: 10.1002/jssc.200900103

31. Schechter Y, Hernaez L, Schlessinger J, Cuatrecasas P. Local aggregation of hormone-receptor complexes is required for activation by epidermal growth factor. *Nature* (1979) 278:835–8. doi: 10.1038/278835a0

32. Shechter Y, Chang KJ, Jacobs S, Cuatrecasas P. Modulation of binding and bioactivity of insulin by anti-insulin antibody: relation to possible role of receptor self-aggregation in hormone action. *Proc Natl Acad Sci USA.* (1979) 76:2720–4. doi: 10.1073/pnas.76.6.2720

33. Aston R, Holder AT, Ivanyi J, Bomford R. Enhancement of bovine growth hormone activity *in vivo* by monoclonal antibodies. *Mol Immunol.* (1987) 24:143–50. doi: 10.1016/0161-5890(87)90086-1

34. Holder AT, Aston R, Preece MA, Ivanyi J. Monoclonal antibody-mediated enhancement of growth hormone activity *in vivo*. *J Endocrinol.* (1985) 107:R9–12. doi: 10.1677/joe.0.107R009

35. Holder AT, Blows JA, Aston R, Bates PC. Monoclonal antibody enhancement of the effects of human growth hormone on growth and body composition in mice. *J Endocrinol.* (1988) 117:85–90. doi: 10.1677/joe.0.1170085

36. Holder AT, Aston R, Rest JR, Hill DJ, Patel N, Ivanyi J. Monoclonal antibodies can enhance the biological activity of thyrotropin. *Endocrinology* (1987) 120:567–73. doi: 10.1210/endo-120-2-567

37. Costagliola S, Bonomi M, Morgenthaler NG, Van Durme J, Panneels V, Refetoff S, et al. Delineation of the discontinuous-conformational epitope of a monoclonal antibody displaying full *in vitro* and *in vivo* thyrotropin activity. *Mol Endocrinol.* (2004) 18:3020–34. doi: 10.1210/me.2004-0231

38. Costagliola S, Franssen JD, Bonomi M, Urizar E, Willnich M, Bergmann A, et al. Generation of a mouse monoclonal TSH receptor antibody with stimulating activity. *Biochem Biophys Res Commun.* (2002) 299:891–6. doi: 10.1016/S0006-291X(02)02762-6

39. Allen WR, Moor RM. The origin of the equine endometrial cups. I. Production of PMSG by fetal trophoblast cells. *J Reprod Fertil.* (1972) 29:313–6. doi: 10.1530/jrf.0.0290313

40. Papkoff H. Chemical and biological properties of the subunits of pregnant mare serum gonadotropin. *Biochem Biophys Res Commun.* (1974) 58:397–404. doi: 10.1016/0006-291X(74)90378-7

41. Sherman GB, Wolfe MW, Farmerie TA, Clay CM, Threadgill DS, Sharp DC, et al. A single gene encodes the beta-subunits of equine luteinizing hormone and chorionic gonadotropin. *Mol Endocrinol.* (1992) 6:951–9.

42. Bousfield GR, Butnev VY, Butnev VY. Identification of twelve O-glycosylation sites in equine chorionic gonadotropin beta and equine luteinizing hormone ss by solid-phase Edman degradation. *Biol Reprod.* (2001) 64:136–47. doi: 10.1095/biolreprod64.1.136

43. Christakos S, Bahl OP. Pregnant mare serum gonadotropin. Purification and physicochemical, biological, and immunological characterization. *J Biol Chem.* (1979) 254:4253–61.

44. Matzuk MM, Hsueh AJ, Lapolt P, Tsafriri A, Keene JL, Boime I. The biological role of the carboxyl-terminal extension of human chorionic gonadotropin [corrected] beta-subunit. *Endocrinology* (1990) 126:376–83. doi: 10.1210/endo-126-1-376

45. McIntosh JE, Moor RM, Allen WR. Pregnant mare serum gonadotrophin: rate of clearance from the circulation of sheep. *J Reprod Fertil.* (1975) 44:95–100. doi: 10.1530/jrf.0.0440095

46. Combarnous Y, Guillou F, Martinat N. Comparison of *in vitro* follicle-stimulating hormone (FSH) activity of equine gonadotropins (luteinizing hormone, FSH, and chorionic gonadotropin) in male and female rats. *Endocrinology* (1984) 115:1821–7. doi: 10.1210/endo-115-5-1821

47. Combarnous Y, Hennen G, Ketelslegers JM. Pregnant mare serum gonadotropin exhibits higher affinity for lutropin than for follitropin receptors of porcine testis. *FEBS Lett.* (1978) 90:65–8. doi: 10.1016/0014-5793(78)80299-3

48. Guillou F, Combarnous Y. Purification of equine gonadotropins and comparative study of their acid-dissociation and receptor-binding specificity. *Biochim Biophys Acta* (1983) 755:229–36. doi: 10.1016/0304-4165(83)90208-8

49. Licht P, Gallo AB, Aggarwal BB, Farmer SW, Castelino JB, Papkoff H. Biological and binding activities of equine pituitary gonadotrophins and pregnant mare serum gonadotrophin. *J Endocrinol.* (1979) 83:311–22. doi: 10.1677/joe.0.0830311

50. Matsui T, Mizuochi T, Titani K, Okinaga T, Hoshi M, Bousfield GR, et al. Structural analysis of N-linked oligosaccharides of equine chorionic gonadotropin and lutropin beta-subunits. *Biochemistry* (1994) 33:14039–48. doi: 10.1021/bi00251a012

51. Smith PL, Bousfield GR, Kumar S, Fiete D, Baenziger JU. Equine lutropin and chorionic gonadotropin bear oligosaccharides terminating with SO4-4-GalNAc and Sia alpha 2,3Gal, respectively. *J Biol Chem.* (1993) 268:795–802.

52. Cole LA. Biological functions of hCG and hCG-related molecules. *Reprod Biol Endocrinol.* (2010) 8:102. doi: 10.1186/1477-7827-8-102

53. Stenman UH, Alfthan H, Hotakainen K. Human chorionic gonadotropin in cancer. *Clin Biochem.* (2004) 37:549–61. doi: 10.1016/j.clinbiochem.2004.05.008

54. Moyle WR, Campbell RK, Myers RV, Bernard MP, Han Y, Wang X. Co-evolution of ligand-receptor pairs. *Nature* (1994) 368:251–5. doi: 10.1038/368251a0

55. Casarini L, Santi D, Brigante G, Simoni M. Two hormones for one receptor: evolution, biochemistry, actions, and pathophysiology of LH and hCG. *Endocr Rev.* (2018) 39:549–92. doi: 10.1210/er.2018-00065

56. Galet C, Ascoli M. The differential binding affinities of the luteinizing hormone (LH)/choriogonadotropin receptor for LH and choriogonadotropin are dictated by different extracellular domain residues. *Mol Endocrinol.* (2005) 19:1263–76. doi: 10.1210/me.2004-0410

57. Casarini L, Lispi M, Longobardi S, Milosa F, La Marca A, Tagliasacchi D, et al. LH and hCG action on the same receptor results in quantitatively and qualitatively different intracellular signalling. *PLoS ONE* (2012) 7:e46682. doi: 10.1371/journal.pone.0046682

58. Riccetti L, De Pascali F, Gilioli L, Poti F, Giva LB, Marino M, et al. Human LH and hCG stimulate differently the early signalling pathways but result in equal testosterone synthesis in mouse Leydig cells *in vitro*. *Reprod Biol Endocrinol.* (2017) 15:2. doi: 10.1186/s12958-016-0224-3

59. De Pascali F, Reiter E. beta-arrestins and biased signaling in gonadotropin receptors. *Minerva Ginecol.* (2018) 70:525–38. doi: 10.23736/S0026-4784.18.04272-7

60. Kara E, Crepieux P, Gauthier C, Martinat N, Piketty V, Guillou F, et al. A phosphorylation cluster of five serine and threonine residues in the C-terminus of the follicle-stimulating hormone receptor is important for desensitization but not for beta-arrestin-mediated ERK activation. *Mol Endocrinol.* (2006) 20:3014–26. doi: 10.1210/me.2006-0098

61. Sun L, Peng Y, Sharrow AC, Iqbal J, Zhang Z, Papachristou DJ, et al. FSH directly regulates bone mass. *Cell* (2006) 125:247–60. doi: 10.1016/j.cell.2006.01.051

62. Cui H, Zhao G, Liu R, Zheng M, Chen J, Wen J. FSH stimulates lipid biosynthesis in chicken adipose tissue by upregulating the expression of its receptor FSHR. *J Lipid Res.* (2012) 53:909–17. doi: 10.1194/jlr.M025403

63. Liu XM, Chan HC, Ding GL, Cai J, Song Y, Wang TT, et al. FSH regulates fat accumulation and redistribution in aging through the Galphai/Ca(2+)/CREB pathway. *Aging Cell* (2015) 14:409–20. doi: 10.1111/acel.12331

64. Zhu LL, Tourkova I, Yuen T, Robinson LJ, Bian Z, Zaidi M, et al. Blocking FSH action attenuates osteoclastogenesis. *Biochem Biophys Res Commun.* (2012) 422:54–8. doi: 10.1016/j.bbrc.2012.04.104

65. Maurel MC, Ban E, Bidart JM, Combarnous Y. Immunochemical study of equine chorionic gonadotropin (eCG/PMSG): antigenic determinants

on alpha- and beta-subunits. *Biochim Biophys Acta* (1992) 1159:74–80. doi: 10.1016/0167-4838(92)90077-Q

66. Chopineau M, Maurel MC, Combarnous Y, Durand P. Topography of equine chorionic gonadotropin epitopes relative to the luteinizing hormone and follicle-stimulating hormone receptor interaction sites. *Mol Cell Endocrinol.* (1993) 92:229–39. doi: 10.1016/0303-7207(93)90013-A

67. Baril G, Leboeuf B, Saumande J. Synchronization of estrus in goats: the relationship between time of occurrence of estrus and fertility following artificial insemination. *Theriogenology* (1993) 40:621–8. doi: 10.1016/0093-691X(93)90414-Z

68. Roy F, Combes B, Vaiman D, Cribiu EP, Pobel T, Deletang F, et al. Humoral immune response to equine chorionic gonadotropin in ewes: association with major histocompatibility complex and interference with subsequent fertility. *Biol Reprod.* (1999) 61:209–18. doi: 10.1095/biolreprod61.1.209

69. Roy F, Maurel MC, Combes B, Vaiman D, Cribiu EP, Lantier I, et al. The negative effect of repeated equine chorionic gonadotropin treatment on subsequent fertility in Alpine goats is due to a humoral immune response involving the major histocompatibility complex. *Biol Reprod.* (1999) 60:805–13. doi: 10.1095/biolreprod60.4.805

70. Herve V, Roy F, Bertin J, Guillou F, Maurel MC. Antiequine chorionic gonadotropin (eCG) antibodies generated in goats treated with eCG for the induction of ovulation modulate the luteinizing hormone and follicle-stimulating hormone bioactivities of eCG differently. *Endocrinology* (2004) 145:294–303. doi: 10.1210/en.2003-0595

71. Wehbi V, Decourtye J, Piketty V, Durand G, Reiter E, Maurel MC. Selective modulation of follicle-stimulating hormone signaling pathways with enhancing equine chorionic gonadotropin/antibody immune complexes. *Endocrinology* (2010) 151:2788–99. doi: 10.1210/en.2009-0892

72. Berger P, Bidart JM, Delves PS, Dirnhofer S, Hoermann R, Isaacs N, et al. Immunochemical mapping of gonadotropins. *Mol Cell Endocrinol* (1996) 125:33–43. doi: 10.1016/S0303-7207(96)03943-3

73. Berger P, Paus E, Hemken PM, Sturgeon C, Stewart WW, Skinner JP, et al. Candidate epitopes for measurement of hCG and related molecules: the second ISOBM TD-7 workshop. *Tumour Biol.* (2013) 34:4033–57. doi: 10.1007/s13277-013-0994-6

74. Bidart JM, Bellet D. Human chorionic gonadotropin Molecular forms, detection, and clinical implications. *Trends Endocrinol Metab.* (1993) 4:285–91. doi: 10.1016/1043-2760(93)90047-I

75. Claustrat B, David L, Faure A, Francois R. Development of anti-human chorionic gonadotropin antibodies in patients with hypogonadotropic hypogonadism. A study of four patients. *J Clin Endocrinol Metab.* (1983) 57:1041–7. doi: 10.1210/jcem-57-5-1041

76. Sokol RZ, McClure RD, Peterson M, Swerdloff RS. Gonadotropin therapy failure secondary to human chorionic gonadotropin-induced antibodies. *J Clin Endocrinol Metab.* (1981) 52:929–32. doi: 10.1210/jcem-52-5-929

77. Amato F, Warnes GM, Kirby CA, Norman RJ. Infertility caused by HCG autoantibody. *J Clin Endocrinol Metab.* (2002) 87:993–7. doi: 10.1210/jcem.87.3.8334

78. Muller V, Ob'edkova K, Krikheli I, Kogan I, Fedorova I, Lesik E, et al. Successful pregnancy outcome in women with recurrent IVF failure and Anti-hCG autoimmunity: a report of three cases. *Case Rep Immunol.* (2016) 2016:4391537. doi: 10.1155/2016/4391537

79. Wass M, McCann K, Bagshawe KD. Isolation of antibodies to HCG/LH from human sera. *Nature* (1978) 274:369–70. doi: 10.1038/274368a0

80. Pala A, Coghi I, Spampinato G, Di Gregorio R, Strom R, Carenza L. Immunochemical and biological characteristics of a human autoantibody to human chorionic gonadotropin and luteinizing hormone. *J Clin Endocrinol Metab.* (1988) 67:1317–21. doi: 10.1210/jcem-67-6-1317

81. Goldman BD, Mahesh VB. A possible role of acute FSH-release in ovulation in the hamster, as demonstrated by utilization of antibodies to LH and FSH. *Endocrinology* (1969) 84:236–43. doi: 10.1210/endo-84-2-236

82. Goldman BD, Mahesh VB. Induction of infertility in male rats by treatment with gonadotropin antiserum during neonatal life. *Biol Reprod.* (1970) 2:444–51. doi: 10.1095/biolreprod2.3.444

83. Ely CA, Schwartz NB. Elucidation of the role of the luteinizing hormone in estrogen secretion and ovulation by use of antigonadotropic sera. *Endocrinology* (1971) 89:1103–8. doi: 10.1210/endo-89-4-1103

84. Schwartz NB. The role of FSH and LH and of their antibodies on follicle growth and on ovulation. *Biol Reprod.* (1974) 10:236–72. doi: 10.1095/biolreprod10.2.236

85. Schwartz NB, Ely CA. Comparison of effects of hypophysectomy, antiserum to ovine LH, and ovariectomy on estrogen secretion during the rat estrous cycle. *Endocrinology* (1970) 86:1420–35. doi: 10.1210/endo-86-6-1420

86. Schwartz NB, Krone K, Talley WL, Ely CA. Administration of antiserum to ovine FSH in the female rat: failure to influence immediate events of cycle. *Endocrinology* (1973) 92:1165–74. doi: 10.1210/endo-92-4-1165

87. Rani CS, Moudgal NR. Examination of the role of FSH in periovulatory events in the hamster. *J Reprod Fertil.* (1977) 50:37–45. doi: 10.1530/jrf.0.0500037

88. Rao AJ, Moudgal NR, Raj HG, Lipner H, Greep RO. The role of FSH and LH in the initiation of ovulation in rats and hamsters: a study using rabbit antisera to ovine FSH and LH. *J Reprod Fertil.* (1974) 37:323–30. doi: 10.1530/jrf.0.0370323

89. Schwartz NB, Cobbs SB, Talley WL, Ely CA. Induction of ovulation by LH and FSH in the presence of antigonadotrophic sera. *Endocrinology* (1975) 96:1171–8. doi: 10.1210/endo-96-5-1171

90. Sheela Rani CS, Moudgal NR. Role of the proestrous surge of gonadotropins in the initiation of follicular maturation in the cyclic hamster: a study using antisera to follicle stimulating hormone and luteinizing hormone. *Endocrinology* (1977) 101:1484–94. doi: 10.1210/endo-101-5-1484

91. Welschen R, Dullaart J. Administration of antiserum against ovine follicle-stimulating hormone or ovine luteinizing hormone at pro-poestrus in the rat: effects on follicular development during the oncoming cycle. *J Endocrinol.* (1976) 70:301–6. doi: 10.1677/joe.0.0700301

92. Rani CS, Moudgal NR. Examination of the role of follicle stimulating hormone in estrogen biosynthesis *in vivo* and *in vitro* in the ovary of the cyclic hamster. *Steroids* (1978) 32:435–51. doi: 10.1016/0039-128X(78)90057-0

93. Sheela Rani CS, Moudgal NR. Effect of follicle-stimulating hormone and its antiserum on the activity of ornithine decarboxylase in the ovary of rat and hamster. *Endocrinology* (1979) 104:1480–3. doi: 10.1210/endo-104-5-1480

94. Ravindranath N, Sheela Rani CS, Martin F, Moudgal NR. Effect of FSH deprivation at specific times on follicular maturation in the bonnet monkey (*Macaca radiata*). *J Reprod Fertil.* (1989) 87:231–41. doi: 10.1530/jrf.0.0870231

95. Aravindan GR, Gopalakrishnan K, Ravindranath N, Moudgal NR. Effect of altering endogenous gonadotrophin concentrations on the kinetics of testicular germ cell turnover in the bonnet monkey (*Macaca radiata*). *J Endocrinol.* (1993) 137:485–95. doi: 10.1677/joe.0.1370485

96. Dym M, Raj HG, Lin YC, Chemes HE, Kotite NJ, Nayfeh SN, et al. Is FSH required for maintenance of spermatogenesis in adult rats? *J Reprod Fertil Suppl.* (1979) 26:175–81.

97. Madhwa Raj HG, Dym M. The effects of selective withdrawal of FSH or LH on spermatogenesis in the immature rat. *Biol Reprod.* (1976) 14:489–94. doi: 10.1093/biolreprod/14.4.489

98. Shetty J, Marathe GK, Dighe RR. Specific immunoneutralization of FSH leads to apoptotic cell death of the pachytene spermatocytes and spermatogonial cells in the rat. *Endocrinology* (1996) 137:2179–82. doi: 10.1210/endo.137.5.8612566

99. Nieschlag E. Reasons for abandoning immunization against FSH as an approach to male fertility regulation. In: Zatuchni GI, Goldsmith A, Spieler JM, Sciarra JJ, editors. *Male contraception: advances and future prospects.* Philadelphia: Harper and Row (1986). p. 395–400.

100. Moudgal NR, Murthy GS, Prasanna Kumar KM, Martin F, Suresh R, Medhamurthy R, et al. Responsiveness of human male volunteers to immunization with ovine follicle stimulating hormone vaccine: results of a pilot study. *Hum Reprod.* (1997) 12:457–63. doi: 10.1093/humrep/12.3.457

101. Haller K, Mathieu C, Rull K, Matt K, Bene MC, Uibo R. IgG, IgA and IgM antibodies against FSH: serological markers of pathogenic autoimmunity or of normal immunoregulation? *Am J Reprod Immunol.* (2005) 54:262–9. doi: 10.1111/j.1600-0897.2005.00306.x

102. Shatavi SV, Llanes B, Luborsky JL. Association of unexplained infertility with gonadotropin and ovarian antibodies. *Am J Reprod Immunol.* (2006) 56:286–91. doi: 10.1111/j.1600-0897.2006.00428.x

103. Haller K, Salumets A, Grigorova M, Talja I, Salur L, Bene MC, et al. Putative predictors of antibodies against follicle-stimulating hormone in female infertility: a study based on *in vitro* fertilization patients. *Am J Reprod Immunol.* (2007) 57:193–200. doi: 10.1111/j.1600-0897.2006.00462.x

104. Haller K, Salumets A, Uibo R. Anti-FSH antibodies associate with poor outcome of ovarian stimulation in IVF. *Reprod Biomed Online* (2008) 16:350–5. doi: 10.1016/S1472-6483(10)60595-0

105. Meyer WR, Lavy G, DeCherney AH, Visintin I, Economy K, Luborsky JL. Evidence of gonadal and gonadotropin antibodies in women with a suboptimal ovarian response to exogenous gonadotropin. *Obstet Gynecol.* (1990) 75:795–9.

106. Reznik Y, Benhaim A, Morello R, Herlicoviez M, Ballet JJ, Mahoudeau J. High frequency of IgG antagonizing follicle-stimulating hormone-stimulated steroidogenesis in infertile women with a good response to exogenous gonadotropins. *Fertil Steril.* (1998) 69:46–52. doi: 10.1016/S0015-0282(97)00430-5

107. Gobert B, Jolivet-Reynaud C, Dalbon P, Barbarino-Monnier P, Faure GC, Jolivet M, et al. An immunoreactive peptide of the FSH involved in autoimmune infertility. *Biochem Biophys Res Commun.* (2001) 289:819–24. doi: 10.1006/bbrc.2001.6059

108. Morte C, Celma C, De Geyter C, Urbancsek J, Coroleu Lletget B, Cometti B. Assessment of the immunogenicity of gonadotrophins during controlled ovarian stimulation. *Am J Reprod Immunol.* (2017) 78:e12675. doi: 10.1111/aji.12675

109. Glencross RG, Lovell RD, Holder AT. Monoclonal antibody enhancement of FSH-induced uterine growth in snell dwarf mice. *J Endocrinol.* (1993) 136:R5–7. doi: 10.1677/joe.0.136R005

110. Ferasin L, Gabai G, Beattie J, Bono G, Holder AT. Enhancement of FSH bioactivity *in vivo* using site-specific antisera. *J Endocrinol.* (1997) 152:355–63. doi: 10.1677/joe.0.1520355

111. Levine HL, Cooney BR. Monoclonal antibodies – the development of therapeutic monoclonal antibody products: a comprehensive guide to CMC activities from clone to clinic. *Drug Dev Deliv.* (2018) 18:32–5.

112. Kaplon H, Reichert JM. Antibodies to watch in 2018. *MAbs* (2018) 10:183–203. doi: 10.1080/19420862.2018.1415671

113. Grilo AL, Mantalaris A. The increasingly human and profitable monoclonal antibody market. *Trends Biotechnol.* (2018) 37:9–16. doi: 10.1016/j.tibtech.2018.05.014

114. Strohl WR. Current progress in innovative engineered antibodies. *Protein Cell* (2018) 9:86–120. doi: 10.1007/s13238-017-0457-8

115. Lopes Dos Santos M, Quintilio W, Manieri TM, Tsuruta LR, Moro AM. Advances and challenges in therapeutic monoclonal antibodies drug development. *Braz J Pharm Sci.* (2018) 54:e01007. doi: 10.1590/s2175-97902018000001007

116. Zhou Y, Marks JD. Mechanism of Action for Therapeutic Antibodies. In: Liu C, Morrow KJ, editors. *Biosimilars of Monoclonal Antibodies: A Practical Guide to Manufacturing, Preclinical, and Clinical Development.* Hoboken, NJ: Wiley (2016). p. 85–111. doi: 10.1002/9781118940648.ch3

117. Nell T, Gielen J. The development of a monoclonal antibody against PMSG for a veterinary application. *Livestock Prod Sci.* (1995) 42:223–8. doi: 10.1016/0301-6226(95)00024-F

118. Van Der Lende T. Generation and applications of monoclonal antibodies for livestock production. *Biotechnol Adv.* (1994) 12:71–87. doi: 10.1016/0734-9750(94)90291-7

119. Dieleman SJ, Bevers MM, Wurth YA, Gielen JT, Willemse AH. Improved embryo yield and condition of donor ovaries in cows after PMSG superovulation with monoclonal anti-PMSG administered shortly after the preovulatory LH peak. *Theriogenology* (1989) 31:473–87. doi: 10.1016/0093-691X(89)90552-9

120. Dielman SJ, Bevers MM, Vos PLAM, De Loos FAM. PMSG/anti-PMSG in cattle: a simple and efficient superovulatory treatment? *Theriogenology* (1993) 39:25–41. doi: 10.1016/0093-691X(93)90022-W

121. Martemucci G, D'Alessandro A, Toteda F, Facciolongo AM, Gambacorta M. Embryo production and endocrine response in ewes superovulated with PMSG, with or without monoclonal anti-PMSG administered at different times. *Theriogenology* (1995) 44:691–703. doi: 10.1016/0093-691X(95)00249-8

122. Pintado B, Gutierrez-Adan A, Perez Llano B. Superovulatory response of Murciana goats to treatments based on PMSG/Anti-PMSG or combined FSH/PMSG administration. *Theriogenology* (1998) 50:357–64. doi: 10.1016/S0093-691X(98)00145-9

123. Talwar GP, Sharma NC, Dubey SK, Salahuddin M, Das C, Ramakrishnan S, et al. Isoimmunization against human chorionic gonadotropin with conjugates of processed beta-subunit of the hormone and tetanus toxoid. *Proc Natl Acad Sci USA.* (1976) 73:218–22. doi: 10.1073/pnas.73.1.218

124. Talwar GP, Sharma NC, Dubey SK, Salahuddin M, Shastri N, Ramakrishnan S. Processing of the preparations of beta-subunit of human chorionic gonadotropin for minimization of cross-reactivity with human luteinizing hormone. *Contraception* (1976) 13:131–9. doi: 10.1016/0010-7824(76)90025-1

125. Stevens VC, Crystle CD. Effects of immunization with hapten-coupled HCG on the human menstrual cycle. *Obstet Gynecol.* (1973) 42:485–95. doi: 10.1097/00006250-197310000-00001

126. Talwar GP, Dubey SK, Salahuddin M, Shastri N. Kinetics of antibody response in animals injected with processed beta-HCG conjugated to tetanus toxoid (Pr- beta-HCG-TT). *Contraception* (1976) 13:153–61. doi: 10.1016/0010-7824(76)90027-5

127. Talwar GP, Singh O, Pal R, Chatterjee N, Sahai P, Dhall K, et al. A vaccine that prevents pregnancy in women. *Proc Natl Acad Sci USA.* (1994) 91:8532–6. doi: 10.1073/pnas.91.18.8532

128. Talwar GP, Nand KN, Gupta JC, Bandivdekar AH, Sharma RS, Lohiya NK. Current status of a unique vaccine preventing pregnancy. *Front Biosci (Elite Ed).* (2017) 9:321–32. doi: 10.2741/e805

129. Ferro VA, Mordini E. Peptide vaccines in immunocontraception. *Curr Opin Mol Ther.* (2004) 6:83–9.

130. Moulton HM, Yoshihara PH, Mason DH, Iversen PL, Triozzi PL. Active specific immunotherapy with a beta-human chorionic gonadotropin peptide vaccine in patients with metastatic colorectal cancer: antibody response is associated with improved survival. *Clin Cancer Res.* (2002) 8:2044–51.

131. Kvirkvelia N, Chikadze N, Makinde J, McBride JD, Porakishvili N, Hills FA, et al. Investigation of factors influencing the immunogenicity of hCG as a potential cancer vaccine. *Clin Exp Immunol.* (2018) 193:73–83. doi: 10.1111/cei.13131

132. Zhu LL, Blair H, Cao J, Yuen T, Latif R, Guo L, et al. Blocking antibody to the beta-subunit of FSH prevents bone loss by inhibiting bone resorption and stimulating bone synthesis. *Proc Natl Acad Sci USA.* (2012) 109:14574–9. doi: 10.1073/pnas.1212806109

133. Liu P, Ji Y, Yuen T, Rendina-Ruedy E, DeMambro VE, Dhawan S, et al. Blocking FSH induces thermogenic adipose tissue and reduces body fat. *Nature* (2017) 546:107–12. doi: 10.1038/nature22342

134. Sponton CH, Kajimura S. Burning fat and building bone by FSH blockade. *Cell Metab.* (2017) 26:285–7. doi: 10.1016/j.cmet.2017.07.018

135. Ji Y, Liu P, Yuen T, Haider S, He J, Romero R, et al. Epitope-specific monoclonal antibodies to FSHbeta increase bone mass. *Proc Natl Acad Sci USA.* (2018) 115:2192–7. doi: 10.1073/pnas.1718144115

136. Zaidi M, Lizneva D, Kim SM, Sun L, Iqbal J, New MI, et al. FSH, bone mass, body fat, and biological aging. *Endocrinology* (2018) 159:3503–14. doi: 10.1210/en.2018-00601

137. Geng W, Yan X, Du H, Cui J, Li L, Chen F. Immunization with FSHbeta fusion protein antigen prevents bone loss in a rat ovariectomy-induced osteoporosis model. *Biochem Biophys Res Commun.* (2013) 434:280–6. doi: 10.1016/j.bbrc.2013.02.116

138. Liu S, Cheng Y, Fan M, Chen D, Bian Z. FSH aggravates periodontitis-related bone loss in ovariectomized rats. *J Dent Res.* (2010) 89:366–71. doi: 10.1177/0022034509358822

139. Qian H, Guan X, Bian Z. FSH aggravates bone loss in ovariectomised rats with experimental periapical periodontitis. *Mol Med Rep.* (2016) 14:2997–3006. doi: 10.3892/mmr.2016.5613

140. Tabatabai LS, Bloom J, Stewart S, Sellmeyer DE. FSH levels predict bone loss in premenopausal women treated for breast cancer more than one year after treatment. *J Clin Endocrinol Metab.* (2016) 101:1257–62. doi: 10.1210/jc.2015-3149

141. Zhu C, Ji Y, Liu S, Bian Z. Follicle-stimulating hormone enhances alveolar bone resorption via upregulation of cyclooxygenase-2. *Am J Transl Res.* (2016) 8:3861–71.

142. Allan CM, Kalak R, Dunstan CR, McTavish KJ, Zhou H, Handelsman DJ, et al. Follicle-stimulating hormone increases bone mass in female mice. *Proc Natl Acad Sci USA.* (2010) 107:22629–34. doi: 10.1073/pnas.1012141108

143. Rouach V, Katzburg S, Koch Y, Stern N, Somjen D. Bone loss in ovariectomized rats: dominant role for estrogen but apparently not for FSH. *J Cell Biochem.* (2011) 112:128–37. doi: 10.1002/jcb.22908

144. Drake MT, McCready LK, Hoey KA, Atkinson EJ, Khosla S. Effects of suppression of follicle-stimulating hormone secretion on bone resorption markers in postmenopausal women. *J Clin Endocrinol Metab.* (2010) 95:5063–8. doi: 10.1210/jc.2010-1103

145. Crawford ED, Schally AV, Pinthus JH, Block NL, Rick FG, Garnick MB, et al. The potential role of follicle-stimulating hormone in the cardiovascular, metabolic, skeletal, and cognitive effects associated with androgen deprivation therapy. *Urol Oncol.* (2017) 35:183–91. doi: 10.1016/j.urolonc.2017.01.025

146. Uihlein AV, Finkelstein JS, Lee H, Leder BZ. FSH suppression does not affect bone turnover in eugonadal men. *J Clin Endocrinol Metab.* (2014) 99:2510–5. doi: 10.1210/jc.2013-3246

147. Finkelstein JS, Lee H, Burnett-Bowie SA, Pallais JC, Yu EW, Borges LF, et al. Gonadal steroids and body composition, strength, and sexual function in men. *N Engl J Med.* (2013) 369:1011–22. doi: 10.1056/NEJMoa1206168

148. Kumar TR. Extragonadal actions of FSH: a critical need for novel genetic models. *Endocrinology* (2018) 159:2–8. doi: 10.1210/en.2017-03118

149. Cummings SR, San Martin J, McClung MR, Siris ES, Eastell R, Reid IR, et al. Denosumab for prevention of fractures in postmenopausal women with osteoporosis. *N Engl J Med.* (2009) 361:756–65. doi: 10.1056/NEJMoa0809493

150. Gupta SK, Talwar GP. Development of hybridomas secreting anti-human chorionic gonadotropin antibodies. *Indian J Exp Biol.* (1980) 18:1361–5.

151. Kathuria S, Sriraman R, Nath R, Sack M, Pal R, Artsaenko O, et al. Efficacy of plant-produced recombinant antibodies against HCG. *Hum Reprod.* (2002) 17:2054–61. doi: 10.1093/humrep/17.8.2054

152. Nand KN, Gupta JC, Panda AK, Jain SK. Development of a recombinant hCG-specific single chain immunotoxin cytotoxic to hCG expressing cancer cells. *Protein Expr Purif.* (2015) 106:10–7. doi: 10.1016/j.pep.2014.10.008

3

Effects of FSH on Sperm DNA Fragmentation: Review of Clinical Studies and Possible Mechanisms of Action

Monica Muratori[1]* and Elisabetta Baldi[2]*

[1] Department of Experimental and Clinical Biomedical Sciences "Mario Serio", University of Florence, Florence, Italy,
[2] Department Experimental and Clinical Medicine, University of Florence, Florence, Italy

*Correspondence:
Monica Muratori
monica.muratori@unifi.it
Elisabetta Baldi
elisabetta.baldi@unifi.it

Sperm DNA fragmentation (sDF) is an important reproductive problem, associated to an increased time-to-pregnancy and a reduced success rate in natural and *in vitro* fertilization. sDF may virtually originate at any time of sperm's life: in the testis, in the epididymis, during transit in the ejaculatory ducts and even following ejaculation. Studies demonstrate that an apoptotic pathway, mainly occurring in the testis, and oxidative stress, likely acting in the male genital tract, are responsible for provoking the DNA strand breaks present in ejaculated spermatozoa. Although several pharmacological anti-oxidants tools have been used to reduce sDF, the efficacy of this type of therapies is questioned. Clearly, anti-apoptotic agents cannot be used because of the ubiquitous role of the apoptotic process in the body. A notable exception is represented by Follicle-stimulating hormone (FSH), which regulates testis development and function and has been demonstrated to exert anti-apoptotic actions on germ cells. Here, we review the existing clinical studies evaluating the effect of FSH administration on sDF and discuss the possible mechanisms through which the hormone may reduce sDF levels in infertile subjects. Although there is evidence for a beneficial effect of the hormone on sDF, further studies with clear and univocal patient inclusion criteria, including sDF cut-off levels and considering the use of a pharmacogenetic approach for patients selection are warranted to draw firm conclusions.

Keywords: testis apoptosis, DNA fragmentation, human spermatozoa, oxidative stress, follicle-stimulating hormone

INTRODUCTION

FSH (follicle-stimulating hormone or follitropin) is the main hormone regulating the development and the functions of male and female gonads. It is a glycoprotein heterodimer consisting of two chains, α (92 amino-acids) and β (111 amino-acids) which are coupled by a non-covalent bond. The hormone acts by binding its receptor (FSHR) which belongs to the superfamily of the seven transmembrane domain G-protein-coupled receptors and is expressed in the gonads. After binding to FSHR, FSH activates the cAMP-protein kinase A cascade, which regulates gene expression through phosphorylation of CREB transcription factors [for a comprehensive review on FSR receptor signaling see (1)]. The action of FSH is influenced by the presence of both polymorphisms of FSHR, affecting the sensitivity of the receptors to the hormone (2), and the β chain of the hormone, which is associated with significantly lower serum FSH levels (3). FSHR and FSHβ polymorphisms influence the response to treatment with FSH in both women (4, 5) and men (6). In particular, in the adult testis, FSH regulates spermatogenesis by acting on Sertoli cells and there is evidence that FSHR polymorphisms are associated with male infertility (7).

FSH is essential for induction of qualitative and quantitative maintenance of spermatogenesis (8), as also demonstrated by studies on FSHR KO animals, which present severe disturbances of testicular function, including small testis and aberrant gametogenesis (9–11). Besides hypogonadotropic hypogonadic men (12), highly purified or recombinant FSH has been proposed for the treatment of infertile normogonadotropic men with idiopathic oligozoospermia or oligoasthenoteratozoospermia (OAT). In human, several trials using FSH to treat men with alterations of spermatogenesis, in particular OAT men, have been published. Although many of these studies report improvement of sperm parameters, such as concentration and motility, the efficacy of FSH treatment for OAT subjects remains controversial (6, 13). Even more controversy exists regarding the effect of FSH treatment on sperm morphology (14–17). Controversy may depend on heterogeneity of the study characteristics, in particular patient inclusion criteria (including FSH basal levels, FSHβ and FSHR genotypes), the dose and the molecule of administered FSH, the length of the treatment and the presence of non-responding men (18). Despite such controversy, a Cochrane meta-analysis (19) including only randomized control trials in which gonadotrophins were compared with placebo or no treatment, suggests a beneficial effect of FSH treatment on live birth and pregnancy after natural conception in men with idiopathic male factor subfertility, but no significant effects after assisted reproduction techniques (ARTs). A more recent meta-analysis (20) evaluating 15 controlled clinical studies [with broader inclusion criteria respect to (19)] with overall 614 men treated with FSH vs. 661 treated with placebo or untreated, confirms the improvement of spontaneous pregnancy and reveals a significant effect also after ARTs, which is independent on the ART methodology. Interestingly, 11 studies evaluated also sperm parameters after FSH treatment and the meta-analysis of these studies indicated that the treatment induced a significant increase of sperm concentration (although with a high degree of heterogeneity of the studies) and a trend to a better progressive sperm motility. However, a meta-regression analysis of the same studies showed no significant correlation between pregnancy rate and sperm parameters (concentration, progressive motility) (20) in line with previous studies demonstrating the poor predictive value of semen parameters for attainment of pregnancy (21, 22). Thus, the improvement of pregnancy rate following treatment of subfertile men with FSH is likely due to effects on other sperm qualities (such as sperm DNA fragmentation (sDF), see below) or on testicular functions leading to an improvement of sperm functions necessary for the process of fertilization which are not evaluated by routine semen analysis (such as hyperactivation motility, ability to undergo acrosome reaction or increased chromatin compaction). In this respect, a recent study (23), demonstrated that treatment with FSH improves the percentage of spermatozoa able to bind hyaluronic acid in FSH responding men (i.e., men increasing total sperm count and total motile sperm count after FSH treatment). As ability to bind hyaluronic acid is indicative of higher sperm maturation (24), the study by Casamonti et al. (23) suggests that FSH may improve such testicular function. Alterations in sperm maturation process are also involved in the generation of sDF (see below).

This review focuses on the effect of FSH administration to idiopathic infertile men on sperm DNA fragmentation levels, discussing the possible mechanisms involved in the action of the hormone.

Sperm DNA Fragmentation (sDF)

The main function of spermatozoa is to deliver DNA to the oocyte at fertilization. Integrity of sperm and oocyte DNA is fundamental for development and quality of embryos. Sperm DNA integrity is often compromised in infertile men and sDF represents the most common DNA abnormality in these men (25). sDF consists in the presence of single and double DNA strand breaks in the sperm nucleus. Such breaks may occur at different levels of the sperm's life, virtually from early steps of spermatogenesis to the site of fertilization. Indeed, there is evidence that sperm DNA breaks may originate in the testis, in the epididymis, during transit in the ejaculatory ducts, following ejaculation and even during in vitro manipulation for ARTs. Many types of insults have been demonstrated to provoke DNA breaks, which act through two main pathways: an apoptotic process, leading to activation of endonucleases and a direct attack to DNA by free radicals which produces both base oxidation and strand breaks (26). The apoptotic process occurs mainly during spermatogenesis, either because of insults impairing the testicular function or because of a derailment of the chromatin condensation process during spermiogenesis (27, 28). Spermatozoa with apoptotic signs (including DNA breaks) are found in the ejaculate because the apoptotic process fails to complete [abortive apoptosis, (29)]. Although free radicals, at low levels, play an important role for sperm functions [such as motility and capacitation (30)], when ROS production overtakes the anti-oxidant defenses of spermatozoa several damages can be produced (31). Excessive ROS production may act virtually at any level during sperm's life (32), although evidence suggests that their action occurs mostly after spermiation (see below) and even during in vitro manipulations for ARTs (33, 34). The occurrence of defects in the process of chromatin compaction renders the spermatozoa particularly vulnerable to ROS attack (35). Muratori et al. (28) has recently reported that a clear overlapping between oxidative damage and DNA breaks was detected only in viable spermatozoa, whereas in the bulk of ejaculated spermatozoa (including viable and non-viable cells and where most DNA fragmented spermatozoa are non-viable) the presence of DNA breaks overlapped highly apoptotic traits. Considering that viable, DNA fragmented spermatozoa are cells where DNA damage developed more recently respect to the ejaculation (28), these results suggest that oxidative stress acts later in sperm's life, most likely during transit in the male genital tract, whereas apoptotic damage occurs earlier, mainly at testicular level. A recent clinical study (36) seems to confirm such hypothesis revealing that sDF in unviable spermatozoa is associated mainly with the presence of ultrasound signs of testicular abnormalities, whereas the DNA fragmented sperm population containing viable spermatozoa was mostly associated with clinical and ultrasound alterations of the prostate and of seminal vesicles, likely due to inflammatory statuses. There is also evidence that DNA damage may occur after ejaculation during in vitro incubations (37–39) or because of in vitro manipulation during sperm selection for ARTs (33, 34, 40). In the latter case, DNA fragmented spermatozoa are highly motile and the damage appears to be induced by the contamination with heavy metals of density gradient preparations (33). Viable sperm with oxidative damage and/or strand breaks in their DNA are, most likely, a very dangerous sperm fraction of the ejaculate: they can actively participate in the fertilization process and give rise to embryos unable to successfully develop if the oocyte does not or only partially repairs the damage.

Many studies (41–43) reported that high levels of sDF are associated with a decrease of natural male fertility and recent meta-analyses confirmed the negative relationship between the amount of sDF and the outcomes of natural or assisted reproduction (44–46). It should be noted that important differences exist among the studies on ART outcomes, especially regarding couple inclusion criteria and methods used to evaluate sDF. Indeed, sDF may be evaluated by several methods [reviewed in (47)], among which TUNEL (Terminal deoxynucleotidyl transferase dUTP nick end labeling), COMET (also known as single-cell gel electrophoresis), SCSA (Sperm Chromatin Structure Assay) and Halosperm assays are the most popular. The problem with these methods is that they likely detect different types of DNA damages (47). In addition, these methods (with the exception of SCSA) are not standardized, thus making difficult to compare results among the studies. Recent meta-analyses grouped the studies according to the methods used to evaluate sDF and reported consistently that TUNEL and COMET methods are those that better reveal the negative association between sDF and pregnancy rate after ARTs (45, 46). TUNEL also resulted the method that better reveals the impact of sperm DNA damage on miscarriage in couples who conceived naturally or after IVF and ICSI (44).

Overall, the bulk of the studies described above suggests that sDF represents a target to treat men with idiopathic infertility. In consideration that apoptosis and oxidative stress are the main mechanisms producing DNA strand breaks (see above) possible therapies to prevent or decrease sDF are antioxidants and anti-apoptotic agents. The former have been used in several clinical studies, but, so far, reported beneficial effects are minimal. Indeed, a recent Cochrane meta-analysis (48) could not draw definitive conclusions regarding the benefit of treatment with anti-oxidant on live birth rates for infertile couples as only four low quality small randomized controlled trials were published at that time. The same meta-analysis reported also data about the effect of antioxidants on sDF levels. Even in this case, no clear conclusions could be drawn

because the two trials included in the meta-analysis utilized different antioxidants in a low number of patients (48). Use of anti-apoptotic agents, on the other hand, is not feasible because of the ubiquitous role of programmed cell death in the body. A notable exception is represented by FSH which has specific anti-apoptotic (or pro-survival) effects at testicular level (49–52).

Effect of Treatment With FSH on sDF Levels

A recent meta-analysis evaluated the effect of FSH on SDF (53) including six studies with overall 383 men with idiopathic infertility treated with FSH. The meta-analysis revealed a slight but significant decrease of sDF after FSH treatment for 3 months but not of other semen parameters such as sperm concentration, motility and morphology. Of note, the studies included in the meta-analysis are extremely heterogeneous, both for inclusion criteria and FSH treatment scheme. Indeed, in three of them patients with severe oligozoospermia (54) or oligoasthenoteratozoospermia (15, 55) were included, in another (56), patients with at least one parameter below the WHO criteria, whereas in the paper by Garolla et al. (57) male partners of infertile couples with any kind of infertility cause (with exclusion of seminal tract infections and antisperm antibodies) were included if sperm count was above 20 millions. The only study where sDF basal levels (at the cut-off level >15%) were comprised in the inclusion criteria was that of Simoni et al. (6). Interestingly, Ruvolo et al. (55), demonstrated that patients with sDF levels >15% were those showing a significant reduction in DNA sperm damage. More recently, Colacurci et al. (58) published results of a multicentric longitudinal trial including 103 infertile men treated with FSH for 3 months: the study demonstrated a slight but significant effect of the hormone on average sDF levels. Interestingly, this study evidenced that the treatment was more effective in the 48 patients showing sDF levels above 17% (median value of the caseload) and demonstrated that lifestyle habits like smoking may decrease the effectiveness of the therapy. The clinical studies included in the meta-analysis of Santi et al. (53) were heterogeneous also regarding the treatment schemes (type and dosage of FSH used) and the methods used to evaluate sDF, even if most studies employed TUNEL assay (6, 15, 54, 55, 57). It should be considered that TUNEL is not a standardized method and it has been reported that even small variations in the different steps of the assay may affect greatly the measures (59). In addition, an important difference regards the detection method: TUNEL positive spermatozoa may be evaluated by flow cytometry in thousands of spermatozoa [as used in the papers by (57) and (6)] or by fluorescence microscopy in few hundreds of spermatozoa [used in (15, 54, 55)]. Discrepancies between the two detection methods are due not only to the different number of analyzed cells but also to the different sensitivity of the procedures. For these reasons, comparison of studies employing flow cytometry or fluorescence microscopy revealed that the former yields greater measures of sDF (60). This methodological issue can explain why the meta-analysis of Santi et al. (53) failed to find

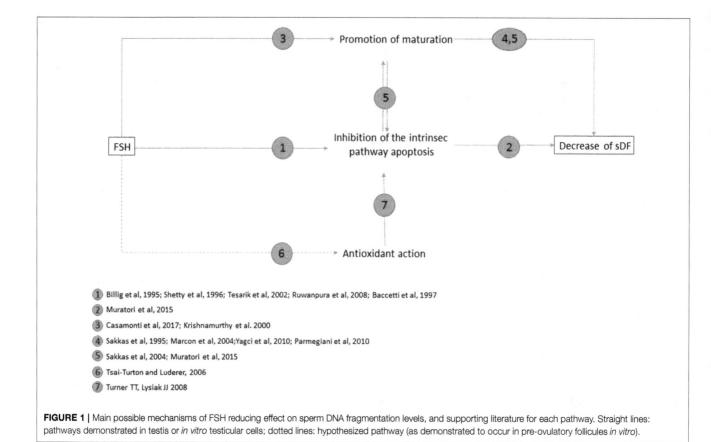

FIGURE 1 | Main possible mechanisms of FSH reducing effect on sperm DNA fragmentation levels, and supporting literature for each pathway. Straight lines: pathways demonstrated in testis or *in vitro* testicular cells; dotted lines: hypothesized pathway (as demonstrated to occur in pre-ovulatory follicules *in vitro*).

a difference in the average sDF levels after treatment when comparing FSH treated and untreated men.

There is also evidence, in the literature, that specific genotypes of FSHR (the polymorphism p.N680s) predicts responsiveness to FSH administration (6) and that the polymorphism of FSH beta-subunit promoter FSHB-211 TT is associated with lower FSH levels and lower sperm counts (61). Overall these studies suggest that the use of pharmacogenetic approaches to select patients, may increase the percentage of responders to the therapy.

Clearly, larger studies are needed to confirm the ameliorative effect of FSH on sDF: such studies should be properly designed, possibly using selection criteria which include a cut-off of sDF basal levels and the above mentioned pharmacogenetic approaches. However, it must be mentioned that, due to lack of international standardized procedures to evaluate sDF, identifying a cut-off value depends strictly on the assay used to measure the parameter. At present, the only possibility is the identification of cut-off values by comparing fertile and infertile subjects in each laboratory using the chosen method to evaluate sDF among those currently available (see above).

Which is(are) the mechanism(s) through which FSH ameliorates sDF levels in the ejaculate? If we consider that most DNA fragmented spermatozoa show signs of apoptosis and chromatin immaturity (28) likely due to a derangement of the spermatogenetic process or of the chromatin maturation process, the most probable mechanisms of action of FSH consist in anti-apoptotic and maturation promoting effects at tubular

level. There is evidence of anti-apoptotic effects of FSH both in the ovary and in the testis. In the ovary, the hormone is a major survival factor for follicles (62) and antagonizes the apoptosis induced by oxidative stress reducing ROS production through stimulation of the antioxidant glutathione (GSH) (63). In the testis, suppression or immunoneutralization of FSH increases apoptotic DNA fragmentation (49–51, 64). FSH suppression induces spermatogonial apoptosis predominantly via the intrinsic pathway, as an increase of caspase activity (52) and a decrease of BCL2 (51) have been demonstrated in spermatogonial cells. Consistently, *in vitro* studies demonstrated up-regulation of the BCL2 family member Bcl2l2 mRNA in spermatogonia of adult mice after FSH treatment (65). However, the molecular details by which FSH deprivation leads to activation of the apoptotic intrinsic pathway in spermatogonia is not fully clarified. In a murine model, upon deprivation of gonadotropins, the initiation of apoptosis was preceded by p38 MAPK activation and induction of iNOS (66) and this seems to be the case also in normal adult men (51, 52). FSH anti-apoptotic effects seems to occur both in Sertoli cells and in germ cells (64) and, in the latter, both before and after meiosis (49, 50, 64). Interestingly, it has been shown that the mechanisms by which gonadotropins promote the survival of germ cells can be different depending on the cell type (51, 52). In Sertoli cells, FSH promotes anti-apoptotic pathways presumably trough activation of protein kinase B/AKT protein (67). These results suggest that FSH may regulate proliferation and development of male germ cells both indirectly, by acting on Sertoli cells, and directly by up-regulating anti-apoptotic pathways in germ cells. There is also evidence for an effect of FSH on sperm maturation. Baccetti et al. (68) reported an improvement of semen quality and ultrastructural characteristics of spermatozoa in men with high levels of apoptosis and immaturity features in their spermatozoa, supporting the anti-apoptotic and pro-maturation role of FSH in human testis. Recently, a role of FSH favoring sperm maturation has been suggested by the above mentioned study of Casamonti et al. (23), which demonstrated that FSH increases the number of spermatozoa binding to Hyaluronic acid. Although the mechanism(s) through which FSH may promote sperm maturation are mostly unknown, interestingly, a disturbance in the normal replacement of histones by protamines during spermiogenesis, leading to poor condensation of spermatid nuclei, has been demonstrated in FSHR KO mice (69). Sperm maturation is closely linked to DNA integrity. Indeed, it is during spermiogenesis that the replacement of histones with protamines occurs and, as mentioned, a derangement of this process may lead to DNA fragmentation due to lack of re-ligation of the nicks necessary for chromatin compaction (70, 71). In addition, there is evidence that a disturbance of the process of chromatin compaction can represent a trigger for induction of apoptosis in the testis (28). Finally, increased ability of sperm to bind to hyaluronic acid has been associated to higher chromatin compaction and decreased DNA fragmentation (24, 72).

As mentioned above, DNA damage can be produced also by a direct attack of ROS. Although, at present, there is no evidence of an anti-oxidant effect of FSH in the testis or in spermatogonial cells *in vitro*, such effect of the hormone cannot be excluded, as it reduces oxidative stress-induced apoptosis in ovarian cells (63).

It should be mentioned that oxidative stress may produce the formation of breaks and stable DNA adducts also through a direct attack to DNA (31) and that such damage could persist following FSH treatment. The main possible mechanisms of FSH-related decrease of sDF levels are summarized in **Figure 1.**

CONCLUSION

Although sDF is an important reproductive problem affecting the outcomes of both natural and assisted reproduction, effective treatments to prevent or limit the sperm DNA damage in men are presently scarce. Treatment with FSH appears promising as there is evidence of a beneficial effect of the treatment on sDF (53). However, the lack of clear and univocal patient inclusion criteria contributes to the high heterogeneity of the clinical studies published so far, which does not allow to draw clear-cut conclusions about the effectiveness of the hormone on sperm DNA damage. Future studies should not only include cut-off values of sDF among patient inclusion criteria but also consider the pharmacogenetic evidence of FSH action to identify subjects that may not have beneficial effects from the therapy.

AUTHOR CONTRIBUTIONS

All authors listed have made a substantial, direct and intellectual contribution to the work, and approved it for publication.

FUNDING

EB is supported by Italian Ministry of University and Research (MIUR) PRIN project 2015.

REFERENCES

1. Ulloa-Aguirre A, Reiter E, Crépieux P. FSH receptor signaling: complexity of interactions and signal diversity. *Endocrinology* (2018) 159:3020–35. doi: 10.1210/en.2018-00452
2. Santi D, Potì F, Simoni M, Casarini L. Pharmacogenetics of G-protein-coupled receptors variants: FSH receptor and infertility treatment. *Best Pract Res Clin Endocrinol Metab.* (2018) 32:189–200. doi: 10.1016/j.beem.2018.01.001
3. Alviggi C, Conforti A, Santi D, Esteves SC, Andersen CY, Humaidan P, et al. Clinical relevance of genetic variants of gonadotrophins and their receptors in controlled ovarian stimulation: a systematic review and meta-analysis. *Hum Reprod Update* (2018) 24:599–614. doi: 10.1093/humupd/dmy019
4. Perez Mayorga M, Gromoll J, Behre HM, Gassner C, Nieschlag E, Simoni M. Ovarian response to follicle-stimulating hormone (FSH) stimulation depends on the FSH receptor genotype. *J Clin Endocrinol Metab.* (2000) 85:3365–9. doi: 10.1210/jcem.85.9.6789
5. Behre HM, Greb RR, Mempel A, Sonntag B, Kiesel L, Kaltwasser P, et al. Significance of a common single nucleotide polymorphism in exon 10 of the follicle-stimulating hormone (FSH) receptor gene for the ovarian response to FSH: a pharmacogenetic approach to controlled ovarian hyperstimulation. *Pharmacogenet Genomics* (2005) 15:451–6. doi: 10.1097/01.fpc.0000167330.92786.5e
6. Simoni M, Santi D, Negri L, Hoffmann I, Muratori M, Baldi E, et al. Treatment with human, recombinant FSH improves sperm DNA fragmentation in idiopathic infertile men depending on the FSH receptor polymorphism p.N680S: a pharmacogenetic study. *Hum Reprod.* (2016) 31:1960–9. doi: 10.1093/humrep/dew167

7. Wu Q, Zhang J, Zhu P, Jiang W, Liu S, Ni M, et al. The susceptibility of FSHB−211G > T and FSHR G-29A, 919A > G, 2039A > G polymorphisms to men infertility: an association study and meta-analysis. *BMC Med Genet.* 18:81. doi: 10.1186/s12881-017-0441-4
8. Nieschlag E, Simoni M, Gromoll J, Weinbauer GF. Role of FSH in the regulation of spermatogenesis: clinical aspects. *Clin Endocrinol.* (1999) 51:139–46. doi: 10.1046/j.1365-2265.1999.00846.x
9. Kumar TR, Wang Y, Lu N, Matzuk MM. Follicle stimulating hormone is required for ovarian follicle maturation but not male fertility. *Nat Genet.* (1997) 15:201–4. doi: 10.1038/ng0297-201
10. Abel MH, Wootton AN, Wilkins V, Huhtaniemi I, Knight PG, Charlton HM. The effect of a null mutation in the follicle-stimulating hormone receptor gene on mouse reproduction. *Endocrinology* (2000) 141:1795–803. doi: 10.1210/endo.141.5.7456
11. Dierich A, Sairam MR, Monaco L, Fimia GM, Gansmuller A, LeMeur M, et al. Impairing follicle-stimulating hormone (FSH) signaling *in vivo*: targeted disruption of the FSH receptor leads to aberrant gametogenesis and hormonal imbalance. *Proc Natl Acad Sci USA.* (1998) 95:13612–7.
12. Kliesch S, Behre HM, Nieschlag E. Recombinant human follicle-stimulating hormone and human chorionic gonadotropin for induction of spermatogenesis in a hypogonadotropic male. *Fertil Steril.* (1995) 63:1326–8. doi: 10.1016/S0015-0282(16)57619-5
13. Shiraishi K, Matsuyama H. Gonadotropin actions on spermatogenesis and hormonal therapies for spermatogenic disorders [Review]. *Endocr J.* (2017) 64:123–31. doi: 10.1507/endocrj.EJ17-0001

14. Baccetti B, Piomboni P, Bruni E, Capitani S, Gambera L, Moretti E, et al. Effect of follicle-stimulating hormone on sperm quality and pregnancy rate. *Asian J Androl.* (2004) 6:133–7.

15. Colacurci N, Monti MG, Fornaro F, Izzo G, Izzo P, Trotta C, et al. Recombinant human FSH reduces sperm DNA fragmentation in men with idiopathic oligoasthenoteratozoospermia. *J Androl.* (2012) 33:588–93. doi: 10.2164/jandrol.111.013326

16. Caroppo E, Niederberger C, Vizziello GM, D'Amato G. Recombinant human follicle-stimulating hormone as a pretreatment for idiopathic oligoasthenoteratozoospermic patients undergoing intracytoplasmic sperm injection. *Fertil Steril.* (2003) 80:1398–403. doi: 10.1016/S0015-0282(03)02202-7

17. Efesoy O, Cayan S, Akbay E. The efficacy of recombinant human follicle-stimulating hormone in the treatment of various types of male-factor infertility at a single university hospital. *J Androl.* (2009) 30:679–84. doi: 10.2164/jandrol.108.007278

18. Barbonetti A, Calogero AE, Balercia G, Garolla A, Krausz C, La Vignera S, et al. The use of follicle stimulating hormone (FSH) for the treatment of the infertile man: position statement from the Italian Society of Andrology and Sexual Medicine (SIAMS). *J Endocrinol Invest.* (2018) 41:1107–22. doi: 10.1007/s40618-018-0843-y

19. Attia AM, Abou-Setta AM, Al-Inany HG. Gonadotrophins for idiopathic male factor subfertility. *Cochrane Database Syst Rev.* (2013) 2013:CD005071. doi: 10.1002/14651858.CD005071.pub4

20. Santi D, Granata AR, Simoni M. FSH treatment of male idiopathic infertility improves pregnancy rate: a meta-analysis. *Endocr Connect.* (2015) 4:R46–58. doi: 10.1530/EC-15-0050

21. Guzick DS, Overstreet JW, Factor-Litvak P, Brazil CK, Nakajima ST, Coutifaris C, et al. Sperm morphology, motility, and concentration in fertile and infertile men. *N Engl J Med.* (2001) 345:1388–93. doi: 10.1056/NEJMoa003005

22. Leushuis E, van der Steeg JW, Steures P, Repping S, Bossuyt PM, Mol BW, et al. Semen analysis and prediction of natural conception. *Hum Reprod.* (2014) 29:1360–7. doi: 10.1093/humrep/deu082

23. Casamonti E, Vinci S, Serra E, Fino MG, Brilli S, Lotti F, et al. Short-term FSH treatment and sperm maturation: a prospective study in idiopathic infertile men. *Andrology* (2017) 5:414–22. doi: 10.1111/andr.12333

24. Yagci A, Murk W, Stronk J, Huszar G. Spermatozoa bound to solid state hyaluronic acid show chromatin structure with high DNA chain integrity: an acridine orange fluorescence study. *J Androl.* (2010) 31:566–72. doi: 10.2164/jandrol.109.008912

25. Tamburrino L, Marchiani S, Montoya M, Elia Marino F, Natali I, Cambi M, et al. Mechanisms and clinical correlates of sperm DNA damage. *Asian J Androl.* (2012) 14:24–31. doi: 10.1038/aja.2011.59

26. Rex AS, Aagaard J, Fedder J. DNA fragmentation in spermatozoa: a historical review. *Andrology* (2017) 5:622–30. doi: 10.1111/andr.12381

27. Sakkas DE, Seli GC, Manicardi M, Nijs W, Ombelet D. Bizzaro: the presence of abnormal spermatozoa in the ejaculate: did apoptosis fail? *Hum Fertil.* (2004) 7:99–103. doi: 10.1080/14647270410001720464

28. Muratori M, Tamburrino L, Marchiani S, Cambi M, Olivito B, Azzari C, et al. Investigation on the origin of sperm DNA fragmentation: role of apoptosis, immaturity and oxidative stress. *Mol Med.* (2015) 21:109–22. doi: 10.2119/molmed.2014.00158

29. Sakkas D, Seli E, Bizzaro D, Tarozzi N, Manicardi GC. Abnormal spermatozoa in the ejaculate: abortive apoptosis and faulty nuclear remodelling during spermatogenesis. *Reprod Biomed Online* (2003) 7:428–32. doi: 10.1016/S1472-6483(10)61886-X

30. O'Flaherty C, Matsushita-Fournier D. Reactive oxygen species and protein modifications in spermatozoa. *Biol Reprod.* (2017) 97:577–85. doi: 10.1093/biolre/iox104

31. Aitken RJ. Reactive oxygen species as mediators of sperm capacitation and pathological damage. *Mol Reprod Dev.* (2017) 84:1039–52. doi: 10.1002/mrd.22871

32. Turner TT, Lysiak JJ. Oxidative stress: a common factor in testicular dysfunction. *J Androl.* (2008) 29:488–98. doi: 10.2164/jandrol.108.005132

33. Aitken RJ, Finnie JM, Muscio L, Whiting S, Connaughton HS, Kuczera L, et al. Potential importance of transition metals in the induction of DNA damage by sperm preparation media. *Hum Reprod.* (2014) 29:2136–47. doi: 10.1093/humrep/deu204

34. Muratori M, Tarozzi N, Cambi M, Boni L, Iorio AL, Passaro C, et al. Variation of DNA fragmentation levels during density gradient sperm selection for assisted reproduction techniques: a possible new male predictive parameter of pregnancy? *Medicine* (2016) 95:e3624. doi: 10.1097/MD.0000000000003624

35. De Iuliis GN, Thomson LK, Mitchell LA, Finnie JM, Koppers AJ, Hedges A, et al. DNA damage in human spermatozoa is highly correlated with the efficiency of chromatin remodeling and the formation of 8-hydroxy-2'-deoxyguanosine, a marker of oxidative stress. *Biol Reprod.* (2009) 81:517–24. doi: 10.1095/biolreprod.109.076836

36. Lotti F, Tamburrino L, Marchiani S, Maseroli E, Vitale P, Forti G, et al. DNA fragmentation in two cytometric sperm populations: relationship with clinical and ultrasound characteristics of the male genital tract. *Asian J Androl.* (2017) 19:272–9. doi: 10.4103/1008-682X.174854

37. Muratori M, Maggi M, Spinelli S, Filimberti E, Forti G, Baldi E. Spontaneous DNA fragmentation in swim-up selected human spermatozoa during long term incubation. *J Androl.* (2003) 24:253–62. doi: 10.1002/j.1939-4640.2003.tb02670.x

38. Toro E, Fernández S, Colomar A, Casanovas A, Alvarez JG, López-Teijón M, et al. Processing of semen can result in increased sperm DNA fragmentation. *Fertil Steril.* (2009) 92:2109–12. doi: 10.1016/j.fertnstert.2009.05.059

39. Gosálvez J, Cortés-Gutiérrez EI, Nuñez R, Fernández JL, Caballero P, López-Fernández C, et al. A dynamic assessment of sperm DNA fragmentation versus sperm viability in proven fertile human donors. *Fertil Steril.* (2009) 92:1915–9. doi: 10.1016/j.fertnstert.2008.08.136

40. Zini A, Nam RK, Mak V, Phang D, Jarvi K. Influence of initial semen quality on the integrity of human sperm DNA following semen processing. *Fertil Steril.* (2000) 74:824–7. doi: 10.1016/S0015-0282(00)01495-3

41. Evenson DP, Jost LK, Marshall D, Zinaman MJ, Clegg E, Purvis K, et al. Utility of the sperm chromatin structure assay as a diagnostic and prognostic tool in the human fertility clinic. *Hum Reprod.* (1999) 14:1039–49. doi: 10.1093/humrep/14.4.1039

42. Giwercman A, Lindstedt L, Larsson M, Bungum M, Spano M, Levine RJ, et al. Sperm chromatin structure assay as an independent predictor of fertility *in vivo*: a case-control study. *Int J Androl.* (2010) 33:e221–7. doi: 10.1111/j.1365-2605.2009.00995.x

43. Muratori M, Marchiani S, Tamburrino L, Cambi M, Lotti F, Natali I, et al. DNA fragmentation in brighter sperm predicts male fertility independently from age and semen parameters. *Fertil Steril.* (2015) 104:582–90.e4. doi: 10.1016/j.fertnstert.2015.06.005

44. Robinson L, Gallos ID, Conner SJ, Rajkhowa M, Miller D, Lewis S, et al. The effect of sperm DNA fragmentation on miscarriage rates: a systematic review and meta-analysis. *Hum Reprod.* (2012) 27:2908–17. doi: 10.1093/humrep/des261

45. Cissen M, Wely MV, Scholten I, Mansell S, Bruin JP, Mol BW, et al. Measuring sperm DNA fragmentation and clinical outcomes of medically assisted reproduction: a systematic review and meta-analysis. *PLoS ONE* (2016) 11:e0165125. doi: 10.1371/journal.pone.0165125

46. Simon L, Zini A, Dyachenko A, Ciampi A, Carrell DT. A systematic review and meta-analysis to determine the effect of sperm DNA damage on *in vitro* fertilization and intracytoplasmic sperm injection outcome. *Asian J Androl.* (2017) 19:80–90. doi: 10.4103/1008-682X.182822

47. Agarwal A, Majzoub A, Esteves SC, Ko E, Ramasamy R, Zini A. Clinical utility of sperm DNA fragmentation testing: practice recommendations based on clinical scenarios. *Transl Androl Urol.* (2016) 5:935–50. doi: 10.21037/tau.2016.10.03

48. Showell MG, Mackenzie-Proctor R, Brown J, Yazdani A, Stankiewicz MT, Hart RJ. Antioxidants for male subfertility. *Cochrane Database Syst Rev.* (2014) 2014:CD007411. doi: 10.1002/14651858.CD007411.pub3

49. Billig H, Furuta I, Rivier C, Tapanainen J, Parvinen M, Hsueh AJ. Apoptosis in testis germ cells: developmental changes in gonadotropin dependence and localization to selective tubule stages. *Endocrinology* (1995) 136:5–12. doi: 10.1210/endo.136.1.7828558

50. Shetty J, Marathe GK, Dighe RR. Specific immunoneutralization of FSH leads to apoptotic cell death of the pachytene spermatocytes and spermatogonial cells in the rat. *Endocrinology* (1996) 137:2179–82. doi: 10.1210/endo.137.5.8612566

51. Ruwanpura SM, McLachlan RI, Stanton PG, Loveland KL, Meachem SJ. Pathways involved in testicular germ cell apoptosis in immature rats

after FSH suppression. *J Endocrinol.* (2008) 197:35–43. doi: 10.1677/JOE-07-0637

52. Ruwanpura SM, McLachlan RI, Stanton PG, Meachem SJ. Follicle-stimulating hormone affects spermatogonial survival by regulating the intrinsic apoptotic pathway in adult rats. *Biol Reprod.* (2008) 78:705–13. doi: 10.1095/biolreprod.107.065912

53. Santi D, Spaggiari G, Simoni M. Sperm DNA fragmentation index as a promisig predictive tool for male infertility diagnosis and treatment management – meta-analyses. *RBMO* (2018) 37:315–26. doi: 10.1016/j.rbmo.2018.06.023

54. Garolla A, Selice R, Engl B, Bertoldo A, Menegazzo M, Finos L, et al. Spermatid count as a predictor of response to FSH therapy. *Reprod Biomed Online* (2014) 29:102–12. doi: 10.1016/j.rbmo.2014.02.014

55. Ruvolo G, Roccheri MC, Brucculeri AM, Longobardi S, Cittadini E, Bosco L. Lower sperm DNA fragmentation after r-FSH administration in functional hypogonadotropic hypogonadism. *J Assist Reprod Genet.* (2013) 30:497–503. doi: 10.1007/s10815-013-9951-y

56. Palomba S, Falbo A, Espinola S, Rocca M, Capasso S, Cappiello F, et al. Effects of highly purified follicle-stimulating hormone on sperm DNA damage in men with male idiopathic subfertility: a pilot study. *J Endocrinol Invest.* (2011) 34:747–52. doi: 10.3275/7745

57. Garolla A, Ghezzi M, Cosci I, Sartini B, Bottacin A, Engl B, et al. FSH treatment in infertile males candidate to assisted reproduction improved sperm DNA fragmentation and pregnancy rate. *Endocrine* (2017) 56:416–25. doi: 10.1007/s12020-016-1037-z

58. Colacurci N, De Leo V, Ruvolo G, Piomboni P, Caprio F, Pivonello R, et al. Recombinant FSH Improves Sperm DNA Damage in Male Infertility: A Phase II Clinical Trial. *Front Endocrinol.* (2018) 9:383. doi: 10.3389/fendo.2018.00383

59. Muratori M, Tamburrino L, Tocci V, Costantino A, Marchiani S, Giachini C, et al. Small variations in crucial steps of TUNEL assay coupled to flow cytometry greatly affect measures of sperm DNA fragmentation. *J Androl.* (2010) 31:336–45. doi: 10.2164/jandrol.109.008508

60. Muratori M, Forti G, Baldi E. Comparing flow cytometry and fluorescence microscopy for analyzing human sperm DNA fragmentation by TUNEL labeling. *Cytometry A* (2008) 73:785–7. doi: 10.1002/cyto.a.20615

61. Ferlin A, Vinanzi C, Selice R, Garolla A, Frigo AC, Foresta C. Toward a pharmacogenetic approach to male infertility: polymorphism of follicle-stimulating hormone beta-subunit promoter. *Fertil Steril.* (2011) 96:1344–9. doi: 10.1016/j.fertnstert.2011.09.034

62. Chun SY, Eisenhauer KM, Minami S, Billig H, Perlas E, Hsueh AJ. Hormonal regulation of apoptosis in early antral follicles: follicle-stimulating hormone as a major survival factor. *Endocrinology* (1996) 137:1447–56. doi: 10.1210/endo.137.4.8625923

63. Tsai-Turton M, Luderer U. Opposing effects of glutathione depletion and follicle-stimulating hormone on reactive oxygen species and apoptosis in cultured preovulatory rat follicles. *Endocrinology* (2006) 147:1224–36. doi: 10.1210/en.2005-1281

64. Tesarik J, Martinez F, Rienzi L, Iacobelli M, Ubaldi F, Mendoza C, et al. *In vitro* effects of FSH and testosterone withdrawal on caspase activation and DNA fragmentation in different cell types of human seminiferous epithelium. *Hum Reprod.* (2002) 17:1811–9. doi: 10.1093/humrep/17.7.1811

65. Meehan T, Loveland KL, de Kretser D, Cory S, Print CG. Developmental regulation of the bcl-2 family during spermatogenesis: insights into the sterility of bcl-w-/- male mice. *Cell Death Differ.* (2001) 8:225–33. doi: 10.1038/sj.cdd.4400799

66. Vera Y, Erkkilä K, Wang C, Nunez C, Kyttänen S, Lue Y, et al. Involvement of p38 mitogen-activated protein kinase and inducible nitric oxide synthase in apoptotic signaling of murine and human male germ cells after hormone deprivation. *Mol Endocrinol.* (2006) 20:1597–609. doi: 10.1210/me.2005-0395

67. Gonzalez-Robayna IJ, Falender AE, Ochsner S, Firestone GL, Richards JS. Follicle-Stimulating hormone (FSH) stimulates phosphorylation and activation of protein kinase B (PKB/Akt) and serum and glucocorticoid-Induced kinase (Sgk): evidence for A kinase-independent signaling by FSH in granulosa cells. *Mol Endocrinol.* (2000) 14:1283–300. doi: 10.1210/mend.14.8.0500

68. Baccetti B, Strehler E, Capitani S, Collodel G, De Santo M, Moretti E, et al. The effect of follicle stimulating hormone therapy on human sperm structure (Notulae seminologicae 11). *Hum Reprod.* (1997) 12:1955–68. doi: 10.1093/humrep/12.9.1955

69. Krishnamurthy H, Danilovich N, Morales CR, Sairam MR. Qualitative and quantitative decline in spermatogenesis of the follicle-stimulating hormone receptor knockout (FORKO) mouse. *Biol Reprod.* (2000) 62:1146-59. doi: 10.1095/biolreprod62.5.1146

70. Sakkas D, Manicardi G, Bianchi PG, Bizzaro D, Bianchi U. Relationship between the presence of endogenous nicks and sperm chromatin packaging in maturing and fertilizing mouse spermatozoa. *Biol Reprod.* (1995) 52:1149–55. doi: 10.1095/biolreprod52.5.1149

71. Marcon L, Boissonneault G. Transient DNA strand breaks during mouse and human spermiogenesis new insights in stage specificity and link to chromatin remodeling. *Biol Reprod.* (2004) 70:910–8. doi: 10.1095/biolreprod.103.022541

72. Parmegiani L, Cognigni GE, Bernardi S, Troilo E, Ciampaglia W, Filicori M. "Physiologic ICSI": hyaluronic acid (HA) favors selection of spermatozoa without DNA fragmentation and with normal nucleus, resulting in improvement of embryo quality. *Fertil Steril.* (2010) 93:598–604. doi: 10.1016/j.fertnstert.2009.03.033

Follicle Stimulating Hormone Receptor (FSHR) Polymorphisms and Polycystic Ovary Syndrome (PCOS)

4

Follicle Stimulating Hormone Receptor (FSHR) Polymorphisms and Polycystic Ovary Syndrome (PCOS)

4

Follicle Stimulating Hormone Receptor (FSHR) Polymorphisms and Polycystic Ovary Syndrome (PCOS)

The typical biochemical features are elevated serum concentrations of testosterone and luteinizing hormone (LH), but PCOS is also associated with a characteristic metabolic disturbance that includes insulin resistance, hyperinsulinaemia, and abnormalities of energy expenditure. Crucially, PCOS is now recognized as a major risk factor for the development of type 2 diabetes (T2D) and cardiovascular disease in later life. Women with PCOS have a 3 to 7-fold increase in risk of T2D (3). At least in part, this reflects the strong associations between PCOS and obesity, with the latter a frequent concomitant, and likely amplifier, of the PCOS state (4).

Finally, it represents the major cause of anovulatory infertility, involving up to 20% of infertile couples. Restoring mono-ovulation is the ultimate goal of ovulation induction strategies. Typically these women do respond to ovulation inducing agents causing their own endogenous follicle-stimulating hormone (FSH) levels to rise and initiate ovulation or inducing the latter by administering exogenous FSH to them (5).

GENETICS OF PCOS

PCOS clusters within families and having a first degree relative suffering from PCOS conveys a 25% risk of either developing the full blown clinical picture or having a 25% risk of sharing characteristics of the syndrome amongst siblings to other siblings (6, 7). Similar results were obtained in several twin studies showing higher rates of concordance in PCOS characteristics between monozygotic twin sisters compared to dizygotic twins (8). Taken together these data strongly suggest a complex genetic basis for PCOS.

Several studies have attempted to explain the high overall prevalence of PCOS among women worldwide despite its link to subfertility and thus constituting an evolutionary paradox. Recently it has been shown that several genetic loci associated with the disease differently modulate the reproductive parameters of men and women. This observation suggests that these genetic variants lead to opposite effects on reproductive success in women and men. Intra-locus sexual conflict as a cause of the persistence of PCOS supports the high prevalence throughout evolution in humans (9).

To date, large numbers of genetic studies have identified over 200 susceptibility genes that might be functionally related to PCOS. However, the vast majority of these have not been replicated in other studies (10). Because PCOS seems to be a complex multigenic disease a more comprehensive, unbiased, non-hypothesis driven approach seems to be more informative. Hence high throughput genome association studies (GWAS) should be performed in order to unravel the genetic background of PCOS.

Recent GWAS have identified up to 18 genetic variants being genome wide significantly associated with PCOS (11–14) (**Figure 1**). Amongst those are variants in or near the LH (LHCGR) and FSH receptor (FSHR) genes as well as a variant in the FSH-β gene. Most of the identified genes have been identified and replicated in Chinese, South-East Asians as well as in Caucasian populations (15). Moreover, Mendelian randomization analyses indicate causal roles in PCOS etiology for higher body mass index (BMI), higher

insulin resistance, and lower serum sex hormone binding globulin concentrations. Furthermore, genetic susceptibility to later menopause is associated with higher PCOS risk and PCOS-susceptibility alleles are associated with higher serum anti-Müllerian hormone concentrations in girls (14). In a recent paper the functional roles of strong PCOS candidate loci focusing on FSHR, LHCGR, insulin receptor (INSR), and the DENND1A gene were reviewed. The authors of this paper propose that these candidates comprise a hierarchical signaling network by which DENN domain containing 1A (DENND1A), LHCGR, INSR, RAS oncogene family member 5B (RAB5B), adapter proteins, and associated downstream signaling cascades converge to regulate theca cell androgen biosynthesis (16).

FSHR POLYMORPHISMS

The FSHR gene is located on chromosome 2 p21-p16 and consists of 10 exons and 9 introns. The first 9 exons encode for the extracellular domain of the receptor, whereas exon 10 encodes for the C-terminal end of the extracellular domain, the entire transmembrane domain and the intracellular domain of the FSHR. Exon 10 is fundamental for signal transduction, but it is not necessary for ligand binding. Up till now around 1,800 SNPs of the FSHR gene have been reported in the National Centre for Biotechnology Information (NCBI) SNP database (http://www.ncbi.nlm.nih.gov). SNPs are located either in the coding regions (exons, 8 SNPs), or within intronic regions of exons. Only 1 SNP is located in the 5′ untranslated region of the FSHR mRNA position−29 (ss2189241). Of the eight SNPs within coding regions 7 are located in exon 10 at codon positions 307, 329, 449, 524, 567, 665, and 680. Six of the latter SNPs eventually result in amino acid substitution and are therefore non-synonymous. The two best characterized polymorphisms as far as their allele frequencies and ethnic distribution is concerned are the Ala307Thr (rs6165) and the Ser680Asn (rs6166). Both of these polymorphisms are linked to each other during recombination in a way that they always occur together (17).

Several studies aimed to correlate the FSHR polymorphism and ovarian function. The polymorphism at position 680 harboring Serine residues at both alleles is associated with higher endogenous FSH serum concentrations and a longer follicular phase length. This suggest that this FSHR variant is less sensitive to FSH. Indeed, women having the Ser/Ser variant needed more exogenous FSH during their ovarian stimulation phase during IVF treatment cycles. Moreover, Asn680Ser polymorphism was not associated with premature ovarian failure (POI). Finally, in women with PCOM the distribution of the two allelic variants greatly varied amongst different studies (17–20).

FSH RECEPTOR POLYMORPHISMS AND PCOS

FSHR Polymorphisms and PCOS Susceptibility

The first study ever which screened the entire coding region of FSHR gene for pathogenic mutations in 124 patients with

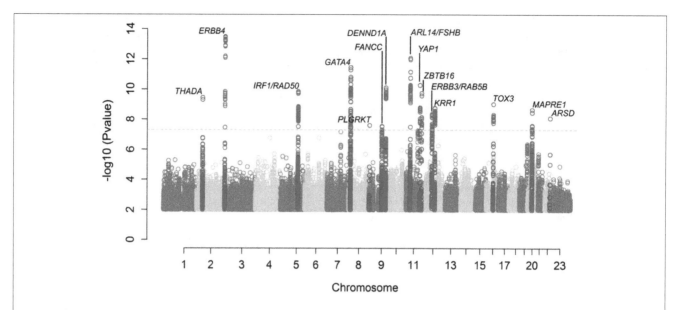

FIGURE 1 | Manhattan plot showing results of meta-analysis for PCOS status, adjusting for age. The inverse log10 of the p value ($-\log10(p)$) is plotted on the Y axis. The green dashed line designates the minimum p value for genome-wide significance ($<5.0 \times 10^{-8}$). Genome wide significant loci are denoted with a label showing the nearest gene to the index SNP at each locus. SNPs with p values $<1.0 \times 10^{-2}$ are not depicted.

PCOS and found no mutations in these patients. The two well-known polymorphisms, Thr307Ala and Ser680Asn showed similar distributions of the allelic variations and protein isoforms in PCOS compared to 236 normal healthy control subjects. It appears from this study that mutations in the coding regions of FSHR gene are not a causative factor for PCOS in Chinese Singapore women (21). Similarly, Fu and co-workers recruited 384 unrelated PCOS patients and 768 healthy individuals from the Shaanxi province in the northern part of China. The Ala307Thr and Ser680Asn polymorphisms were studied together with clinical characteristics of the study subjects in a case-control setting. The frequency of FSHR Ala307Thr and Ser680Asn variants along with the haplotype were not significantly different between the PCOS patients and the controls although the Ser680 variants seemed to be associated with higher levels of endogenous FSH and low estradiol levels. This study suggests that the two variants of the FSHR gene are not a causative factor of PCOS in Northern Chinese Han women (22). In another study in Han Chinese women suffering either from PCOS ($n = 215$) or being healthy controls ($n = 205$) recruited from Shanxi Province in north China the Ala307Thr and Ser680Asn polymorphisms of FSHR were not associated with PCOS. However, the FSHR polymorphisms were related to the endogenous serum concentrations of FSH and Prolactin. No other PCOS-associated endocrine hormones as well as clinical pregnancy rates in PCOS patients were recorded in that study (23). Only one study in Chinese women revealed a significant between FSHR polymorphisms and PCOS. In a case-control sample using 60 PCOS patients and 92 healthy controls all being unrelated Han Chinese from Shanghai the haplotypes covering components Thr307Ala and Asn680Ser were

studied. These authors observed a significant association of both polymorphisms and PCOS (24).

Ten case-control studies were included in the first meta-analysis addressing the relationship between the commonest FSHR polymorphisms and PCOS. This meta-analysis showed no consistent association between either the Thr307Ala polymorphism or the Asn680Ser polymorphism and susceptibility to PCOS. Stratified analysis of ethnicities also showed no association. The authors of this meta-analysis suggested that the FSHR polymorphisms were not associated with an increased risk of PCOS (25). In a second meta-analysis data from 11 studies were analyzed. The pooled odds ratio and 95% confidence interval were calculated using fixed- or random-effect model based on heterogeneity test in 5 genotype models analyses. This analysis showed that the Asn680Ser polymorphism was significantly associated with the reduced susceptibility to PCOS in a dominant model as well as in recessive, homozygote comparison, and allele contrast models. All Odds ratios were similar reducing the chance of having PCOS with about 20%. However, no significant associations were found between Thr307Ala and PCOS (26).

In a Korean study recruiting 235 PCOS patients and 128 control subjects, all within their reproductive age years, from Seoul. The FSHR polymorphisms Ser680Asn and Ala307Thr genotype frequencies were measured. They found that the Ser680Asn of FSHR was significantly more often associated with PCOS. In contrast the Ala307Thr variant was not at all associated with PCOS. However, their haplotype analysis revealed that both the Ser680Asn and Ala307Thr polymorphisms did not constitute a risk factor for PCOS (27). In another study genotyping was performed in 377 women with PCOS and 388 age-matched controls all from South Korean origin. Findings of this study suggest a significant association between FSHR gene polymorphisms Thr307Ala and the Asn680Ser allele frequencies and PCOS. The homozygote variant genotype results in significantly higher risk of PCOS (28). In a population of 522 Japanese women, the overall frequency of Asn/Asn, Asn/Ser, and Ser/Ser was 41.0, 46.9, and 12.1%, respectively. In polycystic ovary patients, the Asn/Ser population was significantly larger when compared with the spontaneously ovulating group (29). In a Pakistani study genomic results from 96 women with PCOS were compared with those from 96 healthy controls from the Punjab region in Pakistan. This study provides evidence of statistically significant associations between susceptibility to PCOS in Pakistani women and the gene polymorphisms in FSHR, the LHHCG-Receptor, LH-β chain and both ER-α and ER-β receptor genes (30). In another study in 386 Thai women with chronic anovulation either without (121 women) or with PCOS (133 women) using 132 known ovulatory fertile women as controls no association between the FSHR gene polymorphism at codons 307 and 680 and PCOS was found (31).

The first published European study assessed the distribution of the two most common FSHR polymorphisms in 148 normogonadotropic anovulatory infertile women and in 30 normo-ovulatory controls. Normogonadotropic anovulatory infertile patients have a different FSH receptor genotype than do normo-ovulatory controls (32). In another study in Dutch women with PCOS FSHR variants were strongly associated with the severity of clinical features of PCOS. The findings in a discovery cohort of 240 women with PCOS were replicated in another independent sample of 185 women suffering from PCOS and showed that the Ser/Ser genotype was associated with higher endogenous levels of FSH, LH and testosterone (19, 20).

In a study in Turkish adolescent girls the possible association between SNPs of the FSHR was studied. Samples from 44 adolescent girls with PCOS and 50 healthy controls were compared. Polymorphic loci on the FSHR (A307T, N680S) genes did not reveal any significant differences between cases and controls. These data do not support an association between SNPs of the FSHR and the susceptibility to PCOS in Turkish adolescent girls (33). Another study in Caucasians included 294 premenopausal Caucasian patients with PCOS, and 78 women with regular menorrhea and without hirsutism. In this study in Polish women no differences in genotype and allele frequencies of the Ser680Asn and Ala307Thr polymorphisms between the case and the control groups. In addition, the two FSHR variants in exon 10 did not increase the risk for PCOS in Polish women (34).

To assess the cross-ethnic effect a meta-analysis of the Dutch data (703 Dutch PCOS patients and 2,164 Dutch controls) combined with results of previously published studies in PCOS patients from China ($n = 2,254$) and the United States ($n = 2,618$) has been performed. Overall, this study observed for 12 of 17 genetic variants mapping to the Chinese PCOS loci similar effect size and identical direction in PCOS patients from Northern European ancestry, indicating a common genetic risk

profile for PCOS across populations. In this study two previously identified GWAS FSHR polymorphisms, i.e., rs2268361 and rs2349415 were significantly associated with PCOS (15). Another study trying to replicate the Chinese GWAS findings in Caucasians included 905 women with PCOS and 956 control women. The strongest evidence for association mapping to FSHR was observed with rs1922476. Furthermore, markers with the FSHR gene region were associated with FSH levels in women with PCOS. Fine mapping of the chromosome 2p16.3 Chinese PCOS susceptibility locus in a European ancestry cohort provides evidence for association with two independent loci and PCOS. The gene products of the FSHR gene are therefore likely to be important in the etiology of PCOS, regardless of ethnicity (35). An American study tried to replicate the FSHR variants from the Chinese GWA studies in case-control examination in a discovery cohort of 485 women with PCOS and in 407 controls from Boston. Replication was performed in women from 884 PCOS cases and 311 controls from Greece and in an additional cohort from Boston constituting 350 cases and 1,258 controls. One variant, rs2268361-T, in the intron of FSHR was associated with PCOS and lower FSH levels (36). In an effort to replicate the hits for the Chinese GWA studies 845 European subjects with PCOS and 845 controls were recruited into this study. Variants in DENND1A, THADA, the FSHR, and the INS-Receptor were associated with PCOS in Europeans. The genetic risk score, generated for each subject based on the total number of risk alleles, was associated with the diagnosis of PCOS and remained associated even after exclusion of the four variants individually associated with PCOS (37). Finally, in an Arab case-control study, involving 203 women with PCOS, and 211 age- and ethnically-matched control women. Significantly lower frequencies of a heterozygous FSHR variant (rs11692782) genotype carriers were observed between women with PCOS and controls (38). In summary most studies in Chinese and Thai women did not substantiate an increased susceptibility for PCOS based on FSHR polymorphisms. In contrast Studies in Korean and Pakistani women did find an increased susceptibility for PCOS based SNP's in the FSHR. Results from meta-analysis are contradictory whereas most studies in women from Caucasian descent revealed a clear-cut increased susceptibility for PCOS based on the FSHR genotype (**Table 1**).

FSHR Polymorphisms and Clinical Features of PCOS

One study aimed to investigate whether the PCOS related SNPs in the FSHR gene are associated with PCOM. The 447 unrelated Han Chinese PCOS from south China were grouped into PCOM ($n = 384$) and non-PCOM ($n = 63$) women. Significant differences were found in the allele distributions of the GG genotype of rs2268361 between the PCOM and non-PCOM groups while no significant differences were observed in the allele distributions of the GG genotype of rs2349415. When rs2268361 was considered, there were statistically significant differences of serum FSH, estradiol, and sex hormone binding globulin between genotypes in the PCOM group. In case of the rs2349415 SNP, only serum sex hormone binding globulin was statistically different

TABLE 1 | Showing the effect different single nucleotide polymorphisms have on either the prevalence of PCOS or on different phenotypical features of the syndrome.

SNP	Location	Risk for PCOS	Effect	Ethnicity	References
FOLLICLE-STIMULATING HORMONE RECEPTOR (FSHR)					
FSHR	rs6165	Similar	Not reported	Chinese	(21)
	rs6166	Similar	Not reported		
FSHR	rs6165	Similar	No effect	Chinese	(22)
	rs6166	Similar	Higher FSH and lower E_2		
FSHR	rs6165	Similar	Higher FSH and Prl	Chinese	(23)
	rs6166	Similar	Higher FSH and Prl		
FSHR	rs6165	Similar	Not reported	Korean	(27)
	rs6166	Increased	Not reported		
FSHR	rs6165	Increased	No effects on FSH, ovarian or metabolic markers	Korean	(28)
	rs6166	Increased	No effects on FSH, ovarian or metabolic markers		
FSHR	rs6165	Similar	No effect	Japanese	(29)
	rs6166	Increased	Reduced FSH sensitivity		
			Lower E_2 levels at OPU		
FSHR	rs6165	Similar	Not reported	Pakistani	(30)
	rs6166	Increased	Not reported		
FSHR	rs6165	Similar	Not reported	Thai	(31)
	rs6166	Similar	Not reported		
FSHR	rs6165	Similar	No effect	European	(32)
	rs6166	Increased	Higher FSH levels		
FSHR	rs6165	Similar	No effect	European	(19)
	rs6166	Increased	Higher FSH levels		
FSHR	rs6165	Similar	No effect	European	(39)
	rs6166	Increased	Higher FSH and LH and Testosterone levels		
FSHR	rs6165	Similar	No effect	European	(20)
	rs6166	Increased	Higher FSH levels		
FSHR	rs6165	Similar	Not Reported	European	(34)
	rs6166	Similar	Not Reported		
FSHR	rs6165	Similar	No effect	Turkish	(33)
	rs6166	Similar	No effect		
FSHR	rs7562215	Increased	Not reported	Caucasian	(35)
	rs10495960	Increased	Not reported		
	rs2956355	Increased	Not reported		
	rs7562879	Increased	Not reported		
	rs13405728	Increased	Not reported		
FSHR	rs2268361	Increased	Lower FSH serum levels	Caucasian	(36)
FSHR	rs11692782	Decreased	Not reported	Arab	(38)
FSHR	rs2268361	Not reported	More PCOM	Chinese	(40)
	rs2349415	Not reported	Different levels of FSH, E_2 and SHBG		
			Different levels of SHBG		
FSHR	rs6165	Similar	No differences in OI outcome	Caucasian	(41)
	rs6166	Similar	No differences in OI outcome		
FSHR	rs6165	Similar	No differences in OI outcome	Caucasian	(42)
	rs6166	Similar	No differences in OI outcome		
FSHR	rs6165	Increased	Higher ovarian responsiveness in OI	Caucasian	(43)
	rs6166	Similar	Similar ovarian responsiveness in OI		
FSHR	rs6165	Similar	Not reported	Chinese	(25)
	rs6166	Similar	Not reported	(Meta-analysis)	
FSHR	rs6165	Similar	Not reported	Chinese	(26)
	rs6166	Decreased	Not reported	(Meta-analysis)	
FSHR	rs2268361 and	Increased	Not reported	Caucasians and	(15)
	rs2349415	Increased	Not reported	Chinese	
				(Meta-analysis)	
FOLLICLE-STIMULATING HORMONE ß CHAIN POLYMORPHISMS (FSHß)					
FSHß	T to C transition at	Increased in Obese	Higher FSH levels in Accl cariers and No	Chinese	(44)
	codon 76 (Accl)	PCOS women	deifferences in E_2 and LH values		

(Continued)

TABLE 1 | Continued

SNP	Location	Risk for PCOS	Effect	Ethnicity	References
FSHß	rs11031010	Increased	Higher LH serum levels	Chinese	(10)
LUTEINIZING HORMONE- AND HUMAN CHORIOGONADOTROPHIN-RECEPTOR (LHCG) POLYMORPHISMS					
LHCGR	rs7371084 rs4953616	Increased Increased	Not reported	Arab	(38)
LHCGR	rs13405728	Increased	higher serum level of testosterone, triglycerides and low-density lipoproteins	Chinese	(45)
LHCGR	rs13405728 rs7562879	Similar Increased	Not reported Not reported	Caucasians	(35)

between genotypes in the PCOM group (40). Similar findings were reported another study showing that the Ser/Ser genotype had significantly higher basal level of serum FSH was observed as compared with that in the Asn/Ser group (29). A study trying to replicate the GWAS findings of the first two Chinese studies in Caucasians found a similar relationship between FSHR polymorphisms and lower FSH levels (36). Several Dutch studies found similar relationships between the Ser/Ser FSHR variant and higher basal endogenous FSH serum concentrations (19, 20, 39). In one study it was also reported that the Ser/Ser variant was also associated with increased serum concentrations of LH and testosterone (39). There is only limited information available regarding the relationship between FSHR SNP's and the phenotype of PCOS. Some SNP's are associated with the PCOM whereas most data are showing a more strict relationship between higher basal FSH serum levels and the least sensitive FSHR (**Table 1**).

FSH RECEPTOR POLYMORPHISMS AND TREATMENT OUTCOME IN PCOS

In order to determine whether an allelic variant of the FSHR gene affects fertility parameters in women with PCOS a UK group of investigators studied 93 women with PCOS and compared those with 51 healthy controls. The allelic variant Thr307/Ser680 was found to be similarly prevalent in both study groups and had no phenotype in terms of fertility parameters in women with PCOS (41). In a study comparing 58 women with PCOS and 80 healthy ethnically matched female controls there was no evidence that the Asn680Ser FSHR genotypes were neither associated with PCOS nor with the response to clomiphene citrate (42).

In contrast in a population of 522 Japanese women the NS genotype was significantly more prominent in women with PCOS. In women with the SS genotype significantly higher basal serum levels of FSH were observed as compared with the NS group suggesting a lower sensitivity of this particular SNP. Indeed, higher doses of the exogenous FSH was required to achieve ovulation induction in the SS group. Moreover, after hCG administration, estradiol levels at the time of ovum pick-up were significantly lower in the SS group as compared to the other allelic variants. In case the two receptor variants were over expressed in 293T cell line no differences could be found in

either levels of FSH-stimulated cAMP production, PI turnover or ligand-binding affinity. These results suggest some FSHR variants might have clinical implications (29). Similar results have been reported in a large Dutch case control cohort of women with PCOS and healthy controls the Ser/Ser FSHR polymorphism was associated with some clinical features such as FSH and LH serum concentrations. Indeed, the Ser/Ser FSHR polymorphism seemed to be less sensitive to endogenous FSH thereby leading to higher serum concentrations of FSH. Surprisingly this variant was also associated with higher serum LH and testosterone levels (32, 39). In the same study the Dutch group revealed an association with clomiphene citrate resistance during ovulation induction treatment. A pooled analysis showed an 89% higher chance of being CRA in homozygous carriers of the Ser/Ser FSHR variant. Similarly, a lower chance of ongoing pregnancy [hazard ratio 0.51 (95% confidence interval 0.27–0.98)] was observed among these patients during clomiphene citrate treatment in two independent prospective cohorts (39). These data may be used to design a treatment algorithm that is more efficacious and better tailored to the individual patient (20).

Similar results were obtained from another Dutch group retrospectively studying a cohort of 193 patients all diagnosed with PCOS according to Rotterdam criteria and treated with ovulation induction. Significantly more patients with Ser/Ser-polymorphism were resistant to CC compared with the Asn/Ser and Asn/Asn genotypes with an odds ratio for ovulation of 0.44. Patients with higher FSH levels, higher age and lower BMI were significantly more likely to ovulate in univariate analysis. In a multivariate logistic regression model, corrected for age, BMI, mean ovarian, volume, hyperandrogenism, and amenorrhea, only the FSHR genotype and basal FSH serum levels were predictive for ovulation (19). An Italian study compared 40 women with PCOS undergoing *in-vitro* fertilization (IVF) with 66 normo-ovulatory women. That study showed that the heterozygote FSH-R polymorphism Ala307Thr was significantly more frequent in women with PCOS compared to the normo-ovulatory subjects. Moreover, the Ala307Thr SNP was more frequently associated with a higher ovarian responsiveness to exogenous FSH (43). Although smaller studies in Caucasian women did not reveal a clear-cut relationship between FSHR polymorphisms and treatment outcome the larger studies did reveal an increase in clomiphene citrate resistance and the least sensitive FSHR (Ser680Ser variant) (**Table 1**).

OTHER GENETIC VARIANTS GONADOTROPHIC REGULATION THAT MIGHT BE ASSOCIATED WITH PCOS

FSH-β Gene Polymorphisms

In a cohort of 135 patients with PCOS and 105 normal control subjects no missense mutations were found in the functional units of the FSH-β gene in patients with PCOS. However, this study identified a thymine-cytosine substitution in exon 3 (codon 76, TAT to TAC) that led to creation of a so called AccI digestion site. The distribution pattern of this AccI polymorphism in the patients was significantly different from that in the control group since homozygous carriers were more often affected by PCOS. Within the PCOS patient group homozygosity for Accl was also associated with obesity. The latter finding correlated with significantly higher androgen levels in the obese patients. Hence the AccI polymorphism in FSHβ gene may be associated with PCOS in some women, especially those with obesity (44). A meta-analysis of Chinese GWAS data showed that the allele frequency difference of a SNP in the FSH-β gene (rs11031010) between PCOS and controls was genome-wide significant. PCOS women with AA and AC genotypes had a significantly higher LH serum levels compared to women carrying the CC genotype. Hence, variants in FSH-β gene are associated with PCOS and LH levels in Han Chinese women. The FSH-β gene is thus likely to play an important role in the etiology of PCOS, regardless of ethnicity (10) (Table 1).

LHCG-Receptor Polymorphisms

In a retrospective case-control study, involving 203 women with PCOS, and 211 age- and ethnically-matched control women LHCGR genotyping was done by allelic exclusion method. Significantly lower frequencies of heterozygous LHCGR rs7371084 genotype carriers were seen between women with PCOS vs. controls. Furthermore, an increased frequency of heterozygous homozygous LHCGR rs4953616 genotype carriers was detected between women with PCOS compared to control women. The authors of this study observed a significant increase of LHCG-Receptor variants (rs7371084, rs4953616) SNP's in women with PCOS (38). In a case control study in Hui ethnic women from China 51 patients with PCOS and 99 healthy women were involved. The frequencies of the genotype and allele frequency of rs13405728 in LHCG-Receptor gene were significantly different between the PCOS and the control women. Moreover, PCOS cases with TT genotype of the variant rs13405728 had higher serum level of total testosterone, triglycerides, and low-density lipoproteins (LDL) than those with the CC and CT genotypes. The authors concluded that the SNP rs13405728 in the LHCG-Receptor gene was associated with PCOS and some of its clinical features (45). An attempt to replicate the Chinese SNP's in an American cohort revealed that the LHCG-Receptor variant (rs13405728) was not informative in a white Americans from European descent. However, these authors identified and genotyped three markers (rs35960650, rs2956355, and rs7562879) within 5 kb of rs13405728. Of these, rs7562879 was nominally associated with PCOS. The gene products of the LHCRG-Receptor gene are therefore likely to be important in the etiology of PCOS, regardless of ethnicity (35).

In Indian study involving 204 women with PCOS and 204 healthy, sex-, and age-matched controls. This study demonstrated an association between LHCGR (rs2293275) polymorphism and PCOS. Moreover, a significant association of the GG allele with body-mass index, waist to hip ratio, insulin resistance, LH, and LH/FSH ratio was demonstrated in PCOS when compared with controls. Indeed this study also suggests that LHCG-Receptor polymorphism are associated with PCOS (46) (Table 1).

SUMMARY

Data from Chinese studies regarding the relationship between FSHR polymorphisms and PCOS susceptibility are conflicting. Although the majority of data do not substantiate such a relationship (21–23) there is one report suggesting that FSHR might play a role in genetic susceptibility to PCOS (24). Two different meta-analysis revealed also contradictory results. The first one suggested that the FSHR polymorphisms were not associated with an increased risk of PCOS (25) whereas the last one did reveal a decreased susceptibility to PCOS for Thr307Ala variant carriers (26). Several Korean (27, 28) as well as Japanese (29) and Pakistani studies (30) do substantiate the FSHR variants as a susceptibility locus for PCOS. However, a study in Thai women did not reveal such a relationship (31). It seems that data from South-East Asia are different from those generated in Chinese populations. In European women data are similarly conflicting. Some Dutch studies revealed a straight on forward association between FSHR gene polymorphisms and PCOS (19, 20, 39) whereas others did not substantiate such susceptibility (17, 33, 34). Arab women carrying certain FSHR polymorphisms seem to be more often suffering from PCOS too (38). The most convincing evidence comes from larger replication studies and a cross ethnic meta-analysis that revealed a strong relationship between FSHR variants and PCOS susceptibility (15, 35–37).

In conclusion along with these more convincing data observations underpinning the association of FSHR polymorphisms with clinical features indicating differences in sensitivity of the different receptor genotypes. These receptor variants might generate several phenotypes with differences in basal serum FSH, LH, and testosterone concentrations. Some of the data are also pointing in a direction that at least some of these genetic variants have clinical implications in that they determine individual sensitivity for exogenous FSH (19, 29, 32, 39, 42, 43). The observation that treatment outcome is also partially determined by FSHR polymorphisms is another clue that genetic variants might play a role in the pathophysiology of PCOS (19, 20, 29, 39, 42, 43).

In conclusion SNP's in the FSHR gene causing genetic variants in the FSHR on the one hand do determine the susceptibility for PCOS and on the other had do also affect the sensitivity of the receptor for exogenous FSH during ovulation induction therapy. There is also limited evidence showing that SNP's in the LHCG-Receptor as well as those in FSH-β gene might also determine a women's susceptibility for PCOS.

AUTHOR CONTRIBUTIONS

JL delivered a substantial contribution to the conception of the work and the interpretation of data in the literature for the work.

He drafted the work and agrees to be accountable for all aspects of the work in ensuring that questions related to the accuracy or integrity of any part of the work are appropriately investigated and resolved.

REFERENCES

1. Lizneva D, Kirubakaran R, Mykhalchenko K, Suturina L, Chernukha G, Diamond MP, et al. Phenotypes and body mass in women with polycystic ovary syndrome identified in referral versus unselected populations: systematic review and meta-analysis. *Fertil Steril.* (2016) 106:1510–20.e2. doi: 10.1016/j.fertnstert.2016.07.1121

2. Rotterdam ESHRE/ASRM-Sponsored PCOS Consensus Workshop Group. Revised 2003 consensus on diagnostic criteria and long-term health risks related to polycystic ovary syndrome (PCOS). *Hum Reprod.* (2004) 19:41–7. doi: 10.1093/humrep/deh098

3. Azziz R, Carmina E, Chen Z, Dunaif A, Laven JS, Legro RS, et al. Polycystic ovary syndrome. *Nat Rev Dis Primers* (2016) 2:16057. doi: 10.1038/nrdp.2016.57

4. Teede HJ, Misso ML, Costello MF, Dokras A, Laven J, Moran L, et al. Recommendations from the international evidence-based guideline for the assessment and management of polycystic ovary syndrome. *Hum Reprod.* (2018) 110:364–79. doi: 10.1016/j.fertnstert.2018.05.004

5. Thessaloniki ESHRE/ASRM-Sponsored PCOS Consensus Workshop Group. Consensus on infertility treatment related to polycystic ovary syndrome. *Hum Reprod.* (2008) 23:462–77. doi: 10.1093/humrep/dem426

6. Yilmaz B, Vellanki P, Ata B, Yildiz BO. Diabetes mellitus and insulin resistance in mothers, fathers, sisters, and brothers of women with polycystic ovary syndrome: a systematic review and meta-analysis. *Fertil Steril.* (2018) 110:523–33.e14. doi: 10.1016/j.fertnstert.2018.04.024

7. Yilmaz B, Vellanki P, Ata B, Yildiz BO. Metabolic syndrome, hypertension, and hyperlipidemia in mothers, fathers, sisters, and brothers of women with polycystic ovary syndrome: a systematic review and meta-analysis. *Fertil Steril.* (2018) 109:356–64.e32. doi: 10.1016/j.fertnstert.2017.10.018

8. Vink JM, Sadrzadeh S, Lambalk CB, Boomsma DI. Heritability of polycystic ovary syndrome in a Dutch twin-family study. *J Clin Endocrinol Metab.* (2006) 91:2100–4. doi: 10.1210/jc.2005-1494

9. Casarini L, Simoni M, Brigante G. Is polycystic ovary syndrome a sexual conflict? A review. *Reprod Biomed Online* (2016) 32:350–61. doi: 10.1016/j.rbmo.2016.01.011

10. Tian Y, Zhao H, Chen H, Peng Y, Cui L, Du Y, et al. Variants in FSHB are associated with polycystic ovary syndrome and luteinizing hormone level in Han Chinese women. *J Clin Endocrinol Metab.* (2016) 101:2178–84. doi: 10.1210/jc.2015-3776

11. Chen ZJ, Zhao H, He L, Shi Y, Qin Y, Shi Y, et al. Genome-wide association study identifies susceptibility loci for polycystic ovary syndrome on chromosome 2p16.3, 2p21 and 9q33.3. *Nat Genet.* (2011) 43:55–9. doi: 10.1038/ng.732

12. Shi Y, Zhao H, Shi Y, Cao Y, Yang D, Li Z, et al. Genome-wide association study identifies eight new risk loci for polycystic ovary syndrome. *Nat Genet.* (2012) 44:1020–5. doi: 10.1038/ng.2384

13. Hayes MG, Urbanek M, Ehrmann DA, Armstrong LL, Lee JY, Sisk R, et al. Genome-wide association of polycystic ovary syndrome implicates alterations in gonadotropin secretion in European ancestry populations. *Nat Commun.* (2015) 6:7502. doi: 10.1038/ncomms8502

14. Day F, Karaderi T, Jones MR, Meun C, He C, Drong A, et al. Large-scale genome-wide meta-analysis of polycystic ovary syndrome suggests shared genetic architecture for different diagnosis criteria. *PLoS Genet.* (2018) 14:e1007813. doi: 10.1371/journal.pgen.1007813

15. Louwers YV, Stolk L, Uitterlinden AG, Laven JS. Cross-ethnic meta-analysis of genetic variants for polycystic ovary syndrome. *J Clin Endocrinol Metab.* (2013) 98:E2006–12. doi: 10.1210/jc.2013-2495

16. McAllister JM, Legro RS, Modi BP, Strauss JF III. Functional genomics of PCOS: from GWAS to molecular mechanisms. *Trends Endocrinol Metab.* (2015) 26:118–24. doi: 10.1016/j.tem.2014.12.004

17. Simoni M, Tempfer CB, Destenaves B, Fauser BC. Functional genetic polymorphisms and female reproductive disorders: part I: polycystic ovary syndrome and ovarian response. *Hum Reprod Update* (2008) 14:459–84. doi: 10.1093/humupd/dmn024

18. Theron-Gerard L, Pasquier M, Czernichow C, Cedrin-Durnerin I, and Hugues JN. [Follicle-stimulating hormone receptor polymorphism and ovarian function]. *Gynecol Obstet Fertil.* (2007) 35:135–41. doi: 10.1016/j.gyobfe.2006.10.035

19. Overbeek A, Kuijper EA, Hendriks ML, Blankenstein MA, Ketel IJ, Twisk JW, et al. Clomiphene citrate resistance in relation to follicle-stimulating hormone receptor Ser680Ser-polymorphism in polycystic ovary syndrome. *Hum Reprod.* (2009) 24:2007–13. doi: 10.1093/humrep/dep114

20. Valkenburg O, van Santbrink EJ, Konig TE, Themmen AP, Uitterlinden AG, Fauser BC, et al. Follicle-stimulating hormone receptor polymorphism affects the outcome of ovulation induction in normogonadotropic (World Health Organization class 2) anovulatory subfertility. *Fertil Steril.* (2015) 103:1081–88.e3. doi: 10.1016/j.fertnstert.2015.01.002

21. Tong Y, Liao WX, Roy AC, Ng SC. Absence of mutations in the coding regions of follicle-stimulating hormone receptor gene in Singapore Chinese women with premature ovarian failure and polycystic ovary syndrome. *Horm Metab Res.* (2001) 33:221–6. doi: 10.1055/s-2001-14941

22. Fu L, Zhang Z, Zhang A, Xu J, Huang X, Zheng Q, et al. Association study between FSHR Ala307Thr and Ser680Asn variants and polycystic ovary syndrome (PCOS) in Northern Chinese Han women. *J Assist Reprod Genet.* (2013) 30:717–21. doi: 10.1007/s10815-013-9979-z

23. Wu XQ, Xu SM, Liu JF, Bi XY, Wu YX, Liu J. Association between FSHR polymorphisms and polycystic ovary syndrome among Chinese women in north China. *J Assist Reprod Genet.* (2014) 31:371–7. doi: 10.1007/s10815-013-0166-z

24. Du J, Zhang W, Guo L, Zhang Z, Shi H, Wang J, et al. Two FSHR variants, haplotypes and meta-analysis in Chinese women with premature ovarian failure and polycystic ovary syndrome. *Mol Genet Metab.* (2010) 100:292–5. doi: 10.1016/j.ymgme.2010.03.018

25. Chen DJ, Ding R, Cao JY, Zhai JX, Zhang JX, Ye DQ. Two follicle-stimulating hormone receptor polymorphisms and polycystic ovary syndrome risk: a meta-analysis. *Eur J Obstet Gynecol Reprod Biol.* (2014) 182:27–32. doi: 10.1016/j.ejogrb.2014.08.014

26. Qiu L, Liu J, Hei QM. Association between two polymorphisms of follicle stimulating hormone receptor gene and susceptibility to polycystic ovary syndrome: a meta-analysis. *Chin Med Sci J.* (2015) 30:44–50. doi: 10.1016/S1001-9294(15)30008-0

27. Gu BH, Park JM, Baek KH. Genetic variations of follicle stimulating hormone receptor are associated with polycystic ovary syndrome. *Int J Mol Med.* (2010) 26:107–12. doi: 10.3892/ijmm-00000441

28. Kim JJ, Choi YM, Hong MA, Chae SJ, Hwang K, Yoon SH, et al. FSH receptor gene p. Thr307Ala and p. Asn680Ser polymorphisms are associated with the risk of polycystic ovary syndrome. *J Assist Reprod Genet.* (2017) 34:1087–93. doi: 10.1007/s10815-017-0953-z

29. Sudo S, Kudo M, Wada S, Sato O, Hsueh AJ, Fujimoto S. Genetic and functional analyses of polymorphisms in the human FSH receptor gene. *Mol Hum Reprod.* (2002) 8:893–9. doi: 10.1093/molehr/8.10.893

30. Liaqat I, Jahan N, Krikun G, Taylor HS. Genetic polymorphisms in Pakistani women with polycystic ovary syndrome. *Reprod Sci.* (2015) 22:347–57. doi: 10.1177/1933719114542015

31. Singhasena W, Pantasri T, Piromlertamorn W, Samchimchom S, Vutyavanich T. Follicle-stimulating hormone receptor gene polymorphism in chronic anovulatory women, with or without polycystic ovary syndrome: a cross-sectional study. *Reprod Biol Endocrinol.* (2014) 12:86. doi: 10.1186/1477-7827-12-86

32. Laven JS, Mulders AG, Suryandari DA, Gromoll J, Nieschlag E, Fauser BC, et al. Follicle-stimulating hormone receptor polymorphisms in women with normogonadotropic anovulatory infertility. *Fertil Steril.* (2003) 80:986–92. doi: 10.1016/S0015-0282(03)01115-4

33. Unsal T, Konac E, Yesilkaya E, Yilmaz A, Bideci A, Ilke Onen H, et al. Genetic polymorphisms of FSHR, CYP17, CYP1A1, CAPN10, INSR, SERPINE1 genes in adolescent girls with polycystic ovary syndrome. *J Assist Reprod Genet.* (2009) 26:205–16. doi: 10.1007/s10815-009-9308-8

34. Czeczuga-Semeniuk E, Jarzabek K, Galar M, Kozlowski P, Sarosiek NA, Zapolska G, et al. Assessment of FSHR, AMH, and AMHRII variants in women with polycystic ovary syndrome. *Endocrine* (2015) 48:1001–4. doi: 10.1007/s12020-014-0345-4

35. Mutharasan P, Galdones E, Penalver Bernabe B, Garcia OA, Jafari N, Shea LD, et al. Evidence for chromosome 2p16.3 polycystic ovary syndrome susceptibility locus in affected women of European ancestry. *J Clin Endocrinol Metab.* (2013) 98:E185–90. doi: 10.1210/jc.2012-2471

36. Saxena R, Georgopoulos NA, Braaten TJ, Bjonnes AC, Koika V, Panidis D, et al. Han Chinese polycystic ovary syndrome risk variants in women of European ancestry: relationship to FSH levels and glucose tolerance. *Hum Reprod.* (2015) 30:1454–9. doi: 10.1093/humrep/dev085

37. Brower MA, Jones MR, Rotter JI, Krauss RM, Legro RS, Azziz R, et al. Further investigation in europeans of susceptibility variants for polycystic ovary syndrome discovered in genome-wide association studies of Chinese individuals. *J Clin Endocrinol Metab.* (2015) 100:E182–6. doi: 10.1210/jc.2014-2689

38. Almawi WY, Hubail B, Arekat DZ, Al-Farsi SM, Al-Kindi SK, Arekat MR, et al. Leutinizing hormone/choriogonadotropin receptor and follicle stimulating hormone receptor gene variants in polycystic ovary syndrome. *J Assist Reprod Genet.* (2015) 32:607–14. doi: 10.1007/s10815-015-0427-0

39. Valkenburg O, Uitterlinden AG, Piersma D, Hofman A, Themmen AP, de Jong FH, et al. Genetic polymorphisms of GnRH and gonadotrophic hormone receptors affect the phenotype of polycystic ovary syndrome. *Hum Reprod.* (2009) 24:2014–22. doi: 10.1093/humrep/dep113

40. Du T, Duan Y, Li K, Zhao X, Ni R, Li Y, and Yang D. Statistical genomic approach identifies association between FSHR polymorphisms and polycystic ovary morphology in women with polycystic ovary syndrome. *Biomed Res Int.* (2015) 2015:483726. doi: 10.1155/2015/483726

41. Conway GS, Conway E, Walker C, Hoppner W, Gromoll J, Simoni M. Mutation screening and isoform prevalence of the follicle stimulating hormone receptor gene in women with premature ovarian failure, resistant ovary syndrome and polycystic ovary syndrome. *Clin Endocrinol.* (1999) 51:97–9. doi: 10.1046/j.1365-2265.1999.00745.x

42. Mohiyiddeen L, Salim S, Mulugeta B, McBurney H, Newman WG, Pemberton P, et al. PCOS and peripheral AMH levels in relation to FSH receptor gene single nucleotide polymorphisms. *Gynecol Endocrinol.* (2012) 28:375–7. doi: 10.3109/09513590.2011.633649

43. Dolfin E, Guani B, Lussiana C, Mari C, Restagno G, Revelli A. FSH-receptor Ala307Thr polymorphism is associated to polycystic ovary syndrome and to a higher responsiveness to exogenous FSH in Italian women. *J Assist Reprod Genet.* (2011) 28:925–30. doi: 10.1007/s10815-011-9619-4

44. Tong Y, Liao WX, Roy AC, Ng SC. Association of AccI polymorphism in the follicle-stimulating hormone beta gene with polycystic ovary syndrome. *Fertil Steril.* (2000) 74:1233–6. doi: 10.1016/S0015-0282(00)01616-2

45. Ha L, Shi Y, Zhao J, Li T, Chen ZJ. Association study between polycystic ovarian syndrome and the susceptibility genes polymorphisms in Hui Chinese women. *PLoS ONE* (2015) 10:e0126505. doi: 10.1371/journal.pone.0126505

46. Thathapudi S, Kodati V, Erukkambattu J, Addepally U, Qurratulain H. Association of luteinizing hormone chorionic gonadotropin receptor gene polymorphism (rs2293275) with polycystic ovarian syndrome. *Genet Test Mol Biomarkers* (2015) 19:128–32. doi: 10.1089/gtmb.2014.0249

5

FSH Beyond Fertility

Daria Lizneva[1], Alina Rahimova[1], Se-Min Kim[1], Ihor Atabiekov[1], Seher Javaid[1],
Bateel Alamoush[1], Charit Taneja[1], Ayesha Khan[1], Li Sun[1], Ricardo Azziz[2], Tony Yuen[1] and
Mone Zaidi[1*]

[1] The Mount Sinai Bone Program, Department of Medicine, Icahn School of Medicine at Mount Sinai, New York, NY,
United States, [2] Academic Health and Hospital Affairs, State University of New York, Albany, NY, United States

*Correspondence:
Mone Zaidi
mone.zaidi@mssm.edu

The traditional view of follicle-stimulating hormone (FSH) as a reproductive hormone is changing. It has been shown that FSH receptors (FSHRs) are expressed in various extra-gonadal tissues and mediate the biological effects of FSH at those sites. Molecular, animal, epidemiologic, and clinical data suggest that elevated serum FSH may play a significant role in the evolution of bone loss and obesity, as well as contributing to cardiovascular and cancer risk. This review summarizes recent data on FSH action beyond reproduction.

Keywords: FSH, FSHR, obesity, osteoporosis, BMI, cardiovascular risk

INTRODUCTION

Follicle-stimulating hormone (FSH) is long thought to exert its effects in gonadal tissues, mainly limited to Sertoli cells in testes and granulosa cells in ovaries (1). Recently, using methods such as RT-PCR, Sanger sequencing, immunohistochemistry, and competitive binding assays, FSH receptors (FSHRs) have been shown to be expressed in extragonadal tissues, including endothelium, monocytes, developing placenta, endometrium, malignant tissues, bone and fat (2–10).

Our group first demonstrated that by increasing bone resorption by osteoclasts, FSH regulates bone mass in mouse models (11). Moreover, we found that FSH exerts action on adipocytes. In particular, a novel FSH antibody blocks the action of FSH on FSHRs (10, 11), causing an increase in bone mass, a reduction of body fat and induction of beiging of white adipocytes (9). These findings are consistent with large epidemiologic data. Indeed, the Study of Women's Health Across the Nation (SWAN) has shown significant reductions in bone mineral density (BMD) and high resorption rates ~2–3 years prior to menopause, which was also associated with increased body weight and visceral adiposity (12, 13). It is important to note that these changes take place when serum FSH level is increasing and estrogen level remains normal (14). Emerging epidemiologic evidence also suggests a relationship between FSH and several cardiovascular risk factors such as coronary artery calcium deposition, carotid intima-media thickness, and the number of aortic plaques (15–17). In particular, FSH interacts with its receptor on monocytes, up-regulates RANK expression and promotes monocytic infiltration of atherosclerotic plaque (18).

With this new evidence, the view that FSH acts solely as a gonadal hormone has changed rapidly over the past decade. It also provides perspectives on new roles that FSH might have in the pathophysiology of certain diseases and how treatment approaches targeting FSH may open up new possibilities for prevention and treatment. For example, we showed that a FSH blocking antibody could prevent bone loss and visceral adiposity in various mouse models (10). These data provide the foundation for future human studies. Similarly, detection of vascular endothelial FSHR in various types of solid tumors and sarcomas has prompted a debate as to whether an anti-FSH antibody could serve as a treatment modality in future anti-cancer drugs (7, 19).

Here, we review the epidemiologic, molecular and animal data on FSH action in normal physiology and the pathophysiology of osteoporosis, obesity, cardiovascular disorders, and cancer.

The Role of FSH in Reproduction

FSH, luteinizing hormone (LH), thyroid-stimulating hormone (TSH) and human chorionic gonadotropin (hCG) are all glycoprotein hormones, which share the same alpha subunit and differ in their beta polypeptide units, specific for each of aforementioned molecules (20). Pulsatile release of gonadotropin-releasing hormone (GnRH) from the hypothalamus stimulates the release of FSH and LH. Inhibin B and estradiol are the primary inhibitors of FSH secretion (21–23). Several other pituitary-regulatory proteins, such as activin and follistatin, have been implicated in FSH secretion and action (22). The activity of FSH is regulated in part by glycosylation.

FSH exerts its biological action via a G protein-coupled receptor, FSH receptor (FSHR). A stimulatory $G\alpha_s$ protein initiates signal transduction via the cAMP/protein kinase A (PKA) pathway (1, 24). This cascade of events leads to the activation of cAMP regulatory element-binding protein (CREB) (24). In addition to CREB, cAMP-activated PKA activates several other factors such as p38 MAP kinases, p70-S6 kinase and phosphoinositide-3 kinase (PI3K), PKB/Akt and FOXO1 and regulates gene expression in target tissues (25, 26). According to recent data, the effect of FSHR activation is not limited to the classical pathway, but also produces its action through $G\alpha_i$ (27), $G\alpha_q$ (28), and via other molecules, including β-arrestins (29) and an adapter protein having pleckstrin homology and phosphotyrosine binding domains together with a leucine zipper motif (30). In this case, the signal transduction is accomplished though inositol trisphosphate (IP_3), Akt and ERK1/2.

FSH plays a pivotal role in the development and regulation of both the male and female reproductive systems by acting on the FSHR which is predominantly expressed in granulosa and Sertoli cells (24). In females, FSH induces follicular growth and maturation, and contributes to LH-triggered ovulation and luteinization (31–33). In males, FSH regulates the mitotic proliferation of Sertoli cells, supports their growth and maturation and prompts the release of androgen-binding protein, which regulates the overall process of spermatogenesis (34). Moreover, in testis, endothelial FSHR mediates FSH transport across gonadal endothelial barrier (35). Below, we will discuss the role of FSH on bone, fat, cardiovascular system and cancer cells.

Epidemiologic and Clinical Data Supporting FSH Action on Bone

Traditionally, bone loss in peri- and postmenopausal women has been attributed primarily to reduced estrogen production due to ovarian senescence. Estrogen replacement therapy has been considered a logical therapeutic choice in an attempt to slow postmenopausal bone loss and reduce fracture risk (36). However, FSH has been implicated in bone loss in reproductive and non-reproductive age women, as well as in women undergoing menopausal transition (37, 38).

While data from placebo-controlled randomized clinical trials is not available, the multi-center multi-ethnic cohort SWAN showed a compelling correlation between FSH action and bone loss during the menopausal transition. SWAN demonstrated that changes in bone turnover markers and bone mass density (BMD) in perimenopausal women undergoing menopausal transition were independent of serum estradiol, but were inversely related to changes in the FSH level. The levels of serum FSH over a 4-year time period predicted BMD reduction in these women (14, 39). Moreover, lower levels of bone loss in the lumbar spine during perimenopause were noted in women with higher estrogen-to-FSH ratio (40). All of these observations may suggest that bone loss during perimenopause is not solely dependent on estrogen, and may be due in part to FSH action on bone.

Epidemiological data from across the US, Europe, and China further substantiate findings from SWAN (41–46). The US NHANES III cohort study documented the relationship between serum FSH and femoral neck BMD among woman between the ages of 42 and 60 (41). Likewise, using univariate regression analyses, another US cross-sectional study confirmed the inverse relation of FSH to BMD in perimenopausal women (42). The Italian Bone Turnover Range of Normality (BONTURNO) study compared women undergoing menopausal transition, and showed significantly increased bone loss in the group with FSH>30 IU/L vs. age-matched controls, although both had regular menses (43). Yet another cross-sectional study conducted in Spain included 92 postmenopausal female participants and showed a positive correlation between serum FSH and C-terminal telopeptide of type I collagen (CTX) and serum osteocalcin, but no relation to estradiol. Several Chinese studies have reported a negative relationship between bone loss, bone turnover markers and serum FSH levels in perimenopausal women (45–47), with those in the highest quartile of serum FSH showing bone loss at a rate that was 1.3–2.3-fold higher than those in the lowest quartile (48).

The detrimental and deleterious effect of FSH on bone during a woman's reproductive years can be observed in instances of hypergonadotropic conditions. For example, lower lumbar spine bone density was reported in a hypergonadotropic amenorrheic group as compared to hypogonadotropic European patients under 40 years of age (49). Groups did not differ in estradiol or progesterone levels; however, in hypergonadotropic women, FSH levels had a negative relationship with lumbar spine BMD. Interestingly, females diagnosed with functional hypothalamic amenorrhea tend to develop less severe bone loss (50, 51).

Evidence from genetic studies further explores the function of FSHR in humans. In particular, women with an activating $FSHR^{N680S}$ polymorphism have an increased risk of developing postmenopausal osteoporosis, independent of circulating levels of FSH and estrogens (52). Likewise, in a multicenter study of postmenopausal Spanish women two-gene combinations of wild type IVS4 or 3′UTR markers of CYP19A1 with FSHR and BMP15 genes yielded skeletal protection (53). Therefore, epidemiologic data derived from several cross-sectional and cohort studies, together with genetic association studies, suggest a detrimental effect of FSH on bone.

In contrast, a couple of clinical studies in humans using GnRH agonists failed to demonstrate any effect of FSH suppression on bone. For instance, FSH suppression with leuprolide acetate in a group of postmenopausal women has not being associated with any significant changes in bone resorption markers (54). In another study, eugonadal men receiving goserelin acetate combined with daily topical testosterone gel did not demonstrate any changes in serum N-terminal telopeptide, C-terminal telopeptide, and osteocalcin compared to control (55). However, both studies were relatively small and the duration of the intervention was short (approximately 4 months).

Mechanistic Studies on FSH Action on Bone

In 2006, we were the first to observe the direct regulation of bone mass by FSH, which resulted mainly from osteoclastic bone resorption in rodents (11). Accumulating evidence now shows that FSH acts directly on bone via a specific shorter isoform of the FSHR (identified in humans), which then increases osteoclastogenesis and stimulates bone resorption (4, 11, 56–58). Studies failed to identify the expression of FSHRs on osteoclast lineage cells most likely used PCR primers designed to target the full-length gonadal FSHR (59, 60). FSH binding to the bone FSHR has subsequently been proven in vivo through the binding of fluorophore-tagged FSH to gonads and bone. A molar excess of unlabeled FSH displaced tagged FSH underscoring the specificity of FSH binding to bone (10, 61). The level of FSH glycosylation is important, as fully glycosylated (i.e., 24 kD) recombinant FSH isoform has a higher affinity to the bone FSHR, as compared to the partially glycosylated FSH molecule (i.e., 21 kD isoform), which is more active in gonads (62, 63).

FSH acts on FSHRs on osteoclasts, stimulating NFκB, MEK/Erk, and AKT pathways and, thus, promoting osteoclast formation, function and survival. The osteoclastic FSHR is coupled to $G\alpha i_2$, so that its activation causes intracellular cAMP reductions, in contrast to the ovaries where the FSHR couples with a $G\alpha_s$-protein and triggers an increase in cAMP. Blocking the aforementioned pathway or absence of $G\alpha i_2$ leads to bone unresponsiveness to FSH (11). Stimulation of osteoclasts by FSH also occurs via an indirect pathway—the upregulation of receptor activator NFκB (RANK) increases the synthesis of interleukin-1β (IL-1β), interleukin-6 (IL-6) and tumor necrosis factor alpha (TNFα) proportionately to FSHR expression (64, 65). Moreover, FSH can interact with an immunoreceptor tyrosine-based activation motif (ITAM) adapter to enhance osteoclastogenesis (57).

In vivo FSH injection caused enhanced bone loss, whereas FSH inhibitor administration decreased bone resorption in ovariectomized rats (66, 67). Mice with an absent or deficient allele of FSHR or FSHβ had higher bone mass and diminished bone loss, which may be partially explained by high serum androgens (68). However, mice lacking aromatase, despite elevated androgen levels, still showed dramatic bone loss (69). Moreover, when FSH inhibitor was injected into male mice they also developed increased bone mass (9). To prevent confounding, generated by the opposite effects of FSH and estrogens on bone resorption, we developed a specific antibody to FSHβ (70, 71), which was shown to decrease osteoclastogenesis in vitro (10, 71), and decrease bone loss and stimulate bone formation in vivo (11, 70, 71). It is also known that FSH acts via the FSHR on

mesenchymal stem cells to suppress their differentiation into osteoblasts (70).

Epidemiologic and Clinical Data Supporting an Action of FSH on Body Composition

There is strong correlative evidence between high FSH and body fat in postmenopausal women. A Michigan sub-study of the SWAN, which included women undergoing menopausal transition, showed a positive relationship between fat mass and serum FSH. Participants with higher FSH had increased fat mass and waist circumference, even after adjusting for baseline measurements, and lower lean and skeletal muscle mass (72). In addition, the Oklahoma Postmenopausal Health Disparities Study, which included a large group of postmenopausal women, showed that the best predictors of waist-to-hip ratio were serum FSH, estradiol and body mass index (BMI) (73). A similar positive relation between FSH to central obesity in infertile females of reproductive age has also been reported (74).

FSH has also been independently associated with lean mass in 94 postmenopausal participants after adjustment for estrogen, testosterone, LH, parathyroid hormone, sex hormone binding globulin (SHBG) and urine N-telopeptide (75). The Study of Women Entering and in Endocrine Transition (SWEET) found significantly higher lean mass in premenopausal Sub-Saharan African females, as compared to postmenopausal females, with a negative correlation between FSH and lean mass (76).

However, several groups reported an inverse relationship between FSH levels and BMI in women, particularly those in the reproductive age (77–82). This phenomenon can be explained by feedback FSH inhibition by estrogens arising from adipose tissue. For example, a study from France reported that non-obese reproductive-age females undergoing infertility workups had higher levels of gonadotropins and estradiol compared to obese women (78). Another study found an inverse relationship between FSH and BMI in reproductive age females over 326 IVF cycles (77). Overweight/obese fertile women from Italy had lower FSH, LH, estradiol and inhibin B in the early follicular phase (79). The same scenario was reported in post- and perimenopausal females. For instance, Penn Ovarian Aging Study compared abdominal MR images and hormonal levels in women at different time points and demonstrated a positive relationship between estradiol and visceral fat, but a negative one was found between FSH and visceral fat (13). Furthermore, data from the 11-year follow-up SWAN study demonstrated that obesity is associated with low FSH trajectory in women of all ethnicities (80). According to The Pan-Asia Menopause (PAM) Study, gonadotropins and estradiol had a strong positive correlation with BMI. Interestingly, estrogen and LH levels were dependent on age, whereas FSH was not (81). Another study, conducted among 73 postmenopausal Serbian women, found higher FSH in normal weight individuals than in obese females (82).

These observations are consistent with those in girls, particularly among pubertal girls who underwent bioelectric impedance measures of body fat >29%. Sorensen and Juul demonstrated that girls within this cohort had significantly lower LH and FSH levels vs. normal weight comparators (83). Likewise, Bouvattier et al. observed a negative correlation between LH, FSH and GnRH responses regarding body mass index among perimenarchial and young adult girls (84).

No significant correlation between BMI and FSH was identified in observational studies of males regardless of age (85–88), except that one cross-sectional study reported that body mass index was negatively related to FSH, inhibin B, and testosterone levels in adult men (89). However, very recent data from a randomized clinical trial suggest that high serum FSH levels cause an increase in body fat in the absence of changes in other hormones. A two-arm open-label randomized clinical study included 58 men with prostate cancer, who were randomly assigned to orchiectomy or GnRH agonist treatment for 24 weeks (90). Notably, serum FSH levels increased after orchiectomy, while GnRH agonist injections inhibited FSH secretion (91). Men treated with orchiectomy experienced greater increases in total fat mass, subcutaneous adipose tissue mass, and weight at 48 weeks as compared to men treated with GnRH agonist (90). This is the first intervention study to demonstrate that FSH regulates body fat in human.

Limited data also suggests that serum FSH may be related to metabolic syndrome. For example, one cross-sectional study, of 320 Polish women reported FSH to be a better indicator of increased risk for metabolic syndrome than SHBG levels (92). Serum FSH also appeared to be more accurate in metabolic syndrome prediction compared with leptin or C-reactive peptide in menopausal females (93).

The role of FSH in non-alcoholic fatty liver disease (NAFLD) has not been well-established. However, a few studies have reported an association between serum FSH levels and fat deposition in the liver, detected by ultrasonography (94, 95). For example, the 2014 Survey on Prevalence in East China for Metabolic Diseases conducted among women over 55 years of age have revealed that serum FSH levels were negatively associated with NAFLD (94). In an adjusted model for waist circumference and HOMA-IR, FSH levels were not associated with mild hepatic steatosis, however the association of FSH with moderate-severe hepatic steatosis remained evident (P for trend <0.01) (94). Similarly, another cross-sectional study conducted among 71 elderly (i.e., 60 years of age or older) patients from China showed that the "normal" diurnal rhythm of FSH was independently associated with NAFLD (95).

FSH Action on Body Fat in Mice

There is compelling evidence for FSHR expression in chicken, murine and human adipocytes (9, 96, 97). FSH directly stimulates primary murine adipocytes and 3T3-L1 cells through $G\alpha_i$-coupled FSHR (**Figure 1**), resulting in the up-regulation of core fat genes, such as *Fas, Lpl,* and *Pparg,* and the induction of lipid biosynthesis (9). Moreover, FSHR activation leads to cAMP reduction and subsequently UCP1 inactivation in ThermoMouse-derived differentiated brown fat cells (9).

We have fine-mapped the receptor-binding epitope of FSHβ and developed a blocking antibody capable of binding to this

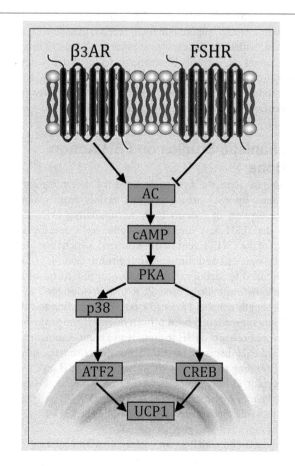

FIGURE 1 | Mechanism of Action of FSH on Adipocytes. The newly described FSH signaling pathway opposes β_3 adrenergic signaling. The latter is known to cause the transdifferentiation of white to beige adipocytes via interaction of the β_3 receptor with a $G\alpha_s$ protein that stimulates cAMP production and activates the MAP kinase p38 and the transcription factor ATF2, which then translocates to the nucleus causing the transcriptional activation of the *Ucp1* gene (98, 99). FSH opposes this action by interacting with a $G\alpha_i$-coupled FSH receptor, also involving CREB-mediated pathway (9, 97).

motif to prevent FSHβ/FSHR interaction (9, 10). Injection of this anti-FSHβ antibody in various murine models, including ovariectomized mice and mice either pair-fed on a high-fat diet or allowed ad libitum access to normal chow, caused a significant reduction in visceral, bone marrow and subcutaneous fat (9). The FSH antibody also significantly increased bone mass in ovariectomized mice (9, 70). These phenotypes were recapitulated in haploinsufficient $Fshr^{+/-}$ mice, indicating a dominant role of FSH in bone and body fat regulation. Interestingly, anti-FSHβ antibody failed to decrease adiposity in $Fshr^{+/-}$ male mice fed on a high-fat diet, proving FSH specificity (9). These observations were reproduced contemporaneously in other centers, using various laboratory methods (9, 100).

FSH blockade in mice also led to the up-regulation of brown adipocyte genes, such as *Cox7, Cox8a, Ucp1,* and *Cidea,* in visceral fat indicating "beiging," which, we found, was occurring independently of sympathetic tone (9). However, it is not clear as to whether the beige adipocytes were the product of transdifferentiation of white adipocytes or if they were formed from a specific precursor (101, 102). Using *in vivo* fluorescence imaging on the IVIS platform, FSH blockade in ThermoMice triggered UCP1 transcription in brown-fat-rich areas initially with increases in white fat-predominant regions. The production of mitochondria-rich, thermogenic "beige" adipose tissue with the anti-FSHβ antibody was further substantiated using PhAM mice, and by documenting elevated basal energy expenditure in metabolic cage studies (9). Interestingly, FSH blockade did not affect glucose or insulin metabolism (92, 93).

Other studies have found a direct correlation between abdominal fat mass and *FSHR* mRNA expression in female chickens (96). FSH was found to alter lipid metabolism by affecting the expression of *Dci, Lpl, RarB, Rdh10, Dgat2,* and *Acsl3* genes, shifting fatty acid and retinol metabolism, and altering PPARγ signaling (96). Interestingly, FSH has also been shown to inhibit hepatic cholesterol metabolism. FSH was found to interact with FSHRs in HepG2 cells, reducing LDLR levels (103). Moreover, FSHR knockdown with specific siRNA in mice demonstrated lower LDLR (103), suggesting that FSH may be indirectly involved in the pathogenesis of NAFLD. Finally, in a Chinese cohort, rising FSH levels correlated positively with serum cholesterol and LDL levels in postmenopausal women (104).

FSH Action on Cardiovascular System

Males receiving androgen deprivation therapy (ADT) for prostate cancer have an increased risk of cardiovascular dysfunction, atherosclerosis and thrombosis (105–107). For example, it has been shown recently that FSH promotes the development of cardiovascular risk in ADT-treated males (18). Moreover, several studies in females have demonstrated effects of FSH on cardiovascular risk measures, such as coronary artery calcium deposition and carotid intima-media thickness. For example, the SWAN study showed that in 856 women who never reported a stroke or a heart attack, FSH trajectory was correlated positively with intima-media thickness(17). Furthermore, a sub-study of the Prospective Army Coronary Calcium project, called the Assessment of the Transition of Hormonal Evaluation with Non-invasive Imaging of Atherosclerosis, showed that serum FSH levels were associated with the number of aortic plaques in 126 women undergoing menopausal transition using contrast-enhanced CT angiography and carotid ultrasound (16). However, a 22-site population-based Survey on Prevalence in East China for Metabolic Diseases and Risk Factors, showed a negative association between FSH levels and cardiovascular risk (108). The study had a cross-sectional design and any causal relationship between FSH levels and cardiovascular risk factor factors could not be established.

Mice receiving ADT have been used to study the relation of serum FSH and cardiovascular disease (CVD) development. The interaction of FSH with FSHR on monocytes has been shown to up-regulate RANK expression and promote monocytic infiltration of atherosclerotic plaques (18). T_h1 helper cells then release RANKL, which activates RANK on monocytes, leading to osteoclast formation. Osteoclasts resorb calcified areas and

provoke atherosclerotic plaque instability, increasing the risk of rupture and thrombosis (18). In a second study, serum FSH levels were also found to be significantly lower in mice treated with GnRH antagonists, as compared to animals getting GnRH agonist or orchiectomized (109). The first group displayed less fat mass, at least a two-fold lower atherosclerotic plaque burden, high levels of high-density lipoproteins (HDL), and reduced serum low-density lipoproteins (LDL) compared to the latter two groups. Although all animals developed fatty changes in the aortic wall, the necrotic regions were dramatically smaller in the first group (109). This suggests that increased CVD risk in ADT cannot be explained solely by hypoandrogenemia, and may relate to changes in serum FSH. Furthermore, it has also been surmised that, as atherosclerotic plaque development is dependent on neovascularization (110), FSH may act by stimulating new vessel formation [as effectively as vascular endothelial growth factor (111, 112)] via FSHR present on vascular endothelial cells (7). The mechanism includes the stimulation of VCAM-1 synthesis by FSHR expressed on endothelial cells. VCAM-1 then recruits monocytes to affect their migration and differentiation into macrophages that accumulate lipid droplets and eventually become foam cells (17, 113). Finally, FSH may elevate production of cytokines, namely IL-6 and TNFα, from macrophages to cause low-grade inflammation, atherosclerosis development and insulin resistance (114). We have documented this direct action in osteoclasts (115).

FSH Action in Oncogenesis

FSH levels are elevated in ovarian cancer (116, 117). Furthermore, epithelial and endothelial FSHRs have been detected in various cancer types, including prostate (118, 119) and ovarian cancers (120–122), as well as in established cancer cell lines, namely prostate cancer cell lines DU145 (118) and PC-3 (118, 119), ovarian cancer cell lines including OVTOKO, CaOV-3, RNG1, OVCAR-3, and TOV-21G (121–126). Endothelial FSHR was detected by immunohistochemical and immunoblotting analysis in samples obtained from >1,000 patients with breast, prostate, colon, pancreas, urinary bladder, kidney, lung, liver, stomach, testis, and ovarian cancer (7). Recent data indicates that these FSHRs are signaling-efficient. In particular, endothelial FSHR expression is associated with vascular remodeling and tumor angiogenesis (6, 7), whereas epithelial FSHR induces cell proliferation (118–120), migration, and cancer cell invasion (127).

Interestingly, murine T-cells directed against FSHR- positive ovarian cancer cells showed increased survival without causing toxicity (122). FSHR stimulation upregulated Oct4 expression via the Erk1/2 pathway in epithelial ovarian cancer (128). Epithelial-to-mesenchymal transition in ovarian cancer was also stimulated through PI3K/Akt-Snail signaling (129). It has been suggested that FSH stimulates ovarian cancer cell proliferation via FSHR isoform 3, which is not coupled with G-proteins and not associated with cAMP production, but activates the Erk pathway in a Ca^{2+}-dependent manner (130, 131).

Cancer cells express abundant receptors to various growth factors, suggesting the potential possibility of restricting cancer growth through antibody-mediated blockade of these receptors (132, 133). Unfortunately, the delivery of antibodies through the endothelium is poor and high doses are prone to cause toxicity (134, 135). To avoid this problem, a different approach, notably targeting the tumor vasculature, has been proposed. However, two major groups of extensively studied agents targeting tumor vessels have proven limitations and lack efficacy. Antiangiogenic agents reduce the action of various growth factors inside the tumor, preventing new blood vessel formation (136–139). Their maximum effect is tumor shrinkage and these agents have failed to improve survival (140, 141). The second group of agents, namely vascular disrupting agents, affect mature vessels, rearranging the endothelial cytoskeleton and increasing vascular wall permeability (142), thus disrupting blood supply and leading to extensive central necrosis of a tumor (143); this nonetheless leaves viable peripheral neoplastic tissue that subsequently repopulates the necrotic area (144–146). A new promising direction for anticancer target therapy is to cause peritumoral infarction using truncated tissue factor (tTF) coupled to ligands that are highly specific for FSHR (147). Antihuman FSHR antibody, conjugated with tTF, binds the FSHR, which is abundant in peritumoral endothelium, initiating blood clotting with subsequent blood supply disruption and tumor necrosis (148). Interestingly, the vasculature of bone and fat has not been shown to express FSHRs: thus, such therapy will most likely cause no issues (8, 149). However, their presence in the female reproductive system may limit anti-FSHR-tTF treatment. This approach still needs extensive investigation in the future and provokes extensive discussion on the development of a cancer therapies based on agents tethered to anti-FSHR antibodies (19).

CONCLUSION

In the transitional phase of a women's reproductive life to menopause, the risk for osteoporosis, obesity and CVDs increase concurrently. Along with declining estrogen levels, sharply rising FSH levels have now been implicated in the pathogenesis of these diseases. It is now well-known that bone loss begins even before estrogen levels are altered in the perimenopause (150).

Several key findings have emerged relating serum FSH to bone loss, obesity, and perhaps even cardiovascular risk and cancer. First, it is clear that FSH directly impacts bone cells—osteoclasts and osteoblast precursors. The underlying mechanisms include a direct action on osteoclasts through the enhancement of RANKL signaling, and indirect actions

to increase the expression of RANK in osteoclasts (151) and stimulate the synthesis of pro-resorptive cytokines, including TNFα, IL1β, and IL-6. Studies also conclusively demonstrate the expression of functional FSHRs on adipose tissue (97), which, when blocked by an FSH antibody, result in a profound reduction of body fat and generation of thermogenic "beige" adipose tissue (152). Together, the studies form the framework for using a humanized FSH antibody for the simultaneous treatment of two public health hazards—obesity and osteoporosis—with a single agent. Admittedly speculative at this stage, an increased risk of cardiovascular event(s) among postmenopausal women may also be in part attributable to subclinical atherosclerosis promoted by sharply rising FSH levels (153). Finally, certain cancers, prominently ovarian tumors in which oncogenic signaling through the FSHR can be proven may be amenable to novel FSH-based therapeutic agents.

Thus, positive correlations between rising FSH levels and a plethora of illnesses like obesity, osteoporosis, cardiovascular pathology, and cancer changes our view of FSH from monogamously associated with fertility to a much broader view of the role of this "gonadotropin" in other medical conditions and in human physiology. It is therefore now conceivable that we question whether FSH is a true aging hormone. By developing new treatment approaches that target this gonadotropin, we may in the future be able to treat multiple age-related diseases perhaps even with a single drug.

AUTHOR CONTRIBUTIONS

DL wrote the manuscript with support from S-MK, AR, IA, SJ, BA, CT, AK, and LS. TY, MZ, and RA helped supervise the project. All authors provided critical feedback and helped shape the manuscript.

FUNDING

Work at Icahn School of Medicine at Mount Sinai was supported by the National Institutes of Health (NIH) by R01 Grants DK113627 to (MZ and LS), AG40132 (to MZ), AR65932 (to MZ), AR67066 (to MZ).

ACKNOWLEDGMENTS

The authors acknowledge Mount Sinai Innovation Partner for their collaboration on the actions of FSH on bone.

REFERENCES

1. Ulloa-Aguirre A, Reiter E, Crepieux P. FSH receptor signaling: complexity of interactions and signal diversity. *Endocrinology*. (2018) 159:3020–35. doi: 10.1210/en.2018-00452

2. Stilley JA, Christensen DE, Dahlem KB, Guan R, Santillan DA, England SK, et al. FSH receptor (FSHR) expression in human extragonadal reproductive tissues and the developing placenta, and the impact of its deletion on pregnancy in mice. *Biol Reprod*. (2014) 91:74. doi: 10.1095/biolreprod.114.118562

3. Ponikwicka-Tyszko D, Chrusciel M, Stelmaszewska J, Bernaczyk P, Sztachelska M, Sidorkiewicz I, et al. Functional expression of FSH receptor

in endometriotic lesions. *J Clin Endocrinol Metab*. (2016) 101:2905–14. doi: 10.1210/jc.2016-1014

4. Robinson LJ, Tourkova I, Wang Y, Sharrow AC, Landau MS, Yaroslavskiy BB, et al. FSH-receptor isoforms and FSH-dependent gene transcription in human monocytes and osteoclasts. *Biochem Biophys Res Commun*. (2010) 394:12–7. doi: 10.1016/j.bbrc.2010.02.112

5. Cannon JG, Kraj B, Sloan G. Follicle-stimulating hormone promotes RANK expression on human monocytes. *Cytokine*. (2011) 53:141–4. doi: 10.1016/j.cyto.2010.11.011

6. Planeix F, Siraj MA, Bidard FC, Robin B, Pichon C, Sastre-Garau X, et al. Endothelial follicle-stimulating hormone receptor expression in invasive breast cancer and vascular remodeling at tumor periphery.

J Exp Clin Cancer Res. (2015) 34:12. doi: 10.1186/s13046-015-0128-7

7. Radu A, Pichon C, Camparo P, Antoine M, Allory Y, Couvelard A, et al. Expression of follicle-stimulating hormone receptor in tumor blood vessels. *N Engl J Med.* (2010) 363:1621–30. doi: 10.1056/NEJMoa1001283

8. Siraj A, Desestret V, Antoine M, Fromont G, Huerre M, Sanson M, et al. Expression of follicle-stimulating hormone receptor by the vascular endothelium in tumor metastases. *BMC Cancer.* (2013) 13:246. doi: 10.1186/1471-2407-13-246

9. Liu P, Ji Y, Yuen T, Rendina-Ruedy E, DeMambro VE, Dhawan S, et al. Blocking FSH induces thermogenic adipose tissue and reduces body fat. *Nature.* (2017) 546:107–12. doi: 10.1038/nature22342

10. Ji Y, Liu P, Yuen T, Haider S, He J, Romero R, et al. Epitope-specific monoclonal antibodies to FSHbeta increase bone mass. *Proc Natl Acad Sci USA.* (2018) 115:2192–7. doi: 10.1073/pnas.1718144115

11. Sun L, Peng Y, Sharrow AC, Iqbal J, Zhang Z, Papachristou DJ, et al. FSH directly regulates bone mass. *Cell.* (2006) 125:247–60. doi: 10.1016/j.cell.2006.01.051

12. Thurston RC, Sowers MR, Sternfeld B, Gold EB, Bromberger J, Chang Y, et al. Gains in body fat and vasomotor symptom reporting over the menopausal transition: the study of women's health across the nation. *Am J Epidemiol.* (2009) 170:766–74. doi: 10.1093/aje/kwp203

13. Senapati S, Gracia CR, Freeman EW, Sammel MD, Lin H, Kim C, et al. Hormone variations associated with quantitative fat measures in the menopausal transition. *Climacteric.* (2014) 17:183–90. doi: 10.3109/13697137.2013.845876

14. Randolph JF Jr, Sowers M, Gold EB, Mohr BA, Luborsky J, Santoro N, et al. Reproductive hormones in the early menopausal transition: relationship to ethnicity, body size, and menopausal status. *J Clin Endocrinol Metab.* (2003) 88:1516–22. doi: 10.1210/jc.2002-020777

15. Celestino Catao Da Silva D, Nogueira De Almeida Vasconcelos A, Cleto Maria Cerqueira J, De Oliveira Cipriano Torres D, Oliveira Dos Santos AC, De Lima Ferreira Fernandes Costa H, et al. Endogenous sex hormones are not associated with subclinical atherosclerosis in menopausal women. *Minerva Ginecol.* (2013) 65:297–302.

16. Munir JA, Wu H, Bauer K, Bindeman J, Byrd C, Feuerstein IM, et al. The perimenopausal atherosclerosis transition: relationships between calcified and noncalcified coronary, aortic, and carotid atherosclerosis and risk factors and hormone levels. *Menopause.* (2012) 19:10–5. doi: 10.1097/gme.0b013e318221bc8d

17. El Khoudary SR, Santoro N, Chen HY, Tepper PG, Brooks MM, Thurston RC, et al. Trajectories of estradiol and follicle-stimulating hormone over the menopause transition and early markers of atherosclerosis after menopause. *Eur J Prev Cardiol.* (2016) 23:694–703. doi: 10.1177/2047487315607044

18. Crawford ED, Schally AV, Pinthus JH, Block NL, Rick FG, Garnick MB, et al. The potential role of follicle-stimulating hormone in the cardiovascular, metabolic, skeletal, and cognitive effects associated with androgen deprivation therapy. *Urol Oncol.* (2017) 35:183–91. doi: 10.1016/j.urolonc.2017.01.025

19. Ghinea N. Vascular Endothelial FSH Receptor, a Target of Interest for Cancer Therapy. *Endocrinology.* (2018) 159:3268–74. doi: 10.1210/en.2018-00466

20. Fox KM, Dias JA, Van Roey P. Three-dimensional structure of human follicle-stimulating hormone. *Mol Endocrinol.* (2001) 15:378–89. doi: 10.1210/mend.15.3.0603

21. Demyashkin GA. Inhibin B in seminiferous tubules of human testes in normal spermatogenesis and in idiopathic infertility. *Syst Biol Reprod Med.* (2018) 65:1–9. doi: 10.1080/19396368.2018.1478470

22. Ying SY. Inhibins, activins, and follistatins: gonadal proteins modulating the secretion of follicle-stimulating hormone. *Endocr Rev.* (1988) 9:267–93. doi: 10.1210/edrv-9-2-267

23. Christensen A, Bentley GE, Cabrera R, Ortega HH, Perfito N, Wu TJ, et al. Hormonal regulation of female reproduction. *Horm Metab Res.* (2012) 44:587–91. doi: 10.1055/s-0032-1306301

24. Simoni M, Gromoll J, Nieschlag E. The follicle-stimulating hormone receptor: biochemistry, molecular biology, physiology, and pathophysiology. *Endocr Rev.* (1997) 18:739–73. doi: 10.1210/edrv.18.6.0320

25. Bruser A, Schulz A, Rothemund S, Ricken A, Calebiro D, Kleinau G, et al. The Activation Mechanism of Glycoprotein Hormone Receptors with Implications in the Cause and Therapy of Endocrine Diseases. *J Biol Chem.* (2016) 291:508–20. doi: 10.1074/jbc.M115.701102

26. Herndon MK, Law NC, Donaubauer EM, Kyriss B, Hunzicker-Dunn M. Forkhead box O member FOXO1 regulates the majority of follicle-stimulating hormone responsive genes in ovarian granulosa cells. *Mol Cell Endocrinol.* (2016) 434:116–26. doi: 10.1016/j.mce.2016.06.020

27. Crepieux P, Marion S, Martinat N, Fafeur V, Vern YL, Kerboeuf D, et al. The ERK-dependent signalling is stage-specifically modulated by FSH, during primary Sertoli cell maturation. *Oncogene.* (2001) 20:4696–709. doi: 10.1038/sj.onc.1204632

28. Escamilla-Hernandez R, Little-Ihrig L, Zeleznik AJ. Inhibition of rat granulosa cell differentiation by overexpression of Galphaq. *Endocrine.* (2008) 33:21–31. doi: 10.1007/s12020-008-9064-z

29. Tranchant T, Durand G, Gauthier C, Crepieux P, Ulloa-Aguirre A, Royere D, et al. Preferential beta-arrestin signalling at low receptor density revealed by functional characterization of the human FSH receptor A189 V mutation. *Mol Cell Endocrinol.* (2011) 331:109–18. doi: 10.1016/j.mce.2010.08.016

30. Nechamen CA, Thomas RM, Cohen BD, Acevedo G, Poulikakos PI, Testa JR, et al. Human follicle-stimulating hormone (FSH) receptor interacts with the adaptor protein APPL1 in HEK 293 cells: potential involvement of the PI3K pathway in FSH signaling. *Biol Reprod.* (2004) 71:629–36. doi: 10.1095/biolreprod.103.025833

31. McGee EA, Hsueh AJ. Initial and cyclic recruitment of ovarian follicles. *Endocr Rev.* (2000) 21:200–14. doi: 10.1210/edrv.21.2.0394

32. Howles CM. Role of LH and FSH in ovarian function. *Mol Cell Endocrinol.* (2000) 161:25–30. doi: 10.1016/S0303-7207(99)00219-1

33. Chan WK, Tan CH. Induction of aromatase activity in porcine granulosa cells by FSH and cyclic AMP. *Endocr Res.* (1987) 13:285–99.

34. Simoni M, Weinbauer GF, Gromoll J, Nieschlag E. Role of FSH in male gonadal function. *Ann Endocrinol.* (1999) 60:102–6.

35. Vu Hai MT, Lescop P, Loosfelt H, Ghinea N. Receptor-mediated transcytosis of follicle-stimulating hormone through the rat testicular microvasculature. *Biol Cell.* (2004) 96:133–44. doi: 10.1016/j.biolcel.2003.11.008

36. Lindsay R. Hormones and bone health in postmenopausal women. *Endocrine.* (2004) 24:223–30. doi: 10.1385/ENDO:24:3:223

37. Colaianni G, Cuscito C, Colucci S. FSH and TSH in the regulation of bone mass: the pituitary/immune/bone axis. *Clin Dev Immunol.* (2013) 2013:382698. doi: 10.1155/2013/382698

38. Davis SR, Lambrinoudaki I, Lumsden M, Mishra GD, Pal L, Rees M, et al. Menopause. *Nat Rev Dis Primers.* (2015) 1:15004. doi: 10.1038/nrdp.2015.4

39. Sowers MR, Greendale GA, Bondarenko I, Finkelstein JS, Cauley JA, Neer RM, et al. Endogenous hormones and bone turnover markers in pre- and perimenopausal women: SWAN. *Osteoporos Int.* (2003) 14:191–7. doi: 10.1007/s00198-002-1329-4

40. Crandall CJ, Tseng CH, Karlamangla AS, Finkelstein JS, Randolph JF Jr, Thurston RC, et al. Serum sex steroid levels and longitudinal changes in bone density in relation to the final menstrual period. *J Clin Endocrinol Metab.* (2013) 98:E654–63. doi: 10.1210/jc.2012-3651

41. Gallagher CM, Moonga BS, Kovach JS. Cadmium, follicle-stimulating hormone, and effects on bone in women age 42-60 years, NHANES III. *Environ Res.* (2010) 110:105–11. doi: 10.1016/j.envres.2009.09.012

42. Cannon JG, Cortez-Cooper M, Meaders E, Stallings J, Haddow S, Kraj B, et al. Follicle-stimulating hormone, interleukin-1, and bone density in adult women. *Am J Physiol Regul Integr Comp Physiol.* (2010) 298:R790–8. doi: 10.1152/ajpregu.00728.2009

43. Adami S, Bianchi G, Brandi ML, Giannini S, Ortolani S, DiMunno O, et al. Determinants of bone turnover markers in healthy premenopausal women. *Calcif Tissue Int.* (2008) 82:341–7. doi: 10.1007/s00223-008-9126-5

44. Garcia-Martin A, Reyes-Garcia R, Garcia-Castro JM, Rozas-Moreno P, Escobar-Jimenez F, Munoz-Torres M. Role of serum FSH measurement on bone resorption in postmenopausal women. *Endocrine.* (2012) 41:302–8. doi: 10.1007/s12020-011-9541-7

45. Xu ZR, Wang AH, Wu XP, Zhang H, Sheng ZF, Wu XY, et al. Relationship of age-related concentrations of serum FSH and LH with bone mineral density, prevalence of osteoporosis in native Chinese women. *Clin Chim Acta.* (2009) 400:8–13. doi: 10.1016/j.cca.2008.09.027

46. Wu XY, Wu XP, Xie H, Zhang H, Peng YQ, Yuan LQ, et al. Age-related changes in biochemical markers of bone turnover and gonadotropin levels and their relationship among Chinese adult women. *Osteoporos Int.* (2010) 21:275–85. doi: 10.1007/s00198-009-0943-9

47. Wang B, Song Y, Chen Y, Wang ES, Zheng D, Qu F, et al. Correlation analysis for follicle-stimulating hormone and C-terminal cross-linked telopetides of type i collagen in menopausal transition women with osteoporosis. *Int J Clin Exp Med.* (2015) 8:2417–22.

48. Cheung E, Tsang S, Bow C, Soong C, Yeung S, Loong C, et al. Bone loss during menopausal transition among southern Chinese women. *Maturitas.* (2011) 69:50–6. doi: 10.1016/j.maturitas.2011.01.010

49. Devleta B, Adem B, Senada S. Hypergonadotropic amenorrhea and bone density: new approach to an old problem. *J Bone Miner Metab.* (2004) 22:360–4. doi: 10.1007/s00774-004-0495-1

50. Podfigurna-Stopa A, Pludowski P, Jaworski M, Lorenc R, Genazzani AR, Meczekalski B. Skeletal status and body composition in young women with functional hypothalamic amenorrhea. *Gynecol Endocrinol.* (2012) 28:299–304. doi: 10.3109/09513590.2011.613972

51. Ozbek MN, Demirbilek H, Baran RT, Baran A. Bone Mineral Density in Adolescent Girls with Hypogonadotropic and Hypergonadotropic Hypogonadism. *J Clin Res Pediatr Endocrinol.* (2016) 8:163–9. doi: 10.4274/jcrpe.2228

52. Rendina D, Gianfrancesco F, De Filippo G, Merlotti D, Esposito T, Mingione A, et al. FSHR gene polymorphisms influence bone mineral density and bone turnover in postmenopausal women. *Eur J Endocrinol.* (2010) 163:165–72. doi: 10.1530/EJE-10-0043

53. Mendoza N, Quereda F, Presa J, Salamanca A, Sanchez-Borrego R, Vazquez F, et al. Estrogen-related genes and postmenopausal osteoporosis risk. *Climacteric.* (2012) 15:587–93. doi: 10.3109/13697137.2012.656160

54. Drake MT, McCready LK, Hoey KA, Atkinson EJ, Khosla S. Effects of suppression of follicle-stimulating hormone secretion on bone resorption markers in postmenopausal women. *J Clin Endocrinol Metab.* (2010) 95:5063–8. doi: 10.1210/jc.2010-1103

55. Uihlein AV, Finkelstein JS, Lee H, Leder BZ. FSH suppression does not affect bone turnover in eugonadal men. *J Clin Endocrinol Metab.* (2014) 99:2510–5. doi: 10.1210/jc.2013-3246

56. Sun L, Zhang Z, Zhu LL, Peng Y, Liu X, Li J, et al. Further evidence for direct pro-resorptive actions of FSH. *Biochem Biophys Res Commun.* (2010) 394:6–11. doi: 10.1016/j.bbrc.2010.02.113

57. Wu Y, Torchia J, Yao W, Lane NE, Lanier LL, Nakamura MC, et al. Bone microenvironment specific roles of ITAM adapter signaling during bone remodeling induced by acute estrogen-deficiency. *PLoS ONE.* (2007) 2:e586. doi: 10.1371/journal.pone.0000586

58. Wang J, Zhang W, Yu C, Zhang X, Zhang H, Guan Q, et al. Follicle-Stimulating Hormone Increases the Risk of Postmenopausal Osteoporosis by Stimulating Osteoclast Differentiation. *PLoS ONE.* (2015) 10:e0134986. doi: 10.1371/journal.pone.0134986

59. Ritter V, Thuering B, Saint Mezard P, Luong-Nguyen NH, Seltenmeyer Y, Junker U, et al. Follicle-stimulating hormone does not impact male bone mass *in vivo* or human male osteoclasts *in vitro*. *Calcif Tissue Int.* (2008) 82:383–91. doi: 10.1007/s00223-008-9134-5

60. Allan CM, Kalak R, Dunstan CR, McTavish KJ, Zhou H, Handelsman DJ, et al. Follicle-stimulating hormone increases bone mass in female mice. *Proc Natl Acad Sci USA.* (2010) 107:22629–34. doi: 10.1073/pnas.1012141108

61. Feng Y, Zhu S, Antaris AL, Chen H, Xiao Y, Lu X, et al. Live imaging of follicle stimulating hormone receptors in gonads and bones using near infrared II fluorophore. *Chem Sci.* (2017) 8:3703–11. doi: 10.1039/c6sc04897h

62. Meher BR, Dixit A, Bousfield GR, Lushington GH. Glycosylation Effects on FSH-FSHR Interaction Dynamics: a case study of different fsh glycoforms by molecular dynamics simulations. *PLoS ONE.* (2015) 10:e0137897. doi: 10.1371/journal.pone.0137897

63. Jiang C, Hou X, Wang C, May JV, Butnev VY, Bousfield GR, et al. Hypoglycosylated hFSH has greater bioactivity than fully glycosylated recombinant hfsh in human granulosa cells. *J Clin Endocrinol Metab.* (2015) 100:E852–60. doi: 10.1210/jc.2015-1317

64. Zaidi S, Zhu LL, Mali R, Iqbal J, Yang G, Zaidi M, et al. Regulation of FSH receptor promoter activation in the osteoclast. *Biochem Biophys Res Commun.* (2007) 361:910–5. doi: 10.1016/j.bbrc.2007.07.081

65. Blair HC, Zaidi M. Osteoclastic differentiation and function regulated by old and new pathways. *Rev Endocr Metab Disord.* (2006) 7:23–32. doi: 10.1007/s11154-006-9010-4

66. Liu S, Cheng Y, Fan M, Chen D, Bian Z. FSH aggravates periodontitis-related bone loss in ovariectomized rats. *J Dent Res.* (2010) 89:366–71. doi: 10.1177/0022034509358822

67. Liu S, Cheng Y, Xu W, Bian Z. Protective effects of follicle-stimulating hormone inhibitor on alveolar bone loss resulting from experimental periapical lesions in ovariectomized rats. *J Endod.* (2010) 36:658-63. doi: 10.1016/j.joen.2010.01.011

68. Zaidi M, Sun L, Kumar TR, Sairam MR, Blair HC. Response: both FSH and sex steroids influence bone mass. *Cell.* (2006) 127:1080–1. doi: 10.1016/j.cell.2006.12.003

69. Oz OK, Hirasawa G, Lawson J, Nanu L, Constantinescu A, Antich PP, et al. Bone phenotype of the aromatase deficient mouse. *J Steroid Biochem Mol Biol.* (2001) 79:49–59. doi: 10.1016/S0960-0760(01)00130-3

70. Zhu LL, Blair H, Cao J, Yuen T, Latif R, Guo L, et al. Blocking antibody to the beta-subunit of FSH prevents bone loss by inhibiting bone resorption and stimulating bone synthesis. *Proc Natl Acad Sci USA.* (2012) 109:14574–9. doi: 10.1073/pnas.1206806109

71. Zhu LL, Tourkova I, Yuen T, Robinson LJ, Bian Z, Zaidi M, et al. Blocking FSH action attenuates osteoclastogenesis. *Biochem Biophys Res Commun.* (2012) 422:54–8. doi: 10.1016/j.bbrc.2012.04.104

72. Sowers M, Zheng H, Tomey K, Karvonen-Gutierrez C, Jannausch M, Li X, et al. Changes in body composition in women over six years at midlife: ovarian and chronological aging. *J Clin Endocrinol Metab.* (2007) 92:895–901. doi: 10.1210/jc.2006-1393

73. Gavaler JS, Rosenblum E. Predictors of postmenopausal body mass index and waist hip ratio in the oklahoma postmenopausal health disparities study. *J Am Coll Nutr.* (2003) 22:269–76. doi: 10.1080/07315724.2003.10719303

74. Seth B, Arora S, Singh R. Association of obesity with hormonal imbalance in infertility: a cross-sectional study in north Indian women. *Indian J Clin Biochem.* (2013) 28:342–7. doi: 10.1007/s12291-013-0301-8

75. Gourlay ML, Specker BL, Li C, Hammett-Stabler CA, Renner JB, Rubin JE. Follicle-stimulating hormone is independently associated with lean mass but not BMD in younger postmenopausal women. *Bone.* (2012) 50:311–6. doi: 10.1016/j.bone.2011.11.001

76. Jaff NG, Norris SA, Snyman T, Toman M, Crowther NJ. Body composition in the Study of Women Entering and in Endocrine Transition (SWEET): A perspective of African women who have a high prevalence of obesity and HIV infection. *Metabolism.* (2015) 64:1031–41. doi: 10.1016/j.metabol.2015.05.009

77. Ecochard R, Marret H, Barbato M, Boehringer H. Gonadotropin and body mass index: high FSH levels in lean, normally cycling women. *Obstet Gynecol.* (2000) 96:8–12. doi: 10.1016/S0029-7844(00)00842-5

78. Caillon H, Freour T, Bach-Ngohou K, Colombel A, Denis MG, Barriere P, et al. Effects of female increased body mass index on *in vitro* fertilization cycles outcome. *Obes Res Clin Pract.* (2015) 9:382–8. doi: 10.1016/j.orcp.2015.02.009

79. De Pergola G, Maldera S, Tartagni M, Pannacciulli N, Loverro G, Giorgino R. Inhibitory effect of obesity on gonadotropin, estradiol, and inhibin B levels in fertile women. *Obesity.* (2006) 14:1954–60. doi: 10.1038/oby.2006.228

80. Tepper PG, Randolph JF Jr, McConnell DS, Crawford SL, El Khoudary SR, Joffe H, et al. Trajectory clustering of estradiol and follicle-stimulating hormone during the menopausal transition among women in the Study of Women's Health across the Nation (SWAN). *J Clin Endocrinol Metab.* (2012) 97:2872–80. doi: 10.1210/jc.2012-1422

81. Ausmanas MK, Tan DA, Jaisamrarn U, Tian XW, Holinka CF. Estradiol, FSH and LH profiles in nine ethnic groups of postmenopausal Asian women: the Pan-Asia Menopause (PAM) study. *Climacteric.* (2007) 10:427–37. doi: 10.1080/13697130701610780

82. Simoncig Netjasov A, Tancic-Gajic M, Ivovic M, Marina L, Arizanovic Z, Vujovic S. Influence of obesity and hormone disturbances on sexuality of women in the menopause. *Gynecol Endocrinol.* (2016) 32:762–6. doi: 10.3109/09513590.2016.1161746

83. Sorensen K, Juul A. BMI percentile-for-age overestimates adiposity in early compared with late maturing pubertal children. *Eur J Endocrinol.* (2015) 173:227–35. doi: 10.1530/EJE-15-0239

84. Bouvattier C, Lahlou N, Roger M, Bougneres P. Hyperleptinaemia is associated with impaired gonadotrophin response to GnRH during late puberty in obese girls, not boys. *Eur J Endocrinol.* (1998) 138:653–8.

85. Bieniek JM, Kashanian JA, Deibert CM, Grober ED, Lo KC, Brannigan RE, et al. Influence of increasing body mass index on semen and reproductive hormonal parameters in a multi-institutional cohort of subfertile men. *Fertil Steril.* (2016) 106:1070–5. doi: 10.1016/j.fertnstert.2016.06.041

86. Foresta C, Di Mambro A, Pagano C, Garolla A, Vettor R, Ferlin A. Insulin-like factor 3 as a marker of testicular function in obese men. *Clin Endocrinol.* (2009) 71:722–6. doi: 10.1111/j.1365-2265.2009.03549.x

87. Casimirri F, Pasquali R, Cantobelli S, Melchionda N, Barbara L. [Obesity and adipose tissue distribution in men: relation to sex steroids and insulin]. *Minerva Endocrinol.* (1991) 16:31–5.

88. Yamacake KG, Cocuzza M, Torricelli FC, Tiseo BC, Frati R, Freire GC, et al. Impact of body mass index, age and varicocele on reproductive hormone profile from elderly men. *Int Braz J Urol.* (2016) 42:365–72. doi: 10.1590/S1677-5538.IBJU.2014.0594

89. Pauli EM, Legro RS, Demers LM, Kunselman AR, Dodson WC, Lee PA. Diminished paternity and gonadal function with increasing obesity in men. *Fertil Steril.* (2008) 90:346–51. doi: 10.1016/j.fertnstert.2007.06.046

90. Ostergren PB, Kistorp C, Fode M, Bennedbaek FN, Faber J, Sonksen J. Metabolic consequences of gonadotropin-releasing hormone agonists vs. orchiectomy: a randomized clinical study. *BJU Int.* (2018) doi: 10.1111/bju.14609. [Epub ahead of print].

91. Ostergren PB, Kistorp C, Fode M, Henderson J, Bennedbaek FN, Faber J, et al. Luteinizing Hormone-Releasing Hormone Agonists are Superior to Subcapsular Orchiectomy in Lowering Testosterone Levels of Men with Prostate Cancer: Results from a Randomized Clinical Trial. *J Urol.* (2017) 197:1441–7. doi: 10.1016/j.juro.2016.12.003

92. Stefanska A, Sypniewska G, Ponikowska I, Cwiklinska-Jurkowska M. Association of follicle-stimulating hormone and sex hormone binding globulin with the metabolic syndrome in postmenopausal women. *Clin Biochem.* (2012) 45:703–6. doi: 10.1016/j.clinbiochem.2012.03.011

93. Stefanska A, Ponikowska I, Cwiklinska-Jurkowska M, Sypniewska G. Association of FSH with metabolic syndrome in postmenopausal women: a comparison with CRP, adiponectin and leptin. *Biomark Med.* (2014) 8:921–30. doi: 10.2217/bmm.14.49

94. Wang N, Li Q, Han B, Chen Y, Zhu C, Chen Y, et al. Follicle-stimulating hormone is associated with non-alcoholic fatty liver disease in Chinese women over 55 years old. *J Gastroenterol Hepatol.* (2016) 31:1196–202. doi: 10.1111/jgh.13271

95. Li X, Jing L, Lin F, Huang H, Chen Z, Chen Y, et al. Diurnal rhythm of follicle-stimulating hormone is associated with nonalcoholic fatty liver disease in a Chinese elderly population. *Eur J Obstet Gynecol Reprod Biol.* (2018) 222:166–70. doi: 10.1016/j.ejogrb.2018.01.034

96. Cui H, Zhao G, Liu R, Zheng M, Chen J, Wen J. FSH stimulates lipid biosynthesis in chicken adipose tissue by upregulating the expression of its receptor FSHR. *J Lipid Res.* (2012) 53:909–17. doi: 10.1194/jlr.M025403

97. Liu XM, Chan HC, Ding GL, Cai J, Song Y, Wang TT, et al. FSH regulates fat accumulation and redistribution in aging through the Galphai/Ca(2+)/CREB pathway. *Aging Cell.* (2015) 14:409–20. doi: 10.1111/acel.12331

98. Cohen P, Spiegelman BM. Brown and beige fat: molecular parts of a thermogenic machine. *Diabetes.* (2015) 64:2346–51. doi: 10.2337/db15-0318

99. Wu J, Bostrom P, Sparks LM, Ye L, Choi JH, Giang AH, et al. Beige adipocytes are a distinct type of thermogenic fat cell in mouse and human. *Cell.* (2012) 150:366–76. doi: 10.1016/j.cell.2012.05.016

100. Rosen CJ, Zaidi M. Contemporaneous reproduction of preclinical science: a case study of FSH and fat. *Ann N Y Acad Sci.* (2017) 1404:17–9. doi: 10.1111/nyas.13457

101. Rosenwald M, Perdikari A, Rulicke T, Wolfrum C. Bi-directional interconversion of brite and white adipocytes. *Nat Cell Biol.* (2013) 15:659–67. doi: 10.1038/ncb2740

102. Wang QA, Tao C, Gupta RK, Scherer PE. Tracking adipogenesis during white adipose tissue development, expansion and regeneration. *Nat Med.* (2013) 19:1338–44. doi: 10.1038/nm.3324

103. Song Y, Wang ES, Xing LL, Shi S, Qu F, Zhang D, et al. Follicle-Stimulating Hormone Induces postmenopausal dyslipidemia through inhibiting hepatic cholesterol metabolism. *J Clin Endocrinol Metab.* (2016) 101:254–63. doi: 10.1210/jc.2015-2724

104. Ma L, Song Y, Li C, Wang E, Zheng D, Qu F, et al. Bone turnover alterations across the menopausal transition in south-eastern Chinese women [corrected]. *Climacteric.* (2016) 19:400–5. doi: 10.1080/13697137.2016.1180677

105. Bosco C, Bosnyak Z, Malmberg A, Adolfsson J, Keating NL, Van Hemelrijck M. Quantifying observational evidence for risk of fatal and nonfatal cardiovascular disease following androgen deprivation therapy for prostate cancer: a meta-analysis. *Eur Urol.* (2015) 68:386–96. doi: 10.1016/j.eururo.2014.11.039

106. Tsai HK, D'Amico AV, Sadetsky N, Chen MH, Carroll PR. Androgen deprivation therapy for localized prostate cancer and the risk of cardiovascular mortality. *J Natl Cancer Inst.* (2007) 99:1516–24. doi: 10.1093/jnci/djm168

107. Zhao J, Zhu S, Sun L, Meng F, Zhao L, Zhao Y, et al. Androgen deprivation therapy for prostate cancer is associated with cardiovascular morbidity and mortality: a meta-analysis of population-based observational studies. *PLoS ONE.* (2014) 9:e107516. doi: 10.1371/journal.pone.0107516

108. Wang N, Shao H, Chen Y, Xia F, Chi C, Li Q, et al. Follicle-Stimulating Hormone, Its association with cardiometabolic risk factors, and 10-year risk of cardiovascular disease in postmenopausal women. *J Am Heart Assoc.* (2017) 6:e05918. doi: 10.1161/JAHA.117.005918

109. Hopmans SN, Duivenvoorden WC, Werstuck GH, Klotz L, Pinthus JH. GnRH antagonist associates with less adiposity and reduced characteristics of metabolic syndrome and atherosclerosis compared with orchiectomy and GnRH agonist in a preclinical mouse model. *Urol Oncol.* (2014) 32:1126–34. doi: 10.1016/j.urolonc.2014.06.018

110. Moulton KS, Heller E, Konerding MA, Flynn E, Palinski W, Folkman J. Angiogenesis inhibitors endostatin or TNP-470 reduce intimal neovascularization and plaque growth in apolipoprotein E-deficient mice. *Circulation.* (1999) 99:1726–32.

111. Albertsen PC, Klotz L, Tombal B, Grady J, Olesen TK, Nilsson J. Cardiovascular morbidity associated with gonadotropin releasing hormone agonists and an antagonist. *Eur Urol.* (2014) 65:565–73. doi: 10.1016/j.eururo.2013.10.032

112. Stilley JA, Guan R, Duffy DM, Segaloff DL. Signaling through FSH receptors on human umbilical vein endothelial cells promotes angiogenesis. *J Clin Endocrinol Metab.* (2014) 99:E813–20. doi: 10.1210/jc.2013-3186

113. El Khoudary SR, Wildman RP, Matthews K, Thurston RC, Bromberger JT, Sutton-Tyrrell K. Endogenous sex hormones impact the progression of subclinical atherosclerosis in women during the menopausal transition. *Atherosclerosis.* (2012) 225:180–6. doi: 10.1016/j.atherosclerosis.2012.07.025

114. Choi SH, Hong ES, Lim S. Clinical implications of adipocytokines and newly emerging metabolic factors with relation to insulin resistance and cardiovascular health. *Front Endocrinol.* (2013) 4:97. doi: 10.3389/fendo.2013.00097

115. Iqbal J, Sun L, Kumar TR, Blair HC, Zaidi M. Follicle-stimulating hormone stimulates TNF production from immune cells to enhance osteoblast and osteoclast formation. *Proc Natl Acad Sci USA.* (2006) 103:14925–30. doi: 10.1073/pnas.0606805103

116. Mertens-Walker I, Baxter RC, Marsh DJ. Gonadotropin signalling in epithelial ovarian cancer. *Cancer Lett.* (2012) 324:152–9. doi: 10.1016/j.canlet.2012.05.017

117. Rzepka-Gorska I, Chudecka-Glaz A, Kosmowska B. FSH and LH serum/tumor fluid ratios and malignant tumors of the ovary. *Endocr Relat Cancer.* (2004) 11:315–21. doi: 10.1677/erc.0.0110315

118. Ben-Josef E, Yang SY, Ji TH, Bidart JM, Garde SV, Chopra DP, et al. Hormone-refractory prostate cancer cells express functional follicle-stimulating hormone receptor (FSHR). *J Urol.* (1999) 161:970–6.

119. Mariani S, Salvatori L, Basciani S, Arizzi M, Franco G, Petrangeli E, et al. Expression and cellular localization of follicle-stimulating hormone receptor in normal human prostate, benign prostatic hyperplasia and prostate cancer. *J Urol.* (2006) 175:2072–7; discussion: 7. doi: 10.1016/S0022-5347(06)00273-4

120. Zheng W, Lu JJ, Luo F, Zheng Y, Feng Y, Felix JC, et al. Ovarian epithelial tumor growth promotion by follicle-stimulating hormone and inhibition of the effect by luteinizing hormone. *Gynecol Oncol.* (2000) 76:80–8. doi: 10.1006/gyno.1999.5628

121. Wang J, Lin L, Parkash V, Schwartz PE, Lauchlan SC, Zheng W. Quantitative analysis of follicle-stimulating hormone receptor in ovarian epithelial tumors: a novel approach to explain the field effect of ovarian cancer development in secondary mullerian systems. *Int J Cancer.* (2003) 103:328–34. doi: 10.1002/ijc.10848

122. Perales-Puchalt A, Svoronos N, Rutkowski MR, Allegrezza MJ, Tesone AJ, Payne KK, et al. Follicle-stimulating hormone receptor is expressed by most ovarian cancer subtypes and is a safe and effective immunotherapeutic target. *Clin Cancer Res.* (2017) 23:441–53. doi: 10.1158/1078-0432. CCR-16-0492

123. Urbanska K, Stashwick C, Poussin M, Powell DJ Jr. Follicle-Stimulating hormone receptor as a target in the redirected t-cell therapy for cancer. *Cancer Immunol Res.* (2015) 3:1130–7. doi: 10.1158/2326-6066.CIR-15-0047

124. Modi DA, Sunoqrot S, Bugno J, Lantvit DD, Hong S, Burdette JE. Targeting of follicle stimulating hormone peptide-conjugated dendrimers to ovarian cancer cells. *Nanoscale.* (2014) 6:2812–20. doi: 10.1039/c3nr0 5042d

125. Choi JH, Choi KC, Auersperg N, Leung PC. Gonadotropins activate proteolysis and increase invasion through protein kinase A and phosphatidylinositol 3-kinase pathways in human epithelial ovarian cancer cells. *Cancer Res.* (2006) 66:3912–20. doi: 10.1158/0008-5472.CAN-05-1785

126. Hong H, Yan Y, Shi S, Graves SA, Krasteva LK, Nickles RJ, et al. PET of follicle-stimulating hormone receptor: broad applicability to cancer imaging. *Mol Pharm.* (2015) 12:403–10. doi: 10.1021/mp500766x

127. Sanchez AM, Flamini MI, Russo E, Casarosa E, Pacini S, Petrini M, et al. LH and FSH promote migration and invasion properties of a breast cancer cell line through regulatory actions on the actin cytoskeleton. *Mol Cell Endocrinol.* (2016) 437:22–34. doi: 10.1016/j.mce.2016.08.009

128. Liu L, Zhang J, Fang C, Zhang Z, Feng Y, Xi X. OCT4 mediates FSH-induced epithelial-mesenchymal transition and invasion through the ERK1/2 signaling pathway in epithelial ovarian cancer. *Biochem Biophys Res Commun.* (2015) 461:525–32. doi: 10.1016/j.bbrc.2015.04.061

129. Yang Y, Zhang J, Zhu Y, Zhang Z, Sun H, Feng Y. Follicle-stimulating hormone induced epithelial-mesenchymal transition of epithelial ovarian cancer cells through follicle-stimulating hormone receptor PI3K/Akt-Snail signaling pathway. *Int J Gynecol Cancer.* (2014) 24:1564–74. doi: 10.1097/IGC.0000000000000279

130. Babu PS, Krishnamurthy H, Chedrese PJ, Sairam MR. Activation of extracellular-regulated kinase pathways in ovarian granulosa cells by the novel growth factor type 1 follicle-stimulating hormone receptor. Role in hormone signaling and cell proliferation. *J Biol Chem.* (2000) 275:27615–26. doi: 10.1074/jbc.M003206200

131. Li Y, Ganta S, Cheng C, Craig R, Ganta RR, Freeman LC. FSH stimulates ovarian cancer cell growth by action on growth factor variant receptor. *Mol Cell Endocrinol.* (2007) 267:26–37. doi: 10.1016/j.mce.2006. 11.010

132. Keereweer S, Van Driel PB, Robinson DJ, Lowik CW. Shifting focus in optical image-guided cancer therapy. *Mol Imaging Biol.* (2014) 16:1–9. doi: 10.1007/s11307-013-0688-x

133. Pento JT. Monoclonal antibodies for the treatment of cancer. *Anticancer Res.* (2017) 37:5935–9. doi: 10.21873/anticanres.12040

134. Babiker HM, McBride A, Newton M, Boehmer LM, Drucker AG, Gowan M, et al. Cardiotoxic effects of chemotherapy: a review of both cytotoxic and molecular targeted oncology therapies and their effect on

the cardiovascular system. *Crit Rev Oncol Hematol.* (2018) 126:186–200. doi: 10.1016/j.critrevonc.2018.03.014

135. Hansel TT, Kropshofer H, Singer T, Mitchell JA, George AJ. The safety and side effects of monoclonal antibodies. *Nat Rev Drug Discov.* (2010) 9:325–38. doi: 10.1038/nrd3003

136. Bouis D, Kusumanto Y, Meijer C, Mulder NH, Hospers GA. A review on pro- and anti-angiogenic factors as targets of clinical intervention. *Pharmacol Res.* (2006) 53:89–103. doi: 10.1016/j.phrs.2005.10.006

137. Raica M, Cimpean AM. Platelet-Derived Growth Factor (PDGF)/PDGF Receptors (PDGFR) Axis as target for antitumor and antiangiogenic therapy. *Pharmaceuticals.* (2010) 3:572–99. doi: 10.3390/ph3030572

138. Korc M, Friesel RE. The role of fibroblast growth factors in tumor growth. *Curr Cancer Drug Targets.* (2009) 9:639–51. doi: 10.2174/156800909789057006

139. Holash J, Maisonpierre PC, Compton D, Boland P, Alexander CR, Zagzag D, et al. Vessel cooption, regression, and growth in tumors mediated by angiopoietins and VEGF. *Science.* (1999) 284:1994–8.

140. Barinaga M. Cancer research - Designing therapies that target tumor blood vessels. *Science.* (1997) 275:482–4. doi: 10.1126/science.275.5299.482

141. Jayson GC, Kerbel R, Ellis LM, Harris AL. Antiangiogenic therapy in oncology: current status and future directions. *Lancet.* (2016) 388:518–29. doi: 10.1016/S0140-6736(15)01088-0

142. Tozer GM, Kanthou C, Baguley BC. Disrupting tumour blood vessels. *Nat Rev Cancer.* (2005) 5:423–35. doi: 10.1038/nrc1628

143. Thorpe PE. Vascular targeting agents as cancer therapeutics. *Clin Cancer Res.* (2004) 10:415–27. doi: 10.1158/1078-0432.Ccr-0642-03

144. Neri D, Bicknell R. Tumour vascular targeting. *Nat Rev Cancer.* (2005) 5:436–46. doi: 10.1038/nrc1627

145. Siemann DW, Chaplin DJ, Horsman MR. Realizing the Potential of Vascular targeted therapy: the rationale for combining vascular disrupting agents and anti-angiogenic agents to treat cancer. *Cancer Invest.* (2017) 35:519–34. doi: 10.1080/07357907.2017.1364745

146. Cesca M, Bizzaro F, Zucchetti M, Giavazzi R. Tumor delivery of chemotherapy combined with inhibitors of angiogenesis and vascular targeting agents. *Front Oncol.* (2013) 3:259. doi: 10.3389/fonc.2013. 00259

147. Huang X, Molema G, King S, Watkins L, Edgington TS, Thorpe PE. Tumor infarction in mice by antibody-directed targeting of tissue factor to tumor vasculature. *Science.* (1997) 275:547–50.

148. Thorpe PE, Chaplin DJ, Blakey DC. The first international conference on vascular targeting: meeting overview. *Cancer Res.* (2003) 63:1144–7.

149. Renner M, Goeppert B, Siraj MA, Radu A, Penzel R, Wardelmann E, et al. Follicle-stimulating hormone receptor expression in soft tissue sarcomas. *Histopathology.* (2013) 63:29–35. doi: 10.1111/his.12135

150. Lizneva D, Yuen T, Sun L, Kim SM, Atabiekov I, Munshi LB, et al. Emerging concepts in the epidemiology, pathophysiology, and clinical care of osteoporosis across the menopausal transition. *Matrix Biol.* (2018) 71–72:70–81. doi: 10.1016/j.matbio.2018.05.001

151. Imai Y. Bone metabolism by sex hormones and gonadotropins. *Clin Calcium.* (2014) 24:815–9.

152. Sponton CH, Kajimura S. Burning fat and building bone by FSH blockade. *Cell Metab.* (2017) 26:285–7. doi: 10.1016/j.cmet.2017. 07.018

153. Xu K, Si QJ. Changes of sex hormones and risk factors associated with atherosclerosis in old patients with castrated prostatic cancer. *Zhongguo Ying Yong Sheng Li Xue Za Zhi.* (2013) 29:368–70.

6

Hormonal Regulation of Follicle-Stimulating Hormone Glycosylation in Males

Stella Campo [1], Luz Andreone [1†], Verónica Ambao [1], Mariela Urrutia [1],
Ricardo S. Calandra [2] and Susana B. Rulli [2]*

[1] Centro de Investigaciones Endocrinológicas "Dr. César Bergadá" (CEDIE), Buenos Aires, Argentina, [2] Instituto de Biología y Medicina Experimental (IBYME-CONICET), Buenos Aires, Argentina

*Correspondence:
Stella Campo
scampo@cedie.org.ar

†Present Address:
Luz Andreone,
Instituto de Investigación en Biomedicina de Buenos Aires (IBioBA) - CONICET - Instituto Partner de la Sociedad Max Planck, Buenos Aires, Argentina

The Follicle-Stimulating Hormone plays an important role in the regulation of gametogenesis. It is synthesized and secreted as a family of glycoforms with differing oligosaccharide structure, biological action, and half-life. The presence of these oligosaccharides is absolutely necessary for the full expression of hormone bioactivity at the level of the target cell. The endocrine milieu modulates the glycosylation of this hormone. During male sexual development a progressive increase in FSH sialylation and in the proportion of glycoforms bearing complex oligosaccharides are the main features in this physiological condition. In late puberty, FSH oligosaccharides are largely processed in the medial- and trans-Golgi cisternae of the gonadotrope and remain without changes throughout adult life. In experimental models, the absence of gonads severely affects FSH sialylation; androgen administration is able to restore the characteristics observed under physiological conditions. The expression of ST6 beta-galactoside alpha-2,6-sialyltransferase 1 is hormonally regulated in the male rat; it decreases after short periods of castration but increases markedly at longer periods of androgen deprivation. Although ST3 beta-galactoside alpha-2,3-sialyltransferase 3 is expressed in the male rat pituitary it is not influenced by changes in the endocrine milieu. The oligosaccharide structure of FSH has an impact on the Sertoli cell endocrine activity. In more advanced stages of Sertoli cell maturation, both sialylation and complexity of the oligosaccharides are involved in the regulation of inhibin B production; moreover, FSH glycoforms bearing incomplete oligosaccharides may enhance the stimulatory effect exerted by gonadal growth factors. In this review, we discuss available information on variation of FSH glycosylation and its hormonal regulation under different physiological and experimental conditions, as well as the effect on Sertoli cell endocrine activity.

Keywords: Follicle-stimulating hormone glycosylation, hormonal regulation, male gonad, Sertoli cell, inhibin

INTRODUCTION

Pituitary gonadotropins regulate basic reproductive processes such as gametogenesis, follicular development, and ovulation. Follicle-stimulating hormone (FSH) is synthesized and secreted in multiple molecular forms with different biological characteristics (1–6). Hormone microheterogeneity arises from the post-translational processing of the gonadotropin, which results in molecular variants showing differences in the structure of the oligosaccharides added during glycoprotein biosynthesis (7, 8).

Gonadotropin glycosylation is a highly complex process; a group of glycosidases (glucosidases and mannosidases) as well as glycosyltransferases (N-acetylglucosaminyltransferases, galactosyltransferases, N-acetylgalactosyltransferases, sialyltransferases, and sulfotransferases) are involved. The initial step in N-linked glycosylation is the co-translational transfer of a dolichol-linked oligosaccharide precursor to specific Asn residues (sequence Asn-X-Ser/Thr) of the nascent polypeptide chain (9–11). When the gonadotropin is still in the rough endoplasmic reticulum (RER), three glucose, and one mannose residues are removed to yield the $Man_8GlcNAc_2Asn$ intermediate (**Figure 1**). Then, glycoproteins are transferred to the Golgi apparatus and removal of additional mannose residues occurs in the cis-Golgi cisterna. This high mannose oligosaccharide serves as substrate for the synthesis of hybrid and complex N-glycans precursors in the medial-Golgi by the addition of N-acetylglucosamine (GlcNAc) residues (9–11). Finally, branch elongation of this precursors occurs in the trans-Golgi; if galactose, and sialic acid are sequentially added, then sialylated oligosaccharides are formed. Alternatively, sequential addition of N-acetylgalactosamine (GalNAc) and sulfate produces sulfated oligosaccharides, which account for almost 10% of human FSH (12, 13) (**Figure 1**).

Several techniques were used to isolate FSH glycosylation variants with differences in charge, including isoelectric focusing (14, 15), chromatofocusing (16, 17), and zone electrophoresis (18, 19). Likewise, lectin affinity column chromatography was useful to isolate mix of glycoforms with marked differences in the oligosaccharide complexity; these techniques based on the different affinity of sugar residues for a specific lectin maintain the biological activity of the hormone (17, 20–22). Methods based on high-performance liquid chromatography were used to determine glycoprotein oligosaccharide structure. Mass spectrometry allowed to identify carbohydrate composition in digested fragments of a glycoprotein. Matrix-assisted laser desorption ionization (MALDI) and electrospray ionization (ESI) are other optional ionization techniques used for glycan analysis. More recently, the alternative fragmentation technologies of electron capture dissociation (ECD) and electron transfer dissociation (ETD) have been introduced (23). Bousfield et al. (8, 24) have extensively characterized FSH glycoform preparations using nano-electrospray mass spectrometry.

The presence of the oligosaccharides is absolutely necessary for the full expression of FSH bioactivity at the level of the target cell (25–27). The endocrine milieu modulates the glycosylation of this hormone; variations in the relative abundance of FSH glycoforms, with differences in their oligosaccharide structure, have been reported under physiological, and pathological conditions both in males and females (18, 19, 22, 28–31).

Studies carried out in several experimental models have shown the relevance of FSH oligosaccharide structure, particularly sialylation, and oligosaccharide complexity, in the regulation of ovarian function (32). The biological effects of FSH glycosylation variants have been demonstrated for follicular growth, antral formation, and estradiol secretion; furthermore, a specific balance of these glycoforms seems to be required for optimal follicle development (7, 33, 34). Sialylation and

complexity of FSH oligosaccharides exert a differential effect on human granulosa cell steroid and peptide production; a less sialylated FSH stimulates the secretion of estradiol, progesterone, free inhibin α-subunit, and inhibin A; whereas more acidic counterparts only affect the production of estradiol and free inhibin α-subunit (35). It has also been shown that the structure of FSH oligosaccharides affects the global gene expression of human granulosa cells (36). The expression of a number of genes involved in regulation of important aspects of granulosa cell function seems to be regulated by FSH carbohydrate structure. In fact, FSH glycosylation variants bearing fully processed carbohydrates modulate the expression of genes associated with biological processes, such as homeostasis, cell differentiation, and apoptosis. The expression of genes related to other essential aspects of granulosa cell function, such as ovarian follicle development, ovulation, response to steroid hormone stimulus, and, in particular, steroid biosynthesis is affected by glycoforms bearing incomplete oligosaccharides.

Pioneering studies carried out by Phillips and Wide (37) and Damian-Matsumura et al. (38) demonstrated that the hormonal milieu regulates the synthesis and secretion of FSH glycosylation variants. The gonadotropin-releasing hormone (GnRH) and sex steroids are recognized endocrine factors involved in the regulation of FSH molecular microheterogeneity, both in females and in males (18, 29, 39, 40). As for the biological relevance of FSH oligosaccharide structure in the regulation of male gonadal function, the available information on variations of FSH glycosylation and its hormonal regulation under different physiological and experimental conditions as well as its effect on endocrine activity in the Sertoli cell are discussed in this review, which includes both experimental and clinical studies.

CHANGES IN FSH GLYCOSYLATION DURING MALE SEXUAL DEVELOPMENT
Studies in Experimental Models
Early studies carried out in rats (41), lambs (42), and humans (18, 43), demonstrated that FSH oligosaccharide structure and its biological characteristics vary during sexual development in both males and females. Additional evidence showed that the structure of pituitary FSH oligosaccharides changes in terms of complexity and sialylation in immature, prepubertal, and adult male rats (44). FSH glycosylation variants bearing high mannose and hybrid type oligosaccharides are predominant in the pituitaries of immature rats; however, this proportion progressively decreases, and that of glycoforms bearing more complex, highly branched oligosaccharides increases in prepubertal, and adult animals. These variations are closely related to the increase in circulating testosterone levels; thus, a possible androgen influence as well as a hypothalamic contribution through pulsatile GnRH secretion on the FSH glycosylation process may be relevant. Based on these findings and considering that sialic acid can only be added if a galactose residue is already present in the carbohydrate chain, variations in the extent of pituitary FSH sialylation during sexual development in male rats may be expected. The shift toward a more sialylated FSH during sexual development concomitantly

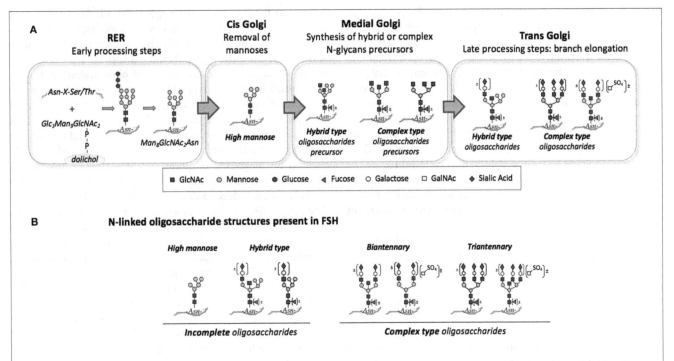

FIGURE 1 | (A) Summary of the N-glycan biosynthetic pathway: N-linked glycosylation begins in the RER with the co-translational transfer of a dolichol-linked Glc₃Man₉GlcNAc₂ to a Asn-X-Ser/Thr motif. In the cis-Golgi cisterna, additional mannose residues are removed. In medial-Golgi, hybrid-, and complex-type precursors are formed by the addition of N-acetylglucosamine (GlcNAc) residues. In the trans-Golgi, sequential addition of galactose, and sialic acid occurs. Alternatively, sequential addition of N-acetylgalactosamine (GalNAc) and sulfate (SO₄) produces sulfated oligosaccharides. **(B)** Some of the N-linked oligosaccharide structures present on human FSH: High mannose and hybrid type N-glycans are incomplete oligosaccharides. Bi- and tri-antennary oligosaccharides are complex type N-glycans. A "bisecting" GlcNAc residue attached to the β-mannose of the core may be present in complex and hybrid-type oligosaccharides. Glycoforms lacking terminal residues such as fucose, galactose, GalNAc, sulfate, and/or sialic acid may also be present.

with the rise in circulating androgen levels has been previously reported (41, 45). Similar results were obtained by Ambao et al. (15); variations in the distribution profiles of FSH charge analogs were observed at the lower pH intervals of the preparative isoelectrofocusing gradient, where the predominant proportion of FSH was isolated.

Studies in Humans

Variations in circulating FSH *in vitro* bioactivity and sialylation extent in prepubertal and pubertal normal boys were clearly shown by Phillips et al. (43) and Olivares et al. (46). These authors reported a significant increment in the proportion of more sialylated FSH at the onset of puberty, and they were not able to detect further changes in advanced puberty and adulthood. Not only changes in hormone sialylation but also variations in the oligosaccharide complexity of circulating FSH were described in normal boys during pubertal development (47). A progressive increase in the proportion of FSH glycoforms bearing highly branched oligosaccharides was observed throughout Tanner stages II to IV-V with a concomitant decrease in those FSH glycosylation variants bearing incomplete carbohydrate chains.

Based on these observations it can be deduced that FSH glycosylation in late puberty, in the presence of adult levels of androgens, is characterized by the predominance of glycoforms

whose oligosaccharides have been completely processed in the medial- and trans-Golgi cisternae of the gonadotrope.

HORMONAL REGULATION OF FSH GLYCOSYLATION IN THE MALE

Considering the evidence showing variations in FSH molecular microheterogeneity associated with changes in the endocrine milieu, the question arises as whether the hypothalamus, and the testis contribute to the regulation of FSH glycosylation. Hormonal factors, mainly GnRH and androgens, are involved in the regulation of FSH oligosaccharide structure, as demonstrated in rodents and humans (37, 48).

STUDIES IN EXPERIMENTAL MODELS

It has been shown that the absence of gonad or the administration of antiandrogens to male golden hamsters and rats increases the proportion of less sialylated FSH in the pituitary gland (40, 49, 50). Studies carried out in the male rat show that castration in prepubertal and adult animals induces changes in the oligosaccharide complexity of pituitary FSH (44). Under these experimental conditions, FSH glycosylation variants bearing incomplete oligosaccharides become predominant as was observed after the administration of the non-steroidal antiandrogen flutamide that blocks androgen action both peripherally and at hypothalamic-pituitary level (51). Interestingly, the proportion of these pituitary FSH glycosylation variants in the absence of androgen action in adults is similar to the one described in the immature male rat. When castrated male rats are treated with dihydrotestosterone, a non-aromatizable androgen, the relative proportion of pituitary FSH glycoforms bearing incomplete oligosaccharides markedly decreases. Concomitantly, a significant increase in FSH glycoforms bearing complex-type oligosaccharides occurs. Thus, androgens are able to restore the characteristic profile of the intact animal. These sex steroids may be needed to regulate the expression of the glycosyltransferases present in the medial Golgi cisternae that determine the FSH oligosaccharide degree of branching.

Not only is the complexity of FSH oligosaccharides altered after castration, but hormone sialylation is also severely affected when testicular function is absent in the male rat. After 4 days of castration a marked decrease in the relative proportion of more sialylated FSH present in the adult pituitary was observed (15). The complete profile of FSH charge analogs shows similar proportions of hormone distributed along the pH gradient of the isoelectrofocusing. Long-term castration further worsens this situation and a considerable amount of hormone is detected at the highest extreme of the pH gradient. The administration of testosterone propionate 2 days after castration is able to restore the physiological distribution profile of pituitary FSH charge analogs characteristic in intact adult animals.

Studies in Humans

Studying anorchid patients enables us to determine serum FSH glycosylation and the effect of regulatory factors (i.e., GnRH and testosterone) under a condition in which testicular function is absent since early life. Not only are FSH serum levels very high, but also the oligosaccharide structure of the hormone may be altered as well as the response to regulatory factors. In these patients, the oligosaccharide structure of FSH is severely affected and no response to classic regulators factors was observed. The profile of FSH glycosylation variants found in serum of prepubertal and pubertal patients is very different in terms of sialylation and complexity of oligosaccharides to that determined in normal boys (47). There is no difference in the distribution pattern of FSH charge analogs between prepubertal and pubertal anorchid patients; the hormone is distributed in similar proportions throughout the isoelectricfocusing pH gradient. The administration of GnRH to prepubertal anorchid patients for diagnostic purposes does not provoke any change in the characteristics of the charge analogs distribution profile; nevertheless, it induces a discreet increase in FSH serum levels. The classic effect of GnRH described in normal boys is secretion of less sialylated hormone, which does not occur in anorchid patients. Similarly, the administration of testosterone enanthate to pubertal patients to maintain secondary sexual characteristics does not provoke any change in serum FSH levels and does not alter the distribution profile of FSH charge analogs. Based on this evidence, it may be proposed that the addition of terminal sugar residues to FSH carbohydrate branches seems to be a sensitive step in oligosaccharide synthesis in the trans-Golgi cisternae, which may be impaired when a functional gonad is not present during the first years of life.

The distribution profile of FSH glycoforms analyzed in terms of oligosaccharide complexity, either in prepubertal or pubertal patients, does not mimic the one determined in normal boys (47). There is a predominant proportion of FSH bearing biantennary; this characteristic is not observed under physiological conditions at any stage of pubertal development. Nevertheless, after testosterone enanthate administration there is a significant increase in the proportion of FSH bearing complex oligosaccharides. These observations suggest that the glycosyltransferases involved in oligosaccharide branching and in the addition of terminal sugar residues to the carbohydrate chain may have a different response to androgen action.

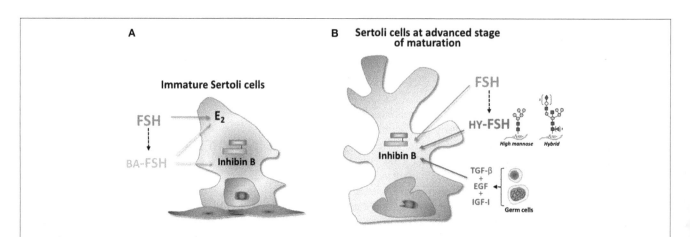

FIGURE 2 | Schematic representation of FSH effect on Sertoli cell endocrine activity at different stages of maturation. **(A)** Immature Sertoli cell: arrows indicate the effects of recombinant human FSH (rhFSH) and basic charge analogs (BA-FSH) isolated at pH 5-7 on estradiol (E₂) and inhibin B production. **(B)** Sertoli cell at advanced stage of maturation: arrows indicate the effects of rhFSH, growth factors produced by germ cells (TGF-β, EGF, IGF-1), and FSH glycoforms bearing high-mannose and hybrid- type oligosaccharides (HY-FSH) on inhibin B production.

ENDOCRINE REGULATION OF PITUITARY SIALYLTRANSFERASE EXPRESSION

Sialic acid content modulates hormone bioactivity; this terminal sugar residue of the oligosaccharide chain determines the half-life of FSH and its metabolic clearance rate (52, 53). On the other hand, more recent studies demonstrated that FSH oligosaccharide structure affects hormone conformation which influences FSHR binding stability and dynamics; thereby, modulates receptor activation and signal transduction (54–57).

It has been described that sialylation of FSH changes under several physiological and pathological conditions concomitantly with variations in the endocrine milieu (18). The question arises as whether the expression of the enzymes that are responsible for sialic acid addition to FSH oligosaccharides may be modulated by endocrine factors. Two sialyltranferases have been identified in the trans-Golgi *cisternae* as responsible for the sialic acid incorporation to FSH carbohydrate chains: ST3 beta-galactoside alpha-2,3-sialyltransferase 3 (ST3GAL3) and ST6 beta-galactoside alpha-2,6-sialyltransferase 1 (ST6GAL1). Damián-Matsumura et al. (38) showed that estradiol modulates mRNA expression of the pituitary *St3gal3* in female rats. The evidence obtained during sexual development and under different experimental conditions in the male rat shows that the pituitary mRNA expression of this enzyme is very low; likewise, very weak staining is observed by immunohistochemistry in tissue sections using a specific antibody (15). Conversely, expression of *St6gal1* is higher than that of *St3gal3* and shows a significant increase in adult rats when compared to immature animals. The effect of castration on *St6gal1* gene expression is intriguing. In the absence of circulating androgens, after 2 days of castration, there is a transient decrease in its mRNA expression. Unexpectedly, at longer periods of castration (5–20 days) there is a progressive increment in the expression of this enzyme. Low mRNA expression for *St3gal3* remains unchanged in all experimental conditions studied. The clear predominance of pituitary FSH glycosylation variants bearing incomplete oligosaccharides after castration may explain the synthesis of less acidic FSH in spite of the presence of the protein and the high expression of *St6gal1* (15). The higher mRNA expression of *St6gal1* than that of *St3gal3* in all the experimental conditions studied further supports the hypothesis that the abundance of FSH charge analogs possessing a 2,6-linked sialic acid is hormonally regulated in male rats.

BIOLOGICAL EFFECTS OF FSH GLYCOSYLATION ON SERTOLI CELL ENDOCRINE ACTIVITY

Sertoli cell function mainly depends on the action of FSH; this hormone is responsible for important structural and functional changes that occur during the maturation process. Under the control of FSH, the Sertoli cell secretes estradiol, and inhibins (58, 59). Based on the effect of FSH oligosaccharide structure on steroid and inhibin production by granulosa cells described by Loreti et al. (35), it becomes possible that a

similar mechanism may operate in the Sertoli cell. Estradiol production is characteristic of the immature Sertoli cell and it is stimulated by FSH; however, during the maturation process the cell progressively loses the ability to synthesize this steroid (60–62). Creus et al. (17) demonstrated that the FSH sialylation modulates estradiol production in cultured immature rat Sertoli cells. FSH charge analogs isolated at pH higher than five and glycoforms bearing complex oligosaccharides were the most potent stimuli for estradiol production.

Inhibin B and Anti- Müllerian hormone (AMH) are considered reliable markers of Sertoli cell function in males (63–68). Although production of these two peptides is regulated by FSH, inhibin B serum levels do not always correlate with those of FSH (65, 66, 69). This evidence suggests that different mechanisms are involved in the regulation of both markers. Recombinant human FSH (rhFSH) is unable to increase inhibin B production in cultured immature Sertoli cells, although it stimulates estradiol and cAMP in a dose-dependent manner (70). Interestingly, less sialylated FSH is the only preparation able to further enhance the high amount of inhibin B that these cells produce under basal conditions (**Figure 2**). As expected, estradiol and cAMP production is markedly stimulated by these charged analogs. Cultured Sertoli cells produce less basal inhibin B than immature cells at advanced stages of maturation (**Figure 2**) (70). Recombinant human FSH stimulates its production in a dose-dependent manner; nevertheless, growth factors secreted by germ cells are absolutely essential to maintain the synthesis of this dimeric form of inhibin. Interestingly, FSH glycoforms bearing incomplete carbohydrate chains are able to further enhance inhibin B production even in the presence of gonadal factors (70). Based on these findings, it may be proposed that the FSH oligosaccharide structure is involved in the regulatory mechanisms of inhibin production, and interacts with factors produced by testicular cells at different stages of Sertoli cell maturation.

There is strong evidence showing that production of AMH is stimulated by FSH (71–73). Studies in prepubertal FSH-deficient mice showed that treatment with recombinant FSH restores normal serum AMH levels and testicular volume (74). Clinical studies in patients with congenital central hypogonadism and low AMH serum levels, according to their Tanner stage, showed that these parameters were increased after treatment with exogenous FSH (72, 73). The possible participation of FSH oligosaccharide structure in the stimulatory effect exerted by this gonadotropin on AMH production by the Sertoli cell has not been explored yet.

CONCLUDING REMARKS AND FUTURE DIRECTIONS

The regulation of FSH glycosylation seems to be a complex mechanism; GnRH and sex steroids may exert their effect through the expression of different glycosyltransferases involved in the addition and removal of sugar residues. The sialylation of FSH and the complexity of its oligosaccharides affect the biological action of the hormone at the level of the target cell. The presence of a fully functioning gonad seems to be necessary to maintain the secretion of adequate FSH glycosylation variants during sexual maturation and in adult life. Further studies would be necessary to elucidate a possible role of FSH glycosylation on other aspects of Sertoli cell function, including global gene expression, peptide production, and activation of different signal transduction pathways.

The development of new methodologies to improve the isolation of glycoforms without altering the bioactivity of the hormone, would allow to use FSH microheterogeneity as a marker of the hypothalamic- pituitary-gonadal axis function.

AUTHOR CONTRIBUTIONS

All authors listed have made a substantial, direct and intellectual contribution to the work, and approved it for publication.

FUNDING

This work was supported by: Consejo Nacional de Investigaciones Científicas y Técnicas (CONICET to SC, RC, SR); Roemmers Foundation (to SC, SR); Agencia Nacional de Promoción Científica y Técnica (to RC, SC).

REFERENCES

1. Chappel SC, Ulloa-Aguirre A, Coutifaris C. Biosynthesis and secretion of follicle-stimulating hormone. *Endocr Rev.* (1983) 4:179–211. doi: 10.1210/edrv-4-2-179
2. Dahl KD, Stone MP. FSH isoforms, radioimmunoassays, bioassays, and their significance. *J Androl.* (1992) 13:11–22.
3. Ulloa-Aguirre A, Midgley AR Jr, Beitins IZ, Padmanabhan V. Follicle-stimulating isohormones: characterization and physiological relevance. *Endocr Rev.* (1995) 16:765–87. doi: 10.1210/edrv-16-6-765
4. Ulloa-Aguirre A, Timossi C, Damián-Matsumura P, Dias JA. Role of glycosylation in function of follicle-stimulating hormone. *Endocrine* (1999) 11:205–15. doi: 10.1385/ENDO:11:3:205
5. Ulloa-Aguirre A, Maldonado A, Damian-Matsumura P, Timossi C. Endocrine regulation of gonadotropin glycosylation. *Arch Med Res.* (2001) 32:520–32. doi: 10.1016/S0188-4409(01)00319-8
6. Wang H, May J, Butnev V, Shuai B, May JV, Bousfield GR, et al. Evaluation of *in vivo* bioactivities of recombinant hypo- (FSH(21/18)) and fully- (FSH(24)) glycosylated human FSH glycoforms in Fshb null mice. *Mol Cell Endocrinol.* (2016) 437:224–36. doi: 10.1016/j.mce.2016.08.031
7. Ulloa-Aguirre A, Timossi C, Barrios-de-Tomasi J, Maldonado A, Nayudu P. Impact of carbohydrate heterogeneity in function of follicle-stimulating hormone: studies derived from *in vitro* and *in vivo* models. *Biol Reprod.* (2003) 69:379–89. doi: 10.1095/biolreprod.103.016915
8. Bousfield GR, May JV, Davis JS, Dias JA, Kumar TR. *In vivo* and *in vitro* impact of carbohydrate variation on human follicle-stimulating hormone function. *Front Endocrinol.* (2018) 9:216. doi: 10.3389/fendo.2018.00216
9. Kornfeld R, Kornfeld S. Assembly of asparagine-linked oligosaccharides. *Annu Rev Biochem.* (1985) 54:631–64. doi: 10.1146/annurev.bi.54.070185.003215
10. Baenziger JU, Green ED. Pituitary glycoprotein hormone oligosaccharides: structure, synthesis and function of the asparagine-linked oligosaccharides on lutropin, follitropin and thyrotropin. *Biochim Biophys Acta* (1988) 947:287–306. doi: 10.1016/0304-4157(88)90012-3
11. Stanley P, Taniguchi, N, Aebi M. Chapter 9: N-Glycans. In: Varki A, Cummings RD, Esko JD, Stanley P, Hart GW, Aebi M, et al. editors. *Essentials of Glycobiology.* 3rd ed. Cold Spring Harbor, NY: Cold Spring Harbor Laboratory Press (2017). p. 2015–17. doi: 10.1101/glycobiology.3e.009
12. Parsons TF, Pierce JG. Oligosaccharide moieties of glycoprotein hormones: bovine lutropin resists enzymatic deglycosylation because of terminal O-sulfated N-acetylhexosamines. *Proc Natl Acad Sci USA.* (1980) 77:7089–93.
13. Dalpathado DS, Irungu J, Go EP, Butnev VY, Norton K, Bousfield GR, et al. Comparative glycomics of the glycoprotein follicle stimulating hormone: glycopeptide analysis of isolates from two mammalian species. *Biochemistry* (2006) 45:8665–73. doi: 10.1021/bi060435k
14. Bedecarras P, Gryngarten M, Ayuso S, Escobar ME, Bergada C, Campo S. Characterization of serum SHBG isoforms in prepubertal and pubertal girls. *Clin Endocrinol.* (1998) 49:603–8. doi: 10.1046/j.1365-2265.1998.00574.x
15. Ambao V, Rulli SB, Carino MH, Cónsole G, Ulloa-Aguirre A, Calandra RS, et al. Hormonal regulation of pituitary FSH sialylation in male rats. *Mol Cell Endocrinol.* (2009) 309:39–47. doi: 10.1016/j.mce.2009.05.002

16. Ulloa-Aguirre A, Damián-Matsumura P, Espinoza R, Dominguez R, Morales L, Flores A. Effects of neonatal androgenization on the chromatofocusing pattern of anterior pituitary FSH in the female rat. *J Endocrinol.* (1990) 126:323–32.
17. Creus S, Chaia Z, Pellizzari EH, Cigorraga SB, Ulloa-Aguirre A, Campo S. Human FSH isoforms: carbohydrate complexity as determinant of *in-vitro* bioactivity. *Mol Cell Endocrinol.* (2001) 174:41–9. doi: 10.1016/S0303-7207(00)00453-6
18. Wide L. Follicle-stimulating hormones in anterior pituitary glands from children and adults differ in relation to sex and age. *J Endocrinol.* (1989) 123:519–29. doi: 10.1677/joe.0.1230519
19. Wide L, Bakos O. More basic forms of both human follicle-stimulating hormone and luteinizing hormone in serum at midcycle compared with the follicular or luteal phase. *J Clin Endocrinol Metab.* (1993) 76:885–9.
20. Ogata S, Muramatsu T, Kobata A. Fractionation of glycopeptides by affinity column chromatography of Concanavalin-A Sepharose. *J Biochem.* (1975) 78:687–96. doi: 10.1093/oxfordjournals.jbchem.a130956
21. Narasimhan S, Wilson JR, Martin E, Schachter H. A structure basis for four distinct elution profiles on concanavalin A-sepharose affinity chromatography of glycopeptides. *Can J Biochem.* (1979) 57:83–96. doi: 10.1139/o79-011
22. Creus S, Pellizzari E, Cigorraga S, Campo S. Human FSH isoforms: bio and immunoactivity in post-menopausal and normal menstruating women. *Clin Endocrinol.* (1996) 44:181–9. doi: 10.1046/j.1365-2265.1996.646467.x
23. Mariño K, Bones J, Kattla JJ, Rudd PM. A systematic approach to protein glycosylation analysis: a path through the maze. *Nat Chem Biol.* (2010) 6:713–23. doi: 10.1038/nchembio.437
24. Bousfield GR, Butnev VY, White WK, Hall AS, Harvey DJ. Comparison of follicle-stimulating hormone glycosylation microheterogenity by quantitative negative mode nano-electrospray mass spectrometry of peptide-N glycanase-released oligosaccharides. *J Glycomics Lipidomics* (2015) 5:129. doi: 10.4172/2153-0637.1000129
25. Chappel SC. Heterogeneity of follicle stimulating hormone: control and physiological function. *Hum Reprod Update* (1995) 1:479–87.
26. Sairam MR, Manjunath P. Studies on pituitary follitropin. XI induction of hormonal antagonistic activity by chemical deglycosylation. *Mol Cell Endocrinol.* (1982) 28:139–50. doi: 10.1016/0303-7207(82)90027-2
27. Manjunath P, Sairam MR, Sairam J. Studies on pituitary follitropin. Biochemical, X, receptor binding and immunological properties of deglycosylated ovine hormone. *Mol Cell Endocrinol.* (1982) 28:125–38. doi: 10.1016/0303-7207(82)90026-0
28. Wide L, Hobson BM. Qualitative difference in follicle-stimulating hormone activity in the pituitaries of young women compared to that of men and elderly women. *J Clin Endocrinol Metab.* (1983) 56:371–5. doi: 10.1210/jcem-56-2-371
29. Padmanabhan V, Lang LL, Sonstein J, Kelch RP, Beitins IZ. Modulation of serum follicle-stimulating hormone bioactivity and isoform distribution by estrogenic steroids in normal women and in gonadal dysgenesis. *J Clin Endocrinol Metab.* (1988) 67:465–73. doi: 10.1210/jcem-67-3-465
30. Velasquez EV, Creus S, Trigo RV, Cigorraga SB, Pellizzari EH, Croxatto HB, et al. Pituitary-ovarian axis during lactational amenorrhoea. II longitudinal assessment of serum FSH polymorphism before and

after recovery of menstrual cycles. *Hum Reprod.* (2006) 21:916–23. doi: 10.1093/humrep/dei411

31. Loreti N, Ambao V, Juliato CT, Machado C, Bahamondes L, Campo S. Carbohydrate complexity and proportion of serum FSH isoforms reflect pituitary-ovarian activity in perimenopausal women and depot medroxyprogesterone acetate users. *Clin Endocrinol.* (2009) 71:558–65. doi: 10.1111/j.1365-2265.2009.03559.x

32. Zambrano E, Barrios-de-Tomasi J, Cárdenas M, Ulloa-Aguirre A. Studies on the relative *in-vitro* biological potency of the naturally-occurring isoforms of intrapituitary follicle stimulating hormone. *Mol Hum Reprod.* (1996) 2:563–71. doi: 10.1093/molehr/2.8.563

33. Barrios-de-Tomasi J, Nayudu PL, Brehm R, Heistermann M, Zarinan T, Ulloa-Aguirre A. Effects of human pituitary FSH isoforms on mouse follicles *in vitro*. *Reprod Biomed Online* (2006) 12:428–41. doi: 10.1016/S1472-6483(10)61995-5

34. Vitt UA, Kloosterboer HJ, Rose UM, Mulders JW, Kiesel PS, Bete S, et al. Isoforms of human recombinant follicle-stimulating hormone: comparison of effects on murine follicle development *in vitro*. *Biol Reprod.* (1998) 59:854–61. doi: 10.1095/biolreprod59.4.854

35. Loreti N, Ambao V, Andreone L, Trigo R, Bussmann U, Campo S. Effect of sialylation and complexity of FSH oligosaccharides on inhibin production by granulosa cells. *Reproduction* (2013) 145:127–35. doi: 10.1530/REP-12-0228

36. Loreti N, Fresno C, Barrera D, Andreone L, Albarran SL, Fernandez EA, et al. The glycan structure in recombinant human FSH affects endocrine activity and global gene expression in human granulosa cells. *Mol Cell Endocrinol.* (2013) 366:68–80. doi: 10.1016/j.mce.2012.11.021

37. Phillips DJ, Wide L. Serum gonadotropin isoforms become more basic after an exogenous challenge of gonadotropin-releasing hormone in children undergoing pubertal development. *J Clin Endocrinol Metab.* (1994) 79:814–9.

38. Damian-Matsumura P, Zaga V, Maldonado A, Sanchez-Hernandez C, Timossi C, Ulloa-Aguirre A. Oestrogens regulate pituitary alpha2,3-sialyltransferase messenger ribonucleic acid levels in the female rat. *J Mol Endocrinol.* (1999) 23:153–65. doi: 10.1677/jme.0.0230153

39. Zarifián T, Olivares A, Söderlund D, Méndez JP, Ulloa-Aguirre A. Changes in the biological:immunological ratio of basal and GnRH-releasable FSH during the follicular, pre-ovulatory and luteal phases of the human menstrual cycle. *Hum Reprod.* (2001) 16:1611–8. doi: 10.1093/humrep/16.8.1611

40. Simoni M, Weinbauer GF, Chandolia RK, Nieschlag E. Microheterogeneity of pituitary follicle-stimulating hormone in male rats: differential effects of the chronic androgen deprivation induced by castration or androgen blockade. *J Mol Endocrinol.* (1992) 92:175–82. doi: 10.1677/jme.0.0090175

41. Ulloa-Aguirre A, Mejia JJ, Dominguez R, Guevara-Aguirre J, Diaz-Sanchez V, Larrea F. Microheterogeneity of anterior pituitary FSH in the male rat: isoelectric focusing pattern throughout sexual maturation. *J Endocrinol.* (1986) 110:539–49. doi: 10.1677/joe.0.1100539

42. Padmanabhan V, Mieher CD, Borondy M, I'Anson H, Wood RI, Landefeld TD, et al. Circulating bioactive follicle-stimulating hormone and less acidic follicle-stimulating hormone isoforms increase during experimental induction of puberty in the female lamb. *Endocrinology* (1992) 131:213–20. doi: 10.1210/endo.131.1.1611999

43. Phillips DJ, Albertsson-Wikland K, Eriksson K, Wide L. Changes in the isoforms of luteinizing hormone and follicle-stimulating hormone during puberty in normal children. *J Clin Endocrinol Metab.* (1997) 82:3103–6. doi: 10.1210/jcem.82.9.4254

44. Rulli SB, Creus S, Pellizzari E, Cigorraga SB, Calandra RS, Campo S. Androgen regulation of immunological and biological activities of pituitary follicle-stimulating hormone isoforms in male rats. *Neuroendocrinology* (1999) 70:255–60. doi: 10.1159/000054484

45. Foulds LM, Robertson DM. Electrofocusing fractionation and characterization of pituitary follicle-stimulating hormone from male and female rats. *Mol Cell Endocrinol.* (1983) 31:117–30. doi: 10.1016/0303-7207(83)90035-7

46. Olivares A, Söderlund D, Castro-Fernández C, Zarifián T, Zambrano E, Méndez JP, et al. Basal and gonadotropin-releasing hormone-releasable serum follicle-stimulating hormone charge isoform distribution and *in vitro* biological-to-immunological ratio in male puberty. *Endocrine* (2004) 23:189–98. doi: 10.1385/ENDO:23:2-3:189

47. Campo S, Ambao V, Creus S, Gottlieb S, Fernandez Vera G, Benencia H, et al. Carbohydrate complexity and proportions of serum FSH isoforms in the male: lectin-based studies. *Mol Cell Endocrinol.* (2007) 260–2:197–204. doi: 10.1016/j.mce.2006.01.020

48. Wide L, Albertsson-Wikland K. Change in electrophoretic mobility of human follicle-stimulating hormone in serum after administration of gonadotropin-releasing hormone. *J Clin Endocrinol Metab.* (1990) 70:271–6. doi: 10.1210/jcem-70-1-271

49. Bogdanove EM, Campbell GT, Peckham WD. FSH pleomorphism in the rat–regulation by gonadal steroids. *Endocr Res Commun.* (1974) 1:87–99. doi: 10.1080/07435807409053818

50. Ulloa-Aguirre A, Chappel SC. Multiple species of follicle-stimulating hormone exist within the anterior pituitary gland of male golden hamsters. *J Endocrinol.* (1982) 95:257–66. doi: 10.1677/joe.0.0950257

51. Rulli SB, Creus S, Pellizzari E, Cigorraga SB, Calandra RS, Campo S. Immunological and biological activities of pituitary FSH isoforms in prepubertal male rats: effect of antiandrogens. *Neuroendocrinology* (1996) 63:514–21. doi: 10.1159/000127080

52. Morell AG, Gregoriadis G, Scheinberg IH, Hickman J, Ashwell G. The role of sialic acid in determining the survival of glycoproteins in the circulation. *J Biol Chem.* (1971) 246:1461–7.

53. Wide L. The regulation of metabolic clearance rate of human FSH in mice by variation of the molecular structure of the hormone. *Acta Endocrinol.* (1986) 112:336–44. doi: 10.1530/acta.0.1120336

54. Jiang X, Dias JA, He X. Structural biology of glycoprotein hormones and their receptors: insights to signaling. *Mol Cell Endocrinol.* (2014) 384:424–51. doi: 10.1016/j.mce.2013.08.021

55. Jiang X, Fischer D, Chen X, McKenna SD, Liu H, Sriraman V, et al. Evidence for follicle-stimulating hormone receptor as a functional trimer. *J Biol Chem.* (2014) 289:14273–82. doi: 10.1074/jbc.M114.549592

56. Meher BR, Dixit A, Bousfield GR, Lushington GH. Glycosylation effects on FSH-FSHR interaction dynamics: a case study of different FSH glycoforms by molecular dynamics simulations. *PLoS ONE* (2015) 10:e0137897. doi: 10.1371/journal.pone.0137897

57. Ulloa-Aguirre A, Zarifián T. The follitropin receptor: matching structure and function. *Mol Pharmacol.* (2016) 90:596–608. doi: 10.1124/mol.116.104398

58. Itman C, Mendis S, Barakat B, Loveland K. All in the family: TGF-beta family action in testis development. *Reproduction* (2006) 132:233–46. doi: 10.1530/rep.1.01075

59. Barakat B, Itman C, Mendis SH, Loveland KL. Activins and inhibins in mammalian testis development: new models, new insights. *Mol Cell Endocrinol.* (2012) 359:66–77. doi: 10.1016/j.mce.2012.02.018

60. Dorrington JH, Fritz IB, Armstrong DT. Control of testicular estrogen synthesis. *Biol Reprod.* (1978) 8:55–64. doi: 10.1095/biolreprod18.1.55

61. Rommerts FF, de Jong FH, Brinkmann AO, van der Molen HJ. Development and cellular localization of rat testicular aromatase activity. *J Reprod Fertil.* (1982) 65:281–8. doi: 10.1530/jrf.0.0650281

62. Le Magueresse B, Jégou B. *In vitro* effects of germ cells on the secretory activity of Sertoli cells recovered from rats of different ages. *Endocrinology* (1988) 122:1672–80. doi: 10.1210/endo-122-4-1672

63. Anawalt BD, Bebb RA, Matsumoto AM, Groome NP, Illingworth PJ, McNeilly AS, et al. Serum inhibin B levels reflect Sertoli cell function in normal men and men with testicular dysfunction. *J Clin Endocrinol Metab.* (1996) 81:3341–5.

64. Crofton PM, Illingworth PJ, Groome NP, Stirling HF, Swanston I, Gow S, et al. Changes in dimeric inhibin A and B during normal early puberty in boys and girls. *Clin Endocrinol.* (1997) 46:109–14. doi: 10.1046/j.1365-2265.1997.d01-1744.x

65. Byrd W, Bennett MJ, Carr BR, Dong Y, Wians F, Rainey W. Regulation of biologically active dimeric inhibin A and B from infancy to adulthood in the male. *J Clin Endocrinol Metab.* (1998) 83:2849–54. doi: 10.1210/jcem.83.8.5008

66. Bergada I, Rojas G, Ropelato G, Ayuso S, Bergada C, Campo S. Sexual dimorphism in circulating monomeric and dimeric inhibins in normal boys and girls from birth to puberty. *Clin Endocrinol.* (1999) 51:455–60. doi: 10.1046/j.1365-2265.1999.00814.x

67. de Kretser DM, Hedger MP, Loveland KL, Phillips DJ. Inhibins, activins and follistatin in reproduction. *Hum Reprod Update* (2002) 8:529–41. doi: 10.1093/humupd/8.6.529

68. de Kretser DM, Buzzard JJ, Okuma Y, O'Connor AE, Hayashi T, Lin SY, et al. The role of activin, follistatin and inhibin in testicular physiology. *Mol Cell Endocrinol.* (2004) 225:57–64. doi: 10.1016/j.mce.2004.07.008

69. Andersson AM, Toppari J, Haavisto AM, Petersen JH, Simell T, Simell O, et al. Longitudinal reproductive hormone profiles in infants: peak of inhibin B levels in infant boys exceeds levels in adult men. *J Clin Endocrinol Metab.* (1998) 83:675–81. doi: 10.1210/jc.83.2.675

70. Andreone L, Ambao V, Pellizzari EH, Loreti N, Cigorraga SB, Campo S. Role of FSH glycan structure in the regulation of Sertoli cell inhibin production. *Reproduction* (2017) 154:711–21. doi: 10.1530/REP-17-0393

71. Al-Attar L, Noël K, Dutertre M, Belville C, Forest MG, Burgoyne PS, et al. Hormonal and cellular regulation of Sertoli cell anti-Müllerian hormone production in the postnatal mouse. *J Clin Invest.* (1997) 100:1335–43. doi: 10.1172/JCI119653

72. Bougnères P, François M, Pantalone L, Rodrigue D, Bouvattier C, Demesteere E, et al. Effects of an early postnatal treatment of hypogonadotropic hypogonadism with a continuous subcutaneous infusion of recombinant follicle-stimulating hormone and luteinizing hormone. *J Clin Endocrinol Metab.* (2008) 93:2202–5. doi: 10.1210/jc.2008-0121

73. Young J, Chanson P, Salenave S, Noël M, Brailly S, O'Flaherty M, et al. Testicular anti-mullerian hormone secretion is stimulated by recombinant human FSH in patients with congenital hypogonadotropic hypogonadism. *J Clin Endocrinol Metab.* (2005) 90:724–8. doi: 10.1210/jc.2004-0542

74. Lukas-Croisier C, Lasala C, Nicaud J, Bedecarrás P, Kumar TR, Dutertre M, et al. Follicle-stimulating hormone increases testicular Anti-Mullerian hormone (AMH) production through Sertoli cell proliferation and a nonclassical cyclic adenosine 5'-monophosphate-mediated activation of the AMH Gene. *Mol Endocrinol.* (2003) 17:550–61. doi: 10.1210/me.2002-0186

7

Pharmacogenetics of FSH Action in the Female

Alessandro Conforti[1]*, Alberto Vaiarelli[2], Danilo Cimadomo[2], Francesca Bagnulo[1],
Stefania Peluso[1], Luigi Carbone[1], Francesca Di Rella[3], Giuseppe De Placido[1],
Filippo Maria Ubaldi[2], Ilpo Huhtaniemi[4] and Carlo Alviggi[1,5]

[1] Department of Neuroscience, Reproductive Science and Odontostomatology, University of Naples Federico II, Naples, Italy,
[2] G.E.N.E.R.A. Centre for Reproductive Medicine, Clinica Valle Giulia, Rome, Italy, [3] Medical Oncology, Department of
Senology, National Cancer Institute, IRCCS Fondazione G. Pascale, Naples, Italy, [4] Department of Surgery and Cancer,
Institute of Reproductive and Developmental Biology, Imperial College London, London, United Kingdom, [5] Istituto per
l'Endocrinologia e l'Oncologia Sperimentale (IEOS) Consiglio Nazionale delle Ricerche, Naples, Italy

*Correspondence:
Alessandro Conforti
confale@hotmail.it

The purpose of a pharmacogenomic approach is to tailor treatment on the basis of an individual human genotype. This strategy is becoming increasingly common in medicine, and important results have been obtained in oncologic and antimicrobial therapies. The rapid technological developments and availability of innovative methodologies have revealed the existence of numerous genotypes that can influence the action of medications and give rise to the idea that a true "individualized" approach could become in the future a reality in clinical practice. Moreover, compared to the past, genotype analyses are now more easily available at accessible cost. Concerning human reproduction, there is ample evidence that several variants of gonadotropins and their receptors influence female reproductive health and ovarian response to exogenous gonadotropins. In more detail, variants in genes of *follicle-stimulating hormone β-chain* (FSH-B) and its *receptor* (FSH-R) seem to be the most promising candidates for a pharmacogenomic approach to controlled ovarian stimulation in assisted reproductive technologies. In the present review, we summarize the evidence regarding FSH-B and FSH-R variants, with special reference to their impact on reproductive health and assisted reproductive technology treatments.

Keywords: FSH, FSH receptor, polymorphisms, mutations, ovarian stimulation, assisted reproductive technology, IVF, genetic variants

INTRODUCTION

Follicle-stimulating hormone (FSH) is a pituitary gonadotropic hormone, which is fundamental for follicle growth in females and spermatogenesis in males. FSH is an heterodimeric molecule belonging to the glycoprotein hormone family. It consists of the common α-subunit shares as with other glycoprotein hormones (LH, hCG, TSH) and the hormone specific β subunit. FSH, when in the ovary and testis, binds to its cognate receptor (FSH-R), which belongs to the superfamily of the G-protein coupled receptors. It is characterized by a long ligand-binding extracellular domain, seven transmembrane domains, mediating the hormonal stimulus, and an intracellular C-terminal domain participating in receptor internalization and desensitization of the signal. Through the interaction with its receptor, FSH activated several intracellular signaling pathways, the most important of them being adenylyl cyclase and β-arrestins (1, 2).

It has recently been demonstrated that FSH exerts its action outside the reproductive tract, including in the placenta, hepatocytes and tumor blood vessels (3, 4). In addition, FSH was demonstrated to be involved in the pathogenesis of endometriotic lesions (5). Focusing on the female reproductive tract, it was also recently demonstrated that FSH could exert its effect on the endometrial glands. In detail, FSH-R was able to increase in these cells intracellular levels of cAMP, leading to induction of steroidogenesis (6). During the menstrual cycle, FSH has several important actions. Firstly, it promotes folliculogenesis by stimulating estradiol production by the aromatase enzyme system, stimulating granulosa cell growth and inducing the expression of luteinizing hormone receptors (1). Together with LH, FSH levels peak in the mid-cycle which induces important actions in the ovulation process, such as the stimulation of proteolytic enzymes essential for follicular wall rupture (7). Finally, in the early follicular phase FSH is involved in the recruitment of new antral follicles for the next cycle of folliculogenesis (8). On the basis of differences in the terminal sialic acid residues in the carbohydrate moieties that are attached to the FSH protein, numerous isoforms of FSH have been identified (9). Acidic isoforms seems to be involved in follicular recruitment at the end of menstrual cycles, while follicle selection and rupture seem to be promoted by basic FSH isoforms (9). Given its biological importance in folliculogenesis, pharmaceutical FSH products are currently adapted for multiple follicular growth in assisted reproductive technology (ART) (10). The ovarian activity, as well as the ovarian response to exogenous gonadotropin appear to be influenced by specific genetic traits involving gonadotropins and their receptors (11–14) (**Table 1**). In the present review, we will summarize the most important evidence concerning variants of FSH and FSH-R and their implication in female reproductive functions.

METHODS

A systematic search was carried out using MEDLINE (Pubmed) AND Scopus databases with no restriction of language or time period. The search strategy consisted in the use of the combinations of the following keywords: "controlled ovarian stimulation," "ART," "IVF," "ICSI," "FIVET," "IUI," "intrauterine insemination," "ovulation induction," "ovarian stimulation," "polymorphism," "SNV," "Single nucleotide variant," "FSH Receptor," "FSHR," "FSH," "follicle-stimulating hormone," "follicle-stimulating hormone," and "beta subunit."

In view of the recent meta-analysis published by our group (15) we updated our research adding also more recent papers in the present review (29–32).

As recommended by Human Genome Variation Society (33) every single nucleotide variants (SNV) illustrated in the present paper was reported indicating Locus Reference Genomic sequence (LRG) and RefSeqGene or transcript (**Table 1**).

Genetic Variants of FSH Beta Subunit

In contrast to LH beta subunit, FSH-B appears to be highly conserved (34). Indeed, few variants of the gene encoding for FSH-B subunit have been identified so far. The first variant

was identified in 1993 in a women with primary amenorrhea, sexual infantilism and infertility (35, 36). This variant consisted in a two-nucleotide deletion in codon 61 that gave rise to premature stop codon. Thereafter, several other inactivating variants have been identified. Most of them induce an alteration of the cysteine knot structure of FSH which is crucial for its biological activity (34). Thus, the majority of variants inactivating FSH-B are characterized by the absence of puberty, infertility and the absence of breast maturation and few of them show partial puberty development (34, 37).

Considering the conserved structure of FSH, very few clinically significant variants have been identified. Among the 24 SNVs identified (18) only the one located in FSH-B chain promoter (*C.-221G>T, RS10835638*) seems to have significant clinical impact on male and female reproduction (38, 39). In the first report by Grigorova et al. T homozygous men showed lower FSH levels and reduced testicular volume than other haplotypes (38). Conversely, in 365 women with normal menses the T homozygotes showed elevated FSH and LH levels with reduced progesterone production (39). In another study, the T allele resulted in longer menstrual cycles [0.16 Standard differences; 95% confidence interval (CI) 0.12–0.20; $P < 0.05$], in delayed age at menopause (0.13 years; 95% CI 0.04–0.22; $P < 0.05$), and greater female nulliparity [odds ratio (OR) = 1.06; 95% CI 1.02–1.11; $P < 0.05$] (26). Interestingly, the same study showed lower risk of endometriosis among T carriers compared with other haplotypes [OR = 0.79; 95% CI 0.69–0.90; $P < 0.05$]. In another study, involving 193 infertile eumenorrheic women, a statistically significant reduction of FSH on cycle day 3 was observed in carriers with the combination of FSH-B *(C-211 G>T, RS10835638)* GT + TT/FSH-R *(C.2039 G>A, RS6166)* AA genotype, compared with the FSH-B GG/FSH-R GG genotype (27). More recently, it was confirmed that the T allele carriers were associated with higher FSH and LH levels and idiopathic infertility (40). The T allele of FSH-B *C-211 G>T, RS10835638* appears to decrease transcriptional activity of the gene (28). Very recently, Trevisan et al. observed in a cross-sectional study involving 140 infertile women (median age 33 years), that women carrying GT genotype ($n = 38$) had a lower response to ovarian stimulation compared to GG (wild type) genotype ($n = 102$) with of number of oocytes retrieved (3.0 vs. 5.0, $p = 0.03$) and a lower number of embryos at the end of stimulation (2 vs. 3, $p = 0.02$) (29).

There is also evidence which suggests that another variant of FSH-B subunit *(C.228 C>T, RS6169)* might be implicated in the development polycystic ovarian syndrome (24, 25). A retrospective analysis of 135 Chinese women between 19 and 38 years of age affected by PCOS with 105 as a normal control, a higher prevalence of homozygous carrier was observed in PCOS than in the control group (12.6 vs. 3.8%) (25). Furthermore, the frequency of this variant was more pronounced in a specific subgroup of PCOS women, namely those with obesity (0.50 and 31.0%, respectively) and hyperandrogenism. These findings support the concept that hyperandrogenic PCOS women could show peculiar characteristics and probably display specific pathogenetic mechanisms (41). In a recent prospective trials involving 30 normogonadotropic women, we did not observe

TABLE 1 | Clinical manifestations and pathogenetic effects of FSH-R and FSH-B subunit most common variants (https://www.ncbi.nlm.nih.gov/snp).

Polymorphisms (reference SNP)	RefSeqGene	Locus reference genomic sequence (LRG)	Variant	Pathogenetic effect	Clinical manifestations	References
FSH-R RS1394205 (likely pathogenic)	NG_008146.1:g.5046 G>A	LRG_536	A	Reduced transcription activity; Reduced protein levels	Higher consumption of gonadotropin during controlled ovarian stimulation; Reduced number of oocytes retrieved	(15) (16) (3) (17)
FSH-R RS6166 (likely pathogenic)	NG_008146.1:g.196710 G>A	LRG_536	G	Impaired ligand sensitivity	Reduced number of oocytes retrieved Higher consumption of gonadotropin during controlled ovarian stimulation	(15) (18) (19) (20) (21)
FSH-R RS6165 (likely pathogenic)	NG_008146.1:g.195590 G>A	LRG_536	G	Impaired ligand sensitivity	Reduced number of oocytes retrieved Higher consumption of gonadotropin during controlled ovarian stimulation Lower number of embryos	(15) (22) (23)
FSH-B RS6169 (uncertain significance)	NG_008144.1:g.7623 C>T	Not available	C	Unknown	Polycystic ovarian syndrome development No effect detected during controlled ovarian stimulation	(24) (13) (25)
FSH-B RS10835638 (likely pathogenic)	NG_008144.1:g.4790 G>T	Not available	T	Decreased transcriptional activity	Reduced FSH basal levels Longer menstrual cycles Delayed menopause	(26) (27) (28)

differences in terms of ovarian response or pregnancy rate when comparing different haplotypes of this variant (13). Despite the low number of patients recruited, our study did not support any implications in terms of ovarian response to exogenous gonadotropin and ART success.

Genetic Variants of FSH Receptor

Several inactivating and activating variants of FSH-R have been identified (42). The majority of the inactivating variants are located on exons 7 and 10 (42). The most typical clinical manifestations are primary amenorrhea, elevated FSH levels, and infertility. Specific inactivating variants were also associated with polycystic ovarian syndrome (43). Also, the majority of activating variants are located in exon 10. The most common clinical manifestation is a spontaneous occurrence of ovarian hyperstimulation syndrome. In general, while activating variants in the FSH-R gene can manifest in heterozygotes, the inactivating variants alter the phenotype only when present in the homozygous or compound heterozygous form Desai et al. (42).

The FSH-R gene carries more than 2000 single nucleotide variants (SNVs) (18). Among them the most widely studied common variants which apparently impact on female reproduction are: -29 G>A. (RS1394205); C.919G>A (RS6165); C.2039G>A (RS6166). Two FSH-R variants with SNVs in the coding region have been identified and well-characterized (44). The SNV known as the Serine680 variant causes the replacement of asparagine (Asn) for serine (Ser) at the 680 position, which is located in the intracellular domain of the FSH-R protein. The RS6165 SNV replaces threonine (Thr) by alanine (Ala). Except in some African populations, the two SNVs are in linkage disequilibrium (19); this means that carriers who possess Thr307 nearly always have Asn680 present on the same allele and carriers who have Ala307 have Ser680

on the same allele (45). The former (RS6166) introduces a potential phosphorylation site and the latter (RS6165) results in a change from a polar to a non-polar hydrophobic amino acid, thereby removing a potential O-linked glycosylation site (19). In vitro studies conducted using human granulosa cells showed that GG carriers of the FSH-R (RS6166) genotype have greater resistance to FSH than do AA carriers (18, 46) and are characterized by slower kinetics of cAMP production, ERK1/2, and CREB phosphorylation (47). Despite the linkage disequilibrium between these two SNVs, several studies suggest that these two variants could influence ovarian stimulation (OS) outcome in different ways. In detail, Achrekar et al. observed that only the FSH-R RS6165 variant could significantly impact the total FSH consumption during OS (3). Discrepancies between FSH-R (RS6166) and FSH-R (RS6166) were also reported by Trevisan et al. in a cross-sectional study involving 149 infertile women, in which a difference in terms of the number of embryos produced was observed only among different FSH-R (RS6165) haplotype (23).

Our findings in a recent systematic review corroborate these previous observations. Indeed, we found that GG FSH-R (RS6166) carriers had higher ovarian resistance to exogenous gonadotropin and, consequently, had fewer oocytes compared with AA carriers (15). These findings were also confirmed in a more recent study (31). In addition, higher FSH basal levels and resistance to clomiphene citrate were observed in G allele carriers, supporting an higher receptorial resistance even to endogenous level of FSH (15, 27, 48, 49). Conversely, A allele carriers show an higher FSH sensitivity as confirmed in a recent retrospective study of 586 infertile women undergoing their first IVF cycle, where an increased risk for developing OHSS syndrome (OR 1.7 95% CI 1.025–2.839, $p = 0.04$) was observed in carriers of this allele (30).

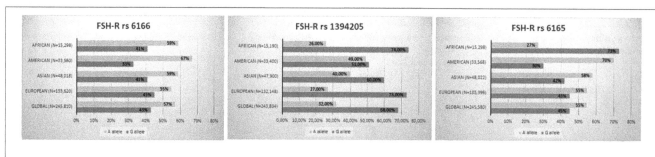

FIGURE 1 | FSH-R variants worldwide distribution (*RS6166; RS1394205; RS6165*) (The Genome Aggregation Database—https://www.ncbi.nlm.nih.gov/snp/).

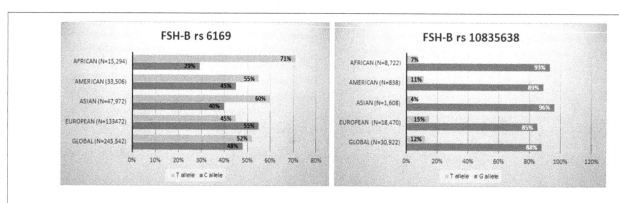

FIGURE 2 | FSH-B subunit variants worldwide distribution (*RS6169; RS10835638*) (The Genome Aggregation Database—https://www.ncbi.nlm.nih.gov/snp/).

The finding of Borgbo et al. that the FSH-R *RS6166* and FSH-R *RS6165* GG carriers had higher *LHCGR* gene expression but lower *Anti-Müllerian hormone receptor-2* expression vs. carriers of the other haplotypes, suggested that these variants could affect the protein expression of human antral follicles (50). Nonetheless, it remains to be established whether FSH-R *RS6166* and *RS6165* influence expression of the FSH-R protein.

The FSH-R−29 G>A (RS1394205) variant is located in the 5′-untranslated region of the gene and is able to influence ovarian response. *In vitro* studies showed that A allele presence is characterized by reduced mRNA transcriptional activity and reduced FSH-R protein level (46, 47).

In ART context, Achrekar et al. reported with homozygous variant genotype AA lower number of oocytes and lower pregnancy rate compared with GG genotype in women who underwent OS (22). This observation was confirmed in a further larger study by Desai et al. involving 100 women (16) where those with the AA genotype at position−29 were at higher risk for poor ovarian response in comparison to the other haplotypes (OR 8.63, 95% CI 1.84–45.79; $P = 0.001$). In contrast, other authors did not confirm significant effects of this variant concerning the ovarian response (31, 32, 51). The evidence regarding the clinical effect of the *FSH-R−29 G>A* (RS1394205) variant on OS was summarized in a recent meta-analysis, which showed that higher exogenous FSH consumption is required in homozygotes for the A allele than carriers of the G allele (15).

Is There Need for a Pharmacogenomic Approach in ART?

Demographic and anthropometric characteristics of women and the ovarian reserve tests do not fully explain the ovarian response to exogenous gonadotropin (52, 53). Indeed, there is a subgroup of women that, despite showing normal ovarian reserve in terms of functional and biochemical markers, have an "unexpected" impaired prognosis to ART and poor or suboptimal number of oocytes at the end of stimulation (54). This ovarian resistance to exogenous gonadotropin is also called "hypo-response," and it was recently included in the new POSEIDON classification of low prognosis patients in ART (55–58).

The fact that several variants could in some way affect the ovarian response to OS opens up the way to a pharmacogenomic approach to ART and might partially explain the hypo-response phenomenon (13, 59). The pharmacogenomic approach is spreading more and more to several fields, and it could provide the explanations for adverse or poor drug effects (60). In the ART scenario, a pharmacogenomic approach to OS could optimize ART treatments, thereby reducing both poor response rates and potentially life-threatening excessive ovarian responses (53). However, although more than 30 studies have already been published, no large randomized clinical trials on this topic have been conducted, indicating that the pharmacogenomic approach to OS is still a largely neglected topic. In addition, it should be underlined that variants, especially those involving FSH receptors are very common in general population (19, 61–63)

(**Figures 1, 2**). Furthermore, the genotype analysis can now be provided at low cost (15). So far, few studies have adopted a pharmacogenomic approach to ART with the FSH-R variant rs6166 being the one most often investigated (2, 20). The first one was conducted by Behre et al. (21). In detail, women undergoing controlled ovarian hyperstimulation for ART, homozygous for the wild-type or for the FSH-R SNV(*C.2039G>A [RS6166]*), were randomly assigned to group I (GG carriers, $n = 24$), receiving an FSH daily dose of 150 U/day, or group II (GG carries, $n = 25$), receiving an FSH dose of 225 U/day. Age- and body mass index-matched AA carriers, receiving a daily dose of 150 IU, served as control group. The wild-type group (AA carriers) had higher estradiol production after treatment with 150 IU/day of FSH compared with the GG carriers who received the same dose. The increment of dosage for 150–225 IU/day was able to compensate for this discrepancy. This finding was confirmed by those reported by Genro et al. (64). The authors showed that the follicle development during OS was not significantly influenced by the presence of *FSH-R RS6166/RS6165* when a high FSH dose (300 IU per day) was administrated during OS (64). These results suggested that increasing FSH dosage during OS could mitigate the negative effect exerted by the FSH-R variant on the ovarian response. Finally, a recent meta-analysis including 4,425 observation concluded that GG allele carriers produced a significantly lower number of oocytes compared with AA (Random Weight Mean Difference: 0.84, 95% CI: 0.19–1.49, $P = 0.01$, $P = 0.03$) and AG carriers (Random Weight Mean Difference: 0.88, 95% CI: 0.12–1.63, $P = 0.02$)

(15). Furthermore, gonadotropin type seems to influence the number of oocytes collected in relation to the FSH-R (*RS6166*) genotype distribution. As a matter of fact, the number of oocytes retrieved was significantly higher in AA carriers than in GG carriers when recombinant FSH was used, but not when urinary FSH formulations with LH activity were used (15). Although this finding suggests that the addition of LH in OS (65–67) could also mitigate the effects of FSH-R *RS6166* variants more data are needed on this issue.

CONCLUSION

In conclusion, increasing evidence indicates that a pharmacogenomic approach to ovarian stimulation could become a clinical reality in the future. So far, specific variants of FSH-B and FSH-R represent promising genetic markers to better standardize controlled ovarian stimulation in women undergoing ART.

AUTHOR CONTRIBUTIONS

AC and CA idealized the paper and wrote the first draft. All authors participated in literature research and paper editing. The senior authors IH and GD supervised the paper and participate in the elaboration of the final version. All authors listed have made intellectual contribution to the work and approved the final version.

REFERENCES

1. Yong EL, Baird DT, Hillier SG. Mediation of gonadotrophin-stimulated growth and differentiation of human granulosa cells by adenosine-3′,5′-monophosphate: one molecule, two messages. *Clin Endocrinol.* (1992) 37:51–8. doi: 10.1111/j.1365-2265.1992.tb02283.x
2. Simoni M, Gromoll J, Nieschlag E. The follicle-stimulating hormone receptor: biochemistry, molecular biology, physiology, and pathophysiology. *Endocr Rev.* (1997) 18:739–73. doi: 10.1210/er.18.6.739
3. Achrekar SK, Modi DN, Desai SK, Mangoli VS, Mangoli RV, Mahale SD. Follicle-stimulating hormone receptor polymorphism (Thr307Ala) is associated with variable ovarian response and ovarian hyperstimulation syndrome in Indian women. *Fertil Steril.* (2009) 91:432–9. doi: 10.1016/j.fertnstert.2007.11.093
4. Radu A, Pichon C, Camparo P, Antoine M, Allory Y, Couvelard A, et al. Expression of follicle-stimulating hormone receptor in tumor blood vessels. *N Engl J Med.* (2010) 363:1621–30. doi: 10.1056/NEJMoa1001283
5. Ponikwicka-Tyszko D, Chrusciel M, Stelmaszewska J, Bernaczyk P, Sztachelska M, Sidorkiewicz I, et al. Functional expression of FSH receptor in endometriotic lesions. *J Clin Endocrinol Metab.* (2016) 101:2905–14. doi: 10.1210/jc.2016-1014
6. Sacchi S, Sena P, Degli Esposti C, Lui J, La Marca A. Evidence for expression and functionality of FSH and LH/hCG receptors in human endometrium. *J Assist Reprod Genet.* (2018) 35:1703–12. doi: 10.1007/s10815-018-1248-8
7. Yoshimura Y, Santulli R, Atlas SJ, Fujii S, Wallach EE. The effects of proteolytic enzymes on *in vitro* ovulation in the rabbit. *Am J Obstet Gynecol.* (1987) 157:468–75. doi: 10.1016/S0002-9378(87)80197-7
8. Roseff SJ, Bangah ML, Kettel LM, Vale W, Rivier J, Burger HG, et al. Dynamic changes in circulating inhibin levels during the luteal-follicular transition of the human menstrual cycle. *J Clin Endocrinol Metab.* (1989) 69:1033–9. doi: 10.1210/jcem-69-5-1033

9. Palermo R. Differential actions of FSH and LH during folliculogenesis. *Reprod Biomed Online.* (2007) 15:326–37. doi: 10.1016/S1472-6483(10)60347-1
10. Leao RB, Esteves SC. Gonadotropin therapy in assisted reproduction: an evolutionary perspective from biologics to biotech. *Clinics.* (2014) 69:279–93. doi: 10.6061/clinics/2014(04)10
11. Alviggi C, Conforti A, Caprio F, Gizzo S, Noventa M, Strina I, et al. In estimated good prognosis patients could unexpected "hyporesponse" to controlled ovarian stimulation be related to genetic polymorphisms of FSH receptor? *Reprod Sci.* (2016) 23:1103–8. doi: 10.1177/1933719116630419
12. Altmae S, Hovatta O, Stavreus-Evers A, Salumets A. Genetic predictors of controlled ovarian hyperstimulation: where do we stand today? *Hum Reprod Update.* (2011) 17:813–28. doi: 10.1093/humupd/dmr034
13. Conforti A, Alfano S, De Rosa P, Alviggi C, De Placido G. The role of gonadotropin polymorphisms and their receptors in assisted reproductive technologies and controlled ovarian stimulation: a prospective observational study. *Italian J Gynaecol Obstetr.* (2017) 29:15–21. doi: 10.14660/2385-0868-67
14. Alviggi C, Clarizia R, Pettersson K, Mollo A, Humaidan P, Strina I, et al. Suboptimal response to GnRHa long protocol is associated with a common LH polymorphism. *Reprod Biomed Online.* (2011) 22(Suppl. 1):S67–72. doi: 10.1016/S1472-6483(11)60011-4
15. Alviggi C, Conforti A, Santi D, Esteves SC, Andersen CY, Humaidan P, et al. Clinical relevance of genetic variants of gonadotrophins and their receptors in controlled ovarian stimulation: a systematic review and meta-analysis. *Hum Reprod Update.* (2018) 24:599–614. doi: 10.1093/humupd/dmy019
16. Desai SS, Achrekar SK, Pathak BR, Desai SK, Mangoli VS, Mangoli RV, et al. Follicle-stimulating hormone receptor polymorphism (G-29A) is associated with altered level of receptor expression in Granulosa cells. *J Clin Endocrinol Metab.* (2011) 96:2805–12. doi: 10.1210/jc.2011-1064
17. Nakayama T, Kuroi N, Sano M, Tabara Y, Katsuya T, Ogihara T, et al. Mutation of the follicle-stimulating hormone receptor gene 5′-untranslated

region associated with female hypertension. *Hypertension*. (2006) 48:512–8. doi: 10.1161/01.HYP.0000233877.84343.d7

18. Casarini L, Santi D, Marino M. Impact of gene polymorphisms of gonadotropins and their receptors on human reproductive success. *Reproduction*. (2015) 150:R175–84. doi: 10.1530/REP-15-0251

19. Simoni M, Casarini L. Mechanisms in endocrinology: genetics of FSH action: a 2014-and-beyond view. *Eur J Endocrinol*. (2014) 170:R91–107. doi: 10.1530/EJE-13-0624

20. Perez Mayorga M, Gromoll J, Behre HM, Gassner C, Nieschlag E, Simoni M. Ovarian response to follicle-stimulating hormone (FSH) stimulation depends on the FSH receptor genotype. *J Clin Endocrinol Metab*. (2000) 85:3365–9. doi: 10.1210/jc.85.9.3365

21. Behre HM, Greb RR, Mempel A, Sonntag B, Kiesel L, Kaltwaßer P, et al. Significance of a common single nucleotide polymorphism in exon 10 of the follicle-stimulating hormone (FSH) receptor gene for the ovarian response to FSH: A pharmacogenetic approach to controlled ovarian hyperstimulation. *Pharmacogenet Genomics*. (2005) 15:451–6. doi: 10.1097/01.fpc.0000167330.92786.5e

22. Achrekar SK, Modi DN, Desai SK, Mangoli VS, Mangoli RV, Mahale SD. Poor ovarian response to gonadotrophin stimulation is associated with FSH receptor polymorphism. *Reprod Biomed Online*. (2009) 18:509–15. doi: 10.1016/S1472-6483(10)60127-7

23. Trevisan CM, Peluso C, Cordts EB, de Oliveira R, Christofolini DM, Barbosa CP, et al. Ala307Thr and Asn680Ser polymorphisms of FSHR gene in human reproduction outcomes. *Cell Physiol Biochem*. (2014) 34:1527–35. doi: 10.1159/000366356

24. Simoni M, Tempfer CB, Destenaves B, Fauser BC. Functional genetic polymorphisms and female reproductive disorders: part I: polycystic ovary syndrome and ovarian response. *Hum Reprod Update*. (2008) 14:459–84. doi: 10.1093/humupd/dmn024

25. Tong Y, Liao WX, Roy AC, Ng SC. Association of AccI polymorphism in the follicle-stimulating hormone beta gene with polycystic ovary syndrome. *Fertil Steril*. (2000) 74:1233–6. doi: 10.1016/S0015-0282(00)01616-2

26. Ruth KS, Beaumont RN, Tyrrell J, Jones SE, Tuke MA, Yaghootkar H, et al. Genetic evidence that lower circulating FSH levels lengthen menstrual cycle, increase age at menopause and impact female reproductive health. *Hum Reprod*. (2016) 31:473–81. doi: 10.1093/humrep/dev318

27. La Marca A, Papaleo E, Alviggi C, Ruvolo G, De Placido G, Candiani M, et al. The combination of genetic variants of the FSHB and FSHR genes affects serum FSH in women of reproductive age. *Hum Reprod*. (2013) 28:1369–74. doi: 10.1093/humrep/det061

28. Hoogendoorn B, Coleman SL, Guy CA, Smith K, Bowen T, Buckland PR, et al. Functional analysis of human promoter polymorphisms. *Hum Mol Genet*. (2003) 12:2249–54. doi: 10.1093/hmg/ddg246

29. Trevisan CM, de Oliveira R, Christofolini DM, Barbosa CP, Bianco B. Effects of a polymorphism in the promoter region of the follicle-stimulating hormone subunit beta (FSHB) gene on female reproductive outcomes. *Genet Test Mol Biomarkers*. (2019) 23:39–44. doi: 10.1089/gtmb.2018.0182

30. Nenonen HA, Lindgren IA, Prahl AS, Trzybulska D, Kharraziha I, Hulten M, et al. The N680S variant in the follicle-stimulating hormone receptor gene identifies hyperresponders to controlled ovarian stimulation. *Pharmacogenet Genomics*. (2019) 29:114–120. doi: 10.1097/FPC.0000000000000374

31. Garcia-Jimenez G, Zarinan T, Rodriguez-Valentin R, Mejia-Dominguez NR, Gutierrez-Sagal R, Hernandez-Montes G, et al. Frequency of the T307A, N680S, and −29G>A single-nucleotide polymorphisms in the follicle-stimulating hormone receptor in Mexican subjects of Hispanic ancestry. *Reprod Biol Endocrinol*. (2018) 16:100. doi: 10.1186/s12958-018-0420-4

32. Zamaniara T, Taheripanah R, Ghaderian SMH, Zamaniara E, Aghabozorgi SSA. Polymorphism FSHR (-29G/A) as a genetic agent together with ESRI (XbaIG/A) in women with poor response to controlled ovarian hyperstimulation. *Hum Antibodies*. (2017) 26:143–7. doi: 10.3233/HAB-180332

33. den Dunnen JT, Dalgleish R, Maglott DR, Hart RK, Greenblatt MS, McGowan-Jordan J, et al. HGVS recommendations for the description of sequence variants: 2016 update. *Hum Mutat*. (2016) 37:564–9. doi: 10.1002/humu.22981

34. Huhtaniemi IT, Themmen AP. Mutations in human gonadotropin and gonadotropin-receptor genes. *Endocrine*. (2005) 26:207–17. doi: 10.1385/ENDO:26:3:207

35. Matthews CH, Borgato S, Beck-Peccoz P, Adams M, Tone Y, Gambino G, et al. Primary amenorrhoea and infertility due to a mutation in the beta-subunit of follicle-stimulating hormone. *Nat Genet*. (1993) 5:83–6. doi: 10.1038/ng0993-83

36. Phillip M, Arbelle JE, Segev Y, Parvari R. Male hypogonadism due to a mutation in the gene for the beta-subunit of follicle-stimulating hormone. *N Engl J Med*. (1998) 338:1729–32. doi: 10.1056/NEJM199806113382404

37. Layman LC, Porto AL, Xie J, da Motta LA, da Motta LD, Weiser W, et al. FSH beta gene mutations in a female with partial breast development and a male sibling with normal puberty and azoospermia. *J Clin Endocrinol Metab*. (2002) 87:3702–7. doi: 10.1210/jcem.87.8.8724

38. Grigorova M, Punab M, Ausmees K, Laan M. FSHB promoter polymorphism within evolutionary conserved element is associated with serum FSH level in men. *Hum Reprod*. (2008) 23:2160–6. doi: 10.1093/humrep/den216

39. Schuring AN, Busch AS, Bogdanova N, Gromoll J, Tuttelmann F. Effects of the FSH-beta-subunit promoter polymorphism−211G->T on the hypothalamic-pituitary-ovarian axis in normally cycling women indicate a gender-specific regulation of gonadotropin secretion. *J Clin Endocrinol Metab*. (2013) 98:E82–6. doi: 10.1210/jc.2012-2780

40. Rull K, Grigorova M, Ehrenberg A, Vaas P, Sekavin A, Nommemees D, et al. FSHB−211 G>T is a major genetic modulator of reproductive physiology and health in childbearing age women. *Hum Reprod*. (2018) 33:954–66. doi: 10.1093/humrep/dey057

41. Alviggi C, Conforti A, De Rosa P, Strina I, Palomba S, Vallone R, et al. The distribution of stroma and antral follicles differs between insulin-resistance and hyperandrogenism-related polycystic ovarian syndrome. *Front Endocrinol*. (2017) 8:117. doi: 10.3389/fendo.2017.00117

42. Desai SS, Roy BS, Mahale SD. Mutations and polymorphisms in FSH receptor: functional implications in human reproduction. *Reproduction*. (2013) 146:R235–48. doi: 10.1530/REP-13-0351

43. Orio F Jr., Ferrarini E, Cascella T, Dimida A, Palomba S, Gianetti E, et al. Genetic analysis of the follicle stimulating hormone receptor gene in women with polycystic ovary syndrome. *J Endocrinol Invest*. (2006) 29:975–82. doi: 10.1007/BF03349210

44. Lalioti MD. Impact of follicle stimulating hormone receptor variants in fertility. *Curr Opin Obstet Gynecol*. (2011) 23:158–67. doi: 10.1097/GCO.0b013e3283455288

45. Alviggi C, Humaidan P, Ezcurra D. Hormonal, functional and genetic biomarkers in controlled ovarian stimulation: tools for matching patients and protocols. *Reprod Biol Endocrinol*. (2012) 10:9. doi: 10.1186/1477-7827-10-9

46. Casarini L, Moriondo V, Marino M, Adversi F, Capodanno F, Grisolia C, et al. FSHR polymorphism p.N680S mediates different responses to FSH *in vitro*. *Mol Cell Endocrinol*. (2014) 393:83–91. doi: 10.1016/j.mce.2014.06.013

47. Riccetti L, De Pascali F, Gilioli L, Santi D, Brigante G, Simoni M, et al. Genetics of gonadotropins and their receptors as markers of ovarian reserve and response in controlled ovarian stimulation. *Best Pract Res Clin Obstet Gynaecol*. (2017) 44:15–25. doi: 10.1016/j.bpobgyn.2017.04.002

48. Laisk-Podar T, Kaart T, Peters M, Salumets A. Genetic variants associated with female reproductive ageing–potential markers for assessing ovarian function and ovarian stimulation outcome. *Reprod Biomed Online*. (2015) 31:199–209. doi: 10.1016/j.rbmo.2015.05.001

49. Overbeek A, Kuijper EA, Hendriks ML, Blankenstein MA, Ketel IJ, Twisk JW, et al. Clomiphene citrate resistance in relation to follicle-stimulating hormone receptor Ser680Ser-polymorphism in polycystic ovary syndrome. *Hum Reprod*. (2009) 24:2007–13. doi: 10.1093/humrep/dep114

50. Borgbo T, Jeppesen JV, Lindgren I, Lundberg Giwercman Y, Hansen LL, Yding Andersen C. Effect of the FSH receptor single nucleotide polymorphisms (FSHR 307/680) on the follicular fluid hormone profile and the granulosa cell gene expression in human small antral follicles. *Mol Hum Reprod*. (2015) 21:255–61. doi: 10.1093/molehr/gau106

51. Tohlob D, Abo Hashem E, Ghareeb N, Ghanem M, Elfarahaty R, Byers H, et al. Association of a promoter polymorphism in FSHR with ovarian reserve and response to ovarian stimulation in women undergoing assisted reproductive treatment. *Reprod Biomed Online*. (2016) 33:391–7. doi: 10.1016/j.rbmo.2016.06.001

52. Alviggi C, Pettersson K, Longobardi S, Andersen CY, Conforti A, De Rosa P, et al. A common polymorphic allele of the LH beta-subunit gene is associated with higher exogenous FSH consumption during controlled

ovarian stimulation for assisted reproductive technology. *Reprod Biol Endocrinol.* (2013) 11:51. doi: 10.1186/1477-7827-11-51

53. Conforti A, Cariati F, Vallone R, Alviggi C, de Placido G. Individualization of treatment in controlled ovarian stimulation: myth or reality? *Biochim Clin.* (2017) 41:294–305. doi: 10.19186/BC_2017.051

54. Alviggi C, Conforti A, Esteves SC, Vallone R, Venturella R, Staiano S, et al. Understanding ovarian hypo-response to exogenous gonadotropin in ovarian stimulation and its new proposed marker-the follicle-to-oocyte (FOI) index. *Front Endocrinol.* (2018) 9:589. doi: 10.3389/fendo.2018.00589

55. Esteves SC, Roque M, Bedoschi GM, Conforti A, Humaidan P, Alviggi C. Defining low prognosis patients undergoing assisted reproductive technology: POSEIDON criteria-the why. *Front Endocrinol.* (2018) 9:461. doi: 10.3389/fendo.2018.00461

56. Alviggi C, Andersen CY, Buehler K, Conforti A, De Placido G, Esteves SC, et al. A new more detailed stratification of low responders to ovarian stimulation: from a poor ovarian response to a low prognosis concept. *Fertil Steril.* (2016) 105:1452–3. doi: 10.1016/j.fertnstert.2016.02.005

57. Esteves SC, Humaidan P, Alviggi C, Fischer R. The novel POSEIDON stratification of 'Low prognosis patients in Assisted Reproductive Technology' and its proposed marker of successful outcome. *F1000Research.* (2016) 5:2911. doi: 10.12688/f1000research.10382.1

58. Conforti A, Esteves SC, Picarelli S, Iorio G, Rania E, Zullo F, et al. Novel approaches for diagnosis and management of low prognosis patients in assisted reproductive technology: the POSEIDON concept. *Panminerva Med.* (2019) 61:24–9. doi: 10.23736/S0031-0808.18.03511-5

59. Alviggi C, Guadagni R, Conforti A, Coppola G, Picarelli S, De Rosa P, et al. Association between intrafollicular concentration of benzene and outcome of controlled ovarian stimulation in IVF/ICSI cycles: a pilot study. *J Ovarian Res.* (2014) 7:67. doi: 10.1186/1757-2215-7-67

60. Sychev DA, Malova EU. Evidence-based pharmacogenetics: Is it possible? *Int J Risk Saf Med.* (2015) 27(Suppl. 1):S97–8. doi: 10.3233/JRS-150706

61. Alviggi C, Conforti A, Fabozzi F, De Placido G. Ovarian stimulation for IVF/ICSI cycles: A pharmacogenomic approach. *Med Ther Med Reproduct Gynecol Endocrinol.* (2009) 11:271–7. doi: 10.1684/mte.2009.0255

62. Alviggi C, Conforti A, Esteves SC. Impact of mutations and polymorphisms of gonadotrophins and their receptors on the outcome of controlled ovarian stimulation. In: Ghumman S, editor. *Principles and Practice of Controlled Ovarian Stimulation in ART.* New Delhi: Springer (2015). p. 147–56. doi: 10.1007/978-81-322-1686-5_14

63. Nilsson C, Pettersson K, Millar RP, Coerver KA, Matzuk MM, Huhtaniemi IT. Worldwide frequency of a common genetic variant of luteinizing hormone: an international collaborative research. International Collaborative Research Group. *Fertil Steril.* (1997) 67:998–1004. doi: 10.1016/S0015-0282(97)81430-6

64. Genro VK, Matte U, De Conto E, Cunha-Filho JS, Fanchin R. Frequent polymorphisms of FSH receptor do not influence antral follicle responsiveness to follicle-stimulating hormone administration as assessed by the Follicular Output RaTe (FORT). *J Assist Reprod Genet.* (2012) 29:657–63. doi: 10.1007/s10815-012-9761-7

65. Alviggi C, Clarizia R, Mollo A, Ranieri A, De Placido G. Who needs LH in ovarian stimulation? *Reproductive BioMedicine Online.* (2006) 12:599–607. doi: 10.1016/S1472-6483(10)61186-8

66. Alviggi C, Mollo A, Clarizia R, De Placido G. Exploiting LH in ovarian stimulation. *Reproduct Bio Med Online.* (2006) 12:221–33. doi: 10.1016/S1472-6483(10)60865-6

67. Alviggi C, Conforti A, Esteves SC, Andersen CY, Bosch E, Bühler K, et al. Recombinant luteinizing hormone supplementation in assisted reproductive technology: a systematic review. *Fertil Steril.* (2018) 109:644–64. doi: 10.1016/j.fertnstert.2018.01.003

8

Small Molecule Follicle-Stimulating Hormone Receptor Agonists and Antagonists

Ross C. Anderson[1]*, Claire L. Newton[2] and Robert P. Millar[2,3]

[1] Centre for Neuroendocrinology, Department of Physiology, Faculty of Health Sciences, University of Pretoria, Pretoria, South Africa, [2] Centre for Neuroendocrinology, Department of Immunology, Faculty of Health Sciences, University of Pretoria, Pretoria, South Africa, [3] Institute of Infectious Disease and Molecular Medicine, Department of Integrative Biomedical Sciences, Faculty of Health Sciences, University of Cape Town, Cape Town, South Africa

*Correspondence:
Ross C. Anderson
ross.anderson@up.ac.za

The follicle-stimulating hormone receptor (FSHR) has been targeted therapeutically for decades, due to its pivotal role in reproduction. To date, only purified and recombinant/biosimilar FSH have been used to target FSHR in assisted reproduction, with the exception of corifollitropin alfa; a modified gonadotropin in which the FSH beta subunit is joined to the C-terminal peptide of the human choriogonadotropin beta subunit, to extend serum half-life. Assisted reproduction protocols usually entail the trauma of multiple injections of FSH to initiate and promote folliculogenesis, which has prompted the development of a number of orally-available low molecular weight (LMW) chemical scaffolds targeting the FSHR. Furthermore, the recently documented roles of the FSHR in diverse extragonadal tissues, including cancer, fat metabolism, and bone density regulation, has highlighted the potential utility of LMW modulators of FSHR activity. Despite these chemical scaffolds encompassing a spectrum of *in vitro* and *in vivo* activities and pharmacological profiles, none have yet reached the clinic. In this review we discuss the major chemical classes of LMW molecules targeting the FSHR, and document their activity profiles and current status of development, in addition to discussing potential clinical applications.

Keywords: follicle-stimulating hormone (FSH), FSH receptor (FSHR), agonists, antagonists, small-molecule, GPCR (G protein-coupled receptors), assisted reproduction (ART)

INTRODUCTION

The hypothalamic-pituitary-gonadal axis comprises hypothalamic kisspeptin and neurokinin B (NKB) driving the secretion of gonadotropin-releasing hormone (GnRH). GnRH subsequently stimulates the pituitary secretion of the gonadotropin hormones luteinizing hormone (LH) and follicle stimulating hormone (FSH), into the general circulation, resulting in gonadal steroidogenesis, and pubertal development via activation of their cognate gonadotropin receptors, FSH receptor (FSHR), and LH receptor (LHR/LHCGR). In this article we review the development and potential clinical application of small molecule/low molecular weight (LMW) modulators of FSHR activity.

The FSHR is a G protein-coupled receptor (GPCR) that belongs to the glycoprotein hormone receptor sub-family of GPCRs that also includes the luteinizing hormone receptor (LHR/LHCGR), and the thyroid-stimulating hormone receptor (TSHR). These GPCRs are characterized by the presence of large extracellular N-terminal ectodomains (ECDs) that bind the heterodimeric glycoprotein hormones, in addition to the classical seven transmembrane domain region (TMD) characteristic of the GPCR superfamily. FSHR predominantly couples to and activates the $G\alpha_s$ class of intracellular G proteins, resulting in adenylyl cyclase stimulation, and a subsequent increase in the second messenger cyclic adenosine monophosphate (cAMP). cAMP then binds to and modulates the activity of a number of cyclic nucleotide-binding proteins, including cAMP-dependent protein kinases, and ion channels.

While $G\alpha_s$ is considered the main effector of FSHR-mediated signaling, $G\alpha_q$-mediated signaling, and β-arrestin mediated (G protein-independent) signaling have also been observed (1–3). These different signaling modalities are responsible for the activation of a multitude of downstream effectors, thus representing a complex network of possible signaling outcomes (2).

It is necessary that the full complement of possible signaling pathways is acknowledged both in the context of gonadal steroidogenesis, but also drug development, as a number of LMW molecules (described in detail below) are emerging with selective signaling profiles (a phenomena referred to as "biased-signaling"). These molecules have greatly informed as to the pathways involved (and required) for successful gonadal steroidogenesis, while simultaneously highlighting the inherent dangers of *in vitro* characterization of LMW molecules targeting the FSHR by measuring cAMP response in isolation.

Despite the successful application of corifollitropin, which comprises a hybrid molecule in which the FSHβ subunit is fused to the C-terminal 24 amino acids of the human chorionic gonadotropin β subunit (hCGβ) to increase serum half-life (marketed under the trade name Elonva) in assisted reproduction (4) and taking into account the signaling complexities discussed above there still remains a drive to develop LMW modulators of the gonadotropin receptors. The utilization of LMW orally-active modulators of FSHR has many theoretical advantages. Multiple injections (and associated site irritation) of polypeptide FSH during assisted reproduction would be avoided. Such classical LMW orally-active pharmaceutical compounds are also potentially superior in their greater stability and uniformity unlike gonadotropin polypeptides which require refrigeration and are subject to variable post-translational glycosylation which might affect half-life and bioactivity (5–8). The desirable properties of LMW analogs would therefore potentially result in more clinically effective treatment regimens. Another advantage of using orally-active gonadotropin analogs is the potential to vary dose which may have an additional benefit in avoiding the vexing and potentially life-threatening condition of ovarian hyperstimulation syndrome (OHSS).

In addition to these potential advantages, orally bioavailable LMW FSH antagonists may have potential as oral contraceptives. Current sex steroid-based contraceptives are administered at supra physiological doses to inhibit ovulation which can increase the risk of side effects, such as cardiovascular thrombosis events associated with estradiol-based contraceptives (9). It is arguable

that some of these side effects would be mitigated by targeting the FSHR, although the potential health risks of increased pituitary FSH release in response to antagonism of FSHR would require investigation. This is in light of the reported links between FSH oversecretion and the progression of certain cancers, bone loss, and increased body fat (10, 11), although it might be predicted that at least some of these effects would be mitigated by the presence of the FSHR antagonist (see *Concluding remarks and future perspectives*).

Despite the theoretical therapeutic potential of LMW modulators of FSHR, a number of substantial challenges needed to be overcome. The FSHR is a leucine-rich repeat containing GPCR, belonging to the glycoprotein hormone receptor family, which also includes the TSHR, and LHR. In addition, there are other GPCRs containing leucine-rich-repeat motifs. These GPCRs share high degrees of sequence conservation with the FSHR suggesting that drug cross-reactivity/specificity could be a potential problem. Moreover, the gonadotropins are large dimeric proteins that contact the gonadotropin receptors via multiple residues that include the glycan moieties, in addition to having a complex mechanism of receptor activation that includes structural movements within the extracellular domain (ECD) and the transmembrane (TM) domains of the receptor. As a result, it appeared that a LMW molecule might not fulfill the requirements of both receptor binding and activation. Nevertheless, these challenges could be successfully addressed in the development of both LHR and FSHR orthosteric agonists and antagonists (whose binding site overlaps with that of the natural ligand), and allosteric analogs which interact with the receptor at a site distinct from the orthosteric ligand binding site (12).

Allosteric GPCR modulators can be categorized based on measures of gonadotropin receptor signaling activity (most frequently measurement of cAMP, but biased modulators have also been described), and fall into three groups; allosteric agonists (allo-agonists) and positive and negative allosteric modulators (PAMs and NAMs). Allosteric agonists have agonist activity, in the absence of gonadotropin, in contrast to PAMs and NAMs whose activity can only be demonstrated in the presence of agonist, usually via modulation of orthosteric hormone binding affinity or altering the ability of the receptor to interact with intracellular signal transducers. In this way, PAMs and NAMs can either augment or diminish the response to orthosteric agonists, respectively. PAMs and NAMs have garnered much interest in the pharmaceutical industry, as these classes of allosteric modulators only have activity in the presence of co-bound endogenous ligand meaning that GPCR activation is limited to the spatio-temporal release of endogenous ligands. This is extremely advantageous, as many of the reproductive neuroendocrine hormones are released/secreted in cyclical patterns or pulses (13).

Structural modeling has been successfully utilized to identify allosteric sites in GPCRs for LMW compounds. Gonadotropin receptor TM domains have been modeled using adenosine receptor crystal structures, and identified two putative allosteric sites within the TM domains, positioned adjacent to the ECL loops (14, 15). These putative TM domain allosteric sites have been confirmed in studies utilizing chimeric trophic hormone receptors, and mutagenesis approaches. These sites have been assigned P1 and P2 (major site and minor site respectively) (14, 16, 17) (**Figure 1**). The P1 site is located between TMs III, IV, V, and VI, and P2 between TMs I, II, III, and VII (15).

Several cell-based screening assays have successfully been employed to identify structural scaffolds that can allosterically bind to the gonadotropin receptors (18). The large array of chemical scaffolds with FSHR activity have revealed a number of interesting and unique activity profiles, both *in vitro* and *in vivo*, with allo-agonists, NAMs, and PAMs identified. While LMW compounds targeting the closely-related, LHR have been identified, most endeavor has been directed toward developing LMW molecules targeting the FSHR. This is predictable, given that ovarian hyperstimulation requires multiple injections of FSH, in contrast to the single administration of LH/hCG (or other stimulus, such as GnRH agonist) needed to induce ovulation. Despite considerable progress in the development of LMW FSH analogs, none have yet entered the clinic. In many cases, this is a result of *in vitro* activity failing to translate into *in vivo* activity, off-target effects/toxicity, synthesis issues, and frequently termination of research programs following pharmaceutical company acquisitions, and differing priorities of the acquiring company. These issues have been previously reviewed in detail (18). Here we review the progress that has been made in developing LMW orally active FSHR analogs, and discuss their potential clinical applications.

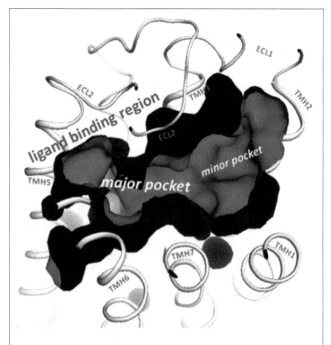

FIGURE 1 | The top view of the LHR with partially removed extracellular loops (ECLs) highlights the two putative allosteric binding sites for LMW gonadotropin receptor ligands (magenta), located within the transmembrane (TM) domains and adjacent to the ECLs. These sites are labeled the P1 (major) site and P2 (minor) site. Reproduced with permission from (10).

FSHR AGONISTS

Thiazolidinones

Thiazolidinone (TZD) core scaffolds have previously been utilized in a number of successful GPCR drug discovery programs, and offer a flexible and versatile platform for compound development (19). Affymax (Cupertino, US) utilized a TZD compound library containing 42,000 molecules, and identified several lead compounds with agonist activity at the FSHR. Several hits with nanomolar (nM) potencies were identified from this screen including a partial agonist (E_{max} 24% of maximal recombinant FSH stimulation) with an EC_{50} of 32 nM (20). This lead compound was subsequently modified by adding γ-lactam congeners and 5-alkyl substituents in an attempt to address stereoselectivity issues with the heterocyclic ring in which the *trans* isomer predominated over the active *cis* isomer during synthesis (21, 22). A parallel drug discovery program run between Affymax and Wyeth [since acquired by Pfizer (New York City, US)] also screened a large compound library representing a spectrum of core scaffolds, with two of the best hits containing TZD core structures. These lead compounds had poor EC_{50}'s of approximately 20 μM, but following parallel synthesis resulted in three promising compounds with nanomolar potencies and full efficacy *in vitro* (1–6 nM) (23). Subsequent studies in which chimeric receptors were created via exchanging of the N-termini and TM domains of the TSHR and FSHR supported the notion that that the analogs bind within the TM domain of the FSHR. The site of interaction of these allo-agonists with the FSHR was further refined to a site located between TM I and ECL2 (23). A compound, (compound 5) (**Figure 2**), was identified and was demonstrated to be capable of stimulating steroid production in FSHR transfected rat primary granulosa cells and mouse adrenal Y1 cells to the same level as FSH, albeit with approximately 1,000-fold lower potency (23). *In vivo* activity was evaluated in a rat ovulation assay, where a dose-dependent increase in the number of ovulated oocytes was observed, however, poor oral bioavailability, and genotoxic effects were noted stalling further development (24).

The pharmacological properties of TZD-containing compounds was further evaluated, and intriguingly it was discovered that minor modification to the core thiazolidine ring, at either an aryl group at position 3 or an acetic acid amide chain at position 5 of the thiazolidine ring resulted in differing pharmacological profiles to the parent compound (25). These activities ranged from agonists (activating $G\alpha_s$) through to NAMs which inhibited estradiol production in rat granulosa cells via $G\alpha_i$ activation ("compound 3"; **Figure 2**) (25). These simple TZD core structures therefore have the potential to deliver a spectrum of LMW allosteric modulators targeting multiple FSHR signaling pathways, should synthesis, bioavailability, and toxicity issues be mitigated.

Diketopiperazines

Pharmacopeia Inc. (now Ligand Pharmaceuticals, San Diego, United States) and Organon [now Merck & Co/Merck Sharpe & Dohme (MSD), Kenilworth, United States] screened a

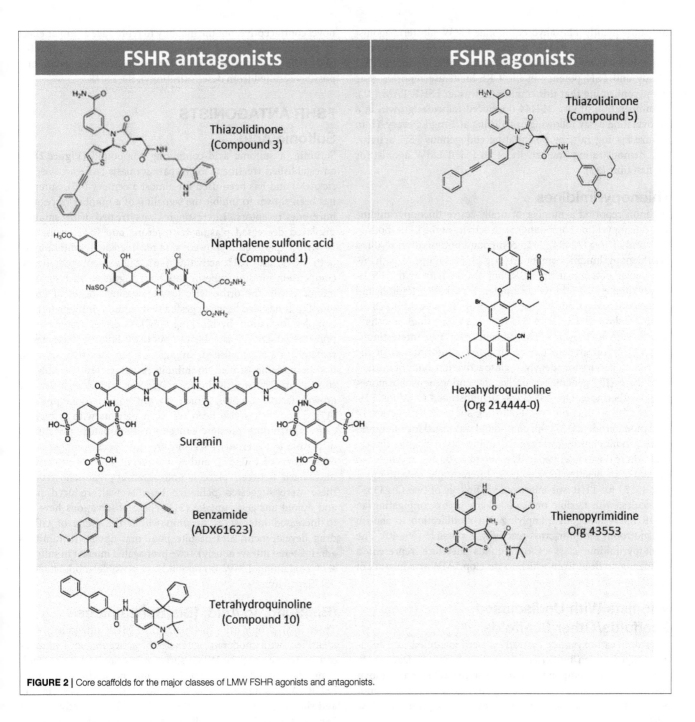

FIGURE 2 | Core scaffolds for the major classes of LMW FSHR agonists and antagonists.

large diketopiperazine compound library. A number of biaryl agonists were identified, with the most potent compounds containing heterocyclic diketopiperazine substituents (26). Lead optimisation, through modification of the diketopiperazine core side chains, led to increased potency of activation, (in the nanomolar range) in a cAMP-response element (CRE)-containing luciferase reporter gene assay, and a cAMP accumulation assay (27). These compounds were apparently not developed further and there is no information on specificity or *in vivo* activity. Interestingly, other piperazine compounds with FSHR activity have been described, and a patent was submitted

by Serono, describing low nanomolar FSHR piperazine agonists (28).

Hexahydroquinolines

Poor oral activity of many LMW compounds has hampered development. Organon demonstrated the first high potency LMW compound with good oral activity targeting the FSHR following the filing of patents on the use of hexahydroquinoline scaffolds (4-phenyl-5-oxo-1,4,5,6,7,8-hexahydroquinolines) as FSHR activators (29, 30). These LMW compounds had potencies of <10 nM in an *in vitro* CRE-luciferase reporter gene assay, and subsequently a hexahydroquinoline LMW allosteric agonist at the FSHR, Org 214444-0 was described (31) (**Figure 2**). Co-incubation with FSH resulted in a substantial increase in FSH affinity and FSH potency in the CRE-luciferase reporter gene assay, confirming that this compound was an FSHR PAM (31). Administration of Org 214444-0 induced follicular growth in a rat ovulation assay following oral dosing at 1 mg/kg every 4 h in mature cycling rats, by potentiating endogenous FSH activity, thus demonstrating oral-activity of an FSHR LMW agonist for the first time (31).

Thienopyrimidines

Organon reported a number of orally-active thienopyrimidine and thienopyridine compounds with activity at the LHR, both *in vitro* and *in vivo* (32–34). Lead compound optimisation resulted in a thienopyrimidine compound (Org 43553; **Figure 2**), with low nanomolar potency at the LHR, but also activity at the FSHR (approximately 10-fold reduced potency vs. LHR). Radioligand dissociation assays and the generation of chimeric LHR/TSHR receptors showed that Org 43553 interacts with a single allosteric site, located in the LHR TM domains (35, 36). Interestingly, Org 43553 appeared to induce an active conformation of the receptor necessary for adenylyl cyclase activation, but not inositol phosphate (IP) generation, unlike the endogenous hormones (36). Furthermore, Org 43553 was demonstrated to inhibit LH-induced IP production (36). Following successful induction of ovulation in rodents (37) this compound was tested for safety and efficacy in humans following oral administration in a pre-clinical trial, where it was tolerated in doses up to 2,700 mg, and induced ovulation in healthy females (38). Interestingly, selectivity of Org 43553 for LHR was improved via linkage of two Org43553 molecules, with flexible or rigid linkers, or by conjugating an FSHR LMW antagonist, implying that modification to abolish gonadotropin receptor cross-reactivity is possible (39, 40). The thienopyrimidine class of compounds therefore represent a promising scaffold from which to develop LMW modulators of FSHR.

Agonists With Undisclosed Scaffolds/Other Scaffolds

Piperidine carboxyamide derivatives were identified in a high-throughput screen by Serono (now Merck KGaA, Darmstadt, Germany). Lead compounds were shown to have low nanomolar potency *in vitro* in a luciferase reporter gene assay, but poor potency in an estradiol production assay utilizing rat granulosa cells (41).

MSD identified two LMW FSHR agonists with undisclosed scaffolds. These agonists had low nanomolar potency at the FSHR, but were notable for their unusual very short-acting profiles with a half-life and T_{max} of approximately 1.5 and 0.5 h respectively) compared to recombinant FSH [half-life approximately 24–48 h (42–44)]. These compounds were subsequently shown to inhibit ovulation, and induce the production of luteinized unruptured follicles in cycling rats when administered orally, with complete reversal of the effect, and resumption of cyclicity following withdrawal of the compounds (44). These compounds may yet form the basis for an effective novel contraceptive, but the inability to reproduce a similar effect in primates has limited their immediate therapeutic potential (44). The mechanism was apparently not investigated and possibly resulted from desensitization of the FSHR.

FSHR ANTAGONISTS

Sulfonic Acid

Suramin, a sulfonic acid-containing compound (**Figure 2**), is an established treatment for trypanosomiasis (African sleeping sickness) and has been used for almost a century (45). Suramin has been shown to inhibit the signaling of a number of peptide hormones/receptors. Interestingly, rats treated with suramin displayed decreased plasma testosterone and FSH levels, and *in vitro* experiments showed suramin-mediated inhibition of both hCG and FSH activities (46). Subsequent radioligand competition-binding experiments have suggested that suramin interacts with the orthosteric ligand binding pocket of FSHR (46, 47). It has also been suggested that suramin inhibits ternary complex formation, by blocking GPCR-G protein interactions, preventing GDP-release (48, 49), but the validity of these claims remains to be established, in light of the fact that suramin has been demonstrated to inhibit receptor tyrosine kinases, such as epidermal growth factor receptor, and platelet-derived growth factor receptor, which do not couple to G proteins (45). Suramin has also been tested in patients with refractory cancers including prostate cancer. In these patients decreases in plasma testosterone, FSH and prostate specific antigen have been observed (50, 51), and while overall survival rates were unchanged between placebo and suramin treatment groups, there were suggested palliative benefits with reduced pain, and opioid analgesic uptake (51). These observations have led to increased interest in suramin within the arena of GPCR drug development, and despite poor oral uptake (suramin is administered intravenously), have propagated interest in sulfonic acid containing LMW compounds as possible modulators of FSHR activity.

(Bis)Sulfonic Acid, (Bis)Benzamides

Three (bis)sulfonic acid, (bis)benzamide FSHR antagonists were identified, with moderate potencies of activation in a number of *in vitro* assays (52). While suramin appears to interact with a number of GPCRs, the (bis)sulfonic acid, (bis)benzamide FSHR LMW antagonists displayed no LHR and TSHR binding and signaling activity up to 100 μM (52). Concurrently, Wyeth identified a naphthalene sulfonic acid compound ("compound 1"; **Figure 2**) that non-competitively inhibited FSH binding to the FSHR, despite binding to the FSHR extracellular domain (ECD), resulting in a reduction of FSH binding sites but not affinity (53). In addition this compound completely abolished the cAMP response to FSH (53). This was substantiated *in vivo* in cycling female rats receiving 100 mg/kg i.p. which inhibited ovulation in all treated animals (53). Issues with oral bioavailability, and safety/off-target effects, including mild inflammation of the ovarian surface epithelium and growth retardation have hindered the successful development and transition of these compounds into the clinic despite promising *in vitro* activity profiles (53).

Modification to improve oral absorption of these compounds was attempted, but carboxylic acid substituents abolished FSHR binding activity (52).

Tetrahydroquinolines

A tetrahydroquinoline (THQ) scaffold containing an amino group at position 6 with modest micromolar FSHR agonistic activity and an efficacy of 85% relative to FSH, was identified by Organon using a CRE-luciferase reporter assay. In a similar vein to the TZD agonists, minor modification of the core structure, in this case introduction of an aromatic group at position 6 of the THQ scaffold, resulted in compounds with completely different pharmacologies. Aromatic groups incorporated at position 6 resulted in a switch from full agonists to full antagonists, with nanomolar IC_{50}'s (compound 10; **Figure 2**) (54). It was established that the binding pocket was likely large and lipophilic, given that large aromatic substituents at position 6 of the THQ scaffold were tolerated (including biphenyl groups), also suggesting that the compounds likely bound in the TM domain. In support of this, competition binding assays showed lack of displacement of FSH binding by these compounds (54). Additionally, it was also shown that these aromatic groups were preferred for antagonistic activity (54). In a mouse *ex vivo* follicular growth assay one of the biphenyl-substituted THQ compounds inhibited follicular growth in the presence of FSH, and substantially inhibited ovulation (up to 78% of follicles) (54).

Benzamide Derivatives

Addex Pharmaceuticals (Geneva, Switzerland) used a homogenous time resolved fluorescence (HTRF) screening assay to screen for FSHR NAMs, and identified a benzamide compound (ADX61623; **Figure 2**) with activity (IC_{50} 0.7 μM with 55% inhibition of FSH EC_{80}). Interestingly, ADX61623 inhibited cAMP and progesterone production in the presence of FSH *in vitro* in a dose-dependent manner, and conversely stimulated estradiol production at high concentrations (55). These results suggest that cAMP signaling is not a requirement for estradiol production. Indeed, it is known that the ovarian functions of FSH (such as estradiol production) are under the control of a number of signaling pathways (see *Introduction*). In an *in vivo* setting, administration of 50 mg/kg ADX61623 s.c. was ineffective in completely inhibiting folliculogenesis and ovulation in rats following sequential treatment with pituitary FSH and hCG, as measured by number of oocytes recovered and ovarian weight (55). The authors postulate that this may be due to the inability of ADX61623 to inhibit the production of estradiol despite inhibition of cAMP. Two additional benzamide analogs, identified by Addex, (ADX68692 and ADX68693) corroborated the antagonistic activity profile of ADX61623, substantiating the requirement for blockade of both arms of the FSHR steroidogenic signaling pathway to inhibit follicular maturation and ovulation in rats (56). Indeed, while subcutaneous or oral administration of ADX68692 (which was demonstrated in primary rat granulosa cells to inhibit progesterone and estradiol production) was shown to disrupt cyclicity in mature female rats, and reduced the number of oocytes recovered, ADX68693 which inhibited progesterone but not estradiol production, had no effect

(56). Interestingly, ADX68692 and ADX68693 demonstrated biased-activity profiles at the LHR as well as the FSHR, with ADX68693 abolishing testosterone and inhibiting progesterone production in rat primary leydig cells while ADX68692 partially inhibited testosterone and potentiated progesterone production (57). Many LMW compound screening strategies assay for a single signaling output, with the benzamide compound series highlighting the inherent dangers of this strategy, and may in part explain the failure of many gonadotropin LMW compounds to translate promising *in vitro* efficacy to *in vivo* bioactivity.

Other FSHR Antagonists

In addition to the compound families described above, acyltryptophanol and pyrrolobenzodiazepine LMW FSHR antagonists have been identified through HTRF and CRE-luciferase screening assays respectively, with a spectrum of IC_{50} concentrations (58, 59). The current status of these programs is unknown.

Additionally, a novel substituted aminoalkylamide series of FSHR modulators have been identified with antagonistic activity. Ortho-McNeil Pharmaceutical discovered two potent compounds (identified in a cAMP screening assay) but they failed to effectively inhibit ovulation and spermatogenesis in Wistar rats (60). To determine whether the inability of the compounds to inhibit FSHR *in vivo* was due to restricted oral bioavailability, poor intestinal absorption, and/or rapid clearance, additional pharmacokinetic data would be required.

CONCLUDING REMARKS AND FUTURE PERSPECTIVES

Natural and recombinant gonadotropins have been the mainstay of infertility treatment in men and women for decades, and are still an essential component of assisted reproductive technologies which have impressively addressed the needs of infertile patients world-wide. However, there is a perceived need to develop gonadotropin analogs and orally-available LMW compounds with gonadotropin receptor activity which would obviate current multiple injection protocols, and importantly, reduce OHSS risk. Modulation of relative FSH and LH activities would also have application in women's health conditions such as polycystic ovarian syndrome (PCOS) and would possibly offer a novel method of contraception. Other potential applications of gonadotropin receptor modulators could include the management of animal reproduction, both as contraceptives in population control, and utilization in assisted reproduction for animal husbandry purposes and in endangered animals. With regards to the latter, IVF and cryopreservation protocols have been applied with varying degrees of success in endangered ungulates, and felid species (61–63).

Although several promising FSHR LMW agonists and antagonists have been shown to have desirable properties in animal models, none have shown efficacy in human clinical studies. This is in contrast to LHR LMW molecules which have been demonstrated to be efficacious in stimulating ovulation in women. One example is MK-8389 (developed by MSD) which had promising activity in a rat model but when tested in an ascending dose study on pituitary-suppressed females, showed an effect on thyroid function, despite no effect on follicular development, or estradiol production (64). Thus, further research endeavors are required to produce efficacious orally-active FSH LMW agonists as substitutes for multiple injections of conventional polypeptide FSH.

Despite these setbacks, the pursuit of FSHR LMW compounds with *in vitro* activity has been highly successful with the impressive development of dozens of allosteric compounds with appropriate properties. The majority of these LMW compounds have arisen from a relatively limited number of core scaffolds, each with distinctive chemistries, and an array of interesting properties. Amongst these allosteric compounds are NAMs and PAMs which have unique properties for exploitation, such as biased-activity profiles, which may be of value in differential stimulation or inhibition of estradiol and progesterone. In view of the diverse structures of molecular scaffolds utilized it is highly likely that following sufficient investment and development, several of these would have the appropriate characteristics and safety profile to be therapeutics.

The acquisition of reproductive health companies by big pharma may have played a significant role in the termination of LMW gonadotropin analog development, due to differing research priorities. For example, the acquisition of Wyeth by Pfizer may have halted development of the TZD FSHR agonist. Encouragingly, a number of small biotech companies are still focussing on the development of LMW modulators of FSHR activity, and we may yet see compounds entering the clinic for a diversity of applications.

An exciting new development in the arena of LMW gonadotropin analogs is the discovery that some of these compounds have gonadotropin receptor "pharmacological chaperone" or "pharmacoperone" activity. These pharmacoperone compounds can restore plasma membrane localization and function to intracellularly-retained GPCRs harboring mutations that result in misfolding and intracellular retention/degradation. LMW LHR allosteric agonists have been shown to act as pharmacoperones, "rescuing" cell surface expression of intracellularly retained mutant LHRs (65) (an outcome of the majority of inactivating point mutations in the LHR) (66). We and others have demonstrated that at high concentrations the LHR LMW molecules are also able to restore cell surface expression to intracellularly retained human

FSHR mutants (67). As there is currently no treatment for patients harboring these mutations, the LMW pharmacoperones potentially represent an exciting novel breakthrough in personalized and precision medicine in reproduction.

It has been suggested that the FSHR is expressed in a number of extragonadal tissues, and current research implies that these receptors may be physiologically important. Indeed, the utilization of LMW gonadotropin analogs targeting the FSHR may extend beyond the current remit of assisted reproduction and may yet herald a new era of gonadotropic therapeutics (68, 69). For example, post-menopausal women have low oestrogens, and elevated FSH, with concomitant bone loss, and increased body fat. It has been implied that FSH as well as low oestrogens may be playing a role, and indeed in ovariectomised mice, an FSHβ neutralizing antibody was found to reduce bone resorption and stimulate bone synthesis (10). In a subsequent publication the neutralizing antibody was demonstrated to induce thermogenic adipose tissue and additionally reduced body fat and increased the lean mass/total mass ratio, compared to control IgG (11). There are, however, opposing views, on the physiological relevance of extragonadal FSHR, and also contradictory findings in *in vivo* studies. The intimate relationship between FSH/FSHR and estradiol frequently confuse and confound the interpretation of data, in addition to the complicated often-opposed effects of the two hormones such as on osteoclasts (and the additional roles of activins in bone). Another area of potential FSHR LMW analog application is in oncology. Reported proliferative effects of FSH and FSHR in prostatic and ovarian cancers alludes to other novel applications for FSHR LMW agonists and antagonists (70–73), although as with other putative extragonadal functions of FSH/FSHR these data are frequently contradictory. Thus, more research is required to fully understand the physiological mechanisms behind these phenomena, and exploit possible therapeutic opportunities.

AUTHOR CONTRIBUTIONS

All authors listed have made a substantial, direct and intellectual contribution to the work, and approved it for publication.

FUNDING

This work is supported by grants from the National Research Foundation (NRF) of South Africa.

REFERENCES

1. Landomiel F, Gallay N, Jégot G, Tranchant T, Durand G, Bourquard T, et al. Biased signalling in follicle stimulating hormone action. *Mol Cell Endocrinol.* (2014) 382:452–9. doi: 10.1016/j.mce.2013.09.035
2. Gloaguen P, Crepieux P, Heitzler D, Poupon A, Reiter E. Mapping the follicle-stimulating hormone-induced signaling networks. *Front Endocrinol (Lausanne).* (2011) 2:45. doi: 10.3389/fendo.2011.00045
3. Hunzicker-Dunn M, Maizels ET. FSH signaling pathways in immature granulosa cells that regulate target gene expression:

branching out from protein kinase A. *Cell Signal.* (2006) 18:1351–9. doi: 10.1016/j.cellsig.2006.02.011
4. Beckers NG, Macklon NS, Devroey P, Platteau P, Boerrigter PJ, Fauser BC. First live birth after ovarian stimulation using a chimeric long-acting human recombinant follicle-stimulating hormone (FSH) agonist (recFSH-CTP) for *in vitro* fertilization. *Fertil Steril.* (2003) 79:621–3. doi: 10.1016/S0015-0282(02)04804-5
5. Mastrangeli R, Satwekar A, Cutillo F, Ciampolillo C, Palinsky W, Longobardi S. *In-vivo* biological activity and glycosylation analysis of a biosimilar recombinant human follicle-stimulating hormone product (bemfola) compared with its reference medicinal product (GONAL-f). *PLoS ONE* (2017) 12:e0184139. doi: 10.1371/journal.pone.0184139

6. Orvieto R, Seifer DB. Biosimilar FSH preparations- are they identical twins or just siblings? *Reprod Biol Endocrinol.* (2016) 14:32. doi: 10.1186/s12958-016-0167-8

7. Riccetti L, Klett D, Ayoub MA, Boulo T, Pignatti E, Tagliavini S, et al. Heterogeneous hCG and hMG commercial preparations result in different intracellular signalling but induce a similar long-term progesterone response in vitro. *Mol Hum Reprod.* (2017) 23:685–97. doi: 10.1093/molehr/gax047

8. Orvieto R, Nahum R, Rabinson J, Ashkenazi J, Anteby EY, Meltcer S. Follitropin-alpha (gonal-F) versus follitropin-beta (puregon) in controlled ovarian hyperstimulation for in vitro fertilization: is there any difference? *Fertil Steril.* (2009) 91(4 Suppl.):1522–5. doi: 10.1016/j.fertnstert.2008.08.112

9. Brynhildsen J. Combined hormonal contraceptives: Prescribing patterns, compliance, and benefits versus risks. *Ther Adv Drug Saf.* (2014) 5:201–13. doi: 10.1177/2042098614548857

10. Zhu LL, Blair H, Cao J, Yuen T, Latif R, Guo L, et al. Blocking antibody to the beta-subunit of FSH prevents bone loss by inhibiting bone resorption and stimulating bone synthesis. *Proc Natl Acad Sci USA.* (2012) 109:14574–9. doi: 10.1073/pnas.1212806109

11. Liu P, Ji Y, Yuen T, Rendina-Ruedy E, DeMambro VE, Dhawan S, et al. Blocking FSH induces thermogenic adipose tissue and reduces body fat. *Nature* (2017) 546:107–12. doi: 10.1038/nature22342

12. Anderson RC, Newton CL, Anderson RA, Millar RP. Gonadotropins and their analogues: current and potential clinical applications. *Endocr Rev.* (2018) 39:911–37. doi: 10.1210/er.2018-00052

13. Wang CI, Lewis RJ. Emerging opportunities for allosteric modulation of G-protein coupled receptors. *Biochem Pharmacol.* (2013) 85:153–62. doi: 10.1016/j.bcp.2012.09.001

14. Heitman LH, Kleinau G, Brussee J, Krause G, Ijzerman AP. Determination of different putative allosteric binding pockets at the lutropin receptor by using diverse drug-like low molecular weight ligands. *Mol Cell Endocrinol.* (2012) 351:326–36. doi: 10.1016/j.mce.2012.01.010

15. Arey BJ. Allosteric modulators of glycoprotein hormone receptors: discovery and therapeutic potential. *Endocrine* (2008) 34:1–10. doi: 10.1007/s12020-008-9098-2

16. Manglik A, Kobilka BK, Steyaert J. Nanobodies to study G protein-coupled receptor structure and function. *Annu Rev Pharmacol Toxicol.* (2017) 57:19–37. doi: 10.1146/annurev-pharmtox-010716-104710

17. Gentry PR, Sexton PM, Christopoulos A. Novel allosteric modulators of G protein-coupled receptors. *J Biol Chem.* (2015) 290:19478–88. doi: 10.1074/jbc.R115.662759

18. Nataraja SG, Yu HN, Palmer SS. Discovery and development of small molecule allosteric modulators of glycoprotein hormone receptors. *Front Endocrinol (Lausanne).* (2015) 6:142. doi: 10.3389/fendo.2015.00142

19. Verma A, Saraf SK. 4-thiazolidinone–a biologically active scaffold. *Eur J Med Chem.* (2008) 43:897–905. doi: 10.1016/j.ejmech.2007.07.017

20. Maclean D, Holden F, Davis AM, Scheuerman RA, Yanofsky S, Holmes CP, et al. Agonists of the follicle stimulating hormone receptor from an encoded thiazolidinone library. *J Comb Chem.* (2004) 6:196–206. doi: 10.1021/cc0300154

21. Wrobel J, Jetter J, Kao W, Rogers J, Di L, Chi J, et al. 5-alkylated thiazolidinones as follicle-stimulating hormone (FSH) receptor agonists. *Bioorg Med Chem.* (2006) 14:5729–41. doi: 10.1016/j.bmc.2006.04.012

22. Pelletier JC, Rogers J, Wrobel J, Perez MC, Shen ES. Preparation of highly substituted gamma-lactam follicle stimulating hormone receptor agonists. *Bioorg Med Chem.* (2005) 13:5986–95. doi: 10.1016/j.bmc.2005.07.025

23. Yanofsky SD, Shen ES, Holden F, Whitehorn E, Aguilar B, Tate E, et al. Allosteric activation of the follicle-stimulating hormone (FSH) receptor by selective, nonpeptide agonists. *J Biol Chem.* (2006) 281:13226–33. doi: 10.1074/jbc.M600601200

24. Sriraman V, Denis D, de Matos D, Yu H, Palmer S, Nataraja S. Investigation of a thiazolidinone derivative as an allosteric modulator of follicle stimulating hormone receptor: evidence for its ability to support follicular development and ovulation. *Biochem Pharmacol.* (2014) 89:266–75. doi: 10.1016/j.bcp.2014.02.023

25. Arey BJ, Yanofsky SD, Claudia Pérez M, Holmes CP, Wrobel J, Gopalsamy A, et al. Differing pharmacological activities of thiazolidinone analogs at the FSH receptor. *Biochem Biophys Res Commun.* (2008) 368:723–8. doi: 10.1016/j.bbrc.2008.01.119

26. Guo T, Adang AE, Dolle RE, Dong G, Fitzpatrick D, Geng P, et al. Small molecule biaryl FSH receptor agonists. part 1: lead discovery via encoded combinatorial synthesis. *Bioorg Med Chem Lett.* (2004) 14:1713–6. doi: 10.1016/j.bmcl.2004.01.042

27. Guo T, Adang AE, Dong G, Fitzpatrick D, Geng P, Ho KK, et al. Small molecule biaryl FSH receptor agonists. part 2: lead optimization via parallel synthesis. *Bioorg Med Chem Lett.* (2004) 14:1717–20. doi: 10.1016/j.bmcl.2004.01.043

28. Magar S, Goutopoulos A, Liao Y, Schwarz M, Russell TJ. *Piperazine Derivatives and Methods of Use.* patent WO2004031182A1. (2002).

29. Poveda PMG, Karstens WFJ, Timmers CM. *4-Phenyl-5-oxo-1,4,5,6,7,8-Hexahydroquinoline Derivatives for the Treatment of Infertility.* patent US8022218B2. (2011).

30. Timmers CM, Karstens WFJ, Grima PPM. *4-Phenyl-5-oxo-1,4,5,6,7,8-Hexahydroquinoline Derivatives as Medicaments for the Treatment of Infertility.* patent WO2006117370A1. (2006).

31. van Koppen CJ, Verbost PM, van de Lagemaat R, Karstens WJ, Loozen HJ, van Achterberg TA, et al. Signaling of an allosteric, nanomolar potent, low molecular weight agonist for the follicle-stimulating hormone receptor. *Biochem Pharmacol.* (2013) 85:1162–70. doi: 10.1016/j.bcp.2013.02.001

32. van Straten NC, Schoonus-Gerritsma GG, van Someren RG, Draaijer J, Adang AE, Timmers CM, et al. The first orally active low molecular weight agonists for the LH receptor: thienopyr(im)idines with therapeutic potential for ovulation induction. *Chembiochem.* (2002) 3:1023–6. doi: 10.1002/1439-7633(20021004)3:10<1023::AID-CBIC1023>3.0.CO;2-9

33. Moore S, Jaeschke H, Kleinau G, Neumann S, Costanzi S, Jiang JK, et al. Evaluation of small-molecule modulators of the luteinizing hormone/choriogonadotropin and thyroid stimulating hormone receptors: Structure-activity relationships and selective binding patterns. *J Med Chem.* (2006) 49:3888–96. doi: 10.1021/jm060247s

34. Jäschke H, Neumann S, Moore S, Thomas CJ, Colson AO, Costanzi S, et al. A low molecular weight agonist signals by binding to the transmembrane domain of thyroid-stimulating hormone receptor (TSHR) and luteinizing hormone/chorionic gonadotropin receptor (LHCGR). *J Biol Chem.* (2006) 281:9841–4. doi: 10.1074/jbc.C600014200

35. Heitman LH, Oosterom J, Bonger KM, Timmers CM, Wiegerinck PH, Ijzerman AP. 3H]org 43553, the first low-molecular-weight agonistic and allosteric radioligand for the human luteinizing hormone receptor. *Mol Pharmacol.* (2008) 73:518–24. doi: 10.1124/mol.107.039875

36. van Koppen CJ, Zaman GJ, Timmers CM, Kelder J, Mosselman S, van de Lagemaat R, et al. A signaling-selective, nanomolar potent allosteric low molecular weight agonist for the human luteinizing hormone receptor. *Naunyn Schmiedebergs Arch Pharmacol.* (2008) 378:503–14. doi: 10.1007/s00210-008-0318-3

37. van de Lagemaat R, Timmers CM, Kelder J, van Koppen C, Mosselman S, Hanssen RG. Induction of ovulation by a potent, orally active, low molecular weight agonist (org 43553) of the luteinizing hormone receptor. *Hum Reprod.* (2009) 24:640–8. doi: 10.1093/humrep/den412

38. Gerrits M, Mannaerts B, Kramer H, Addo S, Hanssen R. First evidence of ovulation induced by oral LH agonists in healthy female volunteers of reproductive age. *J Clin Endocrinol Metab.* (2013) 98:1558–66. doi: 10.1210/jc.2012-3404

39. Bonger KM, Hoogendoorn S, van Koppen CJ, Timmers CM, van der Marel GA, Overkleeft HS. Development of selective LH receptor agonists by heterodimerization with a FSH receptor antagonist. *ACS Med Chem Lett.* (2010) 2:85–9. doi: 10.1021/ml100229v

40. Bonger KM, van den Berg RJ, Knijnenburg AD, Heitman LH, van Koppen CJ, Timmers CM, et al. Discovery of selective luteinizing hormone receptor agonists using the bivalent ligand method. *ChemMedChem.* (2009) 4:1189–95. doi: 10.1002/cmdc.200900058

41. El Tayer N, Reddy A, Buckler D, Magar S. *FSH Mimetics for the Treatment of Infertility.* patent US6235755B1. (2001).

42. Bouloux PM, Handelsman DJ, Jockenhövel F, Nieschlag E, Rabinovici J, Frasa WL, et al. First human exposure to FSH-CTP in hypogonadotrophic hypogonadal males. *Hum Reprod.* (2001) 16:1592–7. doi: 10.1093/humrep/16.8.1592

43. le Contonnec JY, Porchet HC, Beltrami V, Khan A, Toon S, Rowland M. Clinical pharmacology of recombinant human follicle-stimulating hormone.

II. single doses and steady state pharmacokinetics. *Fertil Steril.* (1994) 61:679–86.

44. van de Lagemaat R, van Koppen CJ, Krajnc-Franken MA, Folmer BJ, van Diepen HA, Mulders SM, et al. Contraception by induction of luteinized unruptured follicles with short-acting low molecular weight FSH receptor agonists in female animal models. *Reproduction* (2011) 142:893–905. doi: 10.1530/REP-11-0234

45. Gartrell BA, Tsao CK, Galsky MD. The follicle-stimulating hormone receptor: a novel target in genitourinary malignancies. *Urol Oncol.* (2013) 31:1403–7. doi: 10.1016/j.urolonc.2012.03.005

46. Daugherty RL, Cockett AT, Schoen SR, Sluss PM. Suramin inhibits gonadotropin action in rat testis: Implications for treatment of advanced prostate cancer. *J Urol.* (1992) 147:727–32. doi: 10.1016/S0022-5347(17)37367-6

47. Stevis PE, Deecher DC, Lopez FJ, Frail DE. Pharmacological characterization of soluble human FSH receptor extracellular domain: Facilitated secretion by coexpression with FSH. *Endocrine* (1999) 10:153–60. doi: 10.1385/ENDO:10:2:153

48. Beindl W, Mitterauer T, Hohenegger M, Ijzerman AP, Nanoff C, Freissmuth M. Inhibition of receptor/G protein coupling by suramin analogues. *Mol Pharmacol.* (1996) 50:415–23.

49. Freissmuth M, Boehm S, Beindl W, Nickel P, Ijzerman AP, Hohenegger M, et al. Suramin analogues as subtype-selective G protein inhibitors. *Mol Pharmacol.* (1996) 49:602–11.

50. Danesi R, La Rocca RV, Cooper MR, Ricciardi MP, Pellegrini A, Soldani P, et al. Clinical and experimental evidence of inhibition of testosterone production by suramin. *J Clin Endocrinol Metab.* (1996) 81:2238–46.

51. Small EJ, Meyer M, Marshall ME, Reyno LM, Meyers FJ, Natale RB, et al. Suramin therapy for patients with symptomatic hormone-refractory prostate cancer: results of a randomized phase III trial comparing suramin plus hydrocortisone to placebo plus hydrocortisone. *J Clin Oncol.* (2000) 18:1440–50. doi: 10.1200/JCO.2000.18.7.1440

52. Wrobel J, Green D, Jetter J, Kao W, Rogers J, Pérez MC, et al. Synthesis of (bis)sulfonic acid, (bis)benzamides as follicle-stimulating hormone (FSH) antagonists. *Bioorg Med Chem.* (2002) 10:639–56. doi: 10.1016/S0968-0896(01)00324-8

53. Arey BJ, Deecher DC, Shen ES, Stevis PE, Meade EH, Wrobel J, et al. Identification and characterization of a selective, nonpeptide follicle-stimulating hormone receptor antagonist. *Endocrinology* (2002) 143:3822–9. doi: 10.1210/en.2002-220372

54. van Straten NC, van Berkel TH, Demont DR, Karstens WJ, Merkx R, Oosterom J, et al. Identification of substituted 6-amino-4-phenyltetrahydroquinoline derivatives: potent antagonists for the follicle-stimulating hormone receptor. *J Med Chem.* (2005) 48:1697–700. doi: 10.1021/jm049676l

55. Dias JA, Bonnet B, Weaver BA, Watts J, Kluetzman K, Thomas RM, et al. A negative allosteric modulator demonstrates biased antagonism of the follicle stimulating hormone receptor. *Mol Cell Endocrinol.* (2011) 333:143–50. doi: 10.1016/j.mce.2010.12.023

56. Dias JA, Campo B, Weaver BA, Watts J, Kluetzman K, Thomas RM, et al. Inhibition of follicle-stimulating hormone-induced preovulatory follicles in rats treated with a nonsteroidal negative allosteric modulator of follicle-stimulating hormone receptor. *Biol Reprod.* (2014) 90:19. doi: 10.1095/biolreprod.113.109397

57. Ayoub MA, Yvinec R, Jégot G, Dias JA, Poli SM, Poupon A, et al. Profiling of FSHR negative allosteric modulators on LH/CGR reveals biased antagonism

with implications in steroidogenesis. *Mol Cell Endocrinol.* (2016) 436:10–22. doi: 10.1016/j.mce.2016.07.013

58. Wortmann L, Cleve A, Muhn HP, Langer G, Schrey A, Kuehne R, et al. *Acyltryptophanols for Fertility Control.* patent WO2007017289A2. (2005).

59. Failli A, Heffernan GD, Santilli AA, Quagliato DA, Coghlan RD, Andrae PM, et al. *Pyrrolobenzodiazepine Pyridine Carboxamides and Derivatives as Follicle-Stimulating Hormone Receptor Antagonists.* patent WO2006135687A1. (2005).

60. Coats SJ, Fitzpatrick LJ, Hlasta DJ, Lanter C, Macielag M, Pan K, et al. *Substituted Aminoalkylamide Derivatives as Antagonists of Follicle Stimulating Hormone.* patent US6583179B2. (2003).

61. Cseh S, Solti L. Importance of assisted reproductive technologies in the conservation of wild, rare or indigenous ungulates: review article. *Acta Vet Hung.* (2000) 48:313–23. doi: 10.1556/AVet.48.2000.3.8

62. Swanson WF. Application of assisted reproduction for population management in felids: the potential and reality for conservation of small cats. *Theriogenology* (2006) 66:49–58. doi: 10.1016/j.theriogenology.2006.03.024

63. Comizzoli P, Mermillod P, Mauget R. Reproductive biotechnologies for endangered mammalian species. *Reprod Nutr Dev.* (2000) 40:493–504. doi: 10.1051/rnd:2000113

64. Gerrits MG, Kramer H, el Galta R, van Beerendonk G, Hanssen R, Abd-Elaziz K, et al. Oral follicle-stimulating hormone agonist tested in healthy young women of reproductive age failed to demonstrate effect on follicular development but affected thyroid function. *Fertil Steril.* (2016) 105:1056–62.e4. doi: 10.1016/j.fertnstert.2015.12.017

65. Newton CL, Whay AM, McArdle CA, Zhang M, van Koppen CJ, van de Lagemaat R, et al. Rescue of expression and signaling of human luteinizing hormone G protein-coupled receptor mutants with an allosterically binding small-molecule agonist. *Proc Natl Acad Sci USA.* (2011) 108:7172–6. doi: 10.1073/pnas.1015723108

66. Newton CL, Anderson RC, Katz AA, Millar RP. Loss-of-function mutations in the human luteinizing hormone receptor predominantly cause intracellular retention. *Endocrinology* (2016) 157:4364–77. doi: 10.1210/en.2016-1104

67. Janovick JA, Maya-Núñez G, Ulloa-Aguirre A, Huhtaniemi IT, Dias JA, Verbost P, et al. Increased plasma membrane expression of human follicle-stimulating hormone receptor by a small molecule thienopyr(im)idine. *Mol Cell Endocrinol.* (2009) 298:84–8. doi: 10.1016/j.mce.2008.09.015

68. Zaidi M, New MI, Blair HC, Zallone A, Baliram R, Davies TF, et al. Actions of pituitary hormones beyond traditional targets. *J Endocrinol.* (2018) 237:R83–98. doi: 10.1530/JOE-17-0680

69. Kumar TR. Extragonadal actions of FSH: a critical need for novel genetic models. *Endocrinology* (2018) 159:2–8. doi: 10.1210/en.2017-03118

70. Arslan AA, Zeleniuch-Jacquotte A, Lundin E, Micheli A, Lukanova A, Afanasyeva Y, et al. Serum follicle-stimulating hormone and risk of epithelial ovarian cancer in postmenopausal women. *Cancer Epidemiol Biomarkers Prev.* (2003) 12:1531–5.

71. Zheng W, Lu JJ, Luo F, Zheng Y, Feng Yj, Felix JC, et al. Ovarian epithelial tumor growth promotion by follicle-stimulating hormone and inhibition of the effect by luteinizing hormone. *Gynecol Oncol.* (2000) 76:80–8. doi: 10.1006/gyno.1999.5628

72. Mariani S, Salvatori L, Basciani S, Arizzi M, Franco G, Petrangeli E, et al. Expression and cellular localization of follicle-stimulating hormone receptor in normal human prostate, benign prostatic hyperplasia and prostate cancer. *J Urol.* (2006) 175:2072–7 discussion. doi: 10.1016/S0022-5347(06)00273-4

73. Choi JH, Wong AS, Huang HF, Leung PC. Gonadotropins and ovarian cancer. *Endocr Rev.* (2007) 28:440–61. doi: 10.1210/er.2006-0036

9

The Development of Gonadotropins for Clinical Use in the Treatment of Infertility

Bruno Lunenfeld[1], Wilma Bilger[2], Salvatore Longobardi[3], Veronica Alam[4,5],
Thomas D'Hooghe[3,6,7] and Sesh K. Sunkara[8]*

[1] Faculty of Life Sciences, Bar-Ilan University, Ramat Gan, Israel, [2] Medical Affairs Fertility, Endocrinology and General
Medicine, Merck Serono GmbH, Darmstadt, Germany, [3] Global Medical Affairs Fertility, Merck Healthcare KGaA, Darmstadt,
Germany, [4] Global Clinical Development, EMD Serono, Rockland, MA, United States, [5] A Business of Merck KGaA,
Darmstadt, Germany, [6] Organ Systems, Group Biomedical Sciences, Department of Development and Regeneration, KU
Leuven (University of Leuven), Leuven, Belgium, [7] Department of Obstetrics and Gynecology, Yale University, New Haven, CT,
United States, [8] Assisted Conception Unit, King's College London, Guy's Hospital, London, United Kingdom

*Correspondence:
Bruno Lunenfeld
blunenfeld@gmail.com

The first commercially available gonadotropin product was a human chorionic gonadotropin (hCG) extract, followed by animal pituitary gonadotropin extracts. These extracts were effective, leading to the introduction of the two-step protocol, which involved ovarian stimulation using animal gonadotropins followed by ovulation triggering using hCG. However, ovarian response to animal gonadotropins was maintained for only a short period of time due to immune recognition. This prompted the development of human pituitary gonadotropins; however, supply problems, the risk for Creutzfeld–Jakob disease, and the advent of recombinant technology eventually led to the withdrawal of human pituitary gonadotropin from the market. Urinary human menopausal gonadotropin (hMG) preparations were also produced, with subsequent improvements in purification techniques enabling development of products with standardized proportions of follicle-stimulating hormone (FSH) and luteinizing hormone (LH) activity. In 1962 the first reported pregnancy following ovulation stimulation with hMG and ovulation induction with hCG was described, and this product was later established as part of the standard protocol for ART. Improvements in immunopurification techniques enabled the removal of LH from hMG preparations; however, unidentified urinary protein contaminants remained a problem. Subsequently, monoclonal FSH antibodies were used to produce a highly purified FSH preparation containing <0.1 IU of LH activity and <5% unidentified urinary proteins, enabling the formulation of smaller injection volumes that could be administered subcutaneously rather than intramuscularly. Ongoing issues with gonadotropins derived from urine donations, including batch-to-batch variability and a finite donor supply, were overcome by the development of recombinant gonadotropin products. The first recombinant human FSH molecules received marketing approvals in 1995 (follitropin alfa) and 1996 (follitropin beta). These had superior purity and a more homogenous glycosylation pattern compared with urinary or pituitary FSH. Subsequently recombinant versions of LH and hCG have been developed, and biosimilar versions of follitropin alfa have received marketing authorization. More recent developments include a recombinant FSH produced using a human cell line, and a long-acting FSH preparation. These state of the art products are administered subcutaneously via pen injection devices.

Keywords: recombinant gonadotropin, follicle stimulating hormone, luteinizing hormone, fertility, pregnancy, pre-clinical, clinical

INTRODUCTION

It was observed in 1927, by Ascheim and Zondek, that the blood and urine of pregnant women contained a gonad-stimulating substance, human chorionic gonadotropin (hCG) (1, 2). Seegar-Jones and colleagues demonstrated in the 1940s that hCG was produced by the placenta (3). In 1929, Zondek proposed, based on his experiments and those of Smith, that two hormones were produced by the pituitary gland, both of which stimulated the gonads (4–6). These hormones were described as gonadotropins and subsequently named follicle-stimulating hormone (FSH) and luteinizing hormone (LH), according to their specific actions. The biological activity of gonadotropins suggested that they might be useful for the treatment of patients who were infertile. These observations eventually led to the development of pure gonadotropin products that have enabled the birth of millions of children to people affected by infertility.

This review provides an overview of the major milestones in the development of gonadotropin products (**Figure 1**), as well as issues that may have affected decision making during the development processes, and summarizes the available evidence supporting the use of recombinant gonadotropin products for the treatment of infertility.

HUMAN CHORIONIC GONADOTROPIN

The first commercially available gonadotropin was an hCG extract launched by Organon in 1931 (4). However, the original product was of limited use owing to a lack of reproducibility, in part due to the use of animal units (mouse or rat) to

---

Abbreviations: AMH, anti-Müllerian hormone; ART, assisted reproductive technologies; BMI, body mass index; CHO, Chinese hamster ovary; CI, confidence interval; CLBR, cumulative live birth rate; COS, controlled ovarian stimulation; CPR, clinical pregnancy rate; CTP, carbonyl-terminal peptide; EMA, European Medicine Agency; ESHRE, European Society of Human Reproduction and Embryology; EU, European Union; Fc, Fragment crystallisable; FSH, follicle-stimulating hormone; GnRH, gonadotropin releasing hormone; hCG, human chorionic gonadotropin; HEK, human embryonic kidney; hMG, human menopausal gonadotropin; HPLC, high performance liquid chromatography; ICSH, interstitial cell stimulating hormone; ICSI, intracytoplasmic sperm injection; IgG, immunoglobulin G; IRP, international reference product; IU, international units; IVF, in vitro fertilization; LBR, live birth rate; LH, luteinizing hormone; OHSS, ovarian hyperstimulation syndrome; OPR, ongoing pregnancy rate; OR, odds ratio; PCOS, polycystic ovary syndrome; PD, pharmacodynamics; PK, pharmacokinetics; POR, poor ovarian response; RCT, randomized controlled trial; r-hCG, recombinant human chorionic gonadotropin; r-hFSH, recombinant human follicle-stimulating hormone; r-hLH, recombinant human luteinizing hormone; RR, risk ratio; u-FSH, urinary follicle-stimulating hormone; u-hCG, urinary human chorionic gonadotropin; USA, United States of America; WHO, World Health Organization.

measure bioactivity (7). Reproducibility was greatly improved in 1939 when the League of Nations developed the international standard for hCG; one International Unit (IU) of hCG was defined as the activity contained in 0.1 mg of the reference hCG preparation which was pooled from six sources (8). Following the introduction of this standard, purified hCG preparations extracted from the urine of women during the first half of pregnancy, with bioactivity up to 8,500 IU/mL, became available (9, 10).

Clinical Use

In women, hCG is used during infertility treatment to trigger final follicular maturation and ovulation, as well as for luteal phase support. In men, it is used to stimulate production of testosterone by the Leydig cells in cases of hormone deficiency as well as in male hypogonadism.

ANIMAL PITUITARY GONADOTROPINS

The first animal pituitary gonadotropin was swine pituitary gonadotropin [containing both FSH and LH (11, 12)], followed by hog and sheep pituitary extracts and pregnant mare serum gonadotropin (2, 4, 7, 13). With the availability of both placental and pituitary hormones, the two-step protocol for ovarian stimulation using an animal gonadotropin followed by final maturation and triggering with hCG, was introduced for women in 1941 by Mazer and Ravetz (2, 14). However, owing to their non-human origin, the ovarian response to animal gonadotropins was only maintained in women for a limited duration because of human–animal immune recognition (2, 15).

As a result of the limited clinical value of the animal gonadotropins, human pituitary gonadotropins extracted either post-mortem from human pituitaries or from the urine of postmenopausal women were investigated (2).

CADAVERIC HUMAN PITUITARY GONADOTROPINS

In 1958, Gemzell extracted FSH from pituitaries obtained from human cadavers and reported successful follicle development using this preparation, which was later given to women together with hCG to induce ovulation (16, 17). In 1963, ovarian stimulation with cadaveric human pituitary gonadotropin in hypophysectomised individuals was successfully performed by Bettendorf et al. (7). Owing to their source, these products were produced by several government agencies. Although used successfully for a number of years, these human pituitary

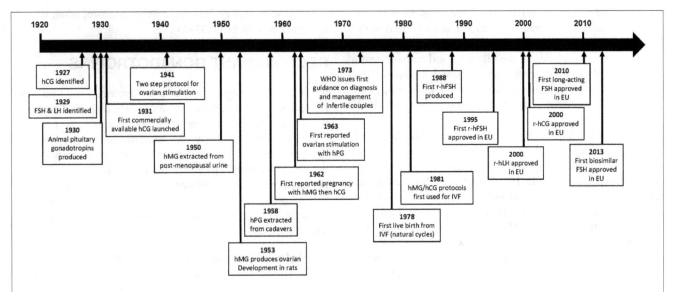

FIGURE 1 | Time line of major events in the development of gonadotropins. CHO, Chinese hamster ovary; FSH, follicle-stimulating hormone; hCG, human chorionic gonadotropin; hMG, human menopausal gonadotropin; LH, luteinizing hormone; r-hCG, recombinant human chorionic gonadotropin; r-hFSH, recombinant human follicle-stimulating hormone; r-hLH, recombinant human luteinizing gonadotropin.

preparations were discontinued in the 1980s because of supply problems and the risk for Creutzfeldt-Jakob disease that resulted from the source of these products (human cadavers) (2, 4, 18–20).

HUMAN MENOPAUSAL GONADOTROPIN

Human menopausal gonadotropin (hMG), which contains two gonadotropin components corresponding to the pituitary-related hormones, FSH and LH, was first successfully extracted from the urine of post-menopausal women in 1950. In 1953 hMG was shown to produce ovarian stimulation in female hypophysectomised infantile rats, and Leydig cell stimulation and full spermatogenesis in male hypophysectomised infantile rats (2, 4, 21). These experiments suggested that hMG would be useful in humans; however, to enable clinical testing, large-scale extraction and purification methods were required, in addition to an agreed standard to enable reproducibility. Furthermore, the starting dose for humans needed to be established. The first hMG preparations were registered by Serono in Italy in 1950, but these were impure in terms of protein content and did not have standardized proportions of FSH and LH. Subsequent preparations contained equal proportions of FSH and LH (for example, Pergonal 75 contained 75 IU FSH and 75 IU LH), in addition to other unwanted urinary proteins (2, 4). Additionally, the bioactivity of the first hMG preparations was measured in "animal" units (mouse or rat); a "rat unit" was the minimum amount of preparation required to induce oestrus in 28-day old female rats ("mouse units" were defined in a similar manner). The bioactivity, therefore, varied depending on the strain of animal used and a uniform standard was required to facilitate clinical use.

The first reference standard for hMG was based upon batches produced by kaolin extraction of menopausal urine (hMG 20, hMG 20a, and hMG 24) and provided by Organon Newhouse

(2, 7). However, by 1959, most of the reference product had been used and further batches could not be provided. At this time, the Serono Institute in Rome offered 50 g of Pergonal 23 (containing equal proportions of FSH and LH) to act as the reference preparation and this material was subsequently used as the International Reference Preparation (IRP) (2, 7, 22). As well as facilitating greater reproducibility in clinical testing, the study of day-to-day variation of gonadotropins and steroid secretion during the normal menstrual cycle and during pregnancy was enabled by the availability of a reference product (2, 4, 7, 23). The aim of these studies was to understand the fundamental variability of gonadotropins in women so that these physiological concepts or patterns could be applied in future clinical tests.

Clinical trials were initiated and, in 1959, hMG (150 U/d for 4 days) was demonstrated to induce the expected, desirable changes in the endometrium and vaginal epithelium (24) and to induce steroid secretion, in women with anovulatory, hypogonadotropic hypopituitary and primary amenorrhea (2, 4, 22, 24–26). This was followed 3 years later by a report from Lunenfeld et al. of the first pregnancy in a patient with hypopituitary hypogonadotropic amenorrhea following ovulation induction with hMG and final oocyte maturation with hCG, no adverse events were reported for this pregnancy (26). This approach subsequently became the standard protocol for ovulation induction treatment of infertility (2, 26, 27).

The World Health Organization (WHO) Expert Committee of Biological Standardization defined, in 1972, the IU for both FSH and LH (then named interstitial cell stimulating hormone [ICSH]) as the respective activities contained in 0.2295 mg of the IRP of hMG (28). The use of IU depends upon determination of the linearity of the bioactivity of the gonadotropin product. The bioactivity of FSH, for example, is determined by the Steelman–Pohley bioassay. This bioassay is based on comparison between the test FSH preparation and the international reference standard (defined by the WHO) of FSH-induced augmentation of ovarian weight in immature female rats co-treated with a high dose of hCG (29). One year later, in 1973, the WHO issued their first guidance on the diagnosis and management of infertile couples, recommending an effective daily dose of 150–225 IU hMG for hypogonadotropic patients (WHO Group I), and 75–150 IU for anovulatory normogonadotropic patients (WHO Group II) (24, 26, 30).

Steptoe and Edwards pioneered *in vitro* fertilization (IVF) procedures using natural cycles, achieving the first live birth in 1978 (31); one pregnancy was reported following 101 attempts (32). However, in 1981, Jones and Jones established hMG/hCG protocols as described by Lunenfeld et al. (26) as the standard approach for ovarian stimulation in assisted reproductive technologies (ART), achieving one pregnancy after three attempts (33, 34). These protocols were later revised when the outcome of ovarian stimulation in ART treatment changed from mono-follicular to multi-follicular development (4).

Improvements in purification techniques enabled the development of an hMG preparation with fewer impurities. However, these extraction steps also removed LH activity (22) and hCG had to be added to re-establish the FSH:LH ratio, resulting in highly purified hMG containing approximately 30% identified impurities that varied from batch to batch (2). Polyclonal immunopurification techniques also resulted in an FSH preparation devoid of LH activity (35). However, this preparation still contained many unwanted urinary proteins. The development of monoclonal FSH antibodies to replace the polyclonal antibodies allowed greater purification of urinary products resulting in a highly purified FSH preparation (Metrodin HP [EU]; Fertinex [USA]; highly purified urofollitropin) containing about 9000 IU of FSH per mg of protein, <0.1 IU LH activity and <5% unidentified urinary proteins. This enabled the formulation of smaller injection volumes and subcutaneous, rather than intramuscular, administration (2). The currently available hMG preparations are considered safe with the most common adverse events, as reported by clinical trials, being ovarian hyperstimulation, abdominal pain, headache, enlarged abdomen, inflammation at the injection site, pain at the injection site and nausea; the incidence rate of these events was 2–7% (36).

Despite these advances in the preparation of urinary gonadotropin products, supplies were limited owing to the finite donor supply, and batch-to-batch variability was an issue because of the source (2). These issues were overcome by the development of recombinant human FSH (r-hFSH) and subsequently recombinant human LH (r-hLH) and hCG (r-hCG) (2).

Clinical Use

hMG is approved for development of a single Graafian follicle in women with anovulation and multifollicular development in women undergoing controlled ovarian hyperstimulation as part of ART treatment. hMG has also been demonstrated to be effective for the induction or restoration of secondary sexual development and fertility due to androgen deficiency

in males with hypogonadotropic hypogonadism, when used in combination with hCG (37–39).

RECOMBINANT GONADOTROPINS

Recombinant biological products are proteins produced using recombinant DNA technology that utilize biological processes to produce large molecule drugs that cannot be produced using synthetic chemistry. Recombinant gonadotropins were developed to avoid the limitations inherent to the earlier urine-derived gonadotropin products, since recombinant products can be produced in large volumes with high purity and without variability in composition. As with hMG, the recombinant products can be used for the treatment of both male and female infertility.

Follicle-Stimulating Hormone

There are currently three r-hFSH products on the market: follitropin alfa, follitropin beta, and follitropin delta. A fourth product, follitropin epsilon, has been reported as being in development (40). Follitropin alfa and follitropin beta are produced in Chinese hamster ovary (CHO) cell lines, whereas follitropin delta is produced in human fetal retinal cells; all these r-hFSH products have an amino acid sequence identical to that of endogenous human FSH. FSH has a relatively short biological half-life of about 1 day (40), necessitating daily administration. There has therefore been interest in long-acting formulations, and one such product is available, the long-acting r-hFSH analog corifollitropin alfa [elimination half-life: corifollitropin alfa, 70 (59–82) hours (41); follitropin alfa, terminal elimination half-life 24 h (42)].

Follitropin Alfa and Follitropin Beta

The originator follitropin alfa (GONAL-f; Merck KGaA, Darmstadt, Germany) was first produced by Serono (a predecessor company of Merck KGaA) in 1988 and received a marketing license for clinical use in both women and men in the EU in 1995 (40) and in the USA in 2004 (42). Subsequently, two biosimilar versions of follitropin alfa have become available, for use in both women and men, Ovaleap (Teva B.V., Haarlem, the Netherlands), which received marketing authorization in Europe in 2013 (43), and Bemfola (Afolia, Finox Biotech AG, Balzers, Liechtenstein), which received marketing authorization in Europe in 2014 (44). The biosimilars are not currently approved in the USA. The safety profile of the biosimilar follitropin alfa preparations is similar to that of the originator product (43, 44). Follitropin beta (Puregon; Merck & Co., Kenilworth, NJ) received marketing authorization in Europe in 1996 and in the USA (Follistim AQ) in 2004 (45, 46). The risk/benefit balance of follitropins alfa and beta are considered positive, with the main adverse events reported being headache, ovarian cysts, local injection site reactions (e.g., pain, erythema, hematoma, swelling, and/or irritation at the site of injection) and mild or moderate OHSS (40, 43, 44).

Although both follitropin alfa and follitropin beta are produced in CHO cells, the vectors used for gene expression differ. Follitropin alfa is produced in CHO cell lines that have been transfected with separate expression vectors for the α- and β-FSH genes, the master cell cultures having been selected to co-amplify both genes (47), whereas follitropin beta (Puregon) is produced in CHO cell lines transfected with a single expression vector containing both α- and β-FSH genes (48). Culture processes also differ, in that large-scale culture of follitropin alfa occurs in a bioreactor, followed by purification of the culture supernatant by an ultrafiltration step and five chromatographic steps, with the main chromatographic purification step achieved through immunoaffinity (using a murine-derived anti-FSH monoclonal antibody) (47). Following large-scale culture of follitropin beta, r-hFSH is isolated from culture supernatant by a series of chromatographic steps including anion and cation exchange chromatography, hydrophobic interaction chromatography and size exclusion chromatography (48).

Owing to differences in the production and purification of follitropin alfa and follitropin beta there are differences in their glycosylation, and they have different sialic acid residue compositions and isoelectric coefficients. The isoelectric point band (pI) for follitropin alfa is narrower than that of follitropin beta (4–5 and 3.5–5.5, respectively), furthermore, follitropin alfa contains fewer isoforms with a pI <4 (9 and <24%, respectively) (49). These variations result in follitropin alfa being slightly more acidic and follitropin beta more basic, which influences their metabolic clearance, half-life (**Table 1**), and biological activity (48, 49, 54). The variance in mean specific FSH activity between follitropin alfa and follitropin beta (13,645 and 7,000–10,000 U/mg protein, respectively) affects the amount of protein required per injection (55). Follitropin alfa was originally dosed in IU based on its bioactivity in the Steelman-Pohley assay. However, owing to the consistency of the preparation it was possible to determine its specific activity, which is the ratio of the bioactivity (IU) to the protein content (mg, determined by size exclusion HPLC). Follitropin alfa can therefore be provided in injection devices filled-by-mass, which resulted in more consist ovarian response and reduced cycle cancelation rate, intra-cycle dose adjustment and repetitive monitoring (56, 57).

Despite the disparities between follitropin alfa and follitropin beta, results of head-to-head clinical studies and retrospective studies comparing the two products for ovarian stimulation in women undergoing IVF have shown no significant differences between the preparations in terms of efficacy or safety (58–61). In the largest randomized prospective comparison, conducted in 172 women treated with follitropin alfa and 172 women treated with follitropin beta, a dose of 150 IU/day resulted in 13.0 and 12.4 oocytes obtained with each treatment (primary outcome), respectively, whereas at a dose of 300 IU/day, numbers were 6.1 and 7.1, respectively (60). Clinical pregnancy rates (secondary outcome) were similar with both preparations; 33.5% per cycle and 37.4% per embryo transfer with follitropin alfa 150 IU/day and 32.9% per cycle and 36.4% per embryo transfer with follitropin beta 150 IU/day (60).

The two biosimilar follitropin alfa products (Ovaleap and Bemfola) are considered to be similar to the reference product, GONAL-f; however, as a result of post-translational modifications, their structures are not identical. This is the result of differences in the processes used for their production and purification, including the cell line (despite all being produced using CHO cells) (43, 44). Specifically, differences in glycosylation were observed between the biosimilars and GONAL-f, with Bemfola showing higher antennarity, higher sialylation and higher batch-to-batch variability in activity compared with GONAL-f (62), whereas Ovaleap has a higher amount of the sialic acid N-glycolyl neuraminic acid compared with GONAL-f (63). For both biosimilars, the differences compared with GONAL-f were considered by regulatory agencies as minor and acceptable. Furthermore, a recent report on validation procedures for the Ovaleap manufacturing process showed the processes to be both robust and consistent, and that the resulting r-hFSH had similar characteristics to GONAL-f when molecular mass, primary structure, secondary structure, biological activity and product-related impurities were considered (64). Nevertheless, the observed differences may have a biological impact, including on FSH receptor activation, which has generated discussion regarding the potential clinical impact of these differences, particularly in "non-ideal" patients (i.e., older, poor or suboptimal responders or with worse prognosis factors), as by their nature there is always variation in biologics (65).

EMA guidelines recommend that, to determine clinical comparability, the efficacy of the reference and the similar biologic should be assessed in a randomized, parallel-group clinical trial, with number of oocytes retrieved as the primary endpoint, and ovarian hyperstimulation syndrome (OHSS) as an adverse reaction of special interest (66). Both Bemfola and Ovaleap have demonstrated equivalence to GONAL-f in terms of the number of oocytes retrieved (primary outcome) in women receiving ART (67, 68). Other outcomes (secondary outcomes), including pregnancy and live birth rate (LBR), have been reported as comparable to, or not statistically significantly different from, the originator product (GONAL-f) (69, 70).

A *post-hoc* pooled analysis of data obtained from randomized controlled trials (RCTs) indicated that treatment with GONAL-f is associated with a higher LBR ($p = 0.037$; primary endpoint) and lower OHSS ($p = 0.011$; secondary endpoint) than treatment with the biosimilars (Bemfola or Ovaleap) (69). However, further meta-analysis of data obtained from RCTs, ongoing post marketing real-world data studies and pharmacovigilance data concerning the use of these biosimilars are needed to ensure comparable clinical efficacy of these therapies to the originator in clinical practice.

Follitropin Delta

Follitropin delta (Rekovelle; Ferring Pharmaceuticals, St. Prex, Switzerland) is produced using a human cell line, PER.C6 human fetal retinal cells, and received a marketing license in Europe in 2016 (51). It has a different glycosylation pattern from both follitropin alfa and follitropin beta (71). Follitropin delta has a higher proportion of tri- and tetra-sialylated glycans than follitropin alfa and also has both α2,3- and α2,6-linked sialic acid whereas follitropin alfa only has α2,3-linked sialic acid (72). *In vitro*, follitropin delta was observed to be equivalent to follitropin alfa in a cell-free FSH-receptor binding assay and in transfected

TABLE 1 | Pharmacokinetics of a single dose of subcutaneous follitropin alfa 150 IU, follitropin beta 150 IU, follitropin delta (individualized dose), follitropin epsilon 150 IU and corifollitropin alfa in healthy women (46, 50–53).

Mean value	Follitropin alfa	Follitropin beta	Follitropin delta	Follitropin epsilon	Corifollitropin alfa
C_{max}	3 IU/L	8 IU/L	_[a]	5.2 IU/L	4.2 ng/mL
t_{max} (h)	16	12	10	22	44
Bioavailability (%)	74	77	64	–	58
$t_{1/2\beta}$ (h)	37	40[b] (IM)	40	29	70
CL (L/h)	0.6[c]	0.01[d]	0.6	–	0.13

[a]Value not reported but specified as being 1.4-fold higher than that of follitropin alfa (GONAL-f).
[b]Measured after intramuscular administration.
[c]Measured after intravenous administration.
[d]Units are l/h/kg.
CL, clearance; C_{max}, maximum plasma concentration; h, hours; $t_{1/2\beta}$, terminal elimination half-life; t_{max}, time to C_{max}.

Human Embryonic Kidney (HEK) 293 cells and cultured human granulosa cells (73). The differing pharmacokinetic (PK) and pharmacodynamic (PD) profiles of follitropin alfa and follitropin delta are likely to contribute to the observed differences in the properties of the two products in women, as well as to influence their efficacy for the treatment of infertility (71). In contrast with follitropin alfa, the bioactivity of follitropin delta determined by the Steelman-Pohley bioassay, which uses an international reference standard of CHO-produced r-hFSH, does not directly predict the PD activity (71). This has been attributed to more rapid clearance of follitropin delta compared with follitropin alfa in rats, resulting in lower apparent potency (73). This means that follitropin delta cannot be dosed according to bioactivity or specific bioactivity, as other follitropins are, and is instead dosed by mass (µg). Additionally, the pharmacological differences between follitropin delta and follitropin alfa suggest that these agents cannot be directly substituted in clinical practice.

The risk/benefit balance of follitropin delta was considered positive by the regulatory agencies and the most frequent adverse reactions reported during clinical trials were headache, pelvic discomfort, OHSS, pelvic pain, nausea, adnexa uteri pain and fatigue (51). In healthy female volunteers, follitropin delta demonstrated higher exposure and lower serum clearance compared with follitropin alfa (72). A phase 3 study (ESTHER-1) compared individualized doses of follitropin delta (fixed-dose throughout treatment; start dose individualized based on BMI and body weight) with follitropin alfa (starting dose of 150 IU, with potential for subsequent adjustment, with a maximum allowed daily dose of 450 IU) for ovarian stimulation in 1,326 women. The starting dose of follitropin delta was 12 µg in patients with AMH <15 pmol/L and 0.10–0.19 µg/kg (maximum daily dose: 12 µg) in patients with AMH ≥15 pmol/L. This study demonstrated non-inferiority of follitropin delta to follitropin alfa for the co-primary endpoints of ongoing pregnancy rate (30.7 and 31.6%, respectively; difference −0.9% [95% confidence interval (CI) −5.9, 4.1%]) and ongoing implantation rate (35.2% and 35.8%, respectively; difference −0.6% [95% CI −6.1, 4.8%]), with fewer women treated with follitropin delta requiring OHSS preventative measures (74). The live birth rate was also similar with follitropin alfa and follitropin delta (29.8 and 30.7%, respectively; difference −0.9% [95% CI −5.8, 4.0%]). However,

the initial follitropin alfa dose allowed in this study (150 IU) was at the lower end of the recommended range in the SmPC for women undergoing multifollicular development prior to ART (150–225 IU daily) (42) and this starting dose could not be individualized, whereas the dose in the follitropin delta arm was individualized according to clinical markers which reduces the comparability of outcomes (75). The EMA assessment report states that, in the ESTHER-1 trial, the non-inferiority of follitropin delta compared with follitropin alfa for ongoing pregnancy can be explained by the heterogeneity of responses in different age groups; non-inferiority was driven by the 15% of the study population aged ≥38 years (75), with non-inferiority not demonstrated for women aged ≤37. It has also been noted that there were a greater number of canceled cycles for poor response in the follitropin delta arm (76).

Follitropin Epsilon

Follitropin epsilon (FSH-GEX; Glycotope, Germany) is a recombinant FSH produced using a human blood cell line derived from a myeloid leukemia cell line and is currently not marketed (77). The cell lines used result in a high degree of bisecting N-acetlyglucosamine, a high antennarity and a high degree of sialylation, in particular after enrichment of the acidic isoforms (78). In addition, follitropin epsilon is highly fucosylated and has a ratio of 2,3 to 2,6 sialylation of about 1:1 (78). This is different from follitropin alfa and follitropin beta, which do not have any bisecting N-acetylgalactosamines or 2,6 sialylation. In phase 1 studies, follitropin epsilon and follitropin alfa had similar PK (**Table 1**), whereas PD activity (follicle growth and serum inhibin B levels) was increased with follitropin epsilon compared with follitropin alfa (77). No Phase III studies have been registered in publicly-available clinical trial repositories for this product.

Corifollitropin Alfa

Due to its short half-life FSH has to be injected daily, which may be inconvenient and an unacceptable burden to patients; longer-acting r-hFSH preparations are, therefore, being investigated (79). The only approved longer acting r-hFSH (FSH-CTP, corifollitropin alfa, Elonva; Merck Sharp Dohme, Kenilworth, NJ, USA) was developed via addition of the carbonyl-terminal peptide (CTP) of the β-subunit of hCG to the β-subunit of FSH, generating a chimeric protein. This prolonged the half-life of the r-hFSH without impacting on assembly with the α-subunit, or the secretion or action of the dimer (50, 80). Corifollitropin alfa received marketing approval in the EU in 2010 for use in women undergoing fertility treatment, it is currently not approved for use in men or in the USA (41). The risk/benefit balance of corifollitropin alfa is considered positive, with the most frequently reported adverse reactions during clinical trials being pelvic discomfort, OHSS, headache, pelvic pain, nausea, fatigue and breast tenderness. Corifollitropin alfa can be administered as a single subcutaneous injection to replace the first 7 days of daily FSH therapy, simplifying treatment, as it has a 2-fold longer half-life and almost four-fold longer time to peak serum level than other available FSH preparations (**Table 1**) (81, 82). Meta-analyses of RCTs comparing corifollitropin alfa and daily injections of r-hFSH in women receiving ART treatment found no significant differences in LBR, ongoing pregnancy rate (OPR) or clinical pregnancy rate (CPR) between the treatments (79, 83, 84). There was evidence of reduced LBR (co-primary endpoint) in women receiving a low dose (60 to 120 μg) of long-acting FSH compared with daily FSH (79). There was no significant increase in OHSS, however, a higher number of oocytes were stimulated with corifollitropin alfa than with r-hFSH, and there was higher cycle cancellation due to overstimulation with corifollitropin alfa (79, 83, 84). Further research is needed to determine whether long-acting FSH is safe and effective for use in hyper-responders and poor ovarian responders and in women with all causes of subfertility (79).

Other methods for prolonging the half-life of FSH have been attempted. These include increasing elimination time by adding the Fc domain of IgG to the FSH molecule (85, 86), addition of new glycosylation sites and N-terminal extensions, which result in larger molecules with increased charge (87) and tethering two copies of the N-linked glycosylation signal sequence between the α- and β-subunits of hFSH, creating a single-chain fusion hormone analog (88).

Differences Between Recombinant and Urinary Follicle-Stimulating Hormone Preparations

Two systematic reviews have compared r-hFSH (any preparation) with urinary gonadotropins (89, 90). The first compared r-hFSH with urinary gonadotropins (hMG, purified urinary FSH [u-FSH] or highly-purified u-FSH) in women undergoing ART, and included 42 trials (9,606 patients); there was no significant difference in LBR (28 trials [7,339 patients]; odds ratio [OR] 0.97, 95% CI 0.87, 1.08) or OHSS incidence (32 trials [7,740 patients]; OR 1.18, 95% CI 0.86, 1.61) between the two types of FSH preparation (89). When only fresh cycles were considered the difference in LBR (25 trials [4,952 patients]; odds ratio [OR] 0.97, 95% CI 0.85, 1.11) remained (89). Similarly, in a comparison of r-hFSH with urinary gonadotropins (hMG or u-FSH) for ovulation induction in patients with polycystic ovary syndrome (PCOS), there was no difference in LBR (co-primary endpoint; five trials [505 patients]; OR 1.21, 95% CI 0.83, 1.78) or

CPR (secondary endpoint; eight trials [1,330 patients]; OR 1.05, 95% CI 0.88, 1.27) with the two FSH preparations (90). There was also no difference in the incidence of OHSS (co-primary endpoint) between r-hFSH and u-FSH (10 trials [1,565 patients]; OR 1.52, 95% CI 0.81, 2.84) or between r-hFSH and hMG (two trials [52 patients]; OR 9.95, 95% CI 0.47, 210.19) (90). Although authors of both reviews concluded that there was likely to be little if any clinical difference between r-hFSH and urinary gonadotropins (89, 90), authors of the latter review considered the available evidence to be of low or very low quality (90).

These results are in general agreement with those of a meta-analysis that compared r-hFSH with highly-purified hMG in ART using data from a total of 16 studies (4,040 patients) (91). When adjusted for baseline conditions, hMG treatment was associated with fewer oocytes (primary endpoint; −2.10, 95% CI −2.83, −1.36) and a higher required dose (secondary endpoint; mean difference 235 IU, 95% CI: 16.62, 454.30) but a similar pregnancy rate (secondary endpoint; risk ratio [RR] 1.10, 95% CI 0.97, 1.25) (91).

These meta-analyses predominantly included fresh cycles, for example, the meta-analysis by van Wely et al. only included three trials that studied frozen-thawed embryo transfer in addition to fresh embryo transfer (89). This is because, for many years, IVF success was measured per fresh cycle or embryo transfer. As freezing and thawing technology has improved, this definition has been challenged and it has been suggested that IVF success should instead be evaluated as cumulative live birth rates (CLBR), defined as the first live birth following the use of all fresh and frozen embryos derived from a single ovarian stimulation cycle (92, 93). A positive correlation has been observed between live birth rate per cycle and number of oocytes retrieved, up to 15 oocytes ($p < 0.001$ for comparison between age groups) (94–97). When the association between CLBR and number of oocytes was evaluated, the association remained (98–100). For example, in an analysis by Polyzos et al. the OR (95% CI) for live birth in the second and third cycle was 1.18 (1.07–1.30) for women with 4–9 aspirated oocytes in the first cycle, 1.41 (1.27–1.57) for women with 10–15 aspirated oocytes and 1.63 (1.42–1.88) for women with more than 15 aspirated oocytes compared with patients with 0–3 aspirated oocytes. In several studies a greater number of oocytes were retrieved when r-hFSH rather than urinary gonadotropins were used (101). This suggests that owing to the higher number of oocytes retrieved with r-hFSH compared with urinary gonadotropins, CLBR might be higher when r-hFSH is used.

In clinical trials comparing originator follitropin alfa (GONAL-f) with highly-purified u-FSH (Metrodin HP) in women undergoing ART, the mean number of oocytes obtained with r-hFSH was significantly higher than that obtained with u-FSH (102, 103). There was no difference in CPR (secondary endpoint; 45 and 48%, respectively) (102) or LBR (secondary endpoint; 36 and 36%, respectively) (103), but singleton pregnancies were more common with u-FSH (102, 103). When follitropin beta (Puregon) and highly-purified u-FSH (Metrodin HP) were compared in women undergoing IVF, the mean number of oocytes (primary endpoint; 9.7 vs. 8.9; 95% CI for the difference: −1.7, 3.2) and CPRs did not differ significantly between treatment groups (secondary endpoints; per attempt, 35.4 vs. 26.6%, respectively [95% CI for the difference: −12.1, 29.6]; per transfer, 40.8 vs. 28.6%, respectively [95% CI for the difference: −10.3, 34.8]) (104).

r-hFSH for the Treatment of Male Infertility

FSH plays an important role in spermatogenesis, stimulating the Sertoli cells to facilitate germ cell differentiation. Follitropin alfa and follitropin beta are approved for clinical use in males who have congenital or acquired hypogonadotropic hypogonadism, for the stimulation of spermatogenesis with concomitant hCG therapy (42, 46). In a small study ($N = 8$), r-hFSH (follitropin alfa) was observed to induce testicular growth, spermatogenesis and fertility, with acceptable tolerability, in men with gonadotropin deficiency; the magnitude of effect was considered to be similar to that achieved historically with u-FSH when used to restore normal fertility in men with gonadotropin deficiency (105). In a second larger study, 15 of 19 men treated with r-hFSH and hCG achieved spermatogenesis (106). A Cochrane review evaluating gonadotropins for idiopathic male factor subfertility, identified six RCTs including 456 patients, and observed a higher spontaneous pregnancy rate per couple with gonadotropin treatment compared with placebo/no treatment (five studies [412 patients]; OR 4.94, 95% CI 2.13, 11.44) (107). This review noted that reporting of adverse event data was sparse. However, the risk/benefit balance in males is considered positive (40).

Human Chorionic Gonadotropin

Recombinant hCG (r-hCG) is produced in a CHO cell line in a similar manner to r-hFSH (55, 108) and is suitable for subcutaneous injection and self-administration (109). In healthy subjects, the PK (**Table 2**) and PD profiles of r-hCG are consistent with endogenous hCG physiology and similar to those seen with urinary hCG (u-hCG) (111). The elimination half-lives of r-hCG and u-hCG are comparable (29–30 h for r-hCG 250 μg vs. 35 h for u-hCG 5000 IU) as are the areas under the concentration-time curve; however, u-hCG tends to be distributed and eliminated slightly slower than r-hCG (111).

In the late 1990s, Duffy et al. observed that r-hCG and u-hCG were equally effective for stimulating steroidogenic and peptidergic activities of the corpus luteum during simulated early pregnancy in rhesus monkeys (112). The equipotency of r-hCG and u-hCG was also demonstrated in macaque monkeys, with the numbers of oocytes resuming meiosis and undergoing IVF being similar in animals treated with either the recombinant or urinary product (113). However, the bioactivity of r-hCG was greater than that of u-hCG, when administered at the same dose (measured in IU), as determined by a mouse Leydig cell bioassay validated for macaque serum ($p < 0.05$) (113). Subsequently, in 2001, r-hCG (choriogonadotropin alfa, Ovitrelle; Merck KGaA, Darmstadt, Germany) was licensed for clinical use as a trigger for final follicular maturation/ovulation and luteinisation after stimulation of follicular growth (109).

Three randomized, double-blind, double-dummy, parallel-group, multicentre trials have confirmed the similar efficacy of

TABLE 2 | Pharmacokinetics of a single dose of subcutaneous choriogonadotropin alfa (r-hCG; dose and population not reported) and lutropin alfa (r-hLH) 75 IU to 40,000 IU in female volunteers (109, 110).

Mean value	r-hCG	r-hLH
Bioavailability (%)	40	60
$t_{1/2\beta}$ (h)	30	≈10–12
CL (L/h)	0.2[a]	2

[a] Measured after intravenous administration.

CL, clearance, C_{max}, maximum plasma concentration; h, hours; $t_{1/2\beta}$, terminal elimination half-life; t_{max}, time to C_{max}.

r-hCG and u-hCG. In one, there were no observed differences following treatment with r-hCG or u-hCG in the number of oocytes retrieved (primary endpoint; mean ± standard deviation [SD] 10.8 ± 4.5 vs. 10.3 ± 5.1) or the number of patients pregnant (secondary endpoint; 10 in each group) and adverse events were generally mild or moderate among the 84 women undergoing IVF or intracytoplasmic sperm injection (ICSI) and embryo transfer (114). Similarly, a multinational study in anovulatory or oligo-ovulatory patients showed that r-hCG administration resulted in the same rates of ovulation and pregnancy as u-hCG administration (115). Overall, 162 of the 177 patients (91.5%) in the per protocol population ovulated (primary endpoint): 95.3% receiving r-hCG and 88.0% receiving u-hCG; however, in this study, r-hCG was better tolerated than u-hCG (115). The European Recombinant Human Chorionic Gonadotropin Study Group compared the efficacy and safety of r-hCG and u-hCG for inducing final follicular maturation and early luteinisation in 172 evaluable women undergoing ovulation induction for ART (116). The primary endpoint, the mean number of oocytes retrieved per patient was not significant between treatments (11.6 for r-HCG and 10.6 for u-hCG; two-sided 90% CI for the difference: −0.841, 1.515). Patients treated with r-hCG demonstrated better outcomes for number of mature oocytes (9.4 and 7.1 with r-hCG and u-hCG, respectively; $p = 0.027$), serum progesterone (day 1 post hCG administration: 30.1 vs. 23.3 nmol/L [$p = 0.04$]; day 6–7 post hCG administration: 391.9 vs. 315.9 nmol/L [$p = 0.03$]) and hCG (day of embryo transfer: 2.1 μg/L vs. 1.6 μg/L [$p = 0.0001$]) levels, CPR (32 [33.0%] and 23 [24.7%] with r-hCG, and u-hCG, respectively), and LBR (26 [26.8%] and 21 [22.6%] with r-hCG and u-hCG, respectively). While both treatments were well tolerated, the incidence of adverse events was significantly higher in patients treated with u-hCG. Injection site reactions being the most common adverse events in with both treatments in these latter two studies (115, 116). Investigators concluded, that for triggering ovulation, r-hCG may have significant advantages over u-hCG (116).

Treatment with r-hCG and u-hCG was also shown to result in similar numbers of oocytes (primary endpoint) and 2PN oocytes (secondary endpoint) obtained in a prospective, open, randomized study in 275 women requiring induction of final follicular maturation and luteinisation for IVF with embryo transfer (117). In this study, the tolerability of r-hCG and u-hCG was similar, with >95% of injections with either hCG producing no adverse reactions. More recently, Bellavia et al.

reported that highly purified u-hCG was not inferior to r-hCG with regard to the mean number of oocytes retrieved (13.3 vs. 12.5), with no differences observed in fertilization rate (57.3% [467/815] vs. 61.3% [482/787]) or tolerability between the hCG preparations (118).

Luteinizing Hormone

Recombinant human luteinizing hormone (r-hLH, lutropin alfa, Luveris; Merck KGaA, Darmstadt, Germany) received marketing authorization for clinical use in 2000 in Europe and 2004 in the US (subsequently withdrawn at Merck KGaA's request in 2016) (110). r-hLH is produced in a similar manner to FSH in CHO cells transfected with vectors encoding the α and β subunits (119), and is suitable for subcutaneous injection and self-administration (110). The PK of r-hLH is almost identical to the LH component of hMG (Pergonal; Laboratoires Serono, Aubonne, Switzerland) with a terminal half-life of ~10–12 h (**Table 2**) (120). It should be highlighted that at the time of this analysis the LH component of hMG preparations was predominantly the LH component of post-menopausal urine, rather than hCG as is more common in later and currently available more highly purified preparations. r-hLH is approved for use in women with severe LH and FSH deficiency, in combination with r-hFSH (121). In specific countries outside Europe (Russia, Mexico) r-hLH is also approved for patients with suboptimal ovarian response in the context of ART treatment (122). To improve convenience, a 2:1 fixed-ratio combination of r-hFSH and r-hLH has also been developed (Pergoveris; Merck KGaA, Darmstadt, Germany), which received marketing approval in Europe in 2007 (123). Pergoveris is not currently approved in the US.

In women with severe FSH and LH deficiency, r-hLH has been shown to support r-hFSH-induced follicular development (124, 125). In an open-label, dose-finding study, in which women with hypogonadotropic hypogonadism were randomized to receive r-hLH in combination with r-hFSH 150 IU, 0, 14.3, 66.7, and 88.0% of women treated with r-hLH 0 IU ($n = 8$), 25 IU ($n = 7$), 75 IU ($n = 9$) and 225 IU ($n = 10$), respectively, had good or excessive follicular growth ($p < 0.01$ by Cochran-Armitage trend test for difference between groups) (125). This study demonstrated that although LH requirements varied, a minimum effective daily dose of 75 IU provides adequate follicular development and steroidogenesis. A second study confirmed that r-hFSH 150 IU plus r-hLH 75 IU is the most appropriate dose schedule for hypogonadotropic anovulatory women, with sufficient follicular growth observed in 94% (79/84) of initiated cycles (five cycles in three patients required a dose increase) and pregnancy achieved by 15 of the 38 treated women (39.5%) (126). A study in 169 women aged 38–42 years randomized to receive a combination of r-hFSH:r-hLH in one of four ratios: 1:0, 1:1, 2:1, or 3:1 (127). The starting dose of r-hFSH was 225 IU, with r-hLH dosed according to the ratio, and the dose of r-hFSH could be adjusted up to 450 IU. A greater mean number of oocytes was retrieved in the group receiving 2:1 r-hFSH:r-hLH compared with those receiving 1:1 and 3:1 r-hFSH:r-hLH (8.4, 7.4, and 7.5, respectively), and the adjusted clinical pregnancy rate was higher in the groups receiving 3:1 or 2:1 r-hFSH:r-hLH (12.2

and 12.0%, respectively) compared with those receiving 1:0 and 1:1 r-hFSH:r-hLH (4.6 and 2.4%, respectively).The 2:1 fixed-ratio is supported by the dose-finding and confirmatory studies in women with hypogonadotropic hypogonadism, as well as the ART study summarized here.

The ESPART study was an RCT evaluating the effect of fixed-ratio (2:1) combination r-hFSH:r-hLH compared with r-hFSH alone for controlled ovarian stimulation in 939 women with POR (128, 129). In the ESPART study, to be defined as having POR, women had to meet at least two of the following criteria: advanced maternal age (≥40–<41 years); a previous ART cycle with ≤3 oocytes retrieved with a conventional stimulation protocol; an abnormal ovarian reserve test characterized by an AMH level between 0.12 and 1.3 ng/ml, inclusive. There were no differences observed in efficacy outcomes (number of oocytes retrieved [primary endpoint]; biochemical pregnancy rate, CPR, OPR; and LBR) between patients receiving r-hFSH/r-hLH and those receiving r-hFSH alone. However, a *post-hoc* analysis of the ESPART study observed a higher live birth rate with r-hLH supplementation in patients with moderate or severe POR, while a higher live birth rate was observed with r-hFSH alone in patients with mild POR (130).

Five recent meta-analyses have evaluated whether supplementation of FSH with LH for controlled ovarian stimulation (COS) might improve ART outcomes (131–135). While LBR is the preferred outcome, reality has shown that LBR is only reported in a small proportion of available studies, and most papers report intermediate pregnancy outcomes (such as CPR or OPR), representing relevant outcomes to measure clinical treatments benefits in reproductive medicine when pregnancy losses are not impacted (136–139). These meta-analyses have reported some conflicting results, despite there being overlap among the studies included.

These meta-analyses have relied on RCTs conducted in the general population, and either suggest that there is no beneficial effect from LH supplementation or that LH supplementation to FSH results in improvements in some outcomes in these patients. A higher number of oocytes were retrieved without LH supplementation (primary endpoint; 29 studies [5,840 patients] standard mean difference −0.20, 95% CI −0.38, −0.02; $p = 0.03$) in one meta-analysis (135), whereas no difference in this endpoint was observed in another meta-analysis (primary endpoint; 43 studies [6,341 patients]; RR 1.17, 95% CI 0.42, 1.92; $p = 0.002$) (133). A higher pregnancy rate (secondary endpoint; 29 studies [5,565 patients] OR 1.20, 95% CI 1.06, 1.37) was observed by one meta-analysis (135), whereas in other meta-analyses a higher CPR (secondary endpoint; 43 studies [6,393 patients]; RR 1.3, 95% CI 1.05, 1.62; $p = 0.016$) (133), higher OPR (secondary endpoint: 19 studies [3,129 patients] OR 1.20, 95% CI 1.01, 1.42) (134) and higher LBR (primary endpoint: 4 studies [499 patients] OR 1.32, 95% CI 0.85, 2.06; secondary endpoint: 39 studies [6,237 patients] RR 1.11, 95% CI 1.01, 1.21) (133, 134) were observed with LH supplementation to FSH compared with FSH alone. These findings may reflect the different characteristics of the pooled populations, depending on the trials included.

It has been suggested that the benefits of LH supplementation may occur in subpopulations characterized by LH insufficiency, including hypo–responders (133, 134). Hypo-response is characterized by an unexpected resistance to ovarian stimulation with standard doses of gonadotropins. This resistance might be diagnosed in women with otherwise normal ovarian reserve during ovarian stimulation who demonstrate an initial slow response and observed through serum estradiol levels and follicular growth or diagnosed retrospectively where higher-than-expected gonadotropin doses have been used (140). In patients with poor ovarian response (POR; including hypo-responders), supplementation with LH results in increased CPR (*post-hoc* analysis: RR 1.3, 95% CI 1.05, 1.62; p=0.016) (133), OPR (subgroup analysis: 3 trials [79 patients] OR 2.06, 95% CI 1.20, 3.53) (134) and LBR (*post-hoc* analysis: RR 1.30, 95% CI 0.95, 1.78) (133).

When only hypo-responders were considered, supplementation with LH did not increase the number of oocytes retrieved (two RCTs and one cohort study [319 patients] OR 1.98, 95% CI 0.17, 3.80; $p = 0.03$), but did increase implantation rate (four RCTS and one cohort study [766 patients] OR 2.62, 95% CI 1.37, 4.99; $p = 0.004$), and CPR (three RCTs and one cohort study [361 patients] OR 2.03, 95% CI 1.27, 3.25; $p = 0.003$) (132) compared with FSH alone. LBR could not be evaluated by this meta-analysis as it was only included as an endpoint in one study (132).

A systematic review (without meta-analysis) that assessed the effect of r-hLH supplementation in COS as part of ART in six different patient populations (prevention of OHSS; women with profoundly suppressed LH levels after administration of a gonadotropin-releasing hormone [GnRH] agonist; women co-treated with a GnRH antagonist; women with a hypo-response to r-hFSH; women of advanced reproductive age; and women with POR, including women meeting the ESHRE Bologna criteria) identified two populations that may benefit from this treatment approach (131). In women with a hypo-response to r-hFSH the evaluated literature suggests that a greater number of oocytes might be retrieved and a higher implantation rate obtained with LH plus FSH compared with FSH alone (based on two studies). In women of advance reproductive age a higher implantation rate may be obtained with LH plus FSH compared with FSH alone (based on four studies). A lower proportion of patients with OHSS were observed with LH supplementation in patients when used for prevention of OHSS. No difference between treatment with LH plus FSH and FSH alone was observed in women with profoundly suppressed LH levels after administration of a GnRH agonist, women co-treated with a GnRH antagonist and poor ovarian responders.

ORAL GONADOTROPINS

All gonadotropin preparations have to be injected, which increases the treatment burden for patients. There has therefore been interest in producing a product that can be dosed orally. It is not possible to dose gonadotropins orally because they are proteins and will not be absorbed, rather they are digested by enzymes. As a result of this, attempts to produce an oral drug for ovarian stimulation have focussed on FSH agonists. One oral

FSH agonist has been evaluated in healthy females but no effect on follicular development was observed, which was eventually attributed to the low doses used (141). Non-conclusive data is available for this option nowadays.

INJECTION DEVICES

Animal-derived and urinary gonadotropin products had to be injected intramuscularly using a syringe and vial, with reconstitution required before injection. Owing to the increased purity of recombinant products, a smaller injection volume is required and these can be injected subcutaneously using smaller gauge needles. In addition, these products have greater stability and liquid formulations of recombinant products have been produced, removing the need for reconstitution before injection. This in turn has enabled the development of pen injection devices, which are designed to improve ease-of-use and patient convenience, including the ability to both select the starting dose with greater precision (in increments as low as 12.5 IU) and adapt the dose during treatment, based on treatment response in small increments (12.5 IU) (142–144).

CONCLUSIONS

ART has come a long way since 1927, when gonadotropins were first identified, and currently available gonadotropin preparations better enable treatment individualization as part of patient-centered care. Patient-centeredness should be an aspect of all consultations and treatment decisions relating to medically assisted reproduction treatment. This should include discussions of whether treatment is appropriate, and if it is appropriate, which treatment would be most favorable. This treatment should be individualized according to the characteristics of the patient(s) and monitored to ensure that effectiveness is optimal, based on treatment response and safety, with treatment adjusted during treatment if it is not. The availability of recombinant products, which provide a pure form of the gonadotropin and can be accurately dosed, has improved the ability of medical practitioners to individualize treatment in this manner. Currently available products can be injected subcutaneously rather than intramuscularly, and pen injection devices are available, improving ease-of-use and more precise dose selection and adaption (in 12.5 IU dose increments). Work to develop new preparations is continuing, and a goal must remain the development of orally active FSH agonists and antagonists.

AUTHOR CONTRIBUTIONS

All authors listed have made a substantial, direct and intellectual contribution to the work, and approved it for publication.

ACKNOWLEDGMENTS

Medical writing support was provided by Alexander Jones of inScience Communications, Springer Healthcare, and was funded by Merck KGaA, Darmstadt, Germany.

REFERENCES

1. Ascheim S, Zondek B. Hypophysenvorderlappenhormone und ovarialhormone im harn von schwangeren. *Klin Wochenschr.* (1927) 6:13. doi: 10.1007/BF01728562

2. Lunenfeld B, Ezcurra D, D'Hooghe T. The development and evolution of gonadotropins in ART. *Fertil Steril.* (2018) 110:255–62. doi: 10.1016/j.fertnstert.2018.06.005

3. Seegar-Jones GE, Gey GO, Ghisletta M. Hormone production by placental cells maintained in continuous culture. *Bull Johns Hopkins Hosp.* (1943) 72:26–38.

4. Lunenfeld B. Gonadotropin stimulation: past, present and future. *Reprod Med Biol.* (2012) 11:11–25. doi: 10.1007/s12522-011-0097-2

5. Smith PE, Engle ET. Experimental evidence of the role of anterior pituitary in development and regulation of gonads. *Am J Anat.* (1927) 40:159. doi: 10.1002/aja.1000400202

6. Zondek B. Weitere untersuchungen zur darstellung, biologie und klinik des hypophysenvorderlappenhormones (Prolan). *Zentralblatt fur Gynakologie.* (1929) 14:834–48.

7. Lunenfeld B. Historical perspectives in gonadotrophin therapy. *Hum Reprod Update.* (2004) 10:453–67. doi: 10.1093/humupd/dmh044

8. D'Amour FE, D'Amour MC. The biologic potency of international standrad chorionic gonadotropin. *Endocrinology.* (1940) 26:93–6. doi: 10.1210/endo-26-1-93

9. Gurin S, Bachman G, Wilson DW. The gonadotropic hormone of urine of pregnancy. ii) Chemical studies of preparations having high biological activity. *J Biol Chem.* (1940) 133:467.

10. Katzman PA, Godfried M, Cain CK, Doisy EA. The preparation of chorionic gonadotrophin by chromatographic adsorption. *J Chem Biol.* (1943) 148:501–7.

11. Greep RO, Van Dyke HB, Chan BF. Gonadotropins of the swine pituitary: various biological effects of purified thylakentrin (FSH) and pure metakentrin (ICSH). *Endocrinolology.* (1942) 30:635–49. doi: 10.1210/endo-30-5-635

12. Steelman SL, Lamont WA, Baltes BJ. Preparation of highly active follicle stimulating hormone from swine pituitaries. *Endocrinology.* (1955) 56:216–7. doi: 10.1210/endo-56-2-216

13. Cole HH, Hart GH. The potency of blood serum of mares in progressive stages of pregnancy in affecting the sexual maturity of the immature rat. *Am J Physiol.* (1930) 93:57. doi: 10.1152/ajplegacy.1930.93.1.57

14. Mazer C, Ravetz E. The effect of combined administration of chorionic gonadotropin and the pituitary synergist on the human ovary. *Am J Obstet Gynaecol.* (1941) 41:474–588. doi: 10.1016/S0002-9378(41)90825-6

15. Leathem JH, Rakoff A. Gonadotrophic hormone therapy in man complicated by antihormone formation. *Am J Obstet Gynecol.* (1948) 56:521–6. doi: 10.1016/0002-9378(48)90638-3

16. Gemzell C. Human pituitary gonadotropins in the treatment of sterility. *Fertil Steril.* (1966) 17:149–59. doi: 10.1016/S0015-0282(16)35880-0

17. Gemzell CA, Diczfalusy E, Tillinger G. Clinical effect of human pituitary follicle-stimulating hormone (FSH). *J Clin Endocrinol Metab.* (1958) 18:1333–48. doi: 10.1210/jcem-18-12-1333

18. Cochius JI, Burns RJ, Blumbergs PC, Mack K, Alderman CP. Creutzfeldt-Jakob disease in a recipient of human pituitary-derived gonadotrophin. *Aust N Z J Med.* (1990) 20:592–3. doi: 10.1111/j.1445-5994.1990.tb01322.x

19. Cochius JI, Hyman N, Esiri MM. Creutzfeldt-Jakob disease in a recipient of human pituitary-derived gonadotrophin: a second case. *J Neurol Neurosurg Psychiatry.* (1992) 55:1094–5. doi: 10.1136/jnnp.55.11.1094

20. Dumble LJ, Klein RD. Creutzfeldt-Jakob legacy for Australian women treated with human pituitary gonadotropins. *Lancet.* (1992) 340:847–8. doi: 10.1016/0140-6736(92)92720-Z

21. Borth R, Lunenfeld B, de Watteville H. Active gonadotrope d'un extrait d'urines de femmes en menopause. *Experientia.* (1954) 10:266–8. doi: 10.1007/BF02157401

22. Albert A. Human Pituitary Gonadotropins- a workshop conference. In: Charles C Thomas, December 1959. Gatlinburg, TN: Springfield (1961).

23. Borth R, Lunenfeld B, De Watteville H. Day-to-day variation in urinary gonadotrophin and steroid levels during the normal menstrual cycle. *Fertil Steril.* (1957) 8:233–54. doi: 10.1016/S0015-0282(16)61356-0

24. Lunenfeld B, Menzi A, Volet B. Clinical effects of human postmenopausal gonadotropin. In: Fuchs F, editor. *Advance Abstracts of Short Communications, 1st International Congress of Endocrinology.* Copenhagen: Periodical (1960).

25. Lunenfeld B, Rabau E, Rumney G, Winkelsberg G. The responsiveness of the human ovary to gonadotropin (Hypophysis III). *Proc Third World Cong Gynecol Obstet.* (1961) 1:22.

26. Lunenfeld B, Sukmovici S, Rabau E, Eshkol A. L'induction de l'ovulation dans les amenorrees hypophysaires par un traitement combini de gonadotrophines unnaires minopausiques et de gonadotrophines chononiques. *CR Soc FT Gynecol.* (1962) 5:1–6.

27. Lunenfeld B. Treatment of anovulation by human gonadotropins. *J Int Fed Gynecol Obstet.* (1963) 1:15. doi: 10.1002/j.1879-3479.1963.tb00335.x

28. World Health Organization. *Expert Committee on Biological Standardization (Chair B.Lunenfeld), Vol 565. Technical Report Series.* Geneva: World Health Organization (1972).

29. Steelman SL, Pohley FM. Assay of the follicle stimulating hormone based on the augmentation with human chorionic gonadotropin. *Endocrinology.* (1953) 53:604–16. doi: 10.1210/endo-53-6-604

30. WHO Expert Committee. *Agents Stimulating Gonadal Function in Human* (Chair B. Lunenfeld). *Technical Report Series.* WHO (1973).

31. Steptoe PC, Edwards RG. Birth after the reimplantation of a human embryo. *Lancet.* (1978) 2:366. doi: 10.1016/S0140-6736(78)92957-4

32. Inge GB, Brinsden PR, Elder KT. Oocyte number per live birth in IVF: were steptoe and edwards less wasteful? *Hum Reprod.* (2005) 20:588–92. doi: 10.1093/humrep/deh655

33. Jones HW Jr. The use of controlled ovarian hyperstimulation (COH) in clinical *in vitro* fertilization: the role of georgeanna seegar jones. *Fertil Steril.* (2008) 90:e1–3. doi: 10.1016/j.fertnstert.2007.07.1333

34. Jones HW Jr, Jones GS, Andrews MC, Acosta A, Bundren C, Garcia J, et al. The program for *in vitro* fertilization at Norfolk. *Fertil steril.* (1982) 38:14–21. doi: 10.1016/S0015-0282(16)46390-9

35. Donini P, Puzzuoli D, D'Alessio I, Lunenfeld B, Eshkol A, Parlow AF. Purification and separation of follicle stimulating hormone (FSH) and luteinizing hormone (LH) from human postmenopausal gonadotrophin (HMG). II. Preparation of biological apparently pure FSH by selective binding of the LH with an anti-HGG serum and subsequent chromatography. *Acta Endocrinol.* (1966) 52:186–98. doi: 10.1530/acta.0.0520186

36. Ferring Pharmaceuticals Ltd. *Menopur 75IU.* (2015). Available online at: https://www.medicines.org.uk/emc/medicine/4322 (accessed March 28, 2019).

37. Howles C, Tanaka T, Matsuda T. Management of male hypogonadotrophic hypogonadism. *Endocr J.* (2007) 54:177–90. doi: 10.1507/endocrj.02-KR-98

38. Lunenfeld B, Mor A, Mani M. Treatment of male infertility. I. human gonadotropins. *Fertil Steril.* (1967) 18:581–92. doi: 10.1016/S0015-0282(16)36421-4

39. Macleod J, Pazianos A, Ray BS. Restoration of human spermatogenesis by menopausal gonadotrophins. *Lancet.* (1964) 1:1196–7. doi: 10.1016/S0140-6736(64)91212-7

40. European Medicines Agency. *GONAL-f.* (2018). Available online at: https://www.ema.europa.eu/en/medicines/human/EPAR/gonal-f (accessed January 29, 2019).

41. Merck Sharp Dohme Limited. *Elonva.* (2019) Available online at: https://www.ema.europa.eu/en/medicines/human/EPAR/elonva (accessed March 26, 2019).

42. EMD Serono I. *Gonal-F.* (2018). Available online at: https://www.drugs.com/pro/gonal-f.html (accessed 2019 26 Mar 2019).

43. European Medicines Agency. *Ovaleap.* (2018). Available online at: https://www.ema.europa.eu/en/medicines/human/EPAR/ovaleap (accessed January 29, 2019).

44. European Medicines Agency. *Bemfola.* (2018). Available online at: https://www.ema.europa.eu/en/medicines/human/EPAR/bemfola (accessed January 29, 2019).

45. Drugs.com. *Follistim AQ Approval History*. (2018). Available online at: https://www.drugs.com/history/follistim-aq.html (accessed March 26, 2019).

46. European Medicines Agency. *Puregon*. (2018). Available online at: https://www.ema.europa.eu/en/medicines/human/EPAR/puregon (accessed January 29, 2019).

47. Howles CM. Genetic engineering of human FSH (Gonal-F). *Hum Reprod Update*. (1996) 2:172–91. doi: 10.1093/humupd/2.2.172

48. Olijve W, de Boer W, Mulders JW, van Wezenbeek PM. Molecular biology and biochemistry of human recombinant follicle stimulating hormone (Puregon). *Mol Hum Reprod*. (1996) 2:371–82. doi: 10.1093/molehr/2.5.371

49. Goa KL, Wagstaff AJ. Follitropin alpha in infertility: a review. *BioDrugs*. (1998) 9:235–60. doi: 10.2165/00063030-199809030-00006

50. European Medicines Agency. *Elonva: Corifollitropin Alfa*. (2015). Available online at: https://www.ema.europa.eu/en/medicines/human/EPAR/elonva (accessed March 10, 2019).

51. European Medicines Agency. *Rekovelle: Follitropin Delta*. (2017). Available online at: http://www.ema.europa.eu/ema/index.jsp?curl=pages/medicines/human/medicines/003994/human_med_002044.jsp&mid=WC0b01ac058001d124 (accessed June 21, 2018).

52. le Contonnec JY, Porchet HC, Beltrami V, Khan A, Toon S, Rowland M. Clinical pharmacology of recombinant human follicle-stimulating hormone. II. single doses and steady state pharmacokinetics. *Fertil Steril*. (1994) 61:679–86. doi: 10.1016/S0015-0282(16)56645-X

53. Voortman G, Mannaerts BM, Huisman JA. A dose proportionality study of subcutaneously and intramuscularly administered recombinant human follicle-stimulating hormone (Follistim*/Puregon) in healthy female volunteers. *Fertil Steril*. (2000) 73:1187–93. doi: 10.1016/S0015-0282(00)00542-2

54. de Leeuw R, Mulders J, Voortman G, Rombout F, Damm J, Kloosterboer L. Structure-function relationship of recombinant follicle stimulating hormone (Puregon). *Mol Hum Reproduct*. (1996) 2:361–9. doi: 10.1093/molehr/2.5.361

55. Leao Rde B, Esteves SC. Gonadotropin therapy in assisted reproduction: an evolutionary perspective from biologics to biotech. *Clinics*. (2014) 69:279–93. doi: 10.6061/clinics/2014(04)10

56. Bassett RM, Driebergen R. Continued improvements in the quality and consistency of follitropin alfa, recombinant human FSH. *Reprod Biomed Online*. (2005) 10:169–77. doi: 10.1016/S1472-6483(10)60937-6

57. Hugues J-N, Durnerin IC. Gonadotrophins – filled-by-mass versus filled-by-bioassay. *Reprod Biomed Online*. (2005) 10:11–7. doi: 10.1016/S1472-6483(11)60385-4

58. Brinsden P, Akagbosu F, Gibbons LM, Lancaster S, Gourdon D, Engrand P, et al. A comparison of the efficacy and tolerability of two recombinant human follicle-stimulating hormone preparations in patients undergoing *in vitro* fertilization-embryo transfer. *Fertil Steril*. (2000) 73:114–6. doi: 10.1016/S0015-0282(99)00450-1

59. Harlin J, Csemiczky G, Wramsby H, Fried G. Recombinant follicle stimulating hormone in *in-vitro* fertilization treatment-clinical experience with follitropin alpha and follitropin beta. *Hum Reprod*. (2000) 15:239–44. doi: 10.1093/humrep/15.2.239

60. Tulppala M, Aho M, Tuuri T, Vilska S, Foudila T, Hakala-Ala-Pietila T, et al. Comparison of two recombinant follicle-stimulating hormone preparations in *in-vitro* fertilization: a randomized clinical study. *Hum Reprod*. (1999) 14:2709–15. doi: 10.1093/humrep/14.11.2709

61. Williams RS, Vensel T, Sistrom CL, Kipersztok S, Rhoton-Vlasak A, Drury K. Pregnancy rates in varying age groups after *in vitro* fertilization: a comparison of follitropin alfa (Gonal F) and follitropin beta (Follistim). *Am J Obstet Gynecol*. (2003) 189:342–6. doi: 10.1067/S0002-9378(03)00728-2

62. Mastrangeli R, Satwekar A, Cutillo F, Ciampolillo C, Palinsky W, Longobardi S. In-vivo biological activity and glycosylation analysis of a biosimilar recombinant human follicle-stimulating hormone product (Bemfola) compared with its reference medicinal product (GONAL-f). *PLoS ONE*. (2017) 12:e0184139. doi: 10.1371/journal.pone.0184139

63. de Mora F, Fauser BCJM. Biosimilars to recombinant human FSH medicines: comparable efficacy and safety to the original biologic. *Reprod Biomed Online*. (2017) 35:81–6. doi: 10.1016/j.rbmo.2017.03.020

64. Winstel R, Wieland J, Gertz B, Mueller A, Allgaier H. Manufacturing of recombinant human follicle-stimulating hormone ovaleap((R)) (XM17), comparability with gonal-f((R)), and performance/consistency. *Drugs R D*. (2017) 17:305–12. doi: 10.1007/s40268-017-0182-z

65. Orvieto R, Seifer DB. Biosimilar FSH preparations- are they identical twins or just siblings? *Reprod Biol Endocrinol*. (2016) 14:32. doi: 10.1186/s12958-016-0167-8

66. European Medicines Agency. *Biosimilars in the EU*. (2017). Available online at: https://www.ema.europa.eu/documents/leaflet/biosimilars-eu-information-guide-healthcare-professionals_en.pdf (accessed January 30, 2019).

67. Rettenbacher M, Andersen AN, Garcia-Velasco JA, Sator M, Barri P, Lindenberg S, et al. A multi-centre phase 3 study comparing efficacy and safety of Bemfola((R)) versus Gonal-f((R)) in women undergoing ovarian stimulation for IVF. *Reprod Biomed Online*. (2015) 30:504–13. doi: 10.1016/j.rbmo.2015.01.005

68. Strowitzki T, Kuczynski W, Mueller A, Bias P. Randomized, active-controlled, comparative phase 3 efficacy and safety equivalence trial of Ovaleap(R) (recombinant human follicle-stimulating hormone) in infertile women using assisted reproduction technology (ART). *Reprod Biol Endocrinol*. (2016) 14:1. doi: 10.1186/s12958-015-0135-8

69. Papsch R, Roeder C, D'Hooghe T, Longobardi S. PMU40 - live birth rate (LBR), ongoing pregnancy rate (OPR) and ovarian hyperstimulation syndrome (OHSS) risk with originator versus biosimilar recombinant follitropin ALFA: a pooled analysis of clinical trial data. *Value Health*. (2018) 21:S314–S5. doi: 10.1016/j.jval.2018.09.1876

70. Strowitzki T, Kuczynski W, Mueller A, Bias P. Safety and efficacy of Ovaleap(R) (recombinant human follicle-stimulating hormone) for up to 3 cycles in infertile women using assisted reproductive technology: a phase 3 open-label follow-up to Main Study. *Reprod Biol Endocrinol*. (2016) 14:31. doi: 10.1186/s12958-016-0164-y

71. Koechling W, Plaksin D, Croston GE, Jeppesen JV, Macklon KT, Andersen CY. Comparative pharmacology of a new recombinant FSH expressed by a human cell line. *Endocrine Connect*. (2017) 6:297–305. doi: 10.1530/EC-17-0067

72. Olsson H, Sandstrom R, Grundemar L. Different pharmacokinetic and pharmacodynamic properties of recombinant follicle-stimulating hormone (rFSH) derived from a human cell line compared with rFSH from a non-human cell line. *J Clin Pharmacol*. (2014) 54:1299–307. doi: 10.1002/jcph.328

73. Therapeutic Goods Administration (TGA) Commonwealth of Australia. *Australian Public Assessment Report (AusPAR) Rekovelle*. (2017). Available online at: https://www.tga.gov.au/sites/default/files/auspar-follitropin-delta-rhu-171025.docx (accessed March 29, 2019).

74. Nyboe Andersen A, Nelson SM, Fauser BCJM, García-Velasco JA, Klein BM, Arce J-C, et al. Individualized versus conventional ovarian stimulation for *in vitro* fertilization: a multicenter, randomized, controlled, assessor-blinded, phase 3 noninferiority trial. *Fertil Steril*. (2017) 107:387–96.e4. doi: 10.1016/j.fertnstert.2016.10.033

75. D'Hooghe T, Longobardi S. *Letter to Editor in Response to: Individualized Versus Conventional Ovarian Stimulation for in vitro Fertilization: A Multicenter, Randomized, Controlled, Assessor-Blinded, Phase 3 Noninferiority Trial*. (2017). Available online at: https://www.fertstertdialog.com/users/16110-fertility-and-sterility/posts/12852--23086. (accessed December 21, 2018).

76. Wilkinson J, Lensen S. Letter to editor in response to: individualized versus conventional ovarian stimulation for *in vitro* fertilization: a multicenter, randomized, controlled, assessor-blinded, phase 3 noninferiority trial (2017) [cited 2019 26 Mar 2019]. Available online at: https://www.fertstertdialog.com/users/16110-fertility-and-sterility/posts/12852--23086.

77. Abd-Elaziz K, Duijkers I, Stöckl L, Dietrich B, Klipping C, Eckert K, et al. A new fully human recombinant FSH (follitropin epsilon): two phase I randomized placebo and comparator-controlled pharmacokinetic and pharmacodynamic trials. *Hum Reprod*. (2017) 32:1639–47. doi: 10.1093/humrep/dex220

78. Glycotope GmbH, inventor; Glycotope GmbH, assignee. *US Patent for Recombinant Human Follicle-Stimulating Hormone Patent*. Patent # 9,527,899. US (2011).

79. Pouwer AW, Farquhar C, Kremer JA. Long-acting FSH versus daily FSH for women undergoing assisted reproduction. *Cochrane Database Syst Rev.* (2015) 2015:CD009577. doi: 10.1002/14651858.CD009577.pub3

80. Fares FA, Suganuma N, Nishimori K, LaPolt PS, Hsueh AJ, Boime I. Design of a long-acting follitropin agonist by fusing the C-terminal sequence of the chorionic gonadotropin beta subunit to the follitropin beta subunit. *Proc Natl Acad Sci USA.* (1992) 89:4304–8. doi: 10.1073/pnas.89.10.4304

81. Fauser BCJM, Alper MM, Ledger W, Schoolcraft WB, Zandvliet A, Mannaerts BMJL. Pharmacokinetics and follicular dynamics of corifollitropin alfa versus recombinant FSH during ovarian stimulation for IVF. *Reprod Biomed Online.* (2010) 21:593–601. doi: 10.1016/j.rbmo.2010.06.032

82. Ledger WL, Fauser BCJM, Devroey P, Zandvliet AS, Mannaerts BMJL. Corifollitropin alfa doses based on body weight: clinical overview of drug exposure and ovarian response. *Reprod Biomed Online.* (2011) 23:150–9. doi: 10.1016/j.rbmo.2011.04.002

83. Fensore S, Di Marzio M, Tiboni GM. Corifollitropin alfa compared to daily FSH in controlled ovarian stimulation for *in vitro* fertilization: a meta-analysis. *J Ovarian Res.* (2015) 8:33. doi: 10.1186/s13048-015-0160-4

84. Mahmoud Youssef MA, van Wely M, Aboulfoutouh I, El-Khyat W, van der Veen F, Al-Inany H. Is there a place for corifollitropin alfa in IVF/ICSI cycles? a systematic review and meta-analysis. *Fertil Steril.* (2012) 97:876–85. doi: 10.1016/j.fertnstert.2012.01.092

85. Low SC, Nunes SL, Bitonti AJ, Dumont JA. Oral and pulmonary delivery of FSH–Fc fusion proteins via neonatal Fc receptor-mediated transcytosis. *Hum Reprod.* (2005) 20:1805–13. doi: 10.1093/humrep/deh896

86. Zhang Y-L, Guo K-P, Ji S-Y, Liu X-M, Wang P, Wu J, et al. Development and characterization of a novel long-acting recombinant follicle stimulating hormone agonist by fusing Fc to an FSH-β subunit. *Hum Reprod.* (2016) 31:169–82. doi: 10.1093/humrep/dev295

87. Perlman S, van den Hazel B, Christiansen J, Gram-Nielsen S, Jeppesen CB, Andersen KV, et al. Glycosylation of an N-terminal extension prolongs the half-life and increases the *in vivo* activity of follicle stimulating hormone. *J Clin Endocrinol Metab.* (2003) 88:3227–35. doi: 10.1210/jc.2002-021201

88. Klein J, Lobel L, Pollak S, Lustbader B, Ogden RT, Sauer MV, et al. Development and characterization of a long acting recombinant hFSH agonist. *Hum Reprod.* (2003) 18:50–6. doi: 10.1093/humrep/deg024

89. van Wely M, Kwan I, Burt AL, Thomas J, Vail A, Van der Veen F, et al. Recombinant versus urinary gonadotrophin for ovarian stimulation in assisted reproductive technology cycles. *Cochrane Database Syst Rev.* (2011) 2011:CD005354. doi: 10.1002/14651858.CD005354.pub2

90. Weiss NS, Kostova E, Nahuis M, Mol BWJ, van der Veen F, van Wely M. Gonadotrophins for ovulation induction in women with polycystic ovary syndrome. *Cochrane Database Syst Rev.* (2019) 1:CD010290. doi: 10.1002/14651858.CD010290.pub3

91. Lehert P, Schertz JC, Ezcurra D. Recombinant human follicle-stimulating hormone produces more oocytes with a lower total dose per cycle in assisted reproductive technologies compared with highly purified human menopausal gonadotrophin: a meta-analysis. *Reprod Biol Endocrinol.* (2010) 8:112. doi: 10.1186/1477-7827-8-112

92. Drakopoulos P, Errazuriz J, Santos-Ribeiro S, Tournaye H, Vaiarelli A, Pluchino N, et al. Cumulative live birth rates in IVF. *Minerva Ginecol.* (2018) 360:236–243. doi: 10.23736/S0026-4784.18.04347-2

93. Maheshwari A, McLernon D, Bhattacharya S. Cumulative live birth rate: time for a consensus? *Hum Reprod.* (2015) 30:2703–7. doi: 10.1093/humrep/dev263

94. Baker VL, Brown MB, Luke B, Conrad KP. Association of number of retrieved oocytes with live birth rate and birth weight: an analysis of 231,815 cycles of in vitro fertilization. *Fertil Steril.* (2015) 103:931–8 e2. doi: 10.1016/j.fertnstert.2014.12.120

95. Briggs R, Kovacs G, MacLachlan V, Motteram C, Baker HW. Can you ever collect too many oocytes? *Hum Reprod.* (2015) 30:81–7. doi: 10.1093/humrep/deu272

96. Steward RG, Lan L, Shah AA, Yeh JS, Price TM, Goldfarb JM, et al. Oocyte number as a predictor for ovarian hyperstimulation syndrome and live birth: an analysis of 256,381 *in vitro* fertilization cycles. *Fertil Steril.* (2014) 101:967–73. doi: 10.1016/j.fertnstert.2013.12.026

97. Sunkara SK, Rittenberg V, Raine-Fenning N, Bhattacharya S, Zamora J, Coomarasamy a. association between the number of eggs and live birth in IVF treatment: an analysis of 400 135 treatment cycles. *Hum Reprod.* (2011) 26:1768–74. doi: 10.1093/humrep/der106

98. Magnusson A, Kallen K, Thurin-Kjellberg A, Bergh C. The number of oocytes retrieved during IVF: a balance between efficacy and safety. *Hum Reprod.* (2018) 33:58–64. doi: 10.1093/humrep/dex334

99. Malchau SS, Henningsen AA, Forman J, Loft A, Nyboe Andersen A, Pinborg A. Cumulative live birth rate prognosis based on the number of aspirated oocytes in previous ART cycles. *Hum Reprod.* (2019) 34:171–80. doi: 10.1093/humrep/dey341

100. Polyzos NP, Drakopoulos P, Parra J, Pellicer A, Santos-Ribeiro S, Tournaye H, et al. Cumulative live birth rates according to the number of oocytes retrieved after the first ovarian stimulation for *in vitro* fertilization/intracytoplasmic sperm injection: a multicenter multinational analysis including approximately 15,000 women. *Fertil Steril.* (2018) 110:661–70 e1. doi: 10.1016/j.fertnstert.2018.04.039

101. Levi Setti PE, Alviggi C, Colombo GL, Pisanelli C, Ripellino C, Longobardi S, et al. Human recombinant follicle stimulating hormone (rFSH) compared to urinary human menopausal gonadotropin (HMG) for ovarian stimulation in assisted reproduction: a literature review and cost evaluation. *J Endocrinol Invest.* (2015) 38:497–503. doi: 10.1007/s40618-014-0204-4

102. Bergh C, Howles CM, Borg K, Hamberger L, Josefsson B, Nilsson L, et al. Recombinant human follicle stimulating hormone (r-hFSH; Gonal-F) versus highly purified urinary FSH (Metrodin HP): results of a randomized comparative study in women undergoing assisted reproductive techniques. *Hum Reprod.* (1997) 12:2133–9. doi: 10.1093/humrep/12.10.2133

103. Frydman R, Howles CM, Truong F. A double-blind, randomized study to compare recombinant human follicle stimulating hormone (FSH; Gonal-F) with highly purified urinary FSH (Metrodin) HP) in women undergoing assisted reproductive techniques including intracytoplasmic sperm injection. The French Multicentre Trialists. *Hum Reprod.* (2000) 15:520–5. doi: 10.1093/humrep/15.3.520

104. Hedon B, Out HJ, Hugues JN, Camier B, Cohen J, Lopes P, et al. Efficacy and safety of recombinant follicle stimulating hormone (Puregon) in infertile women pituitary-suppressed with triptorelin undergoing *in-vitro* fertilization: a prospective, randomized, assessor-blind, multicentre trial. *Hum Reprod.* (1995) 10:3102–6. doi: 10.1093/oxfordjournals.humrep.a135866

105. Liu PY, Turner L, Rushford D, McDonald J, Baker HW, Conway AJ, et al. Efficacy and safety of recombinant human follicle stimulating hormone (Gonal-F) with urinary human chorionic gonadotropin for induction of spermatogenesis and fertility in gonadotrophin-deficient men. *Hum Reprod.* (1999) 14:1540–5. doi: 10.1093/humrep/14.6.1540

106. Bouloux P, Warne DW, Loumaye E. Efficacy and safety of recombinant human follicle-stimulating hormone in men with isolated hypogonadotropic hypogonadism. *Fertil Steril.* (2002) 77:270–3. doi: 10.1016/S0015-0282(01)02973-9

107. Attia AM, Abou-Setta AM, Al-Inany HG. Gonadotrophins for idiopathic male factor subfertility. *Cochrane Database Syst Rev.* (2013) 2013:CD005071. doi: 10.1002/14651858.CD005071.pub4

108. Youssef MA, Abou-Setta AM, Lam WS. Recombinant versus urinary human chorionic gonadotrophin for final oocyte maturation triggering in IVF and ICSI cycles. *Cochrane Database Syst Rev.* (2016) 4:CD003719. doi: 10.1002/14651858.CD003719.pub4

109. European Medicines Agency. *Ovitrelle.* (2018). Available online at: https://www.ema.europa.eu/en/medicines/human/EPAR/ovitrelle (accessed January 30, 2019).

110. European Medicines Agency. *Luveris.* (2018). Available online at: https://www.ema.europa.eu/en/medicines/human/EPAR/luveris (accessed January 30, 2019).

111. Trinchard-Lugan I, Khan A, Porchet HC, Munafo A. Pharmacokinetics and pharmacodynamics of recombinant human chorionic gonadotropin in healthy male and female volunteers. *Reprod Biomed Online.* (2002) 4:106–15. doi: 10.1016/S1472-6483(10)61927-X

112. Duffy DM, Hutchison JS, Stewart DR, Stouffer RL. Stimulation of primate luteal function by recombinant human chorionic gonadotropin and modulation of steroid, but not relaxin, production by an inhibitor of 3 beta-hydroxysteroid dehydrogenase during simulated early pregnancy. *J Clin Endocrinol Metab.* (1996) 81:2307–13. doi: 10.1210/jcem.81.6.8964869

113. Zelinski-Wooten MB, Hutchison JS, Trinchard-Lugan I, Hess DL, Wolf DP, Stouffer RL. Initiation of periovulatory events in gonadotrophin-stimulated macaques with varying doses of recombinant human chorionic gonadotrophin. *Hum Reprod.* (1997) 12:1877–85. doi: 10.1093/humrep/12.9.1877

114. Driscoll GL, Tyler JP, Hangan JT, Fisher PR, Birdsall MA, Knight DC. A prospective, randomized, controlled, double-blind, double-dummy comparison of recombinant and urinary HCG for inducing oocyte maturation and follicular luteinization in ovarian stimulation. *Hum Reprod.* (2000) 15:1305–10. doi: 10.1093/humrep/15.6.1305

115. International Recombinant Human Chorionic Gonadotropin Study Group. Induction of ovulation in World Health Organization group II anovulatory women undergoing follicular stimulation with recombinant human follicle-stimulating hormone: a comparison of recombinant human chorionic gonadotropin (rhCG) and urinary hCG. *Fertil Steril.* (2001) 75:1111–8. doi: 10.1016/S0015-0282(01)01803-9

116. European Recombinant Human Chorionic Gonadotrophin Study Group. Induction of final follicular maturation and early luteinization in women undergoing ovulation induction for assisted reproduction treatment–recombinant HCG versus urinary HCG. the european recombinant human chorionic gonadotropin study group. *Hum Reprod.* (2000) 15:1446–51. doi: 10.1093/humrep/15.7.1446

117. Chang P, Kenley S, Burns T, Denton G, Currie K, DeVane G, et al. Recombinant human chorionic gonadotropin (rhCG) in assisted reproductive technology: results of a clinical trial comparing two doses of rhCG (Ovidrel) to urinary hCG (Profasi) for induction of final follicular maturation in in vitro fertilization-embryo transfer. *Fertil Steril.* (2001) 76:67–74. doi: 10.1016/S0015-0282(01)01851-9

118. Bellavia M, de Geyter C, Streuli I, Ibecheole V, Birkhauser MH, Cometti BP, et al. Randomized controlled trial comparing highly purified (HP-hCG) and recombinant hCG (r-hCG) for triggering ovulation in ART. *Gynecol Endocrinol.* (2013) 29:93–7. doi: 10.3109/09513590.2012.730577

119. Shoham ZMD, Insler VMD. Recombinant technique and gonadotropins production: new era in reproductive medicine. *Fertil Steril.* (1998) 69:3S–15S. doi: 10.1016/S0015-0282(97)00506-2

120. le Cotonnec J-Y, Porchet H, Beltrami V, Munafo A. Clinical pharmacology of recombinant human luteinizing hormone: part I. pharmacokinetics after intravenous administration to healthy female volunteers and comparison with urinary human luteinizing hormone. *Fertil Steril.* (1998) 69:189–94. doi: 10.1016/S0015-0282(97)00501-3

121. Merck Serono. *Luveris Summary of Product Characteristics.* (2018). Available online at: https://www.medicines.org.uk/emc/product/1573/smpc (accessed July 24, 2019).

122. Merck. Pergoveris, Russian Summary of Product Characteristics. (2017).

123. European Medicines Agency. *Pergoveris.* (2018). Available online at: https://www.ema.europa.eu/en/medicines/human/EPAR/pergoveris (accessed January 30, 2019).

124. Dhillon S, Keating GM. Lutropin Alfa. *Drugs.* (2008) 68:1529–40. doi: 10.2165/00003495-200868110-00005

125. The European Recombinant Human LH Study Group. Recombinant human luteinizing hormone (LH) to support recombinant human follicle-stimulating hormone (FSH)-induced follicular development in LH- and FSH-deficient anovulatory women: a dose-finding study. *J Clin Endocrinol Metab.* (1998) 83:1507–14. doi: 10.1210/jc.83.5.1507

126. Burgues S. The effectiveness and safety of recombinant human LH to support follicular development induced by recombinant human FSH in WHO group I anovulation: evidence from a multicentre study in Spain. *Hum Reprod.* (2001) 16:2525–32. doi: 10.1093/humrep/16.12.2525

127. De Moustier B, Brinsden P, Bungum L, Fisch B, Pinkstone S, Warne D, et al. 0-158. The effects of combined treatment of recombinant (r)FSH and rLH in ratios 1:1, 2:1 and 3:1 in women. aged 38–42 years

undergoing IVF-ICSI treatment. *Hum Reprod.* (2002) 17(Suppl 1):55. doi: 10.1093/humrep/17.suppl_1.54

128. Humaidan P, Chin W, Rogoff D, D'Hooghe T, Longobardi S, Hubbard J, et al. Efficacy and safety of follitropin alfa/lutropin alfa in ART: a randomized controlled trial in poor ovarian responders. *Hum Reprod.* (2017) 32:1537–8. doi: 10.1093/humrep/dex208

129. Humaidan P, Chin W, Rogoff D, D'Hooghe T, Longobardi S, Hubbard J, et al. Efficacy and safety of follitropin alfa/lutropin alfa in ART: a randomized controlled trial in poor ovarian responders. *Hum Reprod.* (2017) 32:544–55. doi: 10.1093/humrep/dew360

130. Lehert P, Chin W, Schertz J, D'Hooghe T, Alviggi C, Humaidan P. Predicting live birth for poor ovarian responders: the PROsPeR concept. *Reprod Biomed Online.* (2018) 37:43–52. doi: 10.1016/j.rbmo.2018.03.013

131. Alviggi C, Conforti A, Esteves SC, Andersen CY, Bosch E, Buhler K, et al. Recombinant luteinizing hormone supplementation in assisted reproductive technology: a systematic review. *Fertil Steril.* (2018) 109:644–64. doi: 10.1016/j.fertnstert.2018.01.003

132. Conforti A, Esteves SC, Di Rella F, Strina I, De Rosa P, Fiorenza A, et al. The role of recombinant LH in women with hypo-response to controlled ovarian stimulation: a systematic review and meta-analysis. *Reprod Biol Endocrinol.* (2019) 17:18. doi: 10.1186/s12958-019-0460-4

133. Lehert P, Kolibianakis EM, Venetis CA, Schertz J, Saunders H, Arriagada P, et al. Recombinant human follicle-stimulating hormone (r-hFSH) plus recombinant luteinizing hormone versus r-hFSH alone for ovarian stimulation during assisted reproductive technology: systematic review and meta-analysis. *Reprod Biol Endocrinol.* (2014) 12:17. doi: 10.1186/1477-7827-12-17

134. Mochtar MH, Danhof NA, Ayeleke RO, Van der Veen F, van Wely M. Recombinant luteinizing hormone (rLH) and recombinant follicle stimulating hormone (rFSH) for ovarian stimulation in IVF/ICSI cycles. *Cochrane Database Syst Rev.* (2017) 5:CD005070. doi: 10.1002/14651858.CD005070.pub3

135. Santi D, Casarini L, Alviggi C, Simoni M. Efficacy of follicle-stimulating hormone (FSH) alone, FSH + luteinizing hormone, human menopausal gonadotropin or FSH + human chorionic gonadotropin on assisted reproductive technology outcomes in the "personalized" medicine era: a meta-analysis. *Front Endocrinol.* (2017) 8:114. doi: 10.3389/fendo.2017.00114

136. Braakhekke M, Kamphuis EI, Dancet EA, Mol F, van der Veen F, Mol BW. Ongoing pregnancy qualifies best as the primary outcome measure of choice in trials in reproductive medicine: an opinion paper. *Fertil Steril.* (2014) 101:1203–4. doi: 10.1016/j.fertnstert.2014.03.047

137. Clarke JF, van Rumste MM, Farquhar CM, Johnson NP, Mol BW, Herbison P. Measuring outcomes in fertility trials: can we rely on clinical pregnancy rates? *Fertil Steril.* (2010) 94:1647–51. doi: 10.1016/j.fertnstert.2009.11.018

138. Martins WP, Niederberger C, Nastri CO, Racowsky C. Making evidence-based decisions in reproductive medicine. *Fertil Steril.* (2018) 110:1227–30. doi: 10.1016/j.fertnstert.2018.08.010

139. Mol BW, Bossuyt PM, Sunkara SK, Garcia Velasco JA, Venetis C, Sakkas D, et al. Personalized ovarian stimulation for ART: study design considerations to move from hype to added value for patients. *Fertil Steril.* (2018) 109:968–79. doi: 10.1016/j.fertnstert.2018.04.037

140. Alviggi C, Conforti A, Esteves SC, Vallone R, Venturella R, Staiano S, et al. Understanding ovarian hypo-response to exogenous gonadotropin in ovarian stimulation and its new proposed marker-the follicle-to-oocyte (FOI) index. *Front Endocrinol.* (2018) 9:589. doi: 10.3389/fendo.2018.00589

141. Gerrits MG, Kramer H, el Galta R, van Beerendonk G, Hanssen R, Abd-Elaziz K, et al. Oral follicle-stimulating hormone agonist tested in healthy young women of reproductive age failed to demonstrate effect on follicular development but affected thyroid function. *Fertil Steril.* (2016) 105:1056–62 e4. doi: 10.1016/j.fertnstert.2015.12.017

142. Abbotts C, Salgado-Braga C, Audibert-Gros C. A redesigned follitropin alfa pen injector for infertility: results of a market research study. *Patient Prefer Adherence.* (2011) 5:315–31. doi: 10.2147/PPA.S21421

143. Schertz J, Worton H. Nurse evaluation of the redesigned fertility pen injector: a questionnaire-based observational survey. *Expert Opin Drug Deliv.* (2018) 15:435–42. doi: 10.1080/17425247.2018.1450386

144. Schertz J, Worton H. Patient evaluation of the redesigned follitropin alfa pen injector. *Expert Opin Drug Deliv.* (2017) 14:473–81. doi: 10.1080/17425247.2017.1289174

10

Gain–of–Function Genetic Models to Study FSH Action

Rosemary McDonald [1,2], Carolyn Sadler [1] and T. Rajendra Kumar [1,2,3*]

[1] Division of Reproductive Sciences, Department of Obstetrics and Gynecology, University of Colorado Anschutz Medical Campus, Aurora, IL, United States, [2] Integrated Physiology Graduate Program, University of Colorado Anschutz Medical Campus, Aurora, IL, United States, [3] Division of Reproductive Endocrinology and Infertility, Department of Obstetrics and Gynecology, University of Colorado Anschutz Medical Campus, Aurora, IL, United States

*Correspondence:
T. Rajendra Kumar
raj.kumar@ucdenver.edu

Follicle–stimulating hormone (FSH) is a pituitary-derived gonadotropin that plays key roles in male and female reproduction. The physiology and biochemistry of FSH have been extensively studied for many years. Beginning in the early 1990s, coincident with advances in the then emerging transgenic animal technology, and continuing till today, several gain-of-function (GOF) models have been developed to understand FSH homeostasis in a physiological context. Our group and others have generated a number of FSH ligand and receptor GOF mouse models. An FSH GOF model when combined with *Fshb* null mice provides a powerful genetic rescue platform. In this chapter, we discuss different GOF models for FSH synthesis, secretion and action and describe additional novel genetic models that could be developed in the future to further refine the existing models.

Keywords: pituitary, follicle-stimulating hormone, transgenic mice, testis, ovary

INTRODUCTION

Follicle–Stimulating Hormone (FSH) is a gonadotropin synthesized in gonadotropes of the anterior pituitary gland. FSH is a heterodimeric glycoprotein, consisting of two distinct α- and β (FSHβ) subunits (1–4). The α-subunit is structurally identical to both gonadotropins–luteinizing hormone (LH), and chorionic gonadotropin (CG) as well as thyroid-stimulating hormone (TSH). FSH subunits are encoded by distinct genes. The FSHβ subunit is unique and confers the biological specificity for FSH functions (1–4). The β-subunits exist in comparatively lower amounts within the pituitary than their corresponding α-subunit. FSH subunits are synthesized and assembled non-covalently in gonadotropes (1–4). Non-covalent linkage of the subunits allows for easy separation and hybridization, yet free α and β-subunits are typically expressed by other tissues under a variety of pathological conditions (1–4).

FSH signaling in the hypothalamic-pituitary-gonadal axis (HPG) regulates critical reproductive functions such as steroidogenesis and gametogenesis. In males, FSH contributes to spermatogenesis and testicular development by binding to Sertoli cells and regulating their development and differentiation (5–7). In females, FSH contributes to ovarian follicular development by upregulating aromatase expression in granulosa cells, which results in increased estrogen production. Increased estrogen synthesis is required for normal follicular growth (8).

FSH and LH are synthesized and released in response to gonadotropin-releasing hormone (GnRH) secreted from the hypothalamus. GnRH binds to GnRH- receptors on pituitary gonadotropes (4, 9). Differing GnRH release frequencies favor either FSH or LH synthesis as gonadotropes are sensitive to patterns of GnRH stimulation ad respond by altering hormone-specific subunit gene transcription. LH is secreted in a regulated, pulsatile fashion in response to increased GnRH pulse frequency, whereas FSH is released is mostly constitutive and responds to decreased GnRH pulse frequency (10, 11).

FSH synthesis and release are also regulated by several other proteins, such as follistatin, inhibin, and activin (12–17). Activin exerts positive effects on FSH by stimulating transcription, biosynthesis, and ultimately secretion as well as stimulating GnRH receptor gene expression. In rodents, after activin binds to gonadotrope membrane activin receptors, transcription factors, such as Smad4 are recruited and directly interact with the FSHβ gene promoter to upregulate its expression (15, 18). Another important transcription factor in gonadotropin regulation is the forkhead box (FOX) protein, FoxL2, which is a transcription factor known for its role in folliculogenesis and female sex determination (19). *Foxl2* knockout mice have substantially decreased *Fshb* mRNA and serum FSH levels as well as reduced activin induction of FSHβ (20). Both inhibin and follistatin prevent the stimulatory effects of activin, causing suppression of FSHβ synthesis by blocking activin binding, thereby inhibiting intracellular pathways and subsequent FSHβ transcription (18, 21, 22).

There are several clinical conditions under which FSH expression or signaling via its receptor is increased, resulting in higher circulating levels and ultimately creating a FSH "gain of function" effect. These include ovarian hyperstimulation syndrome (23–26), certain ovarian cancers (27–29), and the recent discovery of non-gonadal FSH actions on bone in transgenic mouse models with elevated human FSH levels (30). GOF effects of FSH in ovaries were also occasionally noted in patients with FSH hypersecreting pituitary adenomas (31). The existence of such conditions highlights the importance of generating animal models that closely mimic human disease phenotypes, allowing us to expand the medical knowledge of these conditions and ultimately providing opportunities to learn how to treat them. While mouse models do not always accurately mimic human pathology, they provide a quick genetic test to address the function of human proteins in a physiological context that cannot be reliably achieved using *in vitro* experimental approaches. In this review, we highlight and describe previously generated FSH gain of function animal models and how they can potentially be used to develop new approaches for treating clinical conditions involving FSH.

GOF Mouse Models for FSH

Several GOF genetic models have been generated and used to study the physiological consequences of FSH. These models are described below in detail and summarized in **Table 1**.

Abbreviations: BAC, Bacterial Artificial Chromosome; cAMP, $3',5'$-cyclic adenosine monophosphate; DCG, Dense Core Granules; E2, Estradiol; FSH, Follicle-stimulating hormone; FSHR, FSH-receptor; FoxL2, Forkhead box L2; FR-I, *Fshb* type - I genetic rescue; FR-II, *Fshb* type - II genetic rescue; GnRH, Gonadotropin releasing hormone; GOF, Gain-of-function; GPCR, G-protein Coupled Receptor; hCG, Human chorionic gonadotropin; HPG, Hypothalamus-Pituitary-Gonadal; *hpg*, Hypogonadal; LH, Luteinizing hormone; LHR, Luteinizing hormone receptor; mMT-1, mouse metallothionein- 1; RIP, Rat insulin II promoter; RT-PCR, Reverse transcription- polymerase chain reaction; T, Testosterone; Tg, Transgenic; TSH, Thyroid-stimulating hormone; m, mouse; h, human; p, porcine; o, ovine; WT, Wild-type.

Expression of Human *FSHB in vivo*

A transgenic mouse model harboring a 10 kb *HFSHB* transgene was the first mouse model generated to test cell-specific expression of FSH in gonadotrope cells and to identify that species-specific differences exist in FSH regulation (32). The *HFSHB* transgene was cloned into an *EcoR1-Sph1* genomic fragment and microinjected into fertilized one-cell embryos. The resulting transgenic mice exhibit only pituitary-specific *HFSHB* transgene expression, with no ectopic expression in non-pituitary tissues (32). Expression of hFSHβ was found to be localized to only gonadotrope cells in the anterior pituitary gland. The FSH heterodimer presumably incorporated the mouse-α subunit, creating an interspecies hybrid heterodimer with hFSHβ, because no free hFSHβ was detected in serum (32). FSH dimer secretion and pituitary *HFSHB* mRNA expression were higher in both transgenic and normal males than in their female counterparts. The retention of normal gonadotrope-specific expression of FSH and its function in mice expressing hFSHβ demonstrates conservation of regulatory elements and transcription factors for this subunit gene in both mice and humans (32). This mouse model provided a novel approach for studying molecular mechanisms and regulatory elements that are involved in control of the human FSHβ-encoding gene and its expression.

Gonadal Steroid Regulation of *HFSHB*

The same transgenic mouse model described above was also used for experiments designed to analyze steroid regulation of *HFSHB in vivo* (32, 33). This study included several experimental groups including castrated male and ovariectomized female mice. Castration resulted in elevated serum FSH levels in both normal controls and transgenic males. Similarly, increased serum FSH levels were observed in ovariectomized normal and transgenic females (33). Testosterone replacement after castration in male transgenic mice resulted in suppressed serum FSH levels. Estradiol (E2) replacement in ovariectomized females similarly resulted in suppressed serum and tissue FSH content. The sexually dimorphic pattern previously observed, in which both normal and transgenic males exhibiting greater tissue and serum FSH levels than the corresponding females, was also observed in these studies (33). These studies highlight the species-specific differences and suggest that the elements responsible for continued synthesis and secretion of hFSHβ in response to androgens are not present in the mouse pituitary environment (32, 33).

GnRH-Independent Androgen Inhibition of *HFSHB* Transgene

To further elucidate the direct roles that steroid hormones play in regulation of hFSHβ at the pituitary level, *HFSHB* transgenic mice were used to observe the effect of androgen in the presence or absence of gonadotropin-releasing hormone (GnRH) using both *in vitro* and *in vivo* approaches (34). Since there was an apparent species-specific difference in FSH secretion and molecular mechanisms in response to androgens, GnRH was identified as a possible key regulatory site in the androgen response of human FSHβ. For *in vitro* studies, primary pituitary cultures were obtained from GnRH-deficient *hypogonadal* (*hpg*)

TABLE 1 | Major phenotypes of FSH gain-of-function genetic models.

Model	Promoter/mutation	Major phenotypes	Implications	References
10 kb hFSHβ targeted expression (pituitary)	HFSHB promoter (Transgenic line)	**Both:** • Sexually dimorphic expression • Gonadectomy resulted in elevated FSH levels in serum, elevated h/m FSHβ mRNA • Treatment with GnRH increases expression 4 to10- fold, which is suppressed by testosterone/ estradiol • Truncation of sequences upstream of 5′ promoter region retained expression of hFSHβ • Truncation of poly-A sequences downstream of 3′ stop codon in exon 3 resulted in complete loss of expression • Replacement of 3′ poly-A sequences with heterologous sequence failed to rescue expression **Males:** • Castration: decreased FSH levels in pituitary • Castrated + testosterone treatment: suppressed mRNA content and serum FSH levels (more so than normal littermates) • Intact: increased testicular weights in adults • Intact: higher serum testosterone levels **Females:** • OVX: increased FSH levels in pituitary • OVX + E$_2$ treatment: FSH suppression in pituitary and serum; mRNA suppression • Intact: normal fertility/ litter size/ number of fertilized embryos	Model for study of hFSHβ regulation	(32–35)
Genetic rescue with 10 kb hFSHβ targeted expression (pituitary);	HFSHB promoter, Fshb null genetic background. (Type I rescue; FR-I) (Combination of a Transgenic and a knockout)	**Both:** • Targeted expression of FSH in gonadotropes **Males:** • Fertile; restored testes size and structure/ histology, normal sperm count/motility **Females:** • Fertile (10/10), normal litters, corpora lutea (CL) in rescued ovaries readily apparent	Model to study effects of pituitary gonadotrope-targeted expression of FSH on Fshb null genetic background	(36, 37)
Ectopic FSH (low)	mMT-1 promoter (mouse Metallothionein-1); Fshb null background (Type II rescue, FR-II) (Combination of a Transgenic and a knockout)	**Both:** • Ectopic expression of FSH **Males:** • Fertile; restored testes size and structure/ histology, normal sperm count/motility **Females:** • Partially fertile (3/10), small litters, small antral follicles and corpora lutea (CL) in rescued 2/3 females died postpartum • Thin uteri, folliculogenesis arrested at pre-antral stage in non-rescued mice • Weak expressors themselves were fertile and had no distinguishable phenotypes from normal littermates	Model to study effects of ectopically expressed FSH	(36)
Ectopic FSH (high)	mMT-1 promoter (Transgenic line)	**Both:** • Infertile • Elevated serum steroid hormone levels (i.e., testosterone, estradiol, progesterone) **Males:** • Enlarged seminal vesicles, normal testicular size/development • Increased (epididymal) sperm counts • Castration reduced seminal vesicles to size similar to castrated wild-type littermates **Females:** • Large hemorrhagic/cystic ovaries • Fluid-filled translucent ovaries	Model to study possible role of FSH (and steroid hormones) in human reproductive diseases	(24)

(Continued)

TABLE 1 | Continued

Model	Promoter/mutation	Major phenotypes	Implications	References
		• Some follicles halted at pre-antral stage, some developed normally • Large/cystic kidneys, abnormal kidney development • Die 6–13 weeks due to urinary tract obstruction		
FSH genetic rescue	Ovine FSHβ (*oFshb*) promoter; *Fshb* null background (Combination of a Transgenic and a knockout)	*Double N-glycosylation mutant hFSH compared to WT hFSH* • Low levels in serum (both) • Readily detectable (mutant) FSH levels in pituitary as subunit monomer but not as FSH heterodimer **Males:** • Fertile • Lower testes weights • No rescue with regard to testes phenotypic characteristics (tubule diameter, and sperm counts) **Females:** • Infertile • No estrus cycles • Hypoplastic ovaries and uteri	Model to study possible therapy for FSH ligand deficiency Model to study role of N-glycans on FSH	(36, 38)
Ectopic *HFSHB* Tg+	Rat insulin II promoter (*RIP II*) (Transgenic line) (Combination of a Transgenic and a natural mutant background)	**Both:** • No significant sexual dimorphism in hFSH levels **Males:** • Similar testosterone levels to controls (non-transgenic *hpg*) • No correlation between hFSH and inhibin B levels • Strong positive correlation between hFSH and testis size (at high serum hFSH levels) • Disorganized testes development • Minimal but incomplete spermatogenesis (no fully differentiated spermatozoa) **Females:** • No apparent estradiol response to hFSH • Strong positive correlation between hFSH and inhibin B levels (similar to WT levels) • Strong positive correlation between serum hFSH and ovaries size • Follicle development to type 7 antral follicles, but no corpora lutea found • *hpg* (Tg+ and non-Tg) body weights lower than WT controls at 9–11 weeks • *hpg* Tg+ ovaries 4x weight increase (compared to non-Tg) • Primordial follicle numbers 2 times higher than in WT and *hpg* non-Tg controls • Secondary follicles restored to normal levels (9–11 weeks) • Number of total antral follicles restored to normal levels (9–11 weeks) • Strong positive correlation between inhibin B and antral follicle count • Increased inhibin A expression (compared to non-Tg) • Dose dependent increase in bone mass (*hpg* and non-*hpg*) • Positive correlation between FSH levels and osteoblast/bone surface area • Negative correlation between FSH levels and osteoclast/bone surface area • Ovariectomy of *hpg* mice resulted in: - decrease of serum levels of inhibin A and testosterone - 47% reduction in bone mass	Model to study FSH actions alone	(30, 39–41)

(Continued)

TABLE 1 | Continued

Model	Promoter/mutation	Major phenotypes	Implications	References
		- uterine weights similar to control in *non-hpg* Tg mice • Uterine weights increased compared to control in *hpg* (still lower than *non-hpg*) • No detectable *Fshr* mRNA in bone cells • Age-specific decline in litter production in females due to increased embryo-fetal resorptions without affecting the number of ovulations.		
FSH re-routed	*HFSHB Mut*; on *Fshb* null background (Combination of a Transgenic and a knockout)	**Both:** • Sexually dimorphic expression • Dense core granule and chaperone proteins co-localized in pituitary with mutant hFSHβ (similar to LHβ) • Secretion of mutant hFSH increased 2–4 times in response to GnRH agonist (no significant release in control mice) • Lower levels of serum LH in mice expressing mutant hFSH (comparable *Lhb* mRNA levels to those in pituitaries of *Lhb* $^{+/-}$ mice) **Males:** • No specific phenotypes **Females:** • Ovarian and uterine morphology similar between mutant and wt hFSHβ expressing mice • Aromatase levels restored to normal in mutant and wt hFSHβ expressing mice at 9 weeks (on *Fshb* null background) • High progesterone levels in mice expressing mutant FSH • 6 times more ovulations in mutant FSH (compared to wt hFSH and normal controls) • Identical primordial follicle counts across all groups • Increased pre-antral follicles, CLs, and follicle size in mutant hFSH-expressing mice • Decreased occurrence of atresia in mutant hFSH-expressing mice • Granulosa pro-survival as well as FSH and LH-responsive genes upregulated in mutant hFSH-expressing mice • *Lhb*-null mice not rescued by mutant FSH	Model to study differences in secretion patterns of LH and FSH	(37)
FSH Tg+ in milk	Rat β-casein promoter (Transgenic line)	**Males:** • No phenotypes reported **Females:** • Recombinant bovine FSH detected exclusively in milk	Model to study ectopic expression of FSH in mammary glands	(42)
	Bovine β-casein promoter (Transgenic line)	• Larger lumens in mammary glands of β-casein-*hFSH Tg* mice than wild type controls • hFSH detected in milk fluids and epithelial cells of Tg mice and not in controls • Amount of hFSH detected in milk proportional to transgene copy number • hFSH increased cAMP levels in hFSH-R transfected cells with competitive binding (biologically active) • Transgenic platelet count 2 times more that of WT controls • 26.7% of highest-expressing line displayed both breast and ovarian granulosa cell tumors with hemorrhagic cysts • Mouse FSH and progesterone levels of Tg mice higher in all phases of estrus cycle than non-Tg littermates		(43)

(Continued)

TABLE 1 | Continued

Model	Promoter/mutation	Major phenotypes	Implications	References
Pig FSH Tg	Chinese Erhualian Boar FSHα/β promoter + gene including long range cis-regulatory elements (Transgenic line)	**Males:** • Boars: *TG compared to WT controls:* • Serum FSH levels significantly higher • Semen volume, sperm concentration and motility similar • Germ cells per seminiferous tubule increased • Comparable body weights throughout growth • No significant differences in gut microflora or disease markers **Females:** • Mice: *TG compared to WT controls:* • Significant increase in litter number • Significant increase in CL number (at 14–28 weeks) • Increased serum levels of endogenous mouse FSH and estradiol • Decreased serum levels of LH and testosterone- • Decreased LH mRNA content • Boars: *TG compared to WT controls* • Higher serum FSH levels • Higher pituitary FSHβ content • Smaller litter size • Comparable body weights • No significant difference in serum LH and estradiol	Model to study biological effects of pig FSH	(44) (45) (46)
Inhibin-α KO	Inhibin α-subunit gene deletion (Knockout)	**Both:** • Infertile • Gonadal stromal tumors • Increased serum FSH levels • Die from cachexia-like symptoms **Males:** • Testicular enlargement/ hemorrhage • Decrease in number of Leydig cells • Decreased spermatogenesis proportional to tumor size **Females:** • Ovarian hemorrhage • Decreased folliculogenesis proportional to tumor size	Model to understand and study role of Inhibin/ inhibin-α in development as well as its tumor suppressor activity in gonads	(24, 47)
Inhibin-α / FSH double knockout	Inhibin α-subunit and *Fshb* gene deletion (Double knockout)	**Both:** • Delayed body weight loss compared to inhibin single mutants • Less severe cachexia in double mutants compared to mice lacking only inhibin **Males:** • Compared to inhibin single knockouts, double mutants live longer • Testicular tumors in double mutants are less hemorrhagic **Females:** • Compared to inhibin single knockouts, double mutants live longer • Ovarian tumors are less aggressive • Folliculogenesis is not disrupted at early stages but eventually hemorrhagic ovarian tumors develop	Model to study how FSH acts as a modifier factor to regulate gonadal tumors in the absence of inhibin	(24)
FSHR gain of function	Rat androgen binding protein promoter (*rABP*) on *hpg* background	**Males:** • Fertile (on non-*hpg* background) • Infertile (on *hpg* background)	Model to study downstream pathways involving FSHR signaling	(48, 49)

(Continued)

TABLE 1 | Continued

Model	Promoter/mutation	Major phenotypes	Implications	References
	(Combination of transgenic and natural mutation) Asp567Gly mutant when compared to *hpg* non-Tg littermates:	• Testis weights increased nearly 2 times • Treatment with testosterone resulted in larger testis • Testis contained small numbers of both round and elongated spermatids, mature Sertoli cells • Increased number of seminiferous tubules (compared to Tg-FSH group) • Slight rise in serum and significant rise in intra-testicular testosterone levels		(50)
	TghFSHRwt	*Compared to non-Tg hpg littermates* • overexpression: • No effect on testis weight/serum testosterone levels • No additive effect on testis weight with testosterone treatment • No change in expression of steroid synthesis genes • No changes in testis structure/cellular morphology • Treatment with FSH increased cAMP levels 2 times more, basal levels remained the same • No TSH or hCG binding		
	TgD567G mutant	• 2 times increase in testis weight • Synergistic effects on testis weight with testosterone treatment • Increased expression of steroid synthesis genes • Later stage spermatogenesis/ post-meiotic elongated spermatids • Treatment with FSH increased cAMP levels (40% as much as *TghFSHwt*), basal levels increased two times more • Binds to TSH and hCG (cAMP levels increased by 40% that of FSH stimulation)		
	Constitutively active FSHR mutants; Human *AMH* promoter driving separately expression of *mFshr D580H* or *D580Y* cDNA transgenes; or a *D580Y* knock-in mouse *Fshr* allele	• Transgenic *Fshr* ^{D580H} female mice demonstrated hemorrhagic and cystic ovaries, loss of immature follicles, increased granulosa cell proliferation, increased E2 production, unruptured and luteinized follicles and occasional teratomas • Most severely affected transgenic *Fshr* ^{D580H} female mice, in addition, displayed increased prolactin levels and mammary gland hyperplasia, pituitary adenoma formation and adrenal defects • Transgenic and knock-in *Fshr* ^{D580Y} mice showed milder ovarian phenotypes with only hemorrhagic cysts		
	Constitutively active FSHR on Lhr null background	*Compared to WT males* • Fertile • Delayed puberty • Mating trials had lower frequency of pregnancy and litter size • 20 times more of *Fshr* mRNA • 40% of serum T levels • Normal spermatogenesis and testis/seminal vesicle size • Treatment with antiandrogen had no effect on spermatogenesis or testis size (though reduced seminal vesicle size) while both were arrested in WT **Females:** • fertile (on non-*hpg* background) • No significant differences in ovarian weights between hpg Tg and non-Tg littermates		(51)

mice (9, 52) carrying the *HFSHB* transgene (34). Testosterone treatment in the absence of GnRH resulted in suppression of *HFSHB* mRNA and confirmed the inhibitory action of androgens directly at the pituitary level independent of GnRH (34). *In vivo* experiments in the *hpg HFSHB* mice included daily GnRH injections, which induced *HFSHB* expression in both males and females. Simultaneous administration of testosterone propionate in males completely blocked the stimulatory effect of GnRH, whereas simultaneous E_2 administration in females only partially inhibited GnRH effects (34). These results demonstrated direct effects of testosterone and E_2 on hFSHβ subunit expression at the pituitary level as well as an indirect suppression of GnRH as an additional regulatory mechanism (34). Additional hypothalamic site of E_2 action cannot also be ruled out based on the above data.

Having established that the 10 kb *HFSHB* transgene is appropriately targeted to and hormonally regulated in mouse gonadotropes, a series of deletions were made on the 10 kb *HFSHB* transgene (35). Several independent transgenic lines expressing 5′ and 3′ truncated versions of *HFSHB* transgene were produced and systematically analyzed. These *in vivo* models helped to identify that truncation of sequences upstream of 5′ promoter region retained expression of hFSHβ in mouse gonadotropes, truncation of poly-A sequences downstream of 3′ stop codon in exon 3 resulted in complete loss of expression. Replacement of 3′ poly-A sequences with heterologous sequences (for example, lacZ reporter sequences) similarly failed to confer expression (35).

Since FSH is normally released from the pituitary in response to GnRH, it is of great interest to observe the physiological response to targeted expression of FSH in non-pituitary tissues. Accordingly, mouse models have been generated that drive expression from either specific or multiple ectopic tissues.

Use of *HFSHB* Transgenes to Achieve Genetic Rescue of *Fshb* Null Mice

An FSH-deficient mouse model was created in 1997 through targeted mutation (*Fshb^{m1}*) in exon 3 of the FSHβ-encoding gene (53). Mice that were homozygous, i.e., *Fshb* null (*Fshb^{m1}/ Fshb^{m1}*), and therefore FSH-deficient, were generated by intercrossing heterozygous mice. *Fshb* null males displayed decreased testis size, yet were fertile (53). Sperm number was decreased by 75%, however, viability remained unchanged. In contrast, *Fshb* null females with the *Fshb^{m1}/ Fshb^{m1}* genotype were infertile, with small ovaries and thin uteri. Ovaries had arrested follicular development at the secondary stage, and lacked any corpora lutea (53).

Genetic rescue of FSH-deficient mice was achieved using two independent methods (36). The type 1 genetic rescue (FR-I) consisted of targeting the previously described 10-kb *HFSHB* transgene specifically to pituitary gonadotrope cells. This genetic strategy resulted in complete rescue of both males and females lacking endogenous *Fshb* (36). Testis size and sperm counts in FR-I males were restored to those observed in wild-type values. Similar results were obtained in FR-1 females, as uterine and ovarian sizes also returned to wild-type values. Normal follicular

development, restored estrous cycles, and production of normal litter sizes were observed in FR-I females.

Low- level ectopic expression of *HFSHB* was achieved in multiple tissues using a mouse metallothionein (mMT-1) gene promoter with the goal of genetically restoring reproductive phenotypes in FSH-deficient mice, designated as type 2 rescue (FR-II) (36). The mMT-1 promoter was used to drive ectopic expression of both a hCGα-encoding minigene and a hFSHβ-encoding gene, thereby resulting in expression of hFSH dimer in multiple tissues (36). Male mice expressing ectopic hFSH (FR-II) showed complete restoration of testis size and sperm counts. However, restoration of normal reproductive phenotypes was incomplete in FR-II females. Only 3 out of 10 FR-II females were able to conceive, and litter sizes were small. Arrested folliculogenesis was frequently observed in FR-II females. The small number of FR-II females that were able to become pregnant produced one litter, had obvious corpora lutea, yet small antral follicles (36). The results with the type 2 genetic rescue suggest that ectopic expression of human FSH can completely rescue *Fshb* null male mice, yet only partially rescue *Fshb* null females (36).

Ectopic Overexpression of HFSH Dimer in Transgenic Mice

Overexpression of FSH may lead to high serum levels and clinical conditions that negatively affect fertility. A transgenic mouse model ectopically expressing human FSHβ using an mMT-1 promoter resulted in male and female mice overexpressing hFSH in several tissues (24). Mice expressing either only transgenic MT-α subunit or only MT-FSHβ were crossed to obtain mice expressing hFSH ectopically (24). Founders expressing hFSH dimer at very high levels were chosen for further analysis. Both males and females were infertile; males showed enlarged seminal vesicles and elevated testosterone levels yet normal testis size and spermatogenesis (24). These high level FSH expressing males were infertile, presumably due to male sexual behavioral deficits secondary to excess testosterone. However, this behavioral phenotype was not tested in these studies. Females displayed arrested folliculogenesis, along with increased serum estrogen, progesterone, and testosterone concentrations. Females also developed urinary tract obstruction and hemorrhagic and cystic ovaries, yet exhibited no signs of tumors (24). Their symptoms were comparable, but not identical to human conditions such as polycystic ovarian and ovarian hyperstimulation syndromes. Most females died between 6 and 13 weeks of age. (24). The overexpression of hFSH in multiple tissues gave insight into these clinical conditions and provided a model that may be used in the future for developing treatments.

Ectopic Expression of FSH in *hpg* Mice

The role of FSH in gonadal physiology was investigated using a mouse model similar to the models described above that carry a *HFSHB* transgene (39). However, this model expressed transgenic human-FSH (tg-FSH) on a gonadotropin-deficient *hypogonadal (hpg)* background to observe FSH effects independent of LH. The *HFSHB* transgene was cloned into a vector containing the rat insulin II promoter (RIP) and injected into mouse oocytes (39). RIP directed ectopic expression of tg-FSH to the pancreas. Hypogonadism was accomplished by breeding tg-FSH mice to an *hpg* strain containing a truncating mutation that caused GnRH depletion, thereby creating tg-FSH+ *hpg* mice (39, 52). Varying serum tg-FSH levels were found in different strains of mice, allowing for analysis of a range of circulating FSH concentrations. Tg-FSH seemed to have no effect on androgen levels in the tg-FSH+ *hpg* mice, which appeared to be due to underdeveloped epididymis and seminal vesicles. In male tg-FSH+ *hpg* mice, testis size increased as compared to non-tg-FSH *hpg* controls, however, this was only observed in males exhibiting high serum FSH levels (>1 IU/liter). Tg-FSH+ *hpg* female mice secreting high levels of FSH exhibited dose-dependent, elevated inhibin B secretion. Ovaries of tg-FSH+ *hpg* females were also enlarged and exhibited increased follicular development to the antral stage (39).

Additional studies were performed using female tg-FSH+ *hpg* mice to determine the effect of FSH alone on primordial follicle reserve and the role of FSH in early follicular development (40). Partial disruption of follicular development was observed in non-tg *hpg* ovaries. Although development past the primary follicle stage occurred, there were small numbers of early antral follicles. In contrast, tg-FSH+ *hpg* females showed advanced follicular development up to the antral stage, although no corpora lutea were observed in any tg-FSH+ or non-tg FSH *hpg* ovaries due to the absence of LH (40). Significant increases in total primordial and secondary follicle numbers were seen in tg-FSH+ *hpg* females as compared with both non-tg *hpg* and wild-type mice. The total antral follicle count was 15-fold higher in tg-FSH+ *hpg* ovaries than non-tg FSH *hpg* levels, which restored values to wild-type levels (40). The findings from this study indicate an important role of FSH in early follicular development, showing an increase in primordial follicle reserve and stimulation of follicle growth.

Interestingly, when tg-FSH+ female mice alone with progressively rising hFSH levels (2.5–10 IU/ml) were monitored across the life span, age-specific phenotypes were observed. Whereas, tg-FSH+ female mice < 22 week of age delivered increased litter sizes, those that were older (>23 week of age) produced decreased litter sizes despite increased ovulations and demonstrated premature infertility due to embryo resorptions and parturition failure. Thus, this model provided a novel *in vivo* scenario in which age-related rise in FSH contributes to female reproductive aging and infertility by a post-implantation defect (embryo-fetal resorption) without directly affecting the ovarian reserve (41).

Contrary to the proposed deleterious and direct effects of FSH on bone osteoclasts in mice (54), ectopic human FSH expression in the above described genetic model caused an increase in bone mass in female mice (30). Similar phenotypes were also observed when the *HFSHB* transgene was expressed on the *hpg* genetic background with a total suppression of endogenous gonadotropins and E2. Expression analysis indicated osteoclasts did not express *Fshr* mRNA and the bone phenotypes manifest only when ovaries were intact. Further studies indicated that bone volume in these transgenic mice positively correlated with ovary-derived inhibin A and androgens. Thus, ectopic human

FSH expression in this model suggests FSH acts indirectly to enhance bone function in an ovary-dependent and LH-independent manner (30). The controversy with regard to non-gonadal actions of FSH is ongoing and has been recently described in detail (55).

Rerouting of FSH Into the LH Secretion Pathway

Transcriptional responses of FSHβ and LHβ encoding genes are different and dependent on GnRH pulse frequencies (10, 11, 56). In immortalized gonadotrope cells, *Fshb* gene transcription is favored by slow GnRH pulses whereas *Lhb* gene transcription is dependent on fast GnRH pulses (10, 11, 56). Once the heterodimers are assembled, FSH is largely released constitutively, while LH is released as pulses via a regulated secretory pathway (10, 11). LH contains a carboxy terminal (C′) heptapeptide that directs its secretion via this regulated pathway. A novel mouse model took advantage of this heptapeptide to observe the physiological response to a mutant FSH that contained this peptide (37). Human transgenes encoding either a wild type (*HFSHB*^{WT}) or mutant (*HFSHB*^{Mut}) FSHβ were introduced onto an *Fshb-null* genetic background.

The presence of interspecies heterodimers of mouse-α-and WT or mutant FSHβ subunits in different mouse lines was confirmed by Western blot analysis (37). LH is stored in dense-core granules (DCG) prior to release (57–59). To determine whether mutant FSH was secreted via the same pathway as LH, co-localization of mutant FSHβ subunit and DCG-specific Rab27 was evaluated in gonadotrope cells. Interestingly, the number of mutant FSHβ subunit and Rab27 co-localized gonadotropes was 6 to 8- fold higher than seen in gonadotropes of control mice, where FSH is secreted via the constitutive pathway (37). Co-localization of mutant FSHβ and a chaperone protein chromogranin-A (Chr-A), which is found in the Golgi network in gonadotropes and important for regulated release of LH, was also examined. Co-localization of mutant FSHβ and Chr-A was higher when compared to both control and *Fshb* null mice expressing a *HFSHB*^{WT} transgene and was similar to levels seen with co-localization of LHβ (37). These results suggest that the engineered mutant FSHβ (containing the C′ heptapeptide normally only found in LH)- containing FSH heterodimer successfully entered the regulated secretory pathway.

As described above, mice deficient in FSH are infertile, have small ovaries and thin uteri, along with disrupted folliculogenesis (53). *HFSHB*^{Mut} transgene was able to genetically rescue *Fshb-null* mice, restoring ovarian and uterine size as well as estrus cycles leading to the presence of antral follicles and corpora lutea in ovaries. Progesterone levels were higher in *HFSHB*^{Mut}-expressing mice than in control and wild-type mice (37). Interestingly, the number of ovulations was increased from 9 to 10 per cycle in control mice to 55 per cycle in mutant FSH–expressing *Fshb* null mice (37). This was accompanied by the presence of more pre-antral follicles and reduced follicular atresia in ovaries. Mice expressing *HFSHB*^{Mut} also demonstrated increased follicle size and enhanced granulosa cell proliferation, leading to a longer reproductive lifespan and follicle survival (37). This mouse model provided a novel approach to studying differential secretory pathways of FSH and LH, and demonstrated a potential role of rerouted FSH in treating age-associated reproductive conditions (37).

Expression of a Transgene Encoding the Non-glycosylated Human FSHβ Subunit

One of the characteristic features of glycoprotein hormones, including FSH is the presence of N-linked sugar chains on both the α- and β-subunits. FSH possesses four (2 on each subunit) potential N-glycan attachment sites (1–4, 60, 61). The presence or absence of both N-glycans on FSHβ subunit contributes to macroheterogeneity, significantly affects serum half–life and may alter bioactivity (60, 61). To genetically determine the role of N-glycans on the human FSHβ subunit, the nucleotides corresponding to two Thr residues following Asn residues on which N-glycans are added, Asn7 and Asn24, were mutated to Ala, thereby abolishing N-glycosylation events at these two sites (38, 60).

The mutant cDNA transgene encoding the N-glycosylation double mutant FSHβ subunit was targeted to gonadotropes in transgenic mice first and the transgene was subsequently introduced onto *Fshb* null genetic background using the well-established genetic rescue scheme. An *HFSHB* ^{WT} transgene similarly was introduced onto *Fshb* null genetic background and the resultant *Fshb* null mice carrying the *HFSHB* ^{WT} transgene were used as positive controls (38, 60). Biochemical studies confirmed that the mutant FSHβ subunit inefficiently assembled with the endogenous mouse α-subunit and very little FSH heterodimer was present in pituitary extracts (38). Moreover, media collected from short term pituitary organ culture experiments and serum from mutant FSHβ-expressing *Fshb* null mice showed very low or undetectable levels of FSH by radioimmunoassays. These data indicated that the double N-glycosylation mutant FSHβ subunit was secretion incompetent (38). Moreover, the mutant transgene, unlike the *HFSHB* ^{WT} transgene, did not rescue *Fshb* null mice, confirming that even if secreted in low levels, the mutant FSHβ-subunit containing FSH dimer was biologically inactive (38). Thus, these studies provided *in vivo* genetic evidence that N-glycosylation on FSHβ subunit is critical for FSH heterodimer assembly, secretion and action (38).

Expression of FSH in the Mammary Gland

Ectopic expression of bovine FSH has been achieved in a model targeting its expression in milk secreted from mouse mammary glands (42). This mouse model was created using a rat β-casein gene promoter driving expression of bovine α and FSHβ subunits. The β-casein promoter drives targeted expression in only the mammary gland, making it possible to observe the effects of ectopic bovine FSH expression in a single tissue (42). Transgenic (Tg) mice expressing the transgene were created either by microinjection of both subunits, or by breeding of mice that expressed each one of them separately (42). The presence of tg-FSH was confirmed by northern blot and radioimmunoassay. Bioactivity of tg-FSH was also confirmed by measuring granulosa cell counts and the ability of the cells to produce estrogen

(42). The amount of tg-FSH positively correlated with granulosa cell number and estrogen production, and therefore suggesting successful bioactivity of the transgene-derived FSH (42). No other overt phenotypes were observed in transgenic mice. This mouse model provided a novel approach for expressing FSH in mammary glands and releasing it into milk.

A similar model was later generated that also ectopically expressed FSH in mammary glands, but in this case, the transgene encoded human FSH. In these studies, the investigators used the bovine β-casein gene promoter to specifically express human FSH in mammary glands of transgenic mice (43). Milk was collected from tg-hFSH mice to determine FSH concentration using an enzyme-linked immunosorbent assay (ELISA). Two mouse lines showed nearly undetectable levels of hFSH, as compared to one line that had high levels (300 mIU/mL). This variation in hFSH concentration in different lines was most likely due to differing transgene copy numbers (43). *In vitro* biological activity of hFSH was determined by measuring cyclic-AMP (cAMP) production after exposing hFSH receptor-transfected cells to sterilized milk from each cell line. Milk containing hFSH increased cAMP production in the assay, indicating receptor binding and intracellular signaling, and therefore, biological activity of hFSH (43).

Blood cell counts were performed to analyze the effects of any hFSH leakage into the circulation. Several of the transgenic lines showed increased white blood cell and platelet levels as compared to normal mice, red blood cells in the affected animals were also smaller in size (43). Ovarian and breast tumors were observed in one transgenic line, along with collapsed alveoli within the lactating glands. Human FSH also seemed to have a stimulatory effect on endogenous mouse FSH, as mFSH levels were higher at all estrus cycle phases in transgenic mice (43). This unique mouse model displayed distinct physiological responses to ectopic expression of hFSH in mammary glands and secretion into milk. Many of them negatively affected blood circulation and reproductive health. Ectopic hFSH leaking into the bloodstream appeared to lead to overproduction of endogenous mouse FSH, possibly contributing to the observed ovarian and breast tumors by increased estrogen production as a secondary consequence (43).

Expression of Porcine FSH in Mice

Transgenic expression of porcine FSH using bacterial artificial chromosome (BAC) methods has been achieved using a gain-of-function mouse model (45). A BAC containing porcine (p) α and β subunits was constructed and isolated from a porcine BAC library from a male Erhualian pig, a highly prolific pig breed. BAC clones containing pFSH α and β were then digested and microinjected into fertilized mouse zygotes (45). Transgenic (Tg) mice expressing pFSH were identified by PCR and Southern blot. After further breeding of Tg mice to wild-type mice, both pFSHβ and pFSHα BACs were transmitted in identical Mendelian ratios to offspring, indicating proper hybridization of the Tg subunits. Expression of Tg pFSH mRNA was confirmed by RT-PCR and northern blot, with expression localized specifically to the pituitary gland. Circulating pFSH was confirmed by evaluation of serum samples by ELISA, showing levels ranging from 6.36 to 19.83 IU/L, which were within the physiological range (45).

Female fecundity was analyzed in both Tg and WT mice. Interestingly, Tg females had litter sizes that were significantly larger than WT females as well as the total number of pups than WT littermates. This increase in fecundity in Tg females seemed to be due to enhanced ovulation, as histological examination revealed a significant increase in the number of corpora lutea at 14 and 28 weeks of age in Tg mice compared to WT. Serum hormone levels were analyzed to determine if increased ovulation was due to differential hormonal regulation (45).

Endogenous mouse FSH levels were elevated in Tg mice, as was estradiol. Serum levels of LH and testosterone were significantly lower in Tg mice compared to WT. Pituitary expression of LHβ mRNA was also lower in Tg mice than in WT mice (45). The increased estradiol levels could be due to greater aromatization of androgens to estrogens due to elevated levels of endogenous mFSH in addition to transgene-derived pFSH (45). This enhanced conversion of testosterone to estrogen as a result of increased aromatase activity could explain the lower serum levels of testosterone. However, the mechanism for reduced LHβ mRNA and serum LH despite low levels of serum testosterone is unclear. The results from this study provided confirmation of successful expression of porcine FSH in a transgenic mouse model with no reproductive effects in males but enhanced ovulation in female Tg mice (45).

Expression of Transgenic Porcine FSH in Large White Boars

Porcine FSH was further analyzed by the same group that produced BAC pFSH subunits from Chinese Erhualian pigs, and introduced them into Large White Boars (44). As the Large White Boar previously showed poor reproductive performance, the investigators sought to determine if overexpression of pFSH from a highly prolific pig breed could improve fertility. Successful integration of pFSH into transgenic (Tg) boars was confirmed using genomic PCR as well as RT-qPCR analysis to determine mRNA expression of porcine FSHα and FSHβ. Expression of FSHα was observed in multiple tissues including heart, liver, spleen, kidney, brain, testis, and epididymis of both Tg and wild type (WT) boars, with higher expression in Tg than WT.

Expression of FSHβ was localized specifically to the pituitary and was significantly higher in Tg than WT boars (44). Higher serum levels of both FSHα and FSHβ were observed in Tg boars suggesting overexpression of pFSH. Male reproductive performance was measured by evaluating semen volume, sperm motility, sperm concentration, and total sperm number per ejaculation (44). There was no significant difference between semen quality parameters of Tg and WT boars. However, the number of germ cells per seminiferous tubule was significantly higher in Tg boars than WT (44). The elevated germ cell counts in seminiferous tubules suggested increased spermatogenesis capacity, but the lack of significant results from semen evaluation leaves room for further analysis to confirm this possibility (44).

In a third study done using the same BAC system containing pFSH α and β, analysis of reproductive phenotypes in female

transgenic (Tg) Large White Boars were analyzed. Methods for pFSH BAC transfer were the same as previously described for this model (44). The specific integration site of pFSH into Large White Boars was determined using whole-genome sequencing, identifying exogenous FSHα/β genes at 140, 646, 456 bp on chromosome 9 (46). The transgene integration site was mapped to perhaps rule out that the integration itself did not result in modification of any endogenous loci that regulate fertility.

Analysis of Tg female boars revealed elevated levels of serum FSH and FSHβ protein in the pituitary, but Tg females produced reduced numbers of total newborn piglets as compared to WT. Reduced expression of *Fshr, Lhr, Esr1,* and *Esr2* was also observed using RT-qPCR in Tg boars as compared to WT at 300 days of age. Reproductive organ weights, blood cell counts, and histological analysis revealed no differences between Tg and WT boars in overall reproductive health (46). The reduced expression of mRNAs encoding receptors for FSH, LH, and estrogen suggest a possible negative effect of pFSH overexpression in female pigs as well as the observation of reduced total newborn piglets (46). Further studies using this model are needed to confirm the effects. However, these studies provided novel information on the physiological role of porcine FSH *in vivo* in the homologous species.

Inhibin Knock Out Mouse Model

Important regulators of FSH production and secretion are gonad-derived dimeric growth factors, activin and inhibin. Inhibin is a heterodimer, consisting of an α and β subunit, whereas activin is a homodimer, consisting of various combinations of the two homologous β subunits (βA and βB) (21). The inhibin and activin subunits are expressed in multiple tissues throughout the body. Inhibins suppress and whereas activins promote FSH synthesis and secretion. To investigate the role of inhibin in reproduction and general physiology, a knockout mouse model with a targeted deletion of the α-inhibin–encoding gene was achieved using homologous recombination technology in mouse embryonic stem cells (47). Targeted deletion of only the α-subunit of inhibin ensured successful inhibin deficiency without unwanted deletion of the activins.

Male and female heterozygous mice produced normal litter sizes and were fertile. However, homozygous males and females proved to be infertile when crossed with wild-type mice, despite developing normal external genitalia (47). In addition to infertility, all homozygous mice tested showed gonadal tumors when examined histologically, which were evident as early as 4 weeks of age. Testicular enlargement was visible in males, along with gradual regression of spermatogenesis and a decrease in Leydig cell count starting at 5–7 weeks of age (47). In females, ovarian tumors disrupted follicular development and morphology from 7 to 16 weeks of age. FSH levels in both males and female homozygous, inhibin-deficient mice were 2- to 3-fold higher when compared to both heterozygous and WT control mice (47). The results of this study suggested a novel secreted tumor suppressor role for inhibin that was highly specific to the gonads. Development of normal external sexual organs and gametes followed by regression and disruption at a later age indicated normal embryogenesis and early sexual development, therefore suggesting gonadal tumors as the cause for infertility (47).

To further investigate the role of inhibin and FSH in gonadal tumorigenesis, a double-mutant knockout approach was taken. Since the inhibin-deficient mice developed aggressive gonadal tumors accompanied by elevated FSH levels, the contribution of FSH to tumorigenesis was directly assessed using a genetic strategy. To achieve this, double-homozygous mutant mice were created by intercrossing heterozygotes for each knockout mutation ($Inha^{m1}$ and $Fshb^{m1}$) to generate mice deficient in both inhibin and FSH ($Inha^{m1}/Inha^{m1}$; $Fshb^{m1}/Fshb^{m1}$) (24). The first parameter examined in the double-knockout mice was weight, as the previous study showed that mice deficient in inhibin only, exhibit a severe cachexia-like syndrome and die by 12 weeks of age (24). Most of double-knockout mutant males survived for 1 year and showed no dramatic weight loss or testis phenotypes. Approximately, 95% of the inhibin-deficient female mice died by 17 weeks. In contrast, double null mutant females, about 70% survived past 17 weeks, but these all eventually died by 39 weeks and all of them exhibited severe weight loss (24).

Gonadal tumor progression was also altered in the double-mutant mice, as development of tumors was slower and less aggressive than in mice deficient in inhibin alone (24). In 12 week old double mutant males, the tumors were small, there were no signs of hemorrhage, and tubule morphology was also unaltered by tumor growth, despite proliferation of tumor cells (24). Beyond 1 year of age, some males showed no tumor development, as compared to inhibin-deficient males which all had tumors as early as 4 weeks (24).

In female double-mutants, ovaries appeared morphologically normal at 12 weeks of age. Histological analysis revealed hemorrhage, cysts, as well as granulosa cell tumors. However, these tumors in the double-knockout females appeared less invasive and developed more slowly than in inhibin-deficient mice. Both male and female double-mutant mice showed reduced serum levels of activin A and estradiol as compared to mice lacking only inhibin (24). In addition to this, aromatase mRNA expression levels were reduced in double-mutant mice compared to those in inhibin-deficient mice. These results confirm the role of inhibin in gonadal tumorigenesis and identify FSH as an important modifier in the progression and aggressive growth of inhibin-deficient gonadal tumors (24).

FSH Receptor Gain of Function

The FSH receptor (FSHR) is a transmembrane, G-protein coupled receptor expressed on testicular Sertoli cells and ovarian granulosa cells in males and females, respectively (2, 4). Signaling via FSHRs results in steroidogenesis (production of

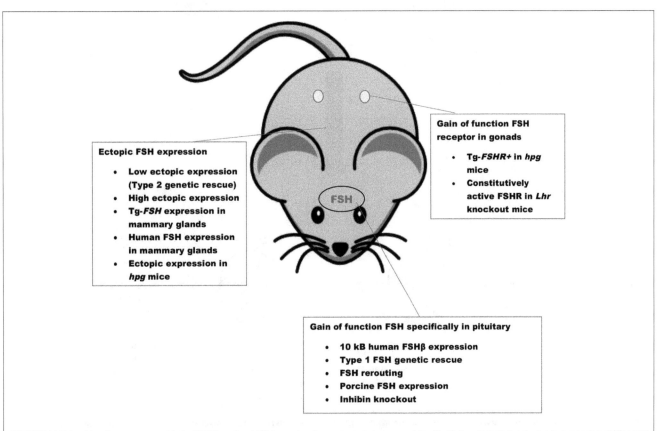

FIGURE 1 | Gain of function mouse models for FSH ligand and FSH receptor. A summary of mouse models with pituitary-targeted and ectopic expression of FSH and gain of function mouse models for FSHR activation. Inhibin knockout mice have high levels of FSH as a result of loss suppression by inhibin.

estrogen) and is essential for gonadal development in both sexes. A novel approach to studying the gain-of-function effects of FSH receptor was undertaken by generating a mouse model exhibiting constitutively active FSH receptor action on an *hpg* genetic background (48). The use of the *hpg* genetic background allowed observation of the effects of active FSHR completely independent of endogenous gonadotropins, FSH and LH.

The gain of function receptor mutation (*FSHR+*) was a single amino acid substitution (Asp567Gly) that was specifically expressed in Sertoli cells by using the rat androgen binding

protein (rABP) promoter (48). Bioactivity of the ligand-independent FSH receptor was confirmed by measuring cAMP production, which was significantly higher in Tg-Sertoli cells than in non-Tg-*hpg* Sertoli cells *in vitro* (48). The *in vivo* effects of the *FSHR+* mutation were first examined by measuring testicular weight. Tg-FSHR+ *hpg* testis weights were increased up to 5-fold, with an average of a 2-fold increase as compared to non-Tg *hpg* controls. Histological examination of *FSHR+* testes showed round and elongated spermatids and signs of Sertoli cell maturation, as compared with non-*FSHR+* *hpg* controls that lacked mature Sertoli cells and exhibited

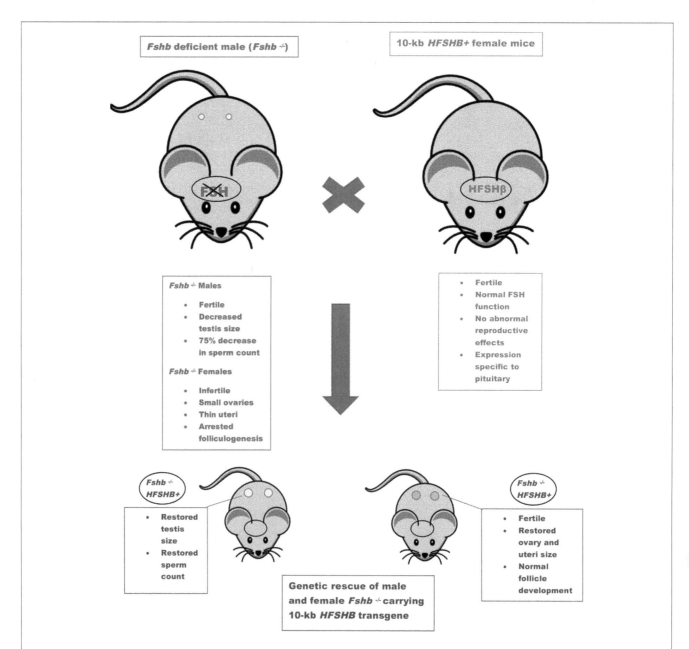

FIGURE 2 | Genetic rescue scheme. Mice lacking *Fshb* show sexually dimorphic phenotypes (red box). The features of *HFSHB+* mice were shown in blue box. *HFSHB+* mice by themselves do not exhibit any overt phenotypes. The *Fshb* null male mice are typically intercrossed with *HFSHB+* transgenic female mice to eventually generate *Fshb$^{-/-}$ HFSHB^{+}* mice. The *HFSHB^{+}* transgene fully rescues both male and female *Fshb* null mice (purple boxes).

blocked spermatogenesis. Tg-FSHR+ mice also had elevated testosterone levels, and undetectable levels of LH and FSH, suggesting that the observed physiological responses to the constitutively active FSH receptor was indeed gonadotropin-independent (48).

To determine whether the results from the FSHR+ mutation were solely due to the amino-acid substitution or if they were in response to overexpression of mutant FSH receptor, a comparative study was performed using the same mouse model in parallel with a transgenically overexpressed wild-type human FSH receptor (TgFSHRwt) (49). Transgenic male and female mice overexpressing TgFSHRwt were created by microinjection of a human FSHR DNA construct into mouse oocytes. Overexpression of TgFSHRwt was confirmed by measuring radioactive ^{125}I-FSH binding to testicular membranes. Significantly elevated ^{125}I-FSH binding was observed in TgFSHRwt testes as compared to non-Tg controls, similar to levels in FSHR+ mice, thereby confirming overexpression.

TgFSHRwt mice displayed no difference in testis weights or serum testosterone (T) levels, as compared to FSHR+ mice, which had larger average testis weights and elevated T concentrations when compared to non-Tg controls. TgFSHRwt Sertoli cells showed higher cAMP activity in vitro, however basal levels did not exhibit the same increased activity as FSHR+ cells (49). Receptor ligand-specificity was decreased in FSHR+ mice, as exposure to human chorionic gonadotropin and TSH resulted in intracellular signaling. However, the same response was not observed in TgFSHRwt mice. Steroidogenic enzyme-encoding mRNAs such as Cyp11a1 and Star, were elevated in FSHR+ mice, suggesting increased steroidogenic potential (49). However, this increase was also not observed in TgFSHRwt mice. Sertoli and germ cell maturation that was observed in FSHR+ mice was also absent in TgFSHRwt mice, as they exhibited immature development similar to non-Tg hpg mice. Together, all of these results suggest that the physiological responses to constitutively active mutant FSH receptors in FSHR+ mice were due to the mutation itself and not the result of receptor overexpression (49).

Activating mutations in human FSHR are very rare. To identify the phenotypic consequences of such mutations in humans, mouse models harboring mutant versions of Fshr were first developed (26, 50). The rationale was that phenotypic analysis of these mice would provide information to look for similar phenotypes in patients carrying analogous mutations. Two independent Fshr point mutants D580H and D580Y were created and expressed using human AMH promoter to achieve ovary-specific expression in transgenic mice. Additionally, an Fshr BAC clone was engineered to carry the D580Y mutation and knocked-in to the endogenous Fshr locus in ES cells first and subsequently, the knock-in mutant mice were generated (26, 50).

Both D580H and D580Y mutants displayed increased basal receptor activity and they both demonstrated FSH binding. D580H mutant FSHR was neither ligand-dependent nor promiscuous toward LH/CG stimulation (26, 50). Granulosa cell-specific expression of mFshr ^{D580H} resulted in multiple ovarian abnormalities in transgenic female mice. Ovaries in the majority of transgenic females displayed hemorrhagic cysts, accelerated loss of immature follicles, increased granulosa cell proliferation and E2 biosynthesis, and luteinized but unruptured follicles, and teratomas (26, 50). A subset of the most severely affected transgenic females were infertile due to disrupted estrus cycles, and decreased gonadotropin, and increased prolactin levels. The increase in E2 and PRL levels led to secondary abnormalities including mammary gland enlargement and hyperplasia, pituitary adenoma formation, and defects in adrenal glands (26, 50). In contrast to phenotypic consequences of mFshr ^{D580H} expression, either transgenic or knock-in expression of mFshr ^{D580Y} mutant resulted in milder phenotypes, mostly hemorrhagic cysts in ovaries (26, 50). Thus, these GOF Fshr mutant mice resulted in distinct changes in ovarian function and proved valuable in the search of similar mutations in humans.

The most recent FSH receptor gain of function model challenged the traditional dogma that testosterone is essential for spermatogenesis (51). A mouse model was created that possessed a constitutively active mutant FSH receptor on an LH receptor null background (Fshr-CAM/Lhr$^{-/-}$) (51). As LH regulates testosterone production via binding of LH receptors (LHRs) in Leydig cells, it was hypothesized that an Lhr knockout approach would eliminate testosterone action. However, testosterone production persisted in the initial Fshr-CAM/Lhr$^{-/-}$ male mice, as serum levels recovered to about 40% of wild-type concentrations. Therefore, the rescue of testicular size and spermatogenesis was probably due to normal testosterone actions (51). To eliminate any basal T activity, a treatment using the antiandrogen, flutamide, was employed. In WT control mice that had no Fshr-CAM, reduction in the size of testes and seminal vesicles was observed as well as arrested spermatogenesis. Interestingly, the Fshr-CAM/Lhr$^{-/-}$ males had only reduced seminal vesicle size after anti-androgen treatment, with no change in testicular size, and normal spermatogenesis (51). In addition to this, expression of androgen-dependent genes (Drd4, Rhox 5, Aqp8, and Eppin) were tested in the Fshr-CAM/Lhr$^{-/-}$ males. Anti-androgen treated WT males showed reduced expression profiles of these genes, whereas mutant Fshr-CAM/Lhr$^{-/-}$ showed no reduction (51). These results suggested that even in the absence of testosterone, constitutively active FSH receptor alone is able to maintain androgen-dependent gene expression as well as normal spermatogenesis and testicular development.

CONCLUSIONS AND FUTURE DIRECTIONS

The first GOF mouse model for FSH was generated by our group more than 25 years ago (32). Since then investigators have used different promoters to achieve gonadotrope-specific as well as ectopic expression of the FSH ligand. Most commonly, human FSHB gene or individual subunit-encoding cDNAs (CGA or FSHB) were used in these experiments. More recently, BACS, or genes encoding porcine FSHβ subunit were also used to create transgenic pigs. GOF models for FSH action were generated using constitutively active FSH receptor–expressing mice and the reproductive consequences were studied either in these models directly or on an *Lhr* null genetic background (**Figure 1**). Combination of *Fshb* null mice and FSH GOF models resulted in genetic rescue that was used as an efficient *in vivo* functional assay for testing bioactivities of FSH and FSH analogs (**Figure 2**). A summary of the major phenotypes observed in each model is listed in **Table 1**.

Promoters used to generate FSH GOF models have also proved useful to express different reporters specifically in the gonadotrope cell lineage (62, 63). Recent advances in temporally regulated gene expression (64–66) will allow us in the future to tightly control FSH expression in desired tissues at desirable times across the life span of a mouse. Such refined genetic models will be useful to identify age-dependent gene/protein networks in FSH target tissues. These genetic models to conditionally "turning on" FSH in desired cells will also allow us to test if FSH receptor expression in non-gonadal cells has any physiological significance (55).

AUTHOR CONTRIBUTIONS

RM wrote the first draft of the manuscript and created the Figures. CS generated the entire Table. TK edited the manuscript, Table, and Figures. He also wrote the abstract, about Glycosylation, and Conclusions, and Future Directions. He created and formatted the entire Bibliography.

FUNDING

Work reported in this Chapter was supported in part by NIH grants CA166557, AG029531, AG056046, HD081162, and The Makowski Endowment (to TK). RM is a Makowski Summer Scholar in the Kumar lab and is a graduate student supported by the Integrated Physiology program at the University of Colorado Anschutz Medical Campus, Aurora, CO, USA.

ACKNOWLEDGMENTS

We thank Dr. George Bousfield for critically reading the manuscript and many helpful suggestions.

REFERENCES

1. Bousfield GR, Jia L, Ward DN. Gonadotropins: chemistry and biosynthesis A2. 3rd ed. In: Neill, Jimmy D, editors. *Knobil and Neill's Physiology of Reproduction*. St Louis, MO: Academic Press (2006). p. 1581–634. doi: 10.1016/B978-012515400-0/50035-X
2. Narayan P, Ulloa-Aguirre A, Dias JA. Gonadotropin hormones and their receptors. In: Strauss J, Barbieri A, Gargiulo A, editors. *Yen & Jaffe's Reproductive Endocrinology*. Philadelphia, PA: Elsevier (2018). p. 25–57.
3. Pierce JG, Parsons TF. Glycoprotein hormones: structure and function. *Annu Rev Biochem*. (1981) 50:465–95. doi: 10.1146/annurev.bi.50.070181.002341
4. Ulloa-Aguirre A, Dias JA, Bousfield GR. Gonadotropins. In: M.SImoni, Huhtaniemi I, editors. *Endocrinology of the Testis and Male Reproduction*. Springer International (2017). p. 1–52.
5. Simoni M, Gromoll J, Nieschlag E. The follicle-stimulating hormone receptor: biochemistry, molecular biology, physiology, and pathophysiology. *Endocr Rev*. (1997) 18:739–73. doi: 10.1210/er.18.6.739
6. Heckert L, Griswold MD. Expression of the FSH receptor in the testis. *Recent Prog Horm Res*. (1993) 48:61–77. doi: 10.1016/B978-0-12-571148-7.50006-3
7. Heckert LL, Griswold MD. The expression of the follicle-stimulating hormone receptor in spermatogenesis. *Recent Prog Horm Res*. (2002) 57:129–48. doi: 10.1210/rp.57.1.129
8. Richards JS, Pangas SA. The ovary: basic biology and clinical implications. *J Clin Invest*. (2010) 120:963–72. doi: 10.1172/JCI41350
9. Mason AJ, Pitts SL, Nikolics K, Szonyi E, Wilcox JN, Seeburg PH, et al. The hypogonadal mouse: reproductive functions restored by gene therapy. *Science* (1986) 234:1372–8. doi: 10.1126/science.3097822
10. Thompson IR, Kaiser UB. GnRH pulse frequency-dependent differential regulation of LH and FSH gene expression. *Mol Cell Endocrinol*. (2014) 385:28–35. doi: 10.1016/j.mce.2013.09.012
11. Stamatiades GA, Kaiser UB. Gonadotropin regulation by pulsatile GnRH: signaling and gene expression. *Mol Cell Endocrinol*. (2018) 463:131–41. doi: 10.1016/j.mce.2017.10.015
12. Bernard DJ, Fortin J, Wang Y, Lamba P. Mechanisms of FSH synthesis: what we know, what we don't, and why you should care. *Fertil Steril*. (2010) 93:2465–85. doi: 10.1016/j.fertnstert.2010.03.034
13. Ciccone NA, Kaiser UB. The biology of gonadotroph regulation. *Curr Opin Endocrinol Diabetes Obes*. (2009) 16:321–7. doi: 10.1097/MED.0b013e32832d88fb
14. Coss D. Regulation of reproduction via tight control of gonadotropin hormone levels. *Mol Cell Endocrinol*. (2018) 463:116–30. doi: 10.1016/j.mce.2017.03.022
15. Coss D, Mellon PL, Thackray VG. A FoxL in the smad house: activin regulation of FSH. *Trends Endocrinol Metab*. (2010) 21:562–8. doi: 10.1016/j.tem.2010.05.006
16. Das N, Kumar TR. Molecular regulation of follicle-stimulating hormone synthesis, secretion and action. *J Mol Endocrinol*. (2018) 60:R131–55. doi: 10.1530/JME-17-0308
17. Matzuk MM, Kumar TR, Shou W, Coerver KA, Lau AL, Behringer RR, et al. Transgenic models to study the roles of inhibins and activins in reproduction, oncogenesis, and development. *Recent Prog Horm Res*. (1996) 51:123–54; discussion 155–27.
18. Fortin J, Ongaro L, Li Y, Tran S, Lamba P, Wang Y, et al. Minireview: activin signaling in gonadotropes: what does the FOX say... to the SMAD? *Mol Endocrinol*. (2015) 29:963–77. doi: 10.1210/me.2015-1004
19. Uhlenhaut NH, Treier M. Forkhead transcription factors in ovarian function. *Reproduction* (2011) 142:489–95. doi: 10.1530/REP-11-0092
20. Thackray VG. Fox tales: regulation of gonadotropin gene expression by forkhead transcription factors. *Mol Cell Endocrinol*. (2014) 385:62–70. doi: 10.1016/j.mce.2013.09.034
21. Gregory SJ, Kaiser UB. Regulation of gonadotropins by inhibin and activin. *Semin Reprod Med*. (2004) 22:253–67. doi: 10.1055/s-2004-831901
22. Fortin J, Boehm U, Deng CX, Treier M, Bernard DJ. Follicle-stimulating hormone synthesis and fertility depend on SMAD4 and FOXL2. *FASEB J*. (2014) 28:3396–410. doi: 10.1096/fj.14-249532
23. Desai SS, Roy BS, Mahale SD. Mutations and polymorphisms in FSH receptor: functional implications in human reproduction. *Reproduction* (2013) 146:R235–48. doi: 10.1530/REP-13-0351
24. Kumar TR, Palapattu G, Wang P, Woodruff TK, Boime I, Byrne MC, et al. Transgenic models to study gonadotropin function: the role of follicle-stimulating hormone in gonadal growth and tumorigenesis. *Mol Endocrinol*. (1999) 13:851–65. doi: 10.1210/mend.13.6.0297
25. Montanelli L, Delbaere A, Di Carlo C, Nappi C, Smits G, Vassart G, et al. A mutation in the follicle-stimulating hormone receptor as a cause of familial

spontaneous ovarian hyperstimulation syndrome. *J Clini Endocrinol Metabol.* (2004) 89:1255–8. doi: 10.1210/jc.2003-031910

26. Peltoketo H, Rivero-Muller A, Ahtiainen P, Poutanen M, Huhtaniemi I. Consequences of genetic manipulations of gonadotrophins and gonadotrophin receptors in mice. *Ann Endocrinol.* (2010) 71:170–6. doi: 10.1016/j.ando.2010.02.022

27. Ghinea N. Vascular endothelial FSH receptor, a target of interest for cancer therapy. *Endocrinology* (2018) 159:3268–74. doi: 10.1210/en.2018-00466

28. Papadimitriou K, Kountourakis P, Kottorou AE, Antonacopoulou AG, Rolfo C, Peeters M, et al. Follicle-stimulating hormone receptor (FSHR): a promising tool in oncology? *Mol Diagn Ther.* (2016) 20:523–30. doi: 10.1007/s40291-016-0218-z

29. Valdelievre C, Sonigo C, Comtet M, Simon C, Eskenazi S, Grynberg M. [Impact of gonadotropins in women suffering from cancer]. *Bull Cancer* (2016) 103:282–8. doi: 10.1016/j.bulcan.2016.01.004

30. Allan CM, Kalak R, Dunstan CR, McTavish KJ, Zhou H, Handelsman DJ, et al. Follicle-stimulating hormone increases bone mass in female mice. *Proc Natl Acad Sci USA.* (2010) 107:22629–34. doi: 10.1073/pnas.1012141108

31. Macchia E, Simoncini T, Raffaelli V, Lombardi M, Iannelli A, Martino E. A functioning FSH-secreting pituitary macroadenoma causing an ovarian hyperstimulation syndrome with multiple cysts resected and relapsed after leuprolide in a reproductive-aged woman. *Gynecol Endocrinol.* (2012) 28:56–9. doi: 10.3109/09513590.2011.588758

32. Kumar TR, Fairchild-Huntress V, Low MJ. Gonadotrope-specific expression of the human follicle-stimulating hormone beta-subunit gene in pituitaries of transgenic mice. *Mol Endocrinol.* (1992) 6:81–90.

33. Kumar TR, Low MJ. Gonadal steroid hormone regulation of human and mouse follicle stimulating hormone beta-subunit gene expression *in vivo. Mol Endocrinol.* (1993) 7:898–906.

34. Kumar TR, Low MJ. Hormonal regulation of human follicle-stimulating hormone-beta subunit gene expression: GnRH stimulation and GnRH-independent androgen inhibition. *Neuroendocrinology* (1995) 61:628–37. doi: 10.1159/000126889

35. Kumar TR, Schuff KG, Nusser KD, Low MJ. Gonadotroph-specific expression of the human follicle stimulating hormone β gene in transgenic mice. *Mol Cell Endocrinol.* (2006) 247:103–15. doi: 10.1016/j.mce.2005. 12.006

36. Kumar TR, Low MJ, Matzuk MM. Genetic rescue of follicle-stimulating hormone beta-deficient mice. *Endocrinology* (1998) 139:3289–95. doi: 10.1210/endo.139.7.6111

37. Wang H, Larson M, Jablonka-Shariff A, Pearl CA, Miller WL, Conn PM, et al. Redirecting intracellular trafficking and the secretion pattern of FSH dramatically enhances ovarian function in mice. *Proc Natl Acad Sci USA.* (2014) 111:5735–40. doi: 10.1073/pnas.1321404111

38. Wang H, Butnev V, Bous GR, Kumar TR. A human FSHB transgene encoding the double N-glycosylation mutant (Asn 7 D Asn 24 D) FSH b subunit fails to rescue Fshb null mice. *Mol Cell Endocrinol.* (2016) 426:113–24. doi: 10.1016/j.mce.2016.02.015

39. Allan CM, Haywood M, Swaraj S, Spaliviero J, Koch A, Jimenez M, et al. A novel transgenic model to characterize the specific effects of follicle-stimulating hormone on gonadal physiology in the absence of luteinizing hormone actions. *Endocrinology* (2001) 142:2213–20. doi: 10.1210/endo.142.6.8092

40. Allan CM, Wang Y, Jimenez M, Marshan B, Spaliviero J, Illingworth P, et al. Follicle-stimulating hormone increases primordial follicle reserve in mature female hypogonadal mice. *J Endocrinol.* (2006) 188:549–57. doi: 10.1677/joe.1.06614

41. McTavish KJ, Jimenez M, Walters KA, Spaliviero J, Groome NP, Themmen AP, et al. Rising follicle-stimulating hormone levels with age accelerate female reproductive failure. *Endocrinology* (2007) 148:4432–39. doi: 10.1210/en.2007-0046

42. Greenberg NM, Anderson JW, Hsueh AJ, Nishimori K, Reeves JJ, deAvila DM, et al. Expression of biologically active heterodimeric bovine follicle-stimulating hormone in milk of transgenic mice. *Proc Natl Acad Sci USA.* (1991) 88:8327–31. doi: 10.1073/pnas.88.19.8327

43. Kim MO, Kim SH, Lee SR, Shin MJ, Min KS, Lee DB, et al. Ectopic expression of tethered human follicle-stimulating hormone (hFSH) gene in

transgenic mice. *Transgenic Res.* (2007) 16:65–75. doi: 10.1007/s11248-006-9031-5

44. Xu P, Li Q, Jiang K, Yang Q, Bi M, Jiang C, et al. BAC mediated transgenic large white boars with FSHalpha/beta genes from Chinese erhualian pigs. *Transgenic Res.* (2016) 25:693–709. doi: 10.1007/s11248-016-9963-3

45. Bi M, Tong J, Chang F, Wang J, Wei H, Dai Y, et al. Pituitary-specific overexpression of porcine follicle-stimulating hormone leads to improvement of female fecundity in BAC transgenic mice. *PLoS ONE* (2012) 7:e42335. doi: 10.1371/journal.pone.0042335

46. Jiang K, Xu P, Li W, Yang Q, Li L, Qiao C, et al. The increased expression of follicle-stimulating hormone leads to a decrease of fecundity in transgenic large white female pigs. *Transgenic Res.* (2017) 26:515–27. doi: 10.1007/s11248-017-0026-1

47. Matzuk MM, Finegold MJ, Su JG, Hsueh AJ, Bradley A. Alpha-inhibin is a tumour-suppressor gene with gonadal specificity in mice. *Nature* (1992) 360:313–9. doi: 10.1038/360313a0

48. Haywood M, Tymchenko N, Spaliviero J, Koch A, Jimenez M, Gromoll J, et al. An activated human follicle-stimulating hormone (FSH) receptor stimulates FSH-like activity in gonadotropin-deficient transgenic mice. *Mol Endocrinol.* (2002) 16:2582–91. doi: 10.1210/me.2002-0032

49. Allan CM, Lim P, Robson M, Spaliviero J, Handelsman DJ. Transgenic mutant D567G but not wild-type human FSH receptor overexpression provides FSH-independent and promiscuous glycoprotein hormone Sertoli cell signaling. *Am J Physiol Endocrinol Metabol.* (2009) 296:E1022–8. doi: 10.1152/ajpendo.90941.2008

50. Peltoketo H, Strauss L, Karjalainen R, Zhang M, Stamp GW, Segaloff DL, et al. Female mice expressing constitutively active mutants of FSH receptor present with a phenotype of premature follicle depletion and estrogen excess. *Endocrinology* (2010) 151:1872–83. doi: 10.1210/en. 2009-0966

51. Oduwole OO, Peltoketo H, Poliandri A, Vengadabady L, Chrusciel M, Doroszko M, et al. Constitutively active follicle-stimulating hormone receptor enables androgen-independent spermatogenesis. *J Clin Invest.* (2018) 128:1787–92. doi: 10.1172/JCI96794

52. Mason AJ, Hayflick JS, Zoeller RT, Young WS, Phillips HS, Nikolics K, et al. A deletion truncating the gonadotropin-releasing hormone gene is responsible for hypogonadism in the hpg mouse. *Science* (1986) 234:1366–71. doi: 10.1126/science.3024317

53. Kumar TR, Wang Y, Lu N, Matzuk MM. Follicle stimulating hormone is required for ovarian follicle maturation but not male fertility. *Nat Genet.* (1997) 15:201–4. doi: 10.1038/ng0297-201

54. Sun L, Peng Y, Sharrow AC, Iqbal J, Zhang Z, Papachristou DJ, et al. FSH directly regulates bone mass. *Cell* (2006) 125:247–60. doi: 10.1016/j.cell.2006.01.051

55. Kumar TR. Extragonadal actions of FSH: a critical need for novel genetic models. *Endocrinology* (2018) 159:2–8. doi: 10.1210/en.2017-03118

56. Stamatiades GA, Carroll RS, Kaiser UB. GnRH-A key regulator of FSH. *Endocrinology* (2019) 160:57–67. doi: 10.1210/en.2018-00889

57. McNeilly AS, Crawford JL, Taragnat C, Nicol L, McNeilly JR. The differential secretion of FSH and LH: regulation through genes, feedback and packaging. *Reprod Suppl.* (2003) 61:463–76.

58. Jablonka-Shariff A, Boime I. Secretory trafficking signal encoded in the carboxyl-terminal region of the CGbeta-subunit. *Mol Endocrinol.* (2009) 23:316–23. doi: 10.1210/me.2008-0351

59. Jablonka-Shariff A, Garcia-Campayo V, Boime I. Evolution of lutropin to chorionic gonadotropin generates a specific routing signal for apical release *in vivo. J Biol Chem.* (2002) 277:879–82. doi: 10.1074/jbc.C100402200

60. Bousfield GR, May JV, Davis JS, Dias JA, Kumar TR. *In Vivo* and *in vitro* impact of carbohydrate variation on human follicle-stimulating hormone function. *Front Endocrinol.* (2018) 9:216. doi: 10.3389/fendo.2018. 00216

61. Kumar TR. Fshb knockout mouse model, two decades later and into the future. *Endocrinology* (2018) 159:1941–9. doi: 10.1210/en.2018-00072

62. Kumar TR. *Mouse Models for the Study of Synthesis, Secretion, and Action of Pituitary Gonadotropins.* New York, NY: Elsevier Inc. (2016). doi: 10.1016/bs.pmbts.2016.08.006

63. Wang H, Hastings R, Miller WL, Kumar TR. Fshb -i Cre mice are efficient and specific Cre deleters for the gonadotrope lineage. *Mol Cell Endocrinol.* (2016) 419:124–38. doi: 10.1016/j.mce.2015.10.006

64. Jeong JH. Inducible mouse models for cancer drug target validation. *J Cancer Prev.* (2016) 21:243–8. doi: 10.15430/JCP.2016.21.4.243

65. Morozov A. Conditional gene expression and targeting in neuroscience research. *Curr Protoc Neurosci.* (2008) 4:4.31. doi: 10.1002/0471142301.ns0431s44

66. Yeh ES, Vernon-Grey A, Martin H, Chodosh LA. Tetracycline-regulated mouse models of cancer. *Cold Spring Harb Protoc.* (2014) 2014:pdb top069823. doi: 10.1101/pdb.top069823

11

Intracellular Follicle-Stimulating Hormone Receptor Trafficking and Signaling

Niamh Sayers and Aylin C. Hanyaloglu *

Department Surgery and Cancer, Institute of Reproductive and Developmental Biology, Imperial College London, London, United Kingdom

Correspondence:
Aylin C. Hanyaloglu
a.hanyaloglu@imperial.ac.uk

Models of G protein-coupled receptor (GPCR) signaling have dramatically altered over the past two decades. Indeed, GPCRs such as the follicle-stimulating hormone receptor (FSHR) have contributed to these new emerging models. We now understand that receptor signaling is highly organized at a spatial level, whereby signaling not only occurs from the plasma membrane but distinct intracellular compartments. Recent studies in the role of membrane trafficking and spatial organization of GPCR signaling in regulating gonadotropin hormone receptor activity has identified novel intracellular compartments, which are tightly linked with receptor signaling and reciprocally regulated by the cellular trafficking machinery. Understanding the impact of these cell biological mechanisms to physiology and pathophysiology is emerging for certain GPCRs. However, for FSHR, the potential impact in both health and disease and the therapeutic possibilities of these newly identified systems is currently unknown, but offers the potential to reassess prior strategies, or unveil novel opportunities, in targeting this receptor.

Keywords: GPCR, FSH receptor, endocytosis, signaling, trafficking, cAMP, endosome

INTRODUCTION

The follicle-stimulating hormone receptor (FSHR) belongs to the superfamily of G protein-coupled receptors (GPCRs). With more than 800 members in humans they represent the largest family of signaling receptors and a major, successful, drug target (1). The canonical model of GPCR signaling is via plasma membrane localized receptors coupling to distinct heterotrimeric G proteins. However, we now understand the signaling pathways activated by GPCRs are much more complex to mediate the many distinct functions these receptors play in all physiological systems, but also equally important to decipher is how such signal pathways are regulated. These novel mechanisms are beginning to open up new avenues for therapeutic exploitation. One mechanism that not only contributes to the diversification of signaling but how cells decode or specify these signals is membrane trafficking. Classically, membrane trafficking was viewed as a mechanism to regulate sensitivity of a tissue to hormone, by altering the level of surface receptor either through ligand-mediated endocytosis in to the cell, and/or reduced biosynthetic trafficking of newly synthesized receptor. However, intracellular membrane compartments have been shown to represent additional signaling platforms for many kinds of receptors, including GPCRs such as FSHR.

This review will discuss our current understanding of the molecular mechanisms and signaling roles of membrane trafficking of FSHR, and how gonadotropin hormone receptors have shed light on novel cell biological pathways potentially applicable to many GPCRs. We will primarily focus on post-endocytic intracellular trafficking, and then discuss how this novel cell biology could shed light on specific facets of FSH/FSHR function and its implications to endocrine function.

CLASSICAL REGULATION OF FSHR SIGNALING PATHWAYS

Pleiotropic G Protein Signal Profiles of FSHR

FSHR is a member of the glycoprotein hormone receptor subfamily of the rhodopsin-like, or Class-A, family of GPCRs, which comprise a unique subgroup within the Class A family due to their leucine-rich repeat-containing extracellular ectodomain. Furthermore, the high glycosylation status of its ligand FSH, like other glycoprotein hormones, makes them the most complex of protein hormones. Glycoprotein hormones are heterodimers that consist of a common α-subunit and a β-subunit that confers hormone specificity. These subunits are linked non-covalently and both subunits are subjected to N-glycosylation that can alter their bioactivity (2). For FSH, two naturally occurring glycoforms have been identified, the hypo-glycosylated FSH$^{21/18}$ and the fully glycosylated FSH^{24} (3), which have distinct activities [recently reviewed in (4)] and may be of significance to the trafficking pathways and intracellular signaling to be discussed below.

FSHR plays critical roles in reproduction, identified via numerous studies in both animal models and disease causing mutations in humans reviewed in Huhtaniemi and Themmen(5) and Jonas (6), but also extragonadal functions in uterus, adipose and bone, have been identified. In the gonads, FSH binds its receptor in testicular Sertoli cells and ovarian granulosa cells, where they regulate follicular development, steroidogenesis and spermatogenesis. Additional roles of FSHR in non-gonadal sites include myometrial contractility, regulation of lipid deposition, beiging and steroidogenesis in adipocytes and bone resorption functions in osteoclasts (7–10). The primary G protein pathway classically associated with the gonadally expressed receptor is the Gα$_s$/cAMP/PKA (11). However, FSHR has also been shown to couple to additional G protein pathways: Gα$_{q/11}$, which leads to activation of phospholipase C, leading to production of diacylglycerol and inositol trisphosphate second messengers, the latter of which leads to increases in intracellular calcium levels. However, coupling of Gα$_{q/11}$ to human FSHR is weaker than rodent FSHR and requires high receptor and hormone levels

(12–14). Recently it was reported that in pregnant myometrium FSHR levels are coupled to Gαs to increase cAMP, a second messenger known to quiesce the myocytes, but during labor FSHR levels increase and the signaling switches to the pro-contractile calcium pathway, possibly by Gαq/11 coupling (7). Other G protein pathways can also be activated by FSHR. In Sertoli cells and osteoclasts FSHR has been reported to couple to Gαi/o family members, such as Gα$_{i2}$, with subsequent MEK/Erk, NF-κB, Akt activation (9, 15, 16). Thus, like many GPCRs, FSHR exhibits the potential to activate G protein signaling in a pleiotropic manner, and such diversity in G protein signaling profiles may be tissue specific (**Figure 1**). The mechanisms underlying this tissue specificity in G protein coupling of FSHR may go beyond alterations in the levels of specific Gα subunits. Indeed, mechanisms such as GPCR homo and heteromerization and plasma membrane organization of receptors and signaling proteins such as in lipid rafts, are known to alter signal profiles of different GPCRs (17–19). FSHR is also subject to such mechanisms of signal diversity (20–22), although its role in directing tissue, or cell specific, responses is unknown.

Arrestin-Dependent Desensitization, Internalization and Signaling

The mechanisms mediating regulation of GPCR/G protein signaling are critical in shaping, or programming, the G protein signal profile from the plasma membrane. Although models of this classic pathway of GPCR signal desensitization and internalization have rapidly evolved in the last 5 years, exhibiting increasing complexity, particularly as application of structural and super-resolution imaging are increasingly applied, the core features of this model (**Figure 1**) are still critical. Signal activation of GPCRs at the plasma membrane is regulated initially via a process of rapid desensitization, followed by internalization via clathrin-coated pits (CCPs). The initial step in this model involves receptor phosphorylation on serine/threonine residues by second messenger-activated kinases and/or GPCR kinases (GRKs). It is both the activated and phosphorylated receptor that enables recruitment of the adaptor protein arrestin from the cytoplasm. Arrestins are a family of adaptor proteins with an increasing array of functions, both for GPCRs and non-GPCR mediated signaling. The family contains four isoforms, where arrestin-1 and−4 are restricted to the visual system and are also termed "visual arrestins" (23, 24), whereas the other two isoforms, arrestin-2 and -3, also called β-arrestin-1 and -2, are ubiquitously distributed and bind many GPCRs (25, 26). The arrestin-bound receptor desensitizes signaling via the uncoupling of receptor from its cognate G protein. Rapid arrestin-dependent internalization occurs by firstly inducing receptor clustering into CCPs, via its ability to bind receptor, clathrin heavy chain and core clathrin adaptor proteins (namely the β2 subunit of AP2) (27). This model, comprehensively described across many reviews, have discussed ways in which GPCRs may employ this system in distinct manners, such as differential phosphorylation of intracellular GPCR domains, primarily at the carboxy terminal tail (C-tail), alters association kinetics of GPCR to arrestin and its subsequent impact on receptor activity (28, 29). However,

---

Abbreviations: APPL1, adaptor protein containing PH domain; PTB domain, and Leucine zipper motif; β1AR, β2AR, beta adrenergic receptor 1 or 2; CCP, clathrin coated pit; EE, early endosome; EGF, epidermal growth factor; EGFR, EGF receptor; ESCRT, endosomal sorting complex required for transport; GIPC, Gαi-interacting protein C terminus; GPCR, G protein-coupled receptor; LHR, luteinizing hormone receptor; PDZ, postsynaptic density 95/disc large/zonula occludens-1; PKA, protein kinase A; VEE, very early endosome.

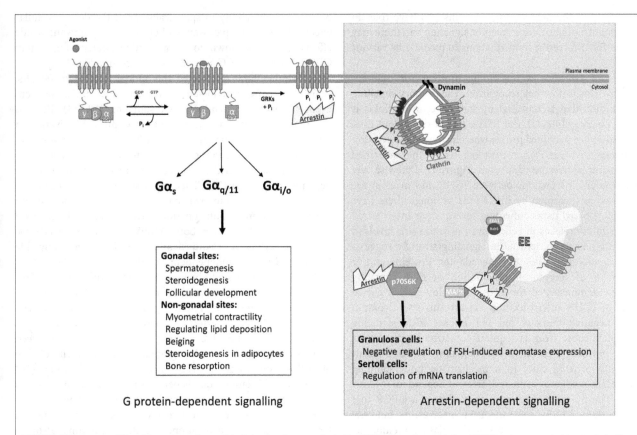

FIGURE 1 | Summary of G protein and arrestin-mediated signal pathways activated by FSHR. Upon ligand binding FSHR has been reported to couple to Gαs, Gαq/11, and Gαi/o heterotrimeric G proteins to mediate its downstream effects, both those in the gonads such as spermatogenesis, steroidogenesis, and follicular development, and more recently at non-gonadal sites, see text for further details. The archetypal view of GPCR signaling occurs in a G protein-dependent manner, however, agonist-activated, phosphorylated receptor recruits arrestin, for G protein signal desensitization and internalization via clathrin-coated pits. Furthermore, arrestin mediates signaling pathways independent of G proteins. This can occur through the scaffolding protein binding signaling proteins such as components of MAPK pathways after G protein activation, or independent of FSHR by complexing and activating ribosomal protein, p70S6K.

more recent structural and functional studies demonstrating the distinct modalities that arrestin can complex with GPCR and the G protein bound GPCR (30–34) have unveiled novel features of regulation that could be highly pertinent for FSHR, and will be discussed below.

FSHR signaling is regulated by this canonical GRK/arrestin model. As discussed above, internalization and desensitization are mediated by GRK phosphorylation, followed by arrestin binding. This is true for FSHR, where a cluster of five serine/threonine residues in its C-tail were identified as the key sites for GRK 2, 5, and 6 phosphorylation (35). Interestingly, while GRK 2 is predominantly involved in FSHR arrestin-mediated desensitization, GRKs 5 and 6 also promote arrestin binding but for scaffolding signaling proteins and signal activation (36). For FSHR, specific threonine residues in the third intracellular loop have been identified to dictate their rate of internalization and arrestin sensitivity, or binding (37). Further, there are differences in how FSHR engages with the GRK/arrestin mechanism between rodent and human receptors and also when compared to its "sister receptor" the LH receptor (LHR) that has unveiled specific structural motifs in FSHR involved in its internalization rate. The rodent

FSHR internalizes faster than the rodent LHR and the human FSHR. Creating chimeras between receptors revealed that six amino-acids in transmembrane 4, intracellular loop 3 and transmembrane 7 determine internalization of rodent FSHR to be 3 times faster than human FSHR, and its sensitivity to arrestins in enhancing receptor internalization (38). In addition, a serine/threonine phosphorylation cluster in the rodent FSHR C-tail is also involved in arrestin binding and arrestin-dependent internalization and desensitization, but not MAPK signaling (36). The importance of the third intracellular loop and C-tail residues in arrestin binding is interesting especially given recent key developments in our molecular understanding of how arrestin engages with GPCRs to mediate its distinct functions. Structural studies have now shown that arrestin engages active receptor in at least three forms, via the phosphorylated C-tail, the receptor core, or both. These forms have helped to explain how arrestin can mediate G protein uncoupling, internalization and yet also facilitate signaling when either as a stable or transient GPCR/arrestin complex (30, 31, 33, 39). These differences in arrestin binding to receptor could suggest that for FSHR core and C-tail interactions with arrestin may mediate its functions in an opposing manner than described for other GPCRs. However, as will be covered in the next section, arrestins also have roles in driving gonadotropin hormone receptor signaling and there may be alternate FSHR/arrestin conformations to mediate its various functions.

The role of arrestins as scaffolding proteins for different signaling proteins is now well recognized. The primary signaling pathway studied that is activated by such arrestin scaffolds is the MAPK pathway (40–42). For FSHR, ligand-dependent ERK signaling exhibits a sustained profile whereby the early activation is dependent on Gαs/PKA activation while the sustained response requires arrestins [(36) and **Figure 1**]. Likewise, the ligand-dependent interactions between FSHR and arrestin are also sustained as measured by BRET (43), although there have been no image-based data confirming sustained, or internalized FSHR/arrestin complexes in cells. Given arrestins are involved in FSHR internalization, its role in signaling strongly suggests additional scaffolding roles of this adaptor protein, and/or a requirement of receptor internalization of ERK signaling as has been demonstrated for LHR (44). However, a partial inhibition of FSHR internalization via arrestin and dynamin dominant negative mutants did not impact ERK signaling (45). Although more work is required to clarify how arrestins mediate G protein-independent FSH signaling, perhaps recent studies could provide clues to a mechanistic understanding of how FSHR mediates sustained arrestin-dependent MAPK responses. The β1-adrenergic receptor (β1AR) is a GPCR that induces a sustained ERK profile mediated by arrestins, but only transiently associates with arrestin at the plasma membrane, while arrestin remains associated within CCPs in order to activate signaling in a sustained manner (46). The authors demonstrated that arrestin transiently binds to the core of β1AR only, which induces a conformational change in arrestin resulting in its capture by binding phosphoinositides in the plasma membrane and clathrin associated adaptor proteins (33). Given the sustained ERK signaling profile of FSHR, that the third intracellular loop residues are involved in arrestin binding, while C-tail sites do not regulate ERK signaling (37, 47, 48) and further similarities in these receptors with the β1AR in their post-endocytic pathways [see section Post-endocytic sorting and endosomal signaling of FSHR from a novel compartment; the very early endosome (VEE)], it is possible that arrestin engages with FSHR in a similar manner. Alternatively, or in addition to this receptor-independent arrestin signaling complex, is the recent elegant report demonstrating that FSHR activates p70S6K within an arrestin complex constitutively assembled with a p70S6K/ribosomal protein S6 (rpS6) to regulate mRNA translation (49). This study supports recent structural findings that arrestin, after its dissociation from receptor, can maintain various active conformations (50), but also suggests that receptor-independent "active" arrestin complexes may not only be a feature of CCPs but also other subcellular locations.

The ability of GPCRs to activate more than one pathway of signaling, such as G protein and arrestin-mediated signaling via the stabilization of a certain active conformation of the receptor, is termed signaling bias (28) and is of high pharmacological interest. Bias can occur through different ligands (ligand bias) or even receptor mutations (receptor bias) (51). From a therapeutic perspective, the ability to specifically target the desired cellular effects, through one pathway, without activating unwanted side effects has been shown to be a feasible strategy for certain GPCRs. In terms of G protein vs. arrestin-mediated signaling, recent studies have challenged this model for certain GPCRs, suggesting that G protein activation is still an essential upstream event of arrestin-dependent ERK signaling (52, 53). Perhaps an argument against a requirement for G protein activation in arrestin-mediated signaling for FSHR is via the observation that lowering expression levels of the receptor to a level where there is no detectable cAMP signaling can induce bias to arrestin-dependent signaling (54). This was first revealed by studies on the A189V FSHR mutant, which is expressed at very low levels on the cell surface and is non-functional with respects to Gαs/cAMP signaling (55). Yet, when both A189V mutant and wild-type FSHR are expressed at equivalent low levels they are only able to trigger G-protein independent MAPK activation (54).

For biased signaling to be therapeutically explored for FSHR, there must be a well characterized understanding of the *in vivo* role of arrestin in FSHR signaling. So far, it has been demonstrated that in Sertoli cells arrestin may regulate mRNA translation and a possible negative regulation of FSH-induced aromatase expression in rodent granulosa cells (via manipulation of GRK6 levels as an upstream step in arrestin binding) (56) (**Figure 1**). This latter study is perhaps corroborated by findings in an immortalized human granulosa tumor cell line, whereby arrestins negatively regulate Gαs/cAMP/PKA pathway, not in terms of classical desensitization, as in these cells gonadotropin-mediated ERK signaling via arrestins was evident in the absence of cAMP signaling. Specifically, FSH, but not LH, dependent apoptosis occurred by cellular depletion of arrestins, due to increases in cAMP/PKA signaling, thus suggesting a role for arrestins in regulating balance between cell proliferation and apoptosis (57). While promising, further work needs to be conducted to evaluate the potential benefit of arrestin-based biased agonism.

Post-endocytic Intracellular Trafficking Pathways of FSHR

Following internalization, GPCRs are trafficked to endosomes where they are sorted to either a plasma membrane recycling pathway, or to the lysosomal pathway for degradation. Such pathways program the temporal profile of G protein signaling, by regulating resensitization/hormone recovery (recycling) or permanent signal termination (degradation), Additionally, the sorting fate of a GPCR pharmacologically manipulated and altered in disease (58). However, we now know that the endocytic system does not only regulate the surface density of receptors but that these divergent, and complex, sorting pathways have direct roles as platforms for signaling, including G protein signaling (59–61). This will be further discussed in section Postendocytic sorting and endosomal signaling of FSHR from a novel compartment; the very early endosome (VEE). The mechanisms that underlie these divergent post-endocytic fates are tightly regulated at multiple levels and are interlinked with the receptors own signaling. These complex mechanisms have recently been reviewed by us and others (61–64) and will not be described in detail here except to illustrate core features that enable discussion of current understanding of FSHR sorting and intracellular signaling.

The textbook model of cargo sorting depicts the Rab5 early endosome (EE) as the common post-endocytic compartment from which receptors are first sorted to opposing fates. GPCRs sorted to a degradative pathway following internalization are trafficked from EEs to Rab7 positive late endosomes. Receptors are involuted into vesicles within the lumen of these endosomes, to form multivesicular bodies (MVBs). MVBs will then fuse with lysosomes resulting in protein degradation. GPCRs will engage with this pathway with distinct kinetics and for those receptors targeted to the recycling pathway, chronic ligand stimulation will reroute receptors to this degradative pathway as part of the mechanism of downregulation. Classically, lysosomal targeting of different receptors is via ubiquitination at lysine residues and engagement with endosomal sorting complex required for transport (ESCRT)-dependent degradation, however, GPCRs exhibit ubiquitin-independent and ESCRT-independence in their mechanisms of degradation [reviewed in (65, 66)]. GPCRs targeted to a rapid recycling pathway are sorted from EEs to Rab4 positive recycling endosomes. An important feature of GPCRs targeted to recycling pathways, is that this is regulated by interactions with specific sequences in the GPCR C-tails, also termed sequence-directed, or regulated, recycling. This mode of recycling is distinct from recycling of other kinds of membrane cargo, e.g., transferrin receptor that does not require its C-tail for recycling and occurs with the bulk membrane flow (default recycling). The distal C-tail receptor sequences are not only essential for recycling, but if fused to the carboxy-terminus of a GPCR sorted to a degradative pathway, it will reroute that GPCR to the recycling pathway. There are no common sequences that determine whether any GPCR undergoes regulated recycling, as they are highly divergent. However, several recycling sequences identified, such as first identified with the β2-adrenergic receptor (β2AR), correspond to a type 1 (PSD95)/discs large (Dlg)/zonula occludens-1 (Zo-1) (PDZ) binding sequence or "PDZ ligand," specifically S/T-X-Φ, (where Φ is any hydrophobic residue) (67, 68). PDZ proteins are scaffold proteins and for GPCRs that bind PDZ proteins, they are often able to bind more than 1 PDZ protein (69), suggesting these sequences and interactions may have additional functions to directing receptors to the recycling pathway. For the β2AR the interacting PDZ-domain containing protein partner responsible for recycling is the endosomally localized PDZ protein, sorting nexin-27 (SNX27) (70). As mentioned above, these recycling sequences are very distinct amongst receptors, so there are several examples of GPCRs targeted to a recycling pathway that do not contain PDZ type 1 ligands or any other recognizable motif, and hence for many their corresponding interacting protein partners are unknown (58, 71). This is also the case for the FSHR whereby both rodent and human FSHR are recycled back to the plasma membrane via specific C-tail sequences that does not indicate any potential binding partners such as a PDZ protein (72). More recently a role for palmitoylation in FSHR sorting has been proposed (73). In FSHR it is known that there are 2 conserved and 1 non-conserved

cysteine in the FSHR C-tail that were all palmitoylated, but only 1 of the conserved cysteines (cysteine 629) affected receptor function by impairing cell surface expression (74). A follow up study demonstrated that mutation of all three cysteines to glycine significantly impaired biosynthetic trafficking of the receptor to the plasma membrane and thus exhibited reduced signaling. Interestingly, the receptor that was transported to the plasma membrane exhibited similar internalization kinetics but impaired recycling, the receptor thus being routed to the degradative pathway (73). This suggests that altering palmitoylation of the receptor changes the ability of the C-tail, and presumably the distal recycling sequence, to interact with key machinery that mediates its sorting, but also indicates that a cell could alter FSHR trafficking, and subsequently signaling responsiveness, through alterations in these post-translation modifications.

While the above describes that the recycling pathway of FSHR, and other GPCRs, involves a one-step mechanism with its recycling sequence and interacting partner, which may be unique to a given GPCR, we now know that both common and receptor-specific post-endocytic mechanisms exist. Furthermore, sequence-directed recycling (and lysosomal sorting) occur via a complex, multi-step system, with the GPCR's own signaling playing a key role in driving receptors to these distinct cellular fates, in addition to trafficking regulating the signal from that receptor. This interconnected property of post-endocytic trafficking and GPCR signaling has been highlighted recently through studies of the gonadotropin hormone receptors and will be discussed next.

POST-ENDOCYTIC SORTING AND ENDOSOMAL SIGNALING OF FSHR FROM A NOVEL COMPARTMENT; THE VERY EARLY ENDOSOME (VEE)

The internalization of GPCRs into the endocytic network is no longer viewed as a mechanism to only control plasma membrane signaling but to also provide additional platforms to continue or reactivate signaling from intracellular compartments, including G protein signaling. Furthermore, this spatial control of signaling has been shown to be important for cells to decode common second messenger signaling molecules, such as cAMP signaling, activated by many GPCRs, into specific downstream cellular functions (59–61). Intracellular signaling is also important for the FSHR, however, it is through studies on human LHR has unveiled how important, and tightly regulated, the compartmentalization of receptors within the complex endomembrane network is to receptor endosomal signaling.

Discovery of the VEE; A Tale of Serendipity
Many GPCRs, including the human FSHR and LHR undergo the regulated recycling pathway described in Section Post-endocytic intracellular trafficking pathways of FSHR. Our studies first identifying the VEE with the gonadotropin hormone receptors were initially driven as way to understand why GPCRs have distinct recycling sequences if there is a common

primary function, i.e., sorting to the recycling pathway. Thus, comparisons were first made between the β2AR and LHR that initially seem quite similar in their signaling and trafficking profiles (44). Both are Gαs-coupled receptors that internalize via arrestin/clathrin pathways and undergo sequence-directed recycling. However, they have distinct C-tail recycling sequences and bind different PDZ proteins for their sorting, SNX27 for β2AR and GIPC (Gαi-interacting protein, C-terminus) for LHR (68, 70). Unexpectedly, when agonist-induced LHR endocytosis was monitored by live confocal microscopy imaging it was evident this receptor trafficked to endosomes closer to the plasma membrane that were approximately a third of the diameter of endosomes containing β2AR. FSHR and the β1AR also internalized to these small endosomes. The identity of this compartment, in terms of the proteins or adaptors that traffic there are poorly understood, except they are distinct from those classically found in the EE and EE intermediates such as EE antigen 1, phosphatidylinositol-3 phosphate (a lipid enriched in the EE membrane) and Rab5 (44). As it was previously established that LHR sorting to the recycling pathway required its C-tail interaction with the PDZ protein GIPC, the hypothesis was that this protein interaction also directed LHR to these small endosomes. Indeed, truncation of the LHR recycling sequence or knockdown of GIPC levels inhibited recycling and also rerouted receptor to the larger EEs (**Figures 2A,B**). As interactions with GIPC occurred only early on during receptor clustering in to CCPs, further supported a model whereby LHR recycling must occur from these small endosomes, we then termed very early endosomes (VEEs) (44). While the discovery of a new cellular compartment was very unexpected, our original aim of understanding the role of these different GPCR recycling sequences was also in part addressed, as it highlights these sorting sequences may encode functions at distinct steps in the endocytic trafficking of a GPCR, and not only sorting from endosomes. In this case, it was sorting to distinct populations of endosomes. It is well known that trafficking regulates signaling, thus what were the signaling functions of the VEE? Surprisingly, when LHR trafficking was rerouted away from VEEs to EEs, via inhibiting interaction with GIPC, the ligand-induced cAMP signaling was not affected but ERK signaling profile was altered from a sustained to a transient one (**Figure 2B**) (44). Given that both acute and sustained ERK signaling was dependent on internalization, suggests that under conditions when GIPC is depleted, the receptor is rapidly routed through the VEE, but not maintained in this compartment due to its trafficking to EEs, hence the altered temporal ERK signaling profile (see **Figure 2B**). It also highlights the interconnectivity of endomembrane systems; indeed, we also demonstrated in this study that the transferrin receptor can internalize through the VEE on its way to the EE. Intriguingly, the ligand-induced ERK signaling of β1AR and FSHR was also affected by GIPC knockdown. While β1AR is known to interact with GIPC via its C-tail (75), this result was unexpected for FSHR since its recycling sequence contains no PDZ ligand and there are no prior reports of its interaction with GIPC. However, FSHR is known to directly interact with the adaptor protein containing PH domain, PTB domain, and leucine zipper motif (APPL1) (12, 76, 77), and so far, APPL1 is the

only protein identified that localizes to a subpopulation of VEEs. Given APPL1 can directly bind GIPC (78) this may underlie the GIPC-dependent nature of ERK signaling by FSHR.

The Role of APPL1 in FSHR and VEE Function

To date, APPL1 is the only known protein present on the VEEs, as the PDZ protein GIPC only associates during the very early steps of endocytosis at the CCP (44). APPL1 is a well-studied adaptor protein comprised by multiple protein and membrane interacting domains (79). Prior studies have shown it localize to EE Rab5 compartment but at an intermediate step prior to conversion of endosomes to EEA1 positive endosomes (80). APPL1 is reported to localize to other compartments including vesicles that do not have Rab5 (81), akin to what we have observed with the gonadotropin hormone receptors and the VEE (44). APPL1 displays multiple, and integrative functions in cargo trafficking and receptor signaling, as evident from the numerous reported interactions including Rabs, receptors such as FSHR, EGF receptor, insulin receptor, adiponectin receptor, androgen receptor, kinases and phosphatases, like protein kinase B and PtdIns(3)P kinase, and PDZ proteins like GIPC (82). Prior to our reports on the VEE, APPL1 was shown to form a complex with FSHR, not via the C-tail but via three specific residues in its first intracellular loop (76). In addition, this complex contained additional adaptor and signaling proteins, including APPL2, Akt, and FOXO1. Such a complex was shown to propagate FSH-induced PI3K/Akt signaling, IP_3 production and calcium release (12, 76, 77, 83). This is consistent with APPL1's roles in positive regulation of signaling (78). These signal pathways in FSHR/APPL1 complexes remain to be studied in the context of the VEE where focus so far has been primarily on cAMP and MAPK.

APPL1 plays critical roles in gonadotropin receptor trafficking and endosomal cAMP signaling from the VEE (84). As described above, interactions with GIPC are essential for directing receptors to the VEE (**Figure 2B**). In contrast, APPL1 is not required for GPCR localization to the VEE but is essential for LHR and FSHR recycling (**Figure 2C**). Interestingly, it is the receptor's own cAMP/PKA signaling that drives this APPL1-dependent recycling (60). The mechanism underlying this requirement is that LH-mediated PKA activation must phosphorylate APPL1 at serine 410 for the receptor to recycle back to the plasma membrane. This raised the possibility that LHR activates signaling from the VEE as it would provide a means for high localized regulation of APPL1 (phosphorylation) at the endomembrane, and perhaps specific populations of APPL1. Inhibiting internalization of LHR almost completely abolished ligand induced increases in cAMP, a finding corroborated using a nanobody biosensor that recognizes active Gαs (85), which localized to a subpopulation of LHR endosomes (84). If the primary location of cAMP signaling from these receptors was the VEE, then inhibition of recycling should enhance cAMP signals. Indeed, this is the case when cellular levels of APPL1 are depleted for all known VEE-targeted receptors (LHR, FSHR, and β1AR, see **Figure 2C**). However,

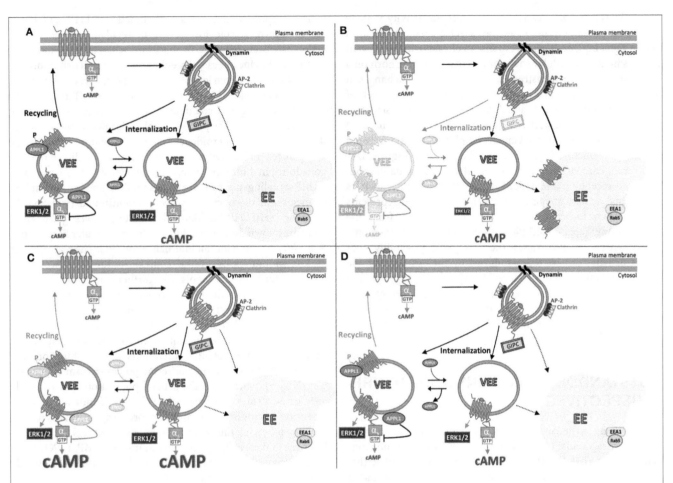

FIGURE 2 | Model summarizing current understanding of gonadotropin hormone receptor post-endocytic pathways and receptor signaling from VEEs. The trafficking of FSHR and LHR to the VEE is inextricably linked to the receptor's signal output, whereby the manipulation of which at distinct steps results in different trafficking and signal profiles. **(A)** Following ligand-activation FSHR internalizes to the very early endosome (VEE). The VEE differs from the early endosome (EE) in its smaller size and neither contain EEA1 nor Rab5, classical markers for the EE. During receptor-mediated endocytosis of FSHR into a clathrin-coated pit, the PDZ domain protein, GIPC, is recruited at the cytosolic interface of the GPCR. Receptor then enters the complex endosomal network where it is primarily localized to the VEE. There are two types of VEE depicted, one contains the adaptor protein, APPL1 (see text), and one is without. GIPC dissociates before FSHR enters the VEE. From the VEE receptor is able to elicit downstream signaling cascades, including cAMP generation and ERK1/2 activation. This cAMP/PKA signal phosphorylates APPL1 on Serine 410. Receptor is trafficked to APPL1 positive VEEs, where the unphosphorylated APPL1 negatively regulates endosomal cAMP signaling. The phosphorylated APPL1 is required for receptor recycling back to the plasma membrane. **(B)** The receptor can be rerouted from the VEE to the EE by the loss of GIPC or disruptions in the receptors ability to interact with this PDZ protein. Loss of GIPC results in the trafficking of the receptor from the VEE pathway to the EE and loss of plasma membrane recycling. While endosomal cAMP signaling is not affected, ERK signaling profile is more transient as the receptor only rapidly passes through the VEE to the EE. **(C)** Loss of APPL1 does not alter the endosomal organization of the receptor but inhibits recycling. The "trapped" receptor in the VEE compartment results in increases in endosomal cAMP signaling due to APPL1's role in negative regulation of G protein signaling, but without impacting ERK signal profile. **(D)** Manipulating the ability of APPL1 to be phosphorylated on Serine 410, either by inhibition of PKA activity or mutation of serine 410 to alanine, specifically inhibits recycling but not cAMP endosomal signaling.

ERK signaling (strength and kinetics) is not affected under these conditions and inhibition of LHR recycling via a PKA inhibitor (as APPL1 phosphorylation is needed for recycling) has no effect on LHR-cAMP signaling. Thus, APPL1 has an additional role in negatively regulating cAMP from VEE targeted GPCRs (84). How APPL1 controls GPCR/Gαs coupling is still unknown, yet intriguingly it is the unphosphorylated form of APPL1 that mediates this, indicating that distinct populations of APPL1, phosphorylated and unphosphorylated forms, have opposing functions on VEE-targeted receptors (**Figure 2**). Furthermore, it highlights that endosomal signaling must be "switched off" prior to receptor recycling, as has been shown in GPCR endosomal

signaling from the EE and the role of the retromer complex (86, 87). Overall, the VEE-network displays exquisite control of signaling and trafficking via the actions of APPL1. There are many outstanding molecular questions for this system, including if there are any roles for the related protein APPL2, which has both common and distinct functions to APPL1, especially as FSHR forms a complex with both adaptor proteins (77). Are other signal pathways that FSHR is known to activate, such as Gαi signaling (see section Classical regulation of FSHR signaling pathways), also regulated at the level of the VEE and by APPL1? Another question these studies have raised is why is such complexity within the endosomal system required? One possibility is that it enables a cell to alter receptor activity at many levels and potentially in a pathway specific manner (location bias in signaling), perhaps in response to physiologically relevant changes in its extracellular environment (e.g., dynamic hormonal environment during menstrual cycle) to pathological changes in disease. This is illustrated in **Figure 2**, whereby altering levels of key adaptor proteins GIPC and APPL1, alters receptor signaling to ERK or cAMP respectively (**Figures 2B,C**), or at the level of APPL1 regulation of PKA mediated phosphorylation, would result in a distinct trafficking and signal phenotype (**Figure 2D**).

Overall, compartmentalization of internalized gonadotropin hormone receptors, and indeed many other GPCRs, mediates their signal activity at specific intracellular sites, and represents a mechanism for cells to diversify signaling even from the same pathway (e.g., cAMP/PKA) to possibly distinct functional consequences. It also raises the intriguing possibility that GPCR activity, can be reprogrammed by the cell to alter the compartment the receptor is targeted to via altering expression of key proteins in this pathway, e.g., GIPC, APPL1 (**Figure 2**). Such a model may explain how FSHR activity in the gonads, commonly mediated by cAMP/PKA, underlies distinct functions but also specificity of this pleiotropically coupled GPCR.

OUTSTANDING QUESTIONS AND FUTURE PERSPECTIVES

These recent advances in FSHR function from its distinct roles in extragonadal tissues and novel cell biological functions demonstrates that FSHR is a good example of a GPCR that achieves signal diversification via multiple strategies and a prototype receptor for understanding novel facets of GPCR function. Whether such pathways are then perturbed in disease and if we can harness these properties of GPCRs therapeutically needs to be addressed.

While much has been uncovered about novel intracellular trafficking systems, there are numerous outstanding questions at the molecular level. A major one to be tackled in the future is the identifying the molecular composition (both protein and lipid content of the membrane) of the VEEs, as so far APPL1 is the only known protein to reside there and is only present in ~50% of the VEE population (84). While not a trivial task to unpick, recent developments in proteomics such as the application of engineered ascorbic acid peroxidase (APEX)-mediated approaches that can capture the local protein network of a receptor with high spatial-temporal resolution as it traffics through the endocytic system (88), may be able to uncover specific VEE proteins and whether such proteins are core to these endosomes, or receptor-specific. A critical outstanding question is understanding the downstream role of VEE targeting, and could there be any clues from disease-causing mutations in the gonadotropin hormone receptors? It is likely that the VEE and APPL1-dependent regulation is a conserved mechanism across cells, as for many membrane trafficking pathways. In primary human endometrial stromal cells, LHR could traffic to VEEs and recycle in an APPL1-dependent manner (84), although the downstream functional role/s in the endometrium,

a tissue reported to express both functional LHR and FSHR are unknown. A role for APPL1 in regulating gonadotropin action has been reported in the ovary whereby knockdown of APPL1 in bovine theca cells enhances LH-mediated androgen production (89). Given loss of APPL1 increases ligand-dependent cAMP signaling in HEK 293 cells (84) (**Figure 2C**), is consistent with this finding and could suggest that deregulated signaling by VEE/APPL1 has key physiological/pathophysiological roles in the ovary such as steroidogenesis and conditions where there is enhanced LH activity e.g., PCOS. Indeed, a direct role for gonadotropin hormone receptor endocytosis in LH-mediated cAMP signaling in the mouse ovarian follicle and the resumption of meiosis in the oocyte has been demonstrated (90). Specific roles for FSH/FSHR function will need to be investigated, given there are known disease causing mutations that alter FSHR signal desensitization and inhibit internalization (91). The reassessment of known mutations in the context of the VEE would be highly informative as tools for further understanding how FSHR engages with these intracellular trafficking and signaling mechanisms. However, such disease-causing mutations are rare, and from a translational perspective there would be value in assessing known single nucleotide polymorphisms that impact FSHR activity for potential alterations in VEE function. For example, the FSHR asparagine/serine polymorphism at position 680 (N680S), whereby in the general population approximately 60% are N680 and 40% S680, while in infertile individuals this is more 50/50. This SNP determines poorer responsiveness to FSH in women bearing the N variant compared to the S carriers that has been linked to temporal alterations in cAMP, ERK1/2 and CREB responses in human granulosa cells, whereby interestingly it is the N variant that exhibits faster signal properties (92, 93). These altered signal properties could result in altered arrestin-mediated signaling and/or altered sorting of FSHR to endosomal compartments. Although any potential alterations in intracellular trafficking at the level of the VEE are unknown, given the C-tail location of the SNP, located upstream of the distal recycling sequence of FSHR (72), one could predict that this variant may modulate interactions with protein partners that bind this distal recycling sequence, resulting in distinct post-endocytic fates and altered endosomal compartmentalization. The faster kinetics in signaling exhibited by the N variant may indicate for example, a lack of APPL1-dependent regulation in signaling and/or inability of GIPC to direct the receptors to the VEE. Given the more widespread functions of FSH that have been reported, this SNP may be predictive of other conditions, such as pre-term birth whereby carriers homozygous for the N variant, as evaluated from placental samples, had a significantly higher risk of pre-term birth than the S variant (94). This variant is not only of significance to female health but also to males. Infertile men carrying the 680N variant compared to the 680S respond better to FSH treatment as assessed by improved DNA fragmentation index of their spermatozoa (95). Furthermore, the increasing reports of FSHR in endothelial cells, bone and adipose (8, 9) may unveil future roles for altered spatial control of FSHR signaling in cancer, obesity, type 2 diabetes and osteoporosis.

The ability to pharmacologically exploit these new GPCR signaling models and target the intracellular signaling receptor specifically has been recently demonstrated for three distinct GPCRs. Employing cholestenol-conjugated antagonists, which accumulate in the lumen of endosomal compartments, can block endosomal signaling from the neurokinin 1 receptor and calcitonin-gene related peptide receptor and has been shown to be an effective nociceptive target in animal models (96, 97). Whilst a similar strategy to inhibit endosomal signaling of the protease-activated receptor 2 prevented hyperexcitability of pain receptors in the colon and thus has been proposed to be of therapeutic value in pain management of irritable bowel syndrome (98). These studies set an important precedent for the likely success of targeting intracellular signaling of GPCRs, however, we know GPCRs including FSHR exhibit pleiotropic signaling and the ability to also target intracellular signaling more specifically, either at a pathway level or endosomal compartment level (e.g., VEE vs. EE) could be valuable. In other words, to create biased intracellularly targeted compounds may offer avenues for more efficacious compounds with less side effects. For FSHR there may already exist avenues to develop such ligands, as a number of small molecule, orally available, and cell permeable, compounds have been produced (99), although their role in altering intracellular signaling of FSHR remain to be determined. It may not always be necessary to target intracellular receptors, and perhaps altering the endosomal fate of a receptor by targeting the plasma membrane receptor prior to its internalization may be advantageous, to also induce location bias. This could even be achieved through native ligands; for FSHR there are known glycovariants of FSH that exhibit distinct activities (4).

In summary, our understanding of the complexity of GPCR signaling pathways via the tight control of their intracellular location has been advanced through studies on the gonadotropin hormone receptors. Such mechanisms have highlighted the interconnected nature of these intracellular systems, and thus a primary future goal is to further understand the significance of these molecular systems to health and disease if they are to be of therapeutic value. The critical nature of intracellular sorting of FSHR to signaling has been demonstrated, so it is not a question of is it important, but rather how the intricacies of modulating receptor from one intracellular compartment to another impact specific functions *in vivo*. This would provide the opportunity to be able to target these intracellular signaling modalities with high precision, in order to create the next generation of therapeutics for reproductive medicine.

AUTHOR CONTRIBUTIONS

All authors listed have made a substantial, direct and intellectual contribution to the work, and approved it for publication.

ACKNOWLEDGMENTS

This work was supported by grants from the Genesis Research Trust (P15844, P67019) and Wellcome Trust (WT087248MA) to AH and an Imperial College London President's scholarship to NS.

REFERENCES

1. Hauser AS, Attwood MM, Rask-Andersen M, Schioth HB, Gloriam DE. Trends in GPCR drug discovery: new agents, targets and indications. *Nat Rev Drug Discov*. (2017) 16:829–42. doi: 10.1038/nrd.2017.178
2. Green ED, Baenziger JU. Asparagine-linked oligosaccharides on lutropin, follitropin, and thyrotropin. II. Distributions of sulfated and sialylated oligosaccharides on bovine, ovine, and human pituitary glycoprotein hormones. *J Biol Chem*. (1988) 263:36–44.
3. Walton WJ, Nguyen VT, Butnev VY, Singh V, Moore WT, Bousfield GR. Characterization of human FSH isoforms reveals a nonglycosylated beta-subunit in addition to the conventional glycosylated beta-subunit. *J Clin Endocrinol Metab*. (2001) 86:3675–85. doi: 10.1210/jcem.86.8.7712
4. Bousfield GR, May JV, Davis JS, Dias JA, Kumar TR. *In vivo* and *in vitro* impact of carbohydrate variation on human follicle-stimulating hormone function. *Front Endocrinol (Lausanne)* (2018) 9:216. doi: 10.3389/fendo.2018.00216
5. Huhtaniemi IT, Themmen AP, Mutations in human gonadotropin and gonadotropin-receptor genes. *Endocrine* (2005) 26:207–17. doi: 10.1385/ENDO:26:3:207
6. Jonas KC, Oduwole OO, Peltoketo H, Rulli SB, Huhtaniemi IT. Mouse models of altered gonadotrophin action: insight into male reproductive disorders, *Reproduction* (2014) 148:R63–70. doi: 10.1530/REP-14-0302
7. Stilley JA, Guan R, Santillan DA, Mitchell BF, Lamping KG, Segaloff DL. Differential regulation of human and mouse myometrial contractile activity by FSH as a function of FSH receptor density. *Biol Reprod*. (2016) 95:36. doi: 10.1095/biolreprod.116.141648
8. Liu P, Ji Y, Yuen T, Rendina-Ruedy E, DeMambro VE, Dhawan S, et al. Blocking FSH induces thermogenic adipose tissue and reduces body fat. *Nature* (2017) 546:107–12. doi: 10.1038/nature22342

9. Sun L, Peng Y, Sharrow AC, Iqbal J, Zhang Z, Papachristou DJ, et al. FSH directly regulates bone mass. *Cell* (2006) 125:247–60. doi: 10.1016/j.cell.2006.01.051
10. Liu XM, Chan HC, Ding GL, Cai J, Song Y, Wang TT, et al. FSH regulates fat accumulation and redistribution in aging through the Galphai/Ca(2+)/CREB pathway. *Aging Cell* (2015) 14:409–20. doi: 10.1111/acel.12331
11. Puett D, Li Y, DeMars G, Angelova K, Fanelli F. A functional transmembrane complex: the luteinizing hormone receptor with bound ligand and G protein. *Mol Cell Endocrinol*. (2007) 260–262:126–36. doi: 10.1016/j.mce.2006.05.009
12. Thomas RM, Nechamen CA, Mazurkiewicz JE, Ulloa-Aguirre A, Dias JA. The adapter protein APPL1 links FSH receptor to inositol 1,4,5-trisphosphate production and is implicated in intracellular Ca(2+) mobilization. *Endocrinology* (2011) 152:1691–701. doi: 10.1210/en.2010-1353
13. Hirsch B, Kudo M, Naro F, Conti M, Hsueh AJ. The C-terminal third of the human luteinizing hormone (LH) receptor is important for inositol phosphate release: analysis using chimeric human LH/follicle-stimulating hormone receptors. *Mol Endocrinol*. (1996) 10:1127–37.
14. Zhu X, Gilbert S, Birnbaumer M, Birnbaumer L. Dual signaling potential is common among Gs-coupled receptors and dependent on receptor density. *Mol Pharmacol*. (1994) 46:460–9.
15. Lin YF, Tseng MJ, Hsu HL, Wu YW Lee YH, Tsai YH. A novel follicle-stimulating hormone-induced G alpha h/phospholipase C-delta1 signaling pathway mediating rat sertoli cell Ca2+-influx. *Mol Endocrinol*. (2006) 20:2514–27. doi: 10.1210/me.2005-0347
16. Crepieux P, Marion S, Martinat N, Fafeur V, Vern YL, Kerboeuf D, et al. The ERK-dependent signalling is stage-specifically modulated by FSH, during primary Sertoli cell maturation. *Oncogene* (2001) 20:4696–709. doi: 10.1038/sj.onc.1204632
17. Jonas KC, Hanyaloglu AC. Impact of G protein-coupled receptor heteromers in endocrine systems. *Mol Cell Endocrinol*. (2017) 449:21–7. doi: 10.1016/j.mce.2017.01.030

18. Ferre S, Casado V, Devi LA, Filizola M, Jockers R, Lohse MJ, et al. G protein-coupled receptor oligomerization revisited: functional and pharmacological perspectives, *Pharmacol Rev.* (2014) 66:413–34. doi: 10.1124/pr.113.008052

19. Patel HH, Murray F, Insel PA. G-protein-coupled receptor-signaling components in membrane raft and caveolae microdomains. *Handb Exp Pharmacol.* (2008) (186):167–84. doi: 10.1007/978-3-540-72843-6_7

20. Feng X, Zhang M, Guan R, Segaloff DL. Heterodimerization between the lutropin and follitropin receptors is associated with an attenuation of hormone-dependent signaling, *Endocrinology* (2013) 154:3925–30. doi: 10.1210/en.2013-1407

21. Jiang X, Fischer D, Chen X, McKenna SD, Liu H, Sriraman V, et al. Evidence for follicle-stimulating hormone receptor as a functional trimer. *J Biol Chem.* (2014) 289:14273–82. doi: 10.1074/jbc.M114.549592

22. Li X, Chen W, Li P, Wei J, Cheng Y, Liu P, et al. Follicular stimulating hormone accelerates atherogenesis by increasing endothelial VCAM-1 expression. *Theranostics* (2017) 7:4671–4688. doi: 10.7150/thno.21216

23. Wilden U, Wust E, Weyand I, Kuhn H. Rapid affinity purification of retinal arrestin (48 kDa protein) via its light-dependent binding to phosphorylated rhodopsin. *FEBS Lett.* (1986) 207:292–5. doi: 10.1016/0014-5793(86)81507-1

24. Craft CM, Whitmore DH, Wiechmann AF. Cone arrestin identified by targeting expression of a functional family. *J Biol Chem.* (1994) 269:4613–9.

25. Attramadal H, Arriza JL, Aoki C, Dawson TM, Codina J, Kwatra MM, et al. Beta-arrestin2, a novel member of the arrestin/beta-arrestin gene family. *J Biol Chem.* (1992) 267:17882–90.

26. Lohse MJ, Benovic JL, Codina J, Caron MG, Lefkowitz RJ. beta-Arrestin: a protein that regulates beta-adrenergic receptor function. *Science* (1990) 248:1547–50. doi: 10.1126/science.2163110

27. Rajagopal S, Shenoy SK. GPCR desensitization: acute and prolonged phases. *Cell Signal.* (2018) 41:9–16. doi: 10.1016/j.cellsig.2017.01.024

28. Reiter E, Ayoub MA, Pellissier LP, Landomiel F, Musnier A, Trefier A, et al. beta-arrestin signalling and bias in hormone-responsive GPCRs. *Mol Cell Endocrinol.* (2017) 449:28–41. doi: 10.1016/j.mce.2017.01.052

29. Liggett SB. Phosphorylation barcoding as a mechanism of directing GPCR signaling. *Sci Signal.* (2011) 4:pe36. doi: 10.1126/scisignal.2002331

30. Shukla AK, Westfield GH, Xiao K, Reis RI, Huang LY, Tripathi-Shukla P, et al. Visualization of arrestin recruitment by a G-protein-coupled receptor. *Nature* (2014) 512:218–22. doi: 10.1038/nature13430

31. Thomsen ARB, Plouffe B, Cahill TJ, Shukla AK, Tarrasch JT, Dosey AM, et al. GPCR-G protein-beta-arrestin super-complex mediates sustained G protein signaling. *Cell* (2016) 166:907–919. doi: 10.1016/j.cell.2016.07.004

32. Cahill TJ III, Thomsen AR, Tarrasch JT, Plouffe B, Nguyen AH, Yang F, et al. Distinct conformations of GPCR-beta-arrestin complexes mediate desensitization, signaling, and endocytosis. *Proc Natl Acad Sci USA.* (2017) 114:2562–2567. doi: 10.1073/pnas.1701529114

33. Eichel K, Jullie D, Barsi-Rhyne B, Latorraca NR, Masureel M, Sibarita JB, et al. Catalytic activation of beta-arrestin by GPCRs. *Nature* (2018) 557:381–386. doi: 10.1038/s41586-018-0079-1

34. Ranjan R, Dwivedi H, Baidya M, Kumar M, Shukla AK. Novel Structural insights into GPCR-beta-arrestin interaction and signaling. *Trends Cell Biol.* (2017) 27:851–862. doi: 10.1016/j.tcb.2017.05.008

35. Troispoux C, Guillou F, Elalouf JM, Firsov D, Iacovelli L, De Blasi A, et al. Involvement of G protein-coupled receptor kinases and arrestins in desensitization to follicle-stimulating hormone action. *Mol Endocrinol.* (1999) 13:1599–614. doi: 10.1210/mend.13.9.0342

36. Kara E, Crepieux P, Gauthier C, Martinat N, Piketty V, Guillou F, et al. A phosphorylation cluster of five serine and threonine residues in the C-terminus of the follicle-stimulating hormone receptor is important for desensitization but not for beta-arrestin-mediated ERK activation. *Mol Endocrinol.* (2006) 20:3014–26. doi: 10.1210/me.2006-0098

37. Bhaskaran RS, Min L, Krishnamurthy H, Ascoli M. Studies with chimeras of the gonadotropin receptors reveal the importance of third intracellular loop threonines on the formation of the receptor/nonvisual arrestin complex. *Biochemistry* (2003) 42:13950–13959. doi: 10.1021/bi034907w

38. Kishi H, Ascoli M. Multiple distant amino acid residues present in the serpentine region of the follitropin receptor modulate the rate of agonist-induced internalization. *J Biol Chem.* (2000) 275:31030–7. doi: 10.1074/jbc.M005528200

39. Kumari P, Srivastava A, Banerjee R, Ghosh E, Gupta P, Ranjan R, et al. Functional competence of a partially engaged GPCR-beta-arrestin complex. *Nat Commun.* (2016) 7:13416. doi: 10.1038/ncomms13416

40. McDonald PH, Chow CW, Miller WE, Laporte SA, Field ME, Lin FT, et al. Beta-arrestin 2: a receptor-regulated MAPK scaffold for the activation of JNK3. *Science* (2000) 290:1574–7. doi: 10.1126/science.290.5496.1574

41. DeFea KA, Zalevsky J, Thoma MS, Dery O, Mullins RD, Bunnett NW. beta-arrestin-dependent endocytosis of proteinase-activated receptor 2 is required for intracellular targeting of activated ERK1/2. *J Cell Biol.* (2000) 148:1267–81. doi: 10.1083/jcb.148.6.1267

42. Terrillon S, Bouvier M. Receptor activity-independent recruitment of betaarrestin2 reveals specific signalling modes. *EMBO J.* (2004) 23:3950–61. doi: 10.1038/sj.emboj.7600387

43. Ayoub MA, Landomiel F, Gallay N, Jegot G, Poupon A, Crepieux P, et al. Assessing gonadotropin receptor function by resonance energy transfer-based assays. *Front Endocrinol (Lausanne)* (2015) 6:130. doi: 10.3389/fendo.2015.00130

44. Jean-Alphonse FG, Bowersox S, Chen S, Beard G, Puthenveedu MA, Hanyaloglu AC. Spatially restricted G protein-coupled receptor activity via divergent endocytic compartments. *J Biol Chem.* (2014) 289:3960–77. doi: 10.1074/jbc.M113.526350

45. Piketty V, Kara E, Guillou F, Reiter E, Crepieux P. Follicle-stimulating hormone (FSH) activates extracellular signal-regulated kinase phosphorylation independently of beta-arrestin- and dynamin-mediated FSH receptor internalization. *Reprod Biol Endocrinol.* (2006) 4:33. doi: 10.1186/1477-7827-4-33

46. Eichel K, Jullie D, von Zastrow M. beta-Arrestin drives MAP kinase signalling from clathrin-coated structures after GPCR dissociation. *Nat Cell Biol.* (2016) 18:303–10. doi: 10.1038/ncb3307

47. Nakamura K, Lazari MF, Li S, Korgaonkar C, Ascoli M. Role of the rate of internalization of the agonist-receptor complex on the agonist-induced down-regulation of the lutropin/choriogonadotropin receptor. *Mol Endocrinol.* (1999) 13:1295–304. doi: 10.1210/mend.13.8.0331

48. Kishi H, Krishnamurthy H, Galet C, Bhaskaran RS, Ascoli M. Identification of a short linear sequence present in the C-terminal tail of the rat follitropin receptor that modulates arrestin-3 binding in a phosphorylation-independent fashion. *J Biol Chem.* (2002) 277:21939–46. doi: 10.1074/jbc.M110894200

49. Trefier A, Musnier A, Landomiel F, Bourquard T, Boulo T, Ayoub MA, et al. G protein-dependent signaling triggers a beta-arrestin-scaffolded p70S6K/ rpS6 module that controls 5'TOP mRNA translation. *FASEB J.* (2018) 32:1154–1169. doi: 10.1096/fj.201700763R

50. Latorraca NR, Wang JK, Bauer B, Townshend RJL, Hollingsworth SA, Olivieri JE, et al. Molecular mechanism of GPCR-mediated arrestin activation. *Nature* (2018) 557:452–456. doi: 10.1038/s41586-018-0077-3

51. Landomiel F, Gallay N, Jégot G, Tranchant T, Durand G, Bourquard T, et al. Biased signalling in follicle stimulating hormone action. *Mol Cell Endocrinol.* (2014) 1:452–459. doi: 10.1016/j.mce.2013.09.035

52. Grundmann M, Merten N, Malfacini D, Inoue A, Preis P, Simon K, et al. Lack of beta-arrestin signaling in the absence of active G proteins, *Nat Commun.* (2018) 1:341. doi: 10.1038/s41467-017-02661-3

53. O'Hayre M, Eichel K, Avino S, Zhao X, Steffen DJ, Feng X, et al. Genetic evidence that beta-arrestins are dispensable for the initiation of beta2-adrenergic receptor signaling to ERK. *Sci Signal.* (2017) 10:eaal3395. doi: 10.1126/scisignal.aal3395

54. Tranchant T, Durand G, Gauthier C, Crepieux P, Ulloa-Aguirre A, Royere D, et al. Preferential beta-arrestin signalling at low receptor density revealed by functional characterization of the human FSH receptor A189 V mutation. *Mol Cell Endocrinol.* (2011) 1:109–18. doi: 10.1016/j.mce.2010.08.016

55. Aittomaki K, Lucena JL, Pakarinen P, Sistonen P, Tapanainen J, Gromoll J, et al. Mutation in the follicle-stimulating hormone receptor gene causes hereditary hypergonadotropic ovarian failure. *Cell* (1995) 1:959–68. doi: 10.1016/0092-8674(95)90275-9

56. Miyoshi T, Otsuka F, Shimasaki S. GRK-6 mediates FSH action synergistically enhanced by estrogen and the oocyte in rat granulosa cells. *Biochem Biophys Res Commun.* (2013) 1:401–6. doi: 10.1016/j.bbrc.2013.04.002

57. Casarini L, Reiter E, Simoni M. beta-arrestins regulate gonadotropin receptor-mediated cell proliferation and apoptosis by controlling different FSHR or

LHCGR intracellular signaling in the hGL5 cell line. *Mol Cell Endocrinol.* (2016) 437:11–21. doi: 10.1016/j.mce.2016.08.005

58. Hanyaloglu AC, von Zastrow M. Regulation of GPCRs by endocytic membrane trafficking and its potential implications. *Annu Rev Pharmacol Toxicol.* (2008) 48:537–68. doi: 10.1146/annurev.pharmtox.48.113006.094830

59. Irannejad R, Tsvetanova NG, Lobingier BT, von Zastrow M. Effects of endocytosis on receptor-mediated signaling. *Curr Opin Cell Biol.* (2015) 35:137–43. doi: 10.1016/j.ceb.2015.05.005

60. Sposini S, Hanyaloglu AC. Spatial encryption of G protein-coupled receptor signaling in endosomes; mechanisms and applications. *Biochem Pharmacol.* (2017) 143:1–9. doi: 10.1016/j.bcp.2017.04.028

61. Pavlos NJ, Friedman PA. GPCR Signaling and trafficking: the long and short of It. *Trends Endocrinol Metab.* (2017) 1:213–26. doi: 10.1016/j.tem.2016.10.007

62. Bowman SL, Puthenveedu MA. Postendocytic Sorting of adrenergic and opioid receptors: new mechanisms and functions. *Prog Mol Biol Transl Sci.* (2015) 132:189–206. doi: 10.1016/bs.pmbts.2015.03.005

63. Sposini S, Hanyaloglu AC. Evolving view of membrane trafficking and signaling systems for g protein-coupled receptors. *Prog Mol Subcell Biol.* (2018) 57:273–99. doi: 10.1007/978-3-319-96704-2_10

64. Hanyaloglu AC. Advances in membrane trafficking and endosomal signaling of g protein-coupled receptors. *Int Rev Cell Mol Biol.* (2018) 339:93–131. doi: 10.1016/bs.ircmb.2018.03.001

65. Hislop JN, von Zastrow M. Role of ubiquitination in endocytic trafficking of G-protein-coupled receptors. *Traffic* (2011) 1:137–48. doi: 10.1111/j.1600-0854.2010.01121.x

66. Kennedy JE, Marchese A, Regulation of GPCR Trafficking by Ubiquitin. *Prog Mol Biol Transl Sci.* (2015) 132:15–38. doi: 10.1016/bs.pmbts.2015.02.005

67. Cao TT, Deacon HW, Reczek D, Bretscher A, von Zastrow M. A kinase-regulated PDZ-domain interaction controls endocytic sorting of the beta2-adrenergic receptor. *Nature* (1999) 401:286–90. doi: 10.1038/45816

68. Hirakawa T, Galet C, Kishi M, Ascoli M. GIPC binds to the human lutropin receptor (hLHR) through an unusual PDZ domain binding motif, and it regulates the sorting of the internalized human choriogonadotropin and the density of cell surface hLHR. *J Biol Chem.* (2003) 1:49348–57. doi: 10.1074/jbc.M306557200

69. He J, Bellini M, Inuzuka H, Xu J, Xiong Y, Yang X, et al. Proteomic analysis of beta1-adrenergic receptor interactions with PDZ scaffold proteins. *J Biol Chem.* (2006) 1:2820–7. doi: 10.1074/jbc.M509503200

70. Lauffer BE, Melero C, Temkin P, Lei C, Hong W, Kortemme T, et al. SNX27 mediates PDZ-directed sorting from endosomes to the plasma membrane. *J Cell Biol.* (2010) 1:565–74. doi: 10.1083/jcb.201004060

71. Marchese A, Paing MM, Temple BR, Trejo J. G protein-coupled receptor sorting to endosomes and lysosomes. *Annu Rev Pharmacol Toxicol.* (2008) 48:601–29. doi: 10.1146/annurev.pharmtox.48.113006.094646

72. Krishnamurthy H, Kishi H, Shi M, Galet C, Bhaskaran RS, Hirakawa T, et al. Postendocytotic trafficking of the follicle-stimulating hormone (FSH)-FSH receptor complex. *Mol Endocrinol.* (2003) 1:2162–76. doi: 10.1210/me.2003-0118

73. Melo-Nava B, Casas-Gonzalez P, Perez-Solis MA, Castillo-Badillo J, Maravillas-Montero JL, Jardon-Valadez E, et al. Role of cysteine residues in the carboxyl-terminus of the follicle-stimulating hormone receptor in intracellular traffic and postendocytic processing. *Front Cell Dev Biol.* (2016) 4:76. doi: 10.3389/fcell.2016.00076

74. Uribe A, Zarinan T, Perez-Solis MA, Gutierrez-Sagal R, Jardon-Valadez E, Pineiro A, et al. Functional and structural roles of conserved cysteine residues in the carboxyl-terminal domain of the follicle-stimulating hormone receptor in human embryonic kidney 293 cells. *Biol Reprod.* (2008) 1:869–82. doi: 10.1095/biolreprod.107.063925

75. Hu LA, Chen W, Martin NP, Whalen EJ, Premont RT, Lefkowitz RJ. GIPC interacts with the beta1-adrenergic receptor and regulates beta1-adrenergic receptor-mediated ERK activation. *J Biol Chem.* (2003) 1:26295–301. doi: 10.1074/jbc.M212352200

76. Nechamen CA, Thomas RM, Cohen BD, Acevedo G, Poulikakos PI, Testa JR, et al. Human follicle-stimulating hormone (FSH) receptor interacts with the adaptor protein APPL1 in HEK 293 cells: potential involvement of the PI3K pathway in FSH signaling. *Biol Reprod.* (2004) 1:629–36. doi: 10.1095/biolreprod.103.025833

77. Nechamen CA, Thomas RM, Dias JA, APPL1, APPL2, Akt2 and FOXO1a interact with FSHR in a potential signaling complex. *Mol Cell Endocrinol.* (2007) 1:93–9. doi: 10.1016/j.mce.2006.08.014

78. Lin DC, Quevedo C, Brewer NE, Bell A, Testa JR, Grimes ML, et al. APPL1 associates with TrkA and GIPC1 and is required for nerve growth factor-mediated signal transduction. *Mol Cell Biol.* (2006) 1:8928–41. doi: 10.1128/MCB.00228-06

79. Liu Z, Xiao T, Peng X, Li G, Hu F. APPLs: more than just adiponectin receptor binding proteins. *Cell Signal* (2017) 32:76–84. doi: 10.1016/j.cellsig.2017.01.018

80. Zoncu R, Perera RM, Balkin DM, Pirruccello M, Toomre D, De Camilli P, A phosphoinositide switch controls the maturation and signaling properties of APPL endosomes. *Cell* (2009) 1:1110–21. doi: 10.1016/j.cell.2009.01.032

81. Kalaidzidis I, Miaczynska M, Brewinska-Olchowik M, Hupalowska A, Ferguson C, Parton RG, et al. APPL endosomes are not obligatory endocytic intermediates but act as stable cargo-sorting compartments. *J Cell Biol.* (2015) 1:123–44. doi: 10.1083/jcb.201311117

82. Diggins NL, Webb DJ, APPL1 is a multifunctional endosomal signaling adaptor protein. *Biochem Soc Trans.* (2017) 1:771–9. doi: 10.1042/BST20160191

83. Dias JA, Mahale SD, Nechamen CA, Davydenko O, Thomas RM, Ulloa-Aguirre A, Emerging roles for the FSH receptor adapter protein APPL1 and overlap of a putative 14-3-3tau interaction domain with a canonical G-protein interaction site. *Mol Cell Endocrinol.* 329 (2010) 17–25. doi: 10.1016/j.mce.2010.05.009

84. Sposini S, Jean-Alphonse FG, Ayoub MA, Oqua A, West C, Lavery S, et al. Integration of GPCR signaling and sorting from very early endosomes via opposing APPL1 Mechanisms. *Cell Rep.* (2017) 1:2855-2867. doi: 10.1016/j.celrep.2017.11.023

85. Irannejad R, Tomshine JC, Tomshine JR, Chevalier M, Mahoney JP, Steyaert J, et al. Conformational biosensors reveal GPCR signalling from endosomes. *Nature* (2013) 495:534–8. doi: 10.1038/nature12000

86. Feinstein TN, Wehbi VL, Ardura JA, Wheeler DS, Ferrandon S, Gardella TJ, et al. Retromer terminates the generation of cAMP by internalized PTH receptors. *Nat Chem Biol.* (2011) 1:278–84. doi: 10.1038/nchembio.545

87. Feinstein TN, Yui N, Webber MJ, Wehbi VL, Stevenson HP, King JD, Jr., et al. Noncanonical control of vasopressin receptor type 2 signaling by retromer and arrestin. *J Biol Chem.* (2013) 1:27849–60. doi: 10.1074/jbc.M112.445098

88. Lobingier BT, Huttenhain R, Eichel K, Miller KB, Ting AY, von Zastrow M, et al. An approach to spatiotemporally resolve protein interaction networks in living cells. *Cell* (2017) 1:350–360 e12. doi: 10.1016/j.cell.2017.03.022

89. Comim FV, Hardy K, Franks S. Adiponectin and its receptors in the ovary: further evidence for a link between obesity and hyperandrogenism in polycystic ovary syndrome. *PLoS ONE* (2013) 1:e80416. doi: 10.1371/journal.pone.0080416

90. Lyga S, Volpe S, Werthmann RC, Gotz K, Sungkaworn T, Lohse MJ, et al. Persistent cAMP Signaling by internalized lh receptors in ovarian follicles. *Endocrinology* (2016) 1:1613–21. doi: 10.1210/en.2015-1945

91. Casas-Gonzalez P, Scaglia HE, Perez-Solis MA, Durand G, Scaglia J, Zarinan T, et al. Normal testicular function without detectable follicle-stimulating hormone. A novel mutation in the follicle-stimulating hormone receptor gene leading to apparent constitutive activity and impaired agonist-induced desensitization and internalization. *Mol Cell Endocrinol.* (2012) 364:71–82. doi: 10.1016/j.mce.2012.08.011

92. Nordhoff V, Sonntag B, von Tils D, Gotte M, Schuring AN, Gromoll J, et al. Effects of the FSH receptor gene polymorphism p.N680S on cAMP and steroid production in cultured primary human granulosa cells. *Reprod Biomed Online* (2011) 1:196–203. doi: 10.1016/j.rbmo.2011.04.009

93. Casarini L, Moriondo V, Marino M, Adversi F, Capodanno F, Grisolia C, et al. FSHR polymorphism p.N680S mediates different responses to FSH in vitro. *Mol Cell Endocrinol.* (2014) 393:83–91. doi: 10.1016/j.mce.2014.06.013

94. Dominguez-Lopez P, Diaz-Cueto L, Arechavaleta-Velasco M, Caldino-Soto F, Ulloa-Aguirre A, Arechavaleta-Velasco F. The follicle-stimulating hormone receptor Asn680Ser polymorphism is associated with preterm birth in Hispanic women. *J Matern Fetal Neonatal Med.* (2018) 1:580–5. doi: 10.1080/14767058.2017.1292245

95. Simoni M, Santi D, Negri L, Hoffmann I, Muratori M, Baldi E, et al. Treatment with human, recombinant FSH improves sperm DNA

fragmentation in idiopathic infertile men depending on the FSH receptor polymorphism p.N680S: a pharmacogenetic study. *Hum Reprod.* (2016) 1:1960–9. doi: 10.1093/humrep/dew167

96. Jensen DD, Lieu T, Halls ML, Veldhuis NA, Imlach WL, Mai QN, et al. Neurokinin 1 receptor signaling in endosomes mediates sustained nociception and is a viable therapeutic target for prolonged pain relief. *Sci Transl Med.* (2017) 9:eaal3447. doi: 10.1126/scitranslmed.aal3447

97. Yarwood RE, Imlach WL, Lieu T, Veldhuis NA, Jensen DD, Klein Herenbrink C, et al. Endosomal signaling of the receptor for calcitonin gene-related peptide mediates pain transmission. *Proc Natl Acad Sci USA.* (2017) 1:12309–14. doi: 10.1073/pnas.1706656114

98. Jimenez-Vargas NN, Pattison LA, Zhao P, Lieu T, Latorre R, Jensen DD, et al. Protease-activated receptor-2 in endosomes signals persistent pain of irritable bowel syndrome. *Proc Natl Acad Sci USA.* (2018) 1:E7438–7447. doi: 10.1073/pnas.1721891115

99. Nataraja SG, Yu HN, Palmer SS. Discovery and development of small molecule allosteric modulators of glycoprotein hormone receptors. *Front Endocrinol.* (2015) 6:142. doi: 10.3389/fendo.2015.00142

12

Individualization of FSH Doses in Assisted Reproduction: Facts and Fiction

*Frank J. Broekmans**

University Medical Center Utrecht, Utrecht, Netherlands

Correspondence:
Frank J. Broekmans
f.broekmans@umcutrecht.nl

The art of ovarian stimulation for IVF/ICSI treatment using exogenous FSH should be balanced against the relative contribution of other steps of the ART process such as the IVF-lab-phase and the Embryo-Transfer. The aim of ovarian stimulation is to obtain a certain number of oocytes, that will enable the best probability of achieving a live birth. It has been suggested that more oocytes will create a better prospect for pregnancy, but studies on the question whether the retrieval of a few oocytes less or more will make the difference are not clearly supportive for this mantra. Personalization strategies have been the subject of many studies over the past 20 years. Creating the optimal response in a patient in terms of live birth prognosis as well as OHSS risks may be based on information from the Ovarian Reserve testing using the Antral Follicle Count or Anti-Mullerian Hormone, the patient's bodyweight, the ovarian response in a previous cycle, and the dosage level of FSH. Taken together, steering the ovarian response into a supposed optimal range may appear difficult as the interrelation for each of these factors with the egg number is weak. Using OR testing for choosing FSH dosage, compared to a standard normal dosage of 150 IU, has been studied in several trials. Dosage individualization, in general, does not appear to improve the prospects for live birth, but the reduction in OHSS risk may be substantial. This implies that the use of high dosages of FSH in predicted LOW responders lacks any cost-benefit for the patient and may be abandoned, while in predicted HIGH responders, reduction of the usual dosage level of 150 IU may create better safety, provided that in case of an unexpected LOW response cancelation of the cycle is refrained from. In view of recent developments in using GnRH agonist triggering of final oocyte maturation, the trend could be that with the Antagonist co-medication system and a standard dosage of 150 IU of FSH, prior ovarian reserve testing may become futile, as safety can be managed well in actual HIGH responders by replacing the high dose hCG trigger.

Keywords: FSH, ovarian response, live birth, safety, OHSS, ovarian reserve testing, dosage individualization, ovarian stimulation

INTRODUCTION

The "ART" of Assisted Reproduction

Infertility is a disease state with potential profound consequences for the quality of life of both women and men. Reproduction is one of the key elements of life and failing to create offspring may lead to lifelong mental and physical health problems. Also, couples faced with infertility are frequently subjected to long-lasting, time consuming, and agonizing treatment schedules, living often between hope, and fear, and frustration. The development of IVF as a tool for solving problems such as tubal disease, severe male factor, anovulation states, and even, although not convincingly proven, conditions like ill-explained infertility, has brought enormous potential to the infertility treatment armamentarium.

Very soon after the development of the IVF technology, the single oocyte system was replaced by the art of ovarian stimulation in order to obtain multiple oocytes. This was aimed at solving two problems: one was the elimination of the risk of having no oocyte at all. The other was the urge to improve efficiency, by obtaining several embryo's and by replacing more than one in order to yield the highest possible probability of a live birth. Ovarian stimulation has thereby become one of the cornerstones of the IVF treatment, next to the *in vitro* handling of gametes and embryos, and the embryo replacement process.

The relative contribution to the overall success of IVF from the ovarian stimulation phase is difficult to assess. Many years of research have aimed at optimizing this specific phase. Issues have been addressed ranging from using urinary FSH products or recombinants, using high or low FSH dosages, triggering with urinary or recombinant, high or low dosage of hCG, adding LH or LH like activity to the FSH as principal drug, management of high, and low responders, adding medication to improve antral follicle availability, etcetera. At the same time, debates have been kept on beliefs like "the more (oocytes) the better," less (mild stimulation) is more (quality), "normal (8–15 oocytes) is the best," and "we need eggs, not ALL the eggs." It seems that agreement on how ovarian stimulation could contribute to the best probability of success is far from settled.

Folliculogenesis

Complex as it seems, the endocrine background for ovarian stimulation is quite straightforward. FSH levels must become elevated above the level that in the normal menstrual cycle will help to select and grow ONE single follicle, out of a group of antral follicles presenting in the FSH "window." During this window period, levels of FSH surpass a certain threshold above which follicle granulosa cells become responsive and start to enhance proliferation, leading to expansion of the granulosa cell mass and the follicle fluid volume This will typically lead to the development of only one follicle, while other potential responsive antral follicles are destined for atresia, as a result of selection mechanisms that are still not fully understood (**Figure 1**). In surpassing the FSH threshold to a greater extent and for a longer period of time, more than one of the antral follicles will become capable of entering the dominant follicle development stage, with the ultimate opportunity of triggering the ovulation process and harvest the eggs within these follicles. Apart from administering FSH as an exogenous drug for the maturation of more than one follicle, other compounds such as selective estradiol receptor blockers, or steroid biosynthesis inhibitors may yield the same effect: increase and prolonged FSH exposure, albeit from an endogenous source.

Pharmacokinetics: FSH Levels

For the drug FSH it has become clear that the one-compartment model with first-order absorption and a transit model for adding a delay in the absorption best describes the process of drug distribution and elimination in the body. This model principally assumes that the human body acts like a single, uniform compartment. When FSH is given in the form of a subcutaneous bolus, the entire dose of the drug enters the bloodstream after a short lag phase and distributes via the circulatory system to potentially all the tissues in the body. The modeled distribution implies that bodyweight, but not other potential confounders such as subject's age, affects the volume of distribution and clearance rate of the FSH medication. Both these effects, however, are small, with substantial variation in FSH serum levels after a standard dosage within bodyweight classes (1).

Pharmacodynamics: FSH Dosage and Number of Oocytes

As indicated, the purpose of ovarian stimulation is to obtain at least one mature oocyte, and in most cases of prolonged supraphysiologic exposure to FSH, the response of the ovaries will be much more intense with a high degree of variation, ranging from 1 to 25 oocytes. The background for this variation may be multifactorial. The number of antral follicles present in the ovaries at any time will be the principal factor. However, under the assumption that these follicles may have different levels of sensitivity to FSH and may be at varying time points in their development through the antral stages, the level of exposure to FSH may be a second factor of importance. From a limited number of sources, it has become apparent that the exogenous FSH dosage will have some degree of positive relation to the oocyte yield, although it may only be true across a narrow range (from ~50 to ~225 IU per day). This relation is, however, far from precise, as actual serum levels of FSH, using a fixed daily dosage, may vary substantially across individuals, with a small contribution of body weight to this variation (2–4) (**Figure 2**). This all means that accurate steering of the oocyte number by the exogenous FSH dosing may not be a very reliable tool for obtaining a certain optimal oocyte number.

OVARIAN RESPONSE

Response Categories

The level of oocyte yield has obtained a differential clinical appreciation, regards items such as success and safety. The "low" ovarian response defined as the yield of <4 oocytes is related to an unfavorable prognosis for live birth, although much of this poor prognosis is in fact dictated by female age and not by the low egg number *per se* (5). At the other side of the spectrum a high response, arbitrarily defined as obtaining more than 15 oocytes at pick up, will jeopardize safety for the patient and may even slightly limit the rates of live birth (6). It is therefore that many clinicians across the world try to foresee the ovarian response category in order to adjust the stimulation protocol with the expectation that the ovarian response can be brought into a "normal range" (5–15 oocytes).

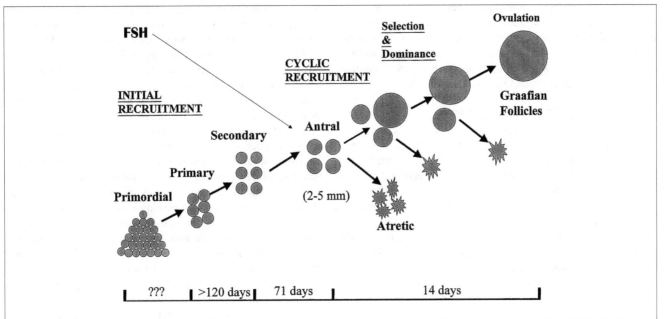

FIGURE 1 | Folliculogenesis in the human ovaries. The antral stages of development provide a continuous target for exogenous or endogenous FSH to drive all or part of the present follicles into dominant follicle growth. It is demonstrated that the ovaries have initial, continuous recruitment with continuously filling, and emptying the pool of antral follicles, a process that is highly independent of control by pituitary hormones. Only during reproductive years, cyclic recruitment from the antral follicle pool occurs resulting in the ovulatory menstrual cycle.

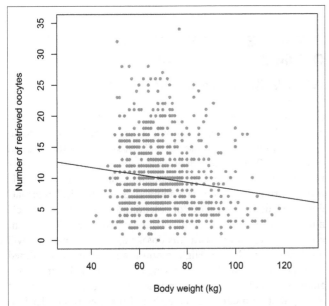

FIGURE 2 | The relation between Bodyweight and Oocyte number in equal dosage (150 IU rec FSH) cases ($n = 900$), showing a weak correlation. With a weight of 60 kg the oocyte number ranges from 1 to 26. In the weight group of 90 kg the variation in oocyte number is not much different: 2–24. Drawn from the Optimist study database (18). It indicates that bodyweight may only have a weak role as a tool for dose assessment in ovarian hyperstimulation.

Factors That Predict Ovarian Response

Prediction of ovarian response category today is mainly applied by using the Antral Follicle Count by transvaginal ultrasound examination or the serum AntiMullerian Hormone level in the early follicle phase. Both relate to the number of antral follicles present at any time in the ovaries. These are the source for the number of dominant follicles that could grow in result to the application of exogenous FSH. As such, these two ovarian response tests (ORTs) have become the standard test for ovarian response prediction, although factors such as female age and, possibly, bodyweight may add to this predictive information.

Both tests may be affected by factors that may make response prediction less reliable. For the AFC ultrasound equipment quality and interobserver variation may be troublesome, as is the exact category of follicles: are only sizes of 2–6 mm or all follicles sized 2–10 mm counted on one of the first days of the cycle (7, 8). AMH assays have been under intense development over the past 15 years, leading to quite some inter-assay variation in results. With the advent of well-controlled automated assay systems many of the procedure problems have now been dealt with, although current available systems may not perfectly overlap (9, 10). It may therefore be noted, that AFC or AMH based predictions will be false positive in some 15–20% of cases, while only 60–70% of truly "out of the normal range" responders will be identified. Basing the FSH stimulation dosage on such predictions therefore may be imprecise practice from the start. Whether this reliability problem arises from imprecise response categorization by the ORT or relates to variation in the ovarian response within the patient to an equivalent dosage of FSH is not fully clear.

Parallel to this, FSH receptor polymorphisms have been long considered as welcome new attributes for response prediction (11). The Asn/Ser allelic variant may reflect a higher FSH sensitivity of follicles, leading to a better and more rapid ovarian response compared to the other two SNP variants. This differential FSH sensitivity may well be overcome by slightly lower or higher FSH dosages, but seems not to impact on live birth rates (12–14). Meaningful application of FSH receptor genomics in dosage personalization is still awaited.

Factors That Predict Success

Success in Assisted Reproduction is defined as the occurrence of an ongoing pregnancy, leading to a healthy live-born, as a result of the IVF procedure. As indicated, the relative contribution of the *ovarian stimulation phase and oocyte retrieval* to this major outcome is not really known. In principle, the *laboratory phase*, with characteristics such as fertilization rate, embryo development rate, and embryo implantation rate, is an important part of the ART process, and must be under rigorous quality control. Also, the *luteal phase with the embryo transfer*, with the endocrine management of endometrium development and timing, and the deposition of the embryo in the uterus with only indirect and incomplete information on the correct "arrival" of the embryo, will contribute greatly to the outcome of the three-step process.

It is assumed that the quality of the oocytes that arrive in the IVF laboratory after follicle aspiration is the important factor. Good quality oocytes handled under optimal laboratory conditions and subsequent good quality embryos placed smoothly and well-timed in the uterine cavity, create the highest chances for having a baby from the ART cycle.

The question is then: will the approach in the stimulation and egg retrieval phase make a difference for the oocyte quality? Many clinicians today follow the idea that more oocytes will lead to a better outcome, especially regarding live birth rates. Such belief is probably not supported by evidence, but strongly suggested by retrospective studies (6, 15). In these studies, the individual patient profiles may be much more relevant than the number of obtained oocytes. The real question here is whether retrieving seven oocytes where potentially the patient could have had 11, creates a disadvantage, or reversely, whether a patient would have a benefit from creating 12 instead of the eight oocytes she obtained in a previous stimulation cycle. The answers here should come from randomizing these two hypothetical patients, and as this is impossible, to rely on group-randomized studies. Such studies seem to indicate that getting oocytes may be more important than striving for a maximal response (2, 7–9). Still, we struggle with a lack of knowledge on whether the hierarchy among the cohort of antral follicles that is capable of responding to elevated FSH levels from exogenous source, is such that the most sensitive follicles will provide the best oocytes in this cohort. From studies where only part of the recruitable follicles are driven into dominant growth and subsequent oocyte retrieval, it has been suggested that this will not create a lower number of good quality eggs compared to maximal stimulation where all follicles present in the FSH sensitive window are captured (2, 16, 17). More specifically, the relation between dosage of recFSH and ovarian response was studied in a randomized design. With increasing dosage, increasing numbers of oocytes were obtained, both in "low" as well as in "high" predicted responders. However,

the cumulative rates of ongoing pregnancies per FSH dosage group, from fresh and frozen replacement cycles, revealed no better outcomes with increasing number of oocytes harvested (2).

Finally, knowing oocyte quality beforehand is to date not possible. We have a clear knowledge gap regarding the question which quality level is present for the oocytes present in the follicle cohort of a specific woman, as well as the quality of the monthly ovulated oocyte. The same is true for a woman entering an ART programme, where we would wish to know whether this woman is a good, poor, or moderate egg quality carrier. It is only after oocyte retrieval that some of this quality information becomes unveiled. More specifically, the retrieval of immature oocytes at aspiration, after well-timed ovarian stimulation and triggering of the ovulation process, does indicate a quality problem that is easily recognized in the lab. The vast majority of oocytes, however, will be mature and have succeeded in getting into the metaphase II stage. How to identify overall quality, and more interestingly, the individual competence of these oocytes to create a viable embryo after fertilization and to move on to the subsequent birth of a baby. Only small pieces of information have recently emerged on factors that may indicate quality in the *in vitro* stage and could become useful as a testing device, such as IL7 (19) and EGF (20). Whether such tools will help only in selecting the best oocyte or may also assist in optimizing the *in vivo* oocyte-follicle maturation during ovarian stimulation remains to become reality.

THE ROLE OF FSH DOSAGE IN OPTIMIZING OUTCOME

What Is the Normal FSH Dosage?

From the limited number of studies that have tried to study the dose response relationship for the drug FSH (2, 2, 21, 22) it has become clear that going from only a single dominant follicle to a maximal ovarian response the FSH dosage needs to be raised from ~50 to 225 IU daily. In order to obtain a reasonable number in between only one and the maximum, a daily dosage of 150 IU is often promoted and in fact adopted as an empirical "normal" dose. Such dosage will allow for obtaining an optimal or "normal" number of 8–15 oocytes in a large part of the ART patient population. However, with this dosage a subset of patients will produce either a Low or High response, and for reasons outlined above, clinicians are keen on trying to prevent such conditions, amongst other by FSH dosage individualization. In fact, the belief is such that with effective correction of the Low responder into a Normal responder the live birth rates will improve. Also, the production of a Normal response in High responders will create a better safety profile, without jeopardizing the outcome live birth. Although such High responder management is very likely to be a real improvement for the patient (23), the low responder may not have any benefit from FSH dose adjustments. This may be true for predicted low responders, as they have no additional follicles available, but also for unexpected low responders, who will have no better prospects in spite of a higher egg number (3, 24).

Today, FSH dosage individualization is based on two components. First, there is a need for an Ovarian Response Test that can predict a woman's response when given a particular dose of FSH. Second, there must be some dose-response relationship, enabling manipulation of the response through adaptation of the dose. With regard to prediction of response, studies have reported that ORT can be used to predict ovarian response to stimulation, with AMH and AFC being superior to bFSH (25–27). Thereby, the effects of FSH dose adjustments in ovarian response categories could be studied.

Is There a Best FSH Preparation?

Compounds containing FSH as primary component are urine derived mixtures of FSH and LH, sometimes enriched with human chorion gonadotropins, urine derived FSH only preparations, recombinant technology based FSH preparations with or without added recombinant LH, and slow release, long acting modifications. Many efforts have been undertaken over the past three decades to demonstrate the benefit of one preparation over the other. Issues like FSH dosage stability and added LH (or hCG) activity for full sustained endocrine support of the follicle have formed most of the backgrounds to propel research, next to cost efficacy needs.

Looking into the current literature there is no evidence of a preference for any of the compounds available today (28–30). This may also be true for application in specific subgroups of patients such as low responders (28, 31), where neither LH/hCG enriched, nor long-acting FSH only compounds have made a difference (32). The only category with a specific and obvious need of ovarian stimulation with both FSH and LH are patients with a hypothalamic amenorrhea.

Higher Dosages in Predicted Low Responders

Several randomized controlled trials have demonstrated that ORT based individualized dosing of FSH will not alter the fate of the predicted low responder. Specifically, in predicted poor responders the actual occurrence of a poor response will mean that the couple is in a prognostic unfavorable category, although female age may be an important additional value for the real prognosis (5). The prognosis for live birth in young predicted low responders may indeed be three times as good compared to old predicted poor responders (33). Thus, the combination of low AMH or AFC, the actual first cycle poor response, and female age may help to decide whether continuation of the ART treatment is really feasible. This theme has been clearly addressed by the POSEIDON group, where both the prior expectation regarding ovarian response, as well as the age of the patient will place her in distinct low responder groups, with potentially differing management and prognosis for live birth (34, 35). It is, however, clear that the use of extremely high dosages of FSH, such as 300–600 IU per day, will not make any difference for the patient, but do have undesirable effects on the costs of treatment (36).

Lower Dosages in Predicted High Responders

The real gain of individualized FSH dosing could be the management of the hyper responding patient. Several studies have indicated that with the use of submaximal dosages of FSH a mitigated response of the ovaries can be obtained, without

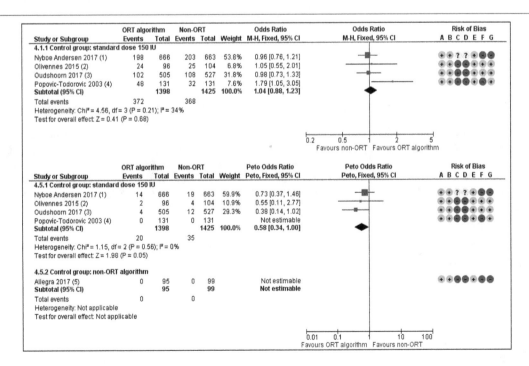

FIGURE 3 | ORT-based vs. Standard dosing of FSH in IVF patients. Effects on Live birth or Ongoing pregnancy per woman randomized (upper panel) and on occurrence of Moderate or Severe OHSS. The individualized dosing has no beneficial effects on the outcome Pregnancy rates but does reduce treatment Risks [Redrawn form Lensen et al. (36)].

jeopardizing efficacy and with a clear improvement of the safety profile, in terms of measures needed to be taken to prevent the OHSS syndrome as well as the actual occurrence of the syndrome (2, 23, 37). This then could be considered as primary preventive management of the OHSS in predicted high responders. At the same time, we may consider whether a standard 150 IU dosage using an antagonist protocol, with the escape of GnRH agonist triggering and with a freeze all strategy as added option, may be the method of secondary OHSS prevention. Such a strategy would bypass imprecise dose picking based on ovarian response tests with moderate accuracy.

Regimens with GnRH antagonist LH peak prevention may, however, be impractical in view of planning issues regards the availability of the IVF laboratory in special cases such as ICSI-PGD or ICSI TESE. Here, OC pretreatment may affect the prognosis for live birth in antagonist cycles, while agonist co-medicated cycles do not seem to have these disadvantages. In the latter, only lower FSH stimulation doses and freeze all are available as safety tools. With lower dosages may arrive conditions where the hyper response is prevented, but in return a low response is observed (37). The fear by clinicians that the patient may then become disadvantaged by collecting fewer oocytes than believed to be optimal is not be supported by current evidence, and thus clinicians may reassure patients at this point (38–40).

The question then remains how ovarian response testing should be embedded in the ART programs. Should we screen every patient and only apply dose adjustments in predicted high responders? Or do we need to scout ovarian reserve status by applying the AFC as a screening test. This could select out patients to undergo an AMH assessment where in predicted high responders either reduced doses of FSH or standard dosing with antagonist co-medication protocols are applied.

For the subgroup of PCOS patients, FSH dosing studies are quite limited in number. In many cases previous cycles of low dose step up FSH ovulation induction will be of help in the right dose picking once entering an IVF programme, in order to manage the substantial risk of extreme hyper response in these patients. Dosages at which mono-follicular follicle growth is obtained may be increased by ~50 units to obtain multi-follicular growth (41). In order to remain within safety limits further parameters such as female age, BMI and AMH level may help in individualizing the dosage levels, which will typically be between 75 and 150 IU per day (42). Needless to state that a GnRH antagonist LH suppression regimen may be preferred in view of secondary options in OHSS prevention (43).

ORT-Based Individualization Studies

Five studies have so far studied the value of ORT based dosage individualization in the general ART population compared to a standard dose of 150 IU (23, 24, 36, 44–46). There is now moderate quality evidence for the absence of a difference between the groups in live birth rate (OR 1.04, 95% CI 0.88 to 1.23) (**Figure 3**). The incidence of moderate to severe OHSS was reduced when compared to a standard dose (OR 0.58, 95% CI 0.34 to 1.00) (**Figure 3**), but this evidence was of also of low quality. So, the promises that individualized dosing based on ovarian reserve markers would positively affect live birth rates in the ART program (46) have not been fulfilled. Yet, the possible gain of FSH dose individualization lies in the better grip on safety for the patient, albeit that dose management may not be the only way forward here. Studies that have compared the use of AMH with the AFC for dose individualization in the general ART patient (47), have not yielded any obvious difference in outcome live birth or OHSS rate. So, there is a strong need for trials recruiting specific patient groups for which a personalized approach would make the relevant difference compared to a standard approach. In such studies, both the added value at the level of oocytes number and good quality embryo's, as well as at the level of children's health need to be considered.

SUMMARIZING CONCLUSIONS

For many years we have held the belief that more oocytes will produce better outcome in terms of live birth rate. The current evidence from well-designed studies has helped us to separate fiction from facts. The facts are that we need more than one oocyte, preferably a number in the range of 8–15. Below that number, but specifically below five oocytes, prognosis for live birth will become jeopardized. Oocyte numbers over 15, and specifically over 20, are undesirable in view of the risk of OHSS occurring. Low responders cannot really be prevented by applying higher than normal dosages, while high responders may benefit from FSH dosage reduction, mainly for the safety issue. So, for that latter purpose, ovarian reserve testing and subsequent dose adjustments could be justified. The high responder patient, however, may also be served by the GnRH antagonist co-medicated stimulation approach: standard dosing with 150 IU, with the option of triggering final oocyte maturation by a GnRH agonist with or without deferred embryo transfer (48–50). With these facts together, we may find that the FSH dose individualization practice may become a realm of the past.

AUTHOR CONTRIBUTIONS

The author confirms being the sole contributor of this work and has approved it for publication.

REFERENCES

1. Rose TH, Röshammar D, Erichsen L, Grundemar L, Ottesen JT. Characterisation of population pharmacokinetics and endogenous follicle-stimulating hormone (FSH) levels after multiple dosing of a recombinant human FSH (FE 999049) in healthy women. *Drugs R D.* (2016) 16:165–72. doi: 10.1007/s40268-016-0126-z

2. Arce JC, Andersen AN, Fernández-Sánchez M, Visnova H, Bosch E, García-Velasco JA, et al. Ovarian response to recombinant human follicle-stimulating hormone: a randomized, antimullerian

hormone-stratified, dose-response trial in women undergoing *in vitro* fertilization/intracytoplasmic sperm injection. *Fertil Steril.* (2014) 102:1633–1640. doi: 10.1016/j.fertnstert.2014.08.013

3. Oudshoorn SC, van Tilborg TC, Hamdine O, Torrance HL, Eijkemans MJC, Lentjes EGWM, et al. Ovarian response to controlled ovarian hyperstimulation: what does serum FSH say? *Hum Reprod.* (2017) 32:1701–9. doi: 10.1093/humrep/dex222

4. McCulloh DH, Maseelall P, Colon JM, McGovern PG. Modeling follicle stimulating hormone levels in serum for controlled ovarian hyperstimulation I: comparing gonadotropin products. *Curr Pharm Biotechnol.* (2012) 13:435–43. doi: 10.2174/138920112799361936

5. Oudendijk JF, Yarde F, Eijkemans MJ, Broekmans FJ, Broer SL. The poor responder in IVF: is the prognosis always poor?: a systematic review. *Hum Reprod Update.* (2012) 18:1–11. doi: 10.1093/humupd/dmr037

6. Sunkara SK, Rittenberg V, Raine-Fenning N, Bhattacharya S, Zamora J, Coomarasamy A. Nomogram for predicting live birth from egg number: an analysis of 400,135 IVF cycles. *Hum Reprod.* (2011) 26:i34. doi: 10.1093/humrep/der106

7. Broekmans FJ, de Ziegler D, Howles CM, Gougeon A, Trew G, Olivennes F. The antral follicle count: practical recommendations for better standardization. *Fertil Steril.* (2010) 94:1044–51. doi: 10.1016/j.fertnstert.2009.04.040

8. Haadsma ML, Bukman A, Groen H, Roeloffzen EM, Groenewoud ER, Heineman MJ, et al. The number of small antral follicles (2–6 mm) determines the outcome of endocrine ovarian reserve tests in a subfertile population. *Hum Reprod.* (2007) 22:1925–31. doi: 10.1093/humrep/dem081

9. Nelson SM, Pastuszek E, Kloss G, Malinowska I, Liss J, Lukaszuk A, et al. Two new automated, compared with two enzyme-linked immunosorbent, antimullerian hormone assays. *Fertil Steril.* (2015) 104:1021.e6. doi: 10.1016/j.fertnstert.2015.06.024

10. Iliodromiti S, Salje B, Dewailly D, Fairburn C, Fanchin R, Fleming R, et al. Non-equivalence of anti-mullerian hormone automated assays-clinical implications for use as a companion diagnostic for individualised gonadotrophin dosing. *Hum Reprod.* (2017) 32:1710–15. doi: 10.1093/humrep/dex219

11. Loutradis D, Patsoula E, Minas V, Koussidis GA, Antsaklis A, Michalas S, et al. FSH receptor gene polymorphisms have a role for different ovarian response to stimulation in patients entering IVF/ICSI-ET programs. *J Assist Reprod Genet.* (2006) 23:177–84. doi: 10.1007/s10815-005-9015-z

12. Mohiyiddeen L, Newman WG, Cerra C, McBurney H, Mulugeta B, Roberts SA, et al. A common Asn680Ser polymorphism in the follicle-stimulating hormone receptor gene is not associated with ovarian response to gonadotropin stimulation in patients undergoing *in vitro* fertilization. *Fertil Steril.* (2013) 99:149–55. doi: 10.1016/j.fertnstert.2012.08.037

13. Desai SS, Roy BS, Mahale SD. Mutations and polymorphisms in FSH receptor: functional implications in human reproduction. *Reproduction.* (2013) 146:235–48. doi: 10.1530/REP-13-0351

14. Desai SS, Achrekar SK, Paranjape SR, Desai SK, Mangoli VS, Mahale SD. Association of allelic combinations of FSHR gene polymorphisms with ovarian response. *Reprod Biomed Online.* (2013) 27:400–6. doi: 10.1016/j.rbmo.2013.07.007

15. Polyzos NP, Drakopoulos P, Parra J, Pellicer A, Santos-Ribeiro S, Tournaye H, et al. Cumulative live birth rates according to the number of oocytes retrieved after the first ovarian stimulation for *in vitro* fertilization/intracytoplasmic sperm injection: a multicenter multinational analysis including approximately 15,000 women. *Fertil Steril.* (2018) 110:670.e1. doi: 10.1016/j.fertnstert.2018.04.039

16. Baart EB, Martini E, Eijkemans MJ, Van Opstal D, Beckers NG, Verhoeff A, et al. Milder ovarian stimulation for *in-vitro* fertilization reduces aneuploidy in the human preimplantation embryo: a randomized controlled trial. *Hum Reprod.* (2007) 22:980–8. doi: 10.1093/humrep/del484

17. Kok JD, Looman CW, Weima SM, te Velde ER. A high number of oocytes obtained after ovarian hyperstimulation for *in vitro* fertilization or intracytoplasmic sperm injection is not associated with decreased pregnancy outcome. *Fertil Steril.* (2006) 85:918–24. doi: 10.1016/j.fertnstert.2005.09.035

18. van Tilborg TC, Oudshoorn SC, Eijkemans MJC, Mochtar MH, van Golde RJT, Hoek A, et al. Individualized FSH dosing based on ovarian reserve testing in women starting IVF/ICSI: a multicentre trial and cost-effectiveness analysis. *Hum Reprod.* (2017) 32:2485–95. doi: 10.1093/humrep/dex321

19. Conti M, Franciosi F. Acquisition of oocyte competence to develop as an embryo: integrated nuclear and cytoplasmic events. *Hum Reprod Update.* (2018) 24:245–66. doi: 10.1093/humupd/dmx040

20. Richani D, Gilchrist RB. The epidermal growth factor network: role in oocyte growth, maturation and developmental competence. *Hum Reprod Update.* (2018) 24:1–14. doi: 10.1093/humupd/dmx029

21. Sterrenburg MD, Veltman-Verhulst SM, Eijkemans MJ, Hughes EG, Macklon NS, Broekmans FJ, et al. Clinical outcomes in relation to the daily dose of recombinant follicle-stimulating hormone for ovarian stimulation in *in vitro* fertilization in presumed normal responders younger than 39 years: a meta-analysis. *Hum Reprod Update.* (2011) 17:184–96. doi: 10.1093/humupd/dmq041

22. van der Meer M, Hompes PG, Scheele F, Schoute E, Veersema S, Schoemaker J. Follicle stimulating hormone (FSH) dynamics of low dose step-up ovulation induction with FSH in patients with polycystic ovary syndrome. *Hum Reprod.* (1994) 9:1612–7. doi: 10.1093/oxfordjournals.humrep.a138761

23. Nyboe Andersen A, Nelson SM, Fauser BC, García-Velasco JA, Klein BM, Arce JC, et al. Individualized versus conventional ovarian stimulation for *in vitro* fertilization: a multicenter, randomized, controlled, assessor-blinded, phase three noninferiority trial. *Fertil Steril.* (2017) 107:396.e4. doi: 10.1016/j.fertnstert.2016.10.033

24. van Tilborg TC, Torrance HL, Oudshoorn SC, Eijkemans MJC, Koks CAM, Verhoeve HR, et al. Individualized versus standard FSH dosing in women starting IVF/ICSI: an RCT. part 1: the predicted poor responder. *Hum Reprod.* (2017) 32:2496–505. doi: 10.1093/humrep/dex318

25. Broer SL, Dólleman M, Opmeer BC, Fauser BC, Mol BW, Broekmans FJ. AMH and AFC as predictors of excessive response in controlled ovarian hyperstimulation: a meta-analysis. *Hum Reprod Update.* (2011) 17:46–54. doi: 10.1093/humupd/dmq034

26. Hamdine O, Eijkemans MJ, Lentjes EW, Torrance HL, Macklon NS, Fauser BC, et al. Ovarian response prediction in GnRH antagonist treatment for IVF using anti-mullerian hormone. *Hum Reprod.* (2015) 30:170–8. doi: 10.1093/humrep/deu266

27. Broer SL, van Disseldorp J, Broeze KA, Dolleman M, Opmeer BC, Bossuyt P, et al. Added value of ovarian reserve testing on patient characteristics in the prediction of ovarian response and ongoing pregnancy: an individual patient data approach. *Hum Reprod Update.* (2013) 19:26–36. doi: 10.1093/humupd/dms041

28. Mochtar MH, Van der Veen, Ziech M, van Wely M. Recombinant luteinizing hormone (rLH) for controlled ovarian hyperstimulation in assisted reproductive cycles. *Cochrane Database Syst Rev.* (2007) 18:CD005070. doi: 10.1002/14651858.CD005070.pub2

29. van Wely M, Kwan I, Burt AL, Thomas J, Vail A, Van der Veen F, et al. Recombinant versus urinary gonadotrophin for ovarian stimulation in assisted reproductive technology cycles. *Cochrane Database Syst Rev.* (2011) 16:CD005354. doi: 10.1002/14651858.CD005354.pub2

30. Lahoud R, Ryan J, Illingworth P, Quinn F, Costello M. Recombinant LH supplementation in patients with a relative reduction in LH levels during IVF/ICSI cycles: a prospective randomized controlled trial. *Eur J Obstet Gynecol Reprod Biol.* (2017) 210:300–5. doi: 10.1016/j.ejogrb.2017.01.011

31. Humaidan P, Chin W, Rogoff D, D'Hooghe T, Longobardi S, Hubbard J, et al. Efficacy and safety of follitropin alfa/lutropin alfa in ART: a randomized controlled trial in poor ovarian responders. *Hum Reprod.* (2017) 32:544–55. doi: 10.1093/humrep/dex208

32. Griesinger G, Boostanfar R, Gordon K, Gates D, McCrary Sisk C, Stegmann BJ. Corifollitropin alfa versus recombinant follicle-stimulating hormone: an individual patient data meta-analysis. *Reprod Biomed Online.* (2016) 33:56–60. doi: 10.1016/j.rbmo.2016.04.005

33. Hamdine O, Eijkemans MJC, Lentjes EGW, Torrance HL, Macklon NS, Fauser BCJM, et al. Antimullerian hormone: prediction of cumulative live birth in gonadotropin-releasing hormone antagonist treatment for *in vitro* fertilization. *Fertil Steril.* (2015) 104:898.e2. doi: 10.1016/j.fertnstert.2015.06.030

34. Esteves SC, Roque M, Bedoschi GM, Conforti A, Humaidan P, Alviggi C. Defining low prognosis patients undergoing assisted reproductive technology: POSEIDON criteria-the why. *Front Endocrinol.* (2018) 9:461. doi: 10.3389/fendo.2018.00461

35. Alviggi C, Conforti A, Esteves SC, Vallone R, Venturella R, Staiano S, et al. Understanding ovarian hypo-response to exogenous gonadotropin in ovarian stimulation and its new proposed marker-the follicle-to-oocyte (FOI) index. *Front Endocrinol.* (2018) 9:589. doi: 10.3389/fendo.2018. 00589

36. Lensen SF, Wilkinson J, Leijdekkers JA, La Marca A, Mol BWJ, Marjoribanks J, et al. Individualised gonadotropin dose selection using markers of ovarian reserve for women undergoing *in vitro* fertilisation plus intracytoplasmic sperm injection (IVF/ICSI). *Cochrane Database Syst Rev.* (2018) 2:CD012693. doi: 10.1002/14651858.CD012693.pub2

37. Oudshoorn SC, van Tilborg TC, Eijkemans MJC, Oosterhuis GJE, Friederich J, van Hooff MHA, et al. Individualized versus standard FSH dosing in women starting IVF/ICSI: an RCT. part 2: the predicted hyper responder. *Hum Reprod.* (2017) 32:2506–14. doi: 10.1093/humrep/dex319

38. Out HJ, Braat DD, Lintsen BM, Gurgan T, Bukulmez O, Gokmen O, et al. Increasing the daily dose of recombinant follicle stimulating hormone (puregon) does not compensate for the age-related decline in retrievable oocytes after ovarian stimulation. *Hum Reprod.* (2000) 15:29–35. doi: 10.1093/humrep/15.1.29

39. Out HJ, Rutherford A, Fleming R, Tay CC, Trew G, Ledger W, et al. A randomized, double-blind, multicentre clinical trial comparing starting doses of 150 and 200 IU of recombinant FSH in women treated with the GnRH antagonist ganirelix for assisted reproduction. *Hum Reprod.* (2004) 19:90–5. doi: 10.1093/humrep/deh044

40. Out HJ, David I, Ron-El R, Friedler S, Shalev E, Geslevich J, et al. A randomized, double-blind clinical trial using fixed daily doses of 100 or 200 IU of recombinant FSH in ICSI cycles. *Hum Reprod.* (2001) 16:1104–9. doi: 10.1093/humrep/16.6.1104

41. Van Der Meer M, Hompes PG, De Boer JA, Schats R, Schoemaker J. Cohort size rather than follicle-stimulating hormone threshold level determines ovarian sensitivity in polycystic ovary syndrome. *J Clin Endocrinol Metab.* (1998) 83:423–6. doi: 10.1210/jc.83.2.423

42. Fischer D, Reisenbüchler C, Rösner S, Haussmann J, Wimberger P, Goeckenjan M. Avoiding OHSS: controlled ovarian low-dose stimulation

in women with PCOS. *Geburtshilfe Frauenheilkd.* (2016) 76:718–26. doi: 10.1055/s-0042-100206

43. Teede HJ, Misso ML, Costello MF, Dokras A, Laven J, Moran L, et al. Erratum. recommendations from the international evidence-based guideline for the assessment and management of polycystic ovary syndrome. *Hum Reprod.* (2018) 34:388. doi: 10.1093/humrep/dey363

44. Allegra A, Marino A, Volpes A, Coffaro F, Scaglione P, Gullo S, et al. A randomized controlled trial investigating the use of a predictive nomogram for the selection of the FSH starting dose in IVF/ICSI cycles. *Reprod Biomed Online.* (2017) 34:429–38. doi: 10.1016/j.rbmo.2017. 01.012

45. Olivennes F, Trew G, Borini A, Broekmans F, Arriagada P, Warne DW, et al. Randomized, controlled, open-label, non-inferiority study of the CONSORT algorithm for individualized dosing of follitropin alfa. *Reprod Biomed Online.* (2015) 30:248–57. doi: 10.1016/j.rbmo.2014.11.013

46. Popovic-Todorovic B, Loft A, Bredkjaeer HE, Bangsbøll S, Nielsen IK, Andersen AN. A prospective randomized clinical trial comparing an individual dose of recombinant FSH based on predictive factors versus a 'standard' dose of 150 IU/day in 'standard' patients undergoing IVF/ICSI treatment. *Hum Reprod.* (2003) 18:2275–82. doi: 10.1093/humrep/ deg472

47. Lan VT, Linh NK, Tuong HM, Wong PC, Howles CM. Anti-mullerian hormone versus antral follicle count for defining the starting dose of FSH. *Reprod Biomed Online.* (2013) 27:390–9. doi: 10.1016/j.rbmo.2013. 07.008

48. Aflatoonian A, Mansoori-Torshizi M, Farid Mojtahedi M, Aflatoonian B, Khalili MA, Amir-Arjmand MH, et al. Fresh versus frozen embryo transfer after gonadotropin-releasing hormone agonist trigger in gonadotropin-releasing hormone antagonist cycles among high responder women: a randomized, multi-center study. *Int J Reprod Biomed.* (2018) 16:9–18. doi: 10.29252/ijrm.16.1.9

49. Dosouto C, Haahr T, Humaidan P. Gonadotropin-releasing hormone agonist (GnRHa) trigger - state of the art. *Reprod Biol.* (2017) 17:1–8. doi: 10.1016/j.repbio.2017.01.004

50. Engmann L, Benadiva C, Humaidan P. GnRH agonist trigger for the induction of oocyte maturation in GnRH antagonist IVF cycles: a SWOT analysis. *Reprod Biomed Online.* (2016) 32:274–285. doi: 10.1016/j.rbmo.2015. 12.007

13

Pharmacogenetics of FSH Action in the Male

Maria Schubert[1], Lina Pérez Lanuza[2] and Jörg Gromoll[2]*

[1] Department of Clinical and Surgical Andrology, Centre of Reproductive Medicine and Andrology, University Hospital Münster, Münster, Germany, [2] Centre of Reproductive Medicine and Andrology, University Hospital Münster, Münster, Germany

*Correspondence:
Jörg Gromoll
Joerg.Gromoll@ukmuenster.de

Male infertility is a major contributor to couple infertility, however in most cases it remains "idiopathic" and putative treatment regimens are lacking. This leads to a scenario in which intra-cytoplasmic spermatozoa injection (ICSI) is widely used in idiopathic male infertility, though the treatment burden is high for the couple and it entails considerable costs and risks. Given the crucial role of the Follicle-stimulating hormone (FSH) for spermatogenesis, FSH has been used empirically to improve semen parameters, but the response to FSH varied strongly among treated infertile men. Single nucleotide polymorphisms (SNPs) within FSH ligand/receptor genes (*FSHB/FSHR*), significantly influencing reproductive parameters in men, represent promising candidates to serve as pharmacogenetic markers to improve prediction of response to FSH. Consequently, several FSH-based pharmacogenetic studies have been conducted within the last years with unfortunately wide divergence concerning selection criteria, treatment and primary endpoints. In this review we therefore outline the current knowledge on single nucleotide polymorphisms (SNPs) in the FSH and FSH receptor genes and their putative functional effects. We compile and critically assess the previously performed pharmacogenetic studies in the male and propose a putative strategy that might allow identifying patients who could benefit from FSH treatment.

Keywords: idiopathic male infertility, FSH, spermatogenesis, genetics, single nucleotide polymorphism (SNP), pharmacogenetic studies

BACKGROUND

Infertility concerns at least 15% of couples in western countries in their reproductive age and in 50% of all cases male factor infertility contributes essentially (1). Several factors such as genetic or oncological causes (e.g., testicular tumors) clearly contribute to impaired spermatogenesis; but a specific cause can only be attributed to 28% of unselected infertile men. This leaves around 72% of men with idiopathic/unexplained infertility or with minor causes, e.g., low grade varicocele, not sufficient to explain their underlying infertility (2) (**Figure 1**). Reduced spermatogenesis is also mirrored in a large fraction of about 60% of infertile men by increased Follicle-stimulating hormone (FSH) and decreased Inhibin levels due to a disturbed feedback loop within the hypothalamic-pituitary–testis axis. Men displaying this endocrine pattern also exhibit reduced testicular volume, decreased serum Testosterone and increased Luteinizing hormone (LH) levels as a general sign for a hypergonadotropic hypogonadism (2). In a small fraction of men, however, this feedback loop is differentially regulated and characterized by lowered testicular volume, reduced sperm count but subnormal to normal FSH levels for so far unknown reasons. This group of idiopathic infertile men could resemble a target group for which a FSH treatment could be beneficial (3). By increasing

FSH serum levels spermatogenesis could be stimulated further, a scenario not valid for the group of hypergonadotropic hypogonadal patients who already have elevated FSH serum levels.

Although the essential role of FSH for spermatogenesis has been recognized for decades (6) and several studies on FSH treatment for infertile men have been conducted, the overall outcome is disappointing. The only significant improvement which could be deduced from the different FSH studies is improved pregnancy rates (7, 8). However, clinical consequences cannot be drawn from these results. According to the recent EAA guidelines, FSH treatment can be offered in selected men [normogonadotropic with idiopathic oligo- or oligo-astheno-teratozoospermia (OAT)], however, with low evidence for success only (9). The Italian Society of Andrology and Sexual Medicine recently suggested in a consensus statement to use FSH to increase sperm concentration and motility in infertile normogonadotropic men with idiopathic oligozoospermia or OAT, with moderate evidence grading. The treatment with FSH is suggested in these men to improve both spontaneous pregnancy as well as pregnancy rates after ART (10). To which extent these recommendations can be adapted by other European countries remains to be seen.

Nowadays in clinical routine, if no causative factor for impaired infertility can be identified and treated, the agreed on procedure for men with idiopathic infertility is to undergo assisted reproduction (ART), which is mainly due to the fact that a clear treatment option cannot be offered or does just not exist. Recent data from the German *in vitro* fertilization (IVF) registry indicates that there is an increasing rate for not only the usage of ART but also for replacing IVF by intracytoplasmic sperm injection (ICSI) treatment (11). This strong tendency can also be observed worldwide, despite the fact that assisted reproduction techniques and treatment is putting the burden on the female side only. Besides the risks for women undergoing ART e.g., ovarian hyperstimulation syndrome, complications by oocyte retrieval and re-implantation, there is also clear evidence that progeny health might be affected by a treatment such as ICSI. In the current literature putative risks of ART for congenital malformations, epigenetic disorders, chromosomal abnormalities, subfertility, cancer and impaired cardio-metabolic profiles are discussed (12). These potential risks may be due to the fact that a routine ICSI procedure circumvents nearly all barriers naturally existing for fertilization such as sperm selection, competition etc.

Taken together, the clear tendency in reproductive medicine to neglect male infertility as a treatable condition and instead to routinely apply ART, demands novel strategies for curing male infertility. The currently most promising approach is to induce full spermatogenesis by FSH treatment. However, it is also clear that FSH treatment is not beneficial for all subfertile/infertile men, and that a personalized treatment regimen which takes into account clinical and genetic factors controlling spermatogenesis might resemble the most promising approach.

In this review we therefore outline the current knowledge on single nucleotide polymorphisms (SNPs) in the FSH beta

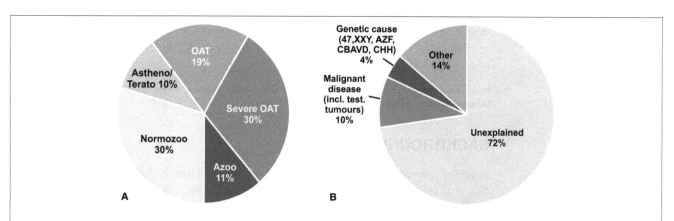

FIGURE 1 | (A) Descriptive diagnoses according to semen analyses of 26,091 men in infertile couples who attended the Center of Reproductive Medicine and Andrology (CeRA), Münster over the last 30 years. **(B)** Clinical diagnoses in the same men. Data from Androbase©, the clinical patient database. Adopted from Tüttelmann et al. (2).

BOX 1 | Pharmacogenetics

The general principle of a pharmacogenetics approach is to optimize drug efficacy, minimize toxic effects based on the inherited genetic variation in each individual. In general genetic variants such as single nucleotide polymorphisms (SNPs) with a frequent prevalence in the population are being used (Minor allele frequency >5%), otherwise the applicability for pharmacogenetic approaches will be limited to individual persons only. For further details on nomenclature of variants, [see (4)].

This personalized medical approach has the potential to identify the most appropriate patient for which a given treatment is really beneficial. Pitfalls of personalized approaches based on genetic information are to which extent variability may be attributed to biological factors (e.g., general health, age etc.) and environmental/behavioral factors (e.g., smoking) giving rise to responders and non-responders. Caution has to be given to the fact that the clinical outcome of a pharmacogenetic study might vary due to either genetically distinct populations or that a subset of unfavorable genetic variants might interfere with the variant being tested and thus bias the expected drug-gene/outcome interaction (5).

and FSH receptor genes, we compile and critically assess the previously performed pharmacogenetic studies in the male and propose a putative selection strategy that might allow identifying patients who could benefit from FSH treatment. Detailed information on pharmacogenetics are comprised in **Box 1**.

Follicle-Stimulating Hormone Action in Sertoli Cells

For qualitative and quantitative normal spermatogenesis an intact hypothalamic-pituitary-gonadal (HPG) axis is essential. Gonadotropin releasing hormone (GnRH) is released by the hypothalamus. In turn, GnRH stimulates the pituitary to secrete LH and FSH. LH stimulates production of testosterone in Leydig cells, which negatively feeds back to the pituitary as well as the hypothalamus in order to modulate the production of GnRH and by this gonadotropin levels (13). FSH synthesis and secretion depends on slow GnRH pulses (every 2–4 h), while rapid GnRH pulses (every 30 min) lead to preferential secretion of LH (14).

During the "mini puberty" (12–18 months of age) the HPG axis is activated for normal genital development, later on during development the HPG axis is again activated with the onset of puberty. During prenatal and prepubertal stage, FSH stimulates Sertoli cell proliferation and by this determines their final number and subsequently testicular size. The proliferation and functional maturation of Sertoli cells is controlled and terminated by thyroid-stimulating hormone (TSH) (15).

Sertoli cells (SCs) are part of the seminiferous tubules of the testes and play a key role in spermatogenesis. They are "nurse cells" as they provide nutritional support for germ cell development. Moreover, they contribute to the spermatogonial stem cell (SSC) niche and are this way indispensable for functional spermatogenesis (16). Sertoli cells and their metabolism are regulated by hormones (17). Some hormone receptors are solely expressed in Sertoli cells which underlines the importance of hormonal signaling for spermatogenesis (17). Thus, Sertoli cells transduce endocrine signals into the paracrine regulation of germ cells (16).

Busch et al. showed that boys with the genotype *FSHB* c.-211GT/TT and *FSHR* c.-29AA entered puberty later, which indicates that the overall endocrine network as well as FSH action might be affected in early phases by SNPs (18). In the adult stage, proliferation is ceased in mature Sertoli cell and FSH stimulates the proliferation of spermatogonia (19). In humans FSH mainly regulates sperm output of the seminiferous epithelium by controlling the expansion of premeiotic germ cells (20). FSH also influences the proliferation of type A spermatogonia upregulating nerve growth factor inducible gene B (NGFI-B, also known as Nur77) which increases the expression of glial cell line-derived neurotrophic factor (GDNF) in SCs (21). GDNF in turn supports the proliferation of germinal stem cells (GSCs) and other undifferentiated spermatogonia (22).

Follicle-Stimulating Hormone Signal Transduction

The FSH receptor (FSHR) belongs to the 7 transmembrane domains receptor (7TMR) family of G-protein coupled receptors and is only expressed in Sertoli cells (23). FSH binding induces

a conformational change of the FSHR especially within the TM domains 5 and 6 which cause intracellularly the dissociation of α- and βγ- subunits of G protein heterotrimer inside the cell. Subsequently, the α-subunit binds to and triggers adenylyl cyclase, which leads to an increase of cAMP levels (24). The main signal transduction pathway for the FSHR is the cAMP-PKA pathway. Its activation leads to a release of the catalytic subunit of protein kinase A (PKA); followed by phosphorylation of enzymes and proteins. Moreover, it targets the cAMP response element binding protein (CREB) which activates transcription of FSH-dependent genes (25). The MAP kinase cascade and extracellular-signal regulated kinase (ERK) get activated most likely via cAMP interactions with guanine nucleotide exchange factors (GEFs) and activation of Ras-like G proteins. By GEFs the phosphatidylinositol 3-kinase (PI3-K) pathway gets activated which leads to an activation of protein kinase B (PBK) (26). The PI3-K pathway plays an important role as it regulates several biological processes e.g., glucose uptake, oxidative burst and mitogenesis (17). Moreover, FSH causes an increase in intracellular calcium mediated by cAMP. Elevated calcium concentrations cause an activation of calmodulin and CaM kinases which result in downstream effects including the phosphorylation of CREB. FSH inducts phospholipase A2 (PLA2) and the release of arachidonic acid (AA) and the activation of eicosanoids (26). These different pathways activate different transcription factors thereby stimulating the transcription of FSH-targeted genes (27). Consequently, Sertoli cells transduce signals from FSH into production of necessary factors for germ cell nutrition and differentiation.

GENETICS OF FOLLICLE-STIMULATING HORMONE/FOLLICLE-STIMULATING HORMONE RECEPTOR

The Follicle-Stimulating Hormone Beta (FSHB) Subunit Gene

FSH is a pituitary derived heterodimeric glycoprotein which consists of an alpha-subunit and a unique beta-subunit that determines biological specificity and provides specificity for receptor binding (14). The human *FSHB* gene (National Center for Biotechnology Information (NCBI) database https://www.ncbi.nlm.nih.gov/gene/2488; GeneID:2488; Locus tag:HGNC:3964) is located on chromosome 11p13 and consist of 3 exons (**Figure 2A**) (30). It encodes the FSH beta-subunit consisting of an 18-amino acid (aa) signal peptide and the 111-aa mature protein (31). The NCBI SNP database (https://www.ncbi.nlm.nih.gov/SNP/) lists 1380 SNPs in the gene region of *FSHB*, 114 SNPs in coding regions. Only very few SNPs have proven clinical relevance. One of them, SNP rs10835638 (c.-211G>T) is located in the 5′untranslated region within an evolutionary conserved element of the *FSHB* promotor (**Table 1**; **Figure 2A**), which leads to an influence on gene transcription (33). This SNP impairs LHX3 binding and induction of *FSHB* transcription. Thus, the SNP rs10835638 reveals significant functional importance (33). The regulation of *FSHB* transcription in gonadotropic cells is essential as the amount of the beta-subunit being transcribed is the rate limiting step in FSHB synthesis and

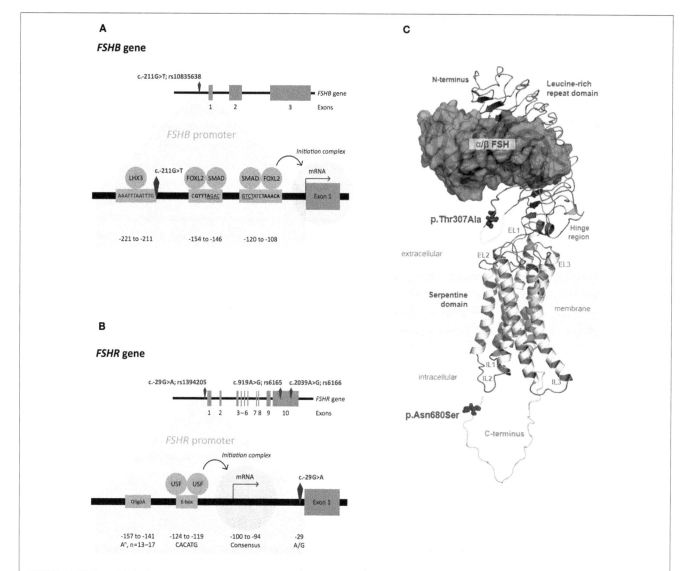

FIGURE 2 | FSHB and FSHR: Gene, promotor and protein structure. **(A)** Structure of the *FSHB* gene and promotor. The *FSHB* gene consists of three exons. The transcription factor LHX3 binds to the *FSHB* promotor as well as FOXL2 (binding sites are bold) and SMAD (binding sites are underlined) (28). The transcription start site is located on exon 1. The SNP rs10835638 (c.-211G>T) is located in the promotor region of the *FSHB* gene. **(B)** Structure of the *FSHR* gene and promotor. The gene consists of 10 exons. The transcription factors USF bind to the E-box and the transcription starts. The SNP rs1294205 is located in the promotor region (c.-29G>A) of the *FSHR* gene. The SNPs rs6165 (c.919A>G) and rs616 (c.2039A>G) are located in exon 10. **(C)** Protein structure of FSH and FSHR. A three-dimensional homology model of the FSH/FSHR complex is shown. The 7 TMD, constituted by transmembrane helices connected by intracellular (IL) and extracellular (EL) loops, was modeled based on the determined active structure-conformation of the β2-adrenergic receptor (29). The (monomeric) extracellular complex between the hinge region, the leucine-rich repeat domain, and FSH were taken as suggested by a structure determined for a fragment (24). The hinge region structurally links the leucine-rich repeat domain with the 7 TMD. The FSHR (backbone white-7 TMD, light blue-hinge, light gray leucine-rich repeat domain) binds the hormone [FSHβ (dark gray) and FSHα (blue), surface representation] at the extracellular side between the leucine-rich repeat domain and the hinge region. The exact orientation between the different components to each other is still unclear. The p.Thr307Al variant is located in the hinge region, where a derived structure is not known yet. The intracellular coiled loop (light green), where also not structural motifs are known yet, harbors the second amino acid variant p.Asn680Ser. The 3-D model of the FSH/FSHR-complex was kindly provided by Gunnar Kleinau (Charité Berlin, Germany).

defines how much mature hormone will eventually be secreted, as the alpha subunit is shared with LH, Thyroid-stimulating hormone (TSH) and human Chorionic Gonadotropin (hCG), and produced in excess. Hence, *FSHB* transcription is directly associated with its translation, secretion and serum levels (14).

The Follicle-Stimulating Hormone Receptor (FSHR) Gene

The 76 kDa FSH receptor (FSHR) is a G protein-coupled receptor, which belongs to the rhodopsin-like receptor subfamily, and consists of 695 amino acids (34). The *FSHR* gene (NCBI database https://www.ncbi.nlm.nih.gov/gene/2492;

TABLE 1 | Minor allele frequencies of the most relevant SNPs within the *FSHB* and *FSHR* genes. Taken from the 1000 Genomes project (32).

Gene	SNP ID	DNA nucleotide	Protein	Minor allele frequency (32)
FSHB	rs10835638	c.-211G>T	Promoter, non-coding	T = 0.0839
FSHR	rs1394205	c.-29G>A	Promoter, non-coding	T = 0.3450
FSHR	rs6165	c.919A>G	p.Thr307Ala	T = 0.4922
FSHR	rs6166	c.2039A>G	p.Asn680Ser	C = 0.4073

GeneID:2492; Locus tag:HGNC:3969) is located on chromosome 2 p21-p16 and consists of 10 exons of which the first nine exons encode the extracellular amino-terminal domain of the receptor (34, 35). Exon 10 encodes the transmembrane and intracellular portions of the protein (**Figure 2B**) (36). Two human isoforms are known, one containing all exons (NM_000145) and the second one lacking exon 6 (NM_181446) (13). The extracellular domain contains a stretch of leucine-rich repeats essential for FSH binding and is encoded by exon 2-9 (**Figure 2C**) (36). The NCBI SNP database (https://www.ncbi.nlm.nih.gov/SNP/) lists 51.677 SNPs in the gene region of *FSHR*, 779 SNPs are located in coding regions. The following SNPs: rs6166 (c.2039A > G, p.N680S) and rs6165 (c.919A > G, p.T307A) (**Table 1**), which are located in exon 10 have been analyzed more thoroughly and are in linkage disequilibrium (LD). The SNP c.919A>G results in an amino acid exchange removing a potential O-linked glycosylation site in the hinge region of the receptor, the SNP c.2039A>G also results in an amino acid exchange causing a potential phosphorylation site in the intracellular domain of the receptor (37, 38). Other known SNPs rs1394205 (c.-29G>A) and rs115357990 [c.-114T>C; MAF 0.0126 (1000 Genomes Project)] are located in the promoter region of the *FSHR* gene (39).

The Impact of *FSHB/FSHR* SNPs on Endocrine Function and Spermatogenesis

Interestingly, data on the putative impact of the several SNPs within the *FSHB* and *FSHR* genes have been mainly and firstly obtained from clinical studies and only later in part paralleled by experimental studies. There are only few *in vitro* studies available concerning the effect of *FSHB* and *FSHR* SNPs on FSH action in the male. This is mainly due to the fact that appropriate read-out systems for studying FSH function and corresponding SNPs functions do not exist. There are neither human gonadotropic nor Sertoli cell lines available. While it is generally believed that mouse gonadotropic cell lines such as the LßT2 cell line are useful and informative for the human as well, the situation for Sertoli cells is worse. The commercial available "Sertoli" cell lines are closer to peritubular cells than to Sertoli cells and therefore of only limited usefulness. Moreover, immortalized Sertoli cells tend to lose their intrinsic FSH receptor expression, making it difficult to study FSH action (40). Some groups have therefore stably transfected Sertoli cell lines with the FSH receptor to regain FSH sensitivity (41). The characteristic

feature of losing FSH receptor during immortalization of testicular somatic cells can also be observed for the female pendant of Sertoli cells, the granulosa cells. One of the reasons for the shut-down of FSH receptor expression might be aberrant methylation of regulatory elements controlling receptor expression (42).

Usage of primary cells as a substitute for lacking immortalized cell lines is at least for adult human Sertoli cells also not an option, since there is currently no protocol available which allows to isolate intact Sertoli cells in sufficient amounts. This is mainly due to the fact that the Sertoli germ cell niche is so tightly interlinked, that most cell separation protocols lead to the destruction of these cells. Thus, there is a great need for cell model systems which would allow studying the impact of SNPs and mutations in the male.

Nevertheless, in the mouse gonadotropic cell line (LßT2) it could be shown that the *FSHB* c.-211G>T polymorphism, located on the promoter region has an effect on the binding of the LHX3 homeodomain transcription factor, which leads to an impaired binding and this way to a 50% decrease in transcriptional promotor activity (33).

The SNP in the promotor region of *FSHR* c.-29G>A, currently used in a number of FSH studies, was analyzed in murine Sertoli cells SK11, but a significant effect could not be shown (39). Conflicting to this result, another group showed that the *FSHR* c.-29G>A decreases transcriptional promoter activity by 56% for the A allele *in vitro* in Chinese hamster ovary (CHO) cells (43). While these results await further confirmation by additional experiments, one should note that there are more SNPs allocated in the core promotor region of the *FSHR* gene such as a highly variable oligo-A stretch and a SNP at position at c.-114T>C. Therefore, a valid investigation on the impact of the c.-29G>A SNP should include the other polymorphic sites as well (39).

The impact of the SNPs in exon 10 in *FSHR* was analyzed *in vivo* showing that a decreased activity of the FSHR has a clinical implication for female infertility (44–46) and *in vitro* (38, 47): Nordhoff and colleagues analyzed the increase of cAMP and Estradiol after FSH stimulation between the variants NN and SS in human granulosa cells and could not show a difference in the mentioned parameters (47). Simoni and Casarini also used human granulosa-lutein cells (hGLC), but analyzed the kinetics of different signal transduction pathways. The p.Asn680Ser FSHR variant led to decreased ERK1/2 activation and the FSHR seemed to be less active (38). Again, no data on the impact of these SNPs on Sertoli cells are available. Hence, there are some *in vitro* studies demonstrating the effect of SNP in *FSHB/FSHR* granulosa cells/cell lines, but more *in vitro* studies targeting the molecular impact of the SNPs on FSH signaling using Sertoli cells are needed.

Clinical Impact of *FSHB/FSHR* SNPs on Spermatogenesis

The essential role of FSH for spermatogenesis is underlined by the identification and clinical characterization of inactivating *FSHB* mutations. Until now five men with such *FSHB* mutations have been described which all showed azoospermia and either very low or absence of FSH serum levels (31). Similar to this,

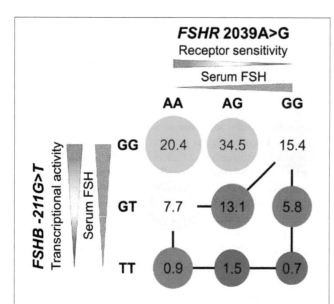

FSHR 2039A>G
Receptor sensitivity

FIGURE 3 | Impact of rs10835638 (*FSHB* c.-211G>T) and rs6166 (*FSHR* c.2039 A>G) on serum FSH, transcriptional activity of *FSHB* and receptor sensitivity of FSHR. Decreasing receptor sensitivity and transcriptional activity of *FSHB* lead to reduced testicular volume shown by circle diameter. The red color indicates unfavorable genotype, the green color a favorable genotype for reproductive fitness. The numbers show the percentage of carriers of combined genotypes in a German population group. The least favorable genotypes are marked with a black line. Men with TT/GG are predicted to show lowest testicular volume. Adopted from Tüttelmann et al. (56).

several mutations and variants of the *FSHR* have already been described in humans (48–50). The first description of a human inactivating *FSHR* mutation (p.Ala189 Val) showed elevated FSH levels and abnormal sperm parameters, but no azoospermia in affected men (51). An activating *FSHR* mutation (p.Asp567Gly) was discovered by Gromoll et al. describing a hypophysectomized man who fathered children being under Testosterone treatment only (52). So far, there have been 11 inactivating - and 7 activating mutations of the *FSHR* described in men and women (53).

Along the findings of completely abolishing FSH action by inactivating mutation, minor genetic changes such as SNPs affecting *FSHB* transcription, FSH binding properties or FSH receptor sensitivity could impact male fertility too. In the *FSHB* gene, the SNP c.-211G>T (rs10835638) has a major effect on serum FSH concentration in men (30). This effect as well as reduced testis size, reduced sperm concentration and lower serum Inhibin B and Testosterone was also shown in a cohort of Italian (54), Baltic (55), and German men (56).

Tüttelmann et al. analyzed the combined effect of a SNP in *FSHB* and *FSHR* on male reproductive parameters. They found a marked dominant effect of *FSHB* c.-211G>T in combination with *FSHR* c.2039A>G on serum FSH and testicular volume. The T allele carriers of the SNP c.-211G>T showed reduced FSH, increased LH, lower testicular volume, lower sperm count and concentrations in comparison to GG homozygotes men (**Figure 3**) (56). A recent study on the impact of *FSHB* c.-211G>T in Italian men from Tamburino et al. described decreased FSH,

LH, Testosterone, sperm count and testicular volumes in men with GT or TT in comparison to GG (57). Additionally, two population-based studies analyzed the effect of *FSHR* c.-29G>A in a Baltic and an Italian men cohort, respectively. Grigorova et al. showed an association between this SNP and FSH levels and Tamburino et al. showed that the *FSHR* c.-29G>A SNP is associated with higher FSH and LH in normozoospermic men. This effect could only be observed in normozoospermic men but not in men with alterations in conventional sperm parameters (58, 59).

The impact of the total phenotypic variance (SNP) was evaluated for the first time in a cohort of young Baltic men by Grigorova et al. (58). The *FSHB* –c.211G>T in combination with the *FSHR* c.-29G>A and the *FSHR* c.2039A>G explained 2,3% of serum FSH variance in young men as well as 1,4% serum Inhibin B, 1% Testosterone and 1,1% total testes volume. Additionally, in a cohort of infertile Estonian men the SNP combination affected 2,3% of serum FSH variance, 2,6% serum Inhibin B and 2% total testes volume (58). In a recent meta-analysis Wu et al. investigated the effect of four SNPs (*FSHB* c.-211G>T, *FSHR* c.-29G>A, *FSHR* c.919A>G, *FSHR* c.2039A>G) on male infertility. It seems that the combination of three SNP genotypes of *FSHR* (*FSHR* c.-29G, c.919A, c.2039A) results in protection against male sterility than either one alone (60).

CLINICAL IMPACT OF FSH IN INFERTILE MEN

Clinical Studies in Infertile Men Using FSH Current Status

In the past multiple clinical studies were carried out on idiopathic infertile men receiving FSH therapy to increase birth and pregnancy rates in the couple. However, results were conflicting. Therefore, a Cochrane Review and a recent meta-analysis were carried out to further elucidate these diverse results (7, 61).

Attia and colleagues analyzed 6 randomized controlled trials (RCTs) in which application of FSH was compared to placebo or no treatment at all. The main results comprise a significant increase in spontaneous pregnancy rate and in live birth rate in couples with FSH treatment in the male. The authors critically conclude that these results are promising, but since number of RCTs and participants is small and the evidence is low, no final clinical conclusions can be drawn (7).

In the most recent meta-analysis Santi et al. evaluated similar endpoints of FSH treatment outcome in idiopathic infertile men in 15 studies. The key finding of this analysis, supporting the prior Cochrane analysis, was the significant improvement in pregnancy rate in FSH-treated men (61). Additionally, an increased pregnancy rate was observed after ART when applying FSH. The pregnancies achieved were independent of FSH preparation and duration of therapy. Interestingly, in the sub-analysis considering the treatment response in terms of sperm parameters, a significant increase was only seen in sperm concentration, whereas other semen parameters did not change.

These are in principle promising results for FSH treatment of idiopathic infertile males, however the most susceptible parameters like FSH serum level or basal sperm count do not contribute to distinguish patients who will benefit from treatment from those who won't; predictive markers are therefore eagerly warranted (61) and a pharmacogenetic approach was suggested by several groups (3, 38).

State of the Art of Pharmacogenetic FSH Studies in Men

To our knowledge, there are currently only 4 studies (54, 62–64), that chose a FSH-based pharmacogenetic approach (**Table 2**). Our literature search was conducted in MEDLINE (PubMed), the Cochrane Library, Scopus and UpToDate. Search was last updated in October 2018.

Records for: FSH/male infertility ($n = 2245$); FSH/male infertility/gene ($n = 292$); *FSHB* gene/male infertility/SNP ($n = 23$); FSH/male infertility/pharmacogenetics ($n = 9$). The four pharmacogenetics studies identified via the literature search are being discussed in terms of study design, selection criteria, treatment, endpoints and results.

Study Design

The four studies have in common a prospective approach, and were, except for the study by Simoni et al, carried out in a monocenter setting. The number of subjects treated with FSH was between $n = 40$–70. Only one study had a 2:1 randomization to a cohort of patients who did not receive treatment and was followed-up (63); all other studies only included subjects that received FSH treatment. No placebo controls were included in any of these studies. Statistical power analyses considering the primary end-point variation was provided by only one study (64).

Selection Criteria

The general selection criteria for the four studies were quite homogenous; more heterogeneity was evident in terms of specific inclusion criteria (see below and **Table 2**). All studies included male patients with idiopathic infertility, excluding major factors affecting spermatogenesis such as karyotype anomalies, Y-chromosomal microdeletions and congenital bilateral aplasia of the vas deferens. (See respective studies for further inclusion and exclusion criteria). FSH was within the regular range (<8IU/l), this was also true for LH, Testosterone, Prolactin, Inhibin B and Estradiol. Heterogeneity exists among inclusion criteria for sperm parameters. This varied from patients with azoospermia or severe OAT, to patients with normozoospermia and "only" increased DNA fragmentation index (DFI). One group selected for hypospermatogenesis (reduced number of germ cells without maturation arrest, via fine needle aspiration) as inclusion criterion (see **Table 2** for details). With respect to the genetic composition the *FSHB* promoter region (c.-211G>T) or the *FSHR* (c.919A>G, c.2039A>G, c.-29G>A) or a combination was chosen. Interestingly, the pharmacogenetic approach in 3 of the 4 studies was performed on *FSHR* SNPs, for which the clinical impact in men is still under debate. In several studies it was shown previously that the impact of the FSHR p.N680S polymorphism only slightly influences reproductive parameters (65–67). Surprisingly, only two studies reported on the female

partners and comprised inclusion (regular ovulation and tubal function) and exclusion criteria (endometriosis, endocrine abnormalities (polycystic ovaries, anovulation, infections). Since female factors present a major factor for pregnancy rates, study results neglecting these parameters should be handled with caution.

FSH Treatment

Great heterogeneity exists among the FSH therapy concerning dosages and time of the application. In the respective studies treatment varied from 75 IU highly purified FSH (hpFSH) every other day to 150 IU recombinant FSH (rFSH) thrice weekly. The treatment period was 3 months in all studies, some accompanied by a follow-up (wash-out) period of further 3 months. In the most recent meta-analysis Santi et al. conclude that the positive effect of FSH (on spontaneous pregnancies and pregnancies after ART) was not dependent on the kind of FSH: hpFSH or rFSH (61). In the current EAA guidelines on the management of OAT treatment with "FSH can be suggested with low evidence in selected men with idiopathic oligozoospermia or OAT" (9). However, no further information on the dosages and the time of application is given.

Endpoints

The primary endpoints chosen were either sperm parameters like total sperm count (TSC), functional sperm tests like DFI or sperm-HBA (hyaluronic acid binding capacity). The latter being a biomarker for complete spermatogenesis, as suggested by the authors (62), since only mature spermatozoa, which have correctly completed spermiogenesis, express receptors for hyaluronic acid (68). DFI was chosen as endpoint, since it can be a predictor of the probability for conception. By using the TUNEL method, a distinction between viable cells (brighter DFI fraction) and dead cells (dimmer fraction of DFI) could be made (69, 70).

Considering the improvement of impaired fertility parameters in patients with idiopathic infertility by FSH as primary objective, one would rather see known and commonly accepted sperm parameters (i.e., TSC, motility) or pregnancy rate as directly linked parameters, rather than functional sperm tests. Especially tests such as DFI and HAB are interesting, but not reliable measures that are accepted as norms and/or standards in evaluation of fertility. These measures reveal further relevant information, but should therefore rather be considered as secondary endpoints. In the four studies the secondary endpoints were quite homogenous, reflecting hormonal parameters (i.e., FSH, LH, Testosterone), sperm parameters (TSC, sperm concentration, motility, morphology), clinical parameters (testicular volume) and pregnancy rate (**Table 2**).

Study Results

Selice et al. having the only study that included a control group (without treatment), showed significant increase in TSC, sperm concentration, motility and morphology in subjects with at least one serine in position 680, whereas patients homozygous for TN/TN showed no significant change in any semen parameters (**Table 2**) (63). However, the authors did not compare these

TABLE 2 | Overview of the current FSH-based pharmacogenetic studies.

Study	Study type	Study size	Female factor	SNP selection	Inclusion criteria	FSH	Prim. end-point	Pharmaco-genetic results
Selice et al. (63)	Prospective RCT Single center	70/35	/	FSHR p.T307A p.N680S (**AS/AS, TN/AS, TN/TN**)	FSH 1-8IU/l, sperm conc.: <20 × 10⁶/ml, testicular cytology: hypo-spermatogenesis	rFSH/ 150IU thrice weekly/ 3 months	TSC	**AS/AS**: ↑ **TN/AS**: ↑ **TN/TN**: −
Ferlin et al. (54)	Prospective Single center	67/0	no etiology for female infertility	*FSHB* c.-211G>T (**GG, GT, TT**)	FSH ≤8IU/l TSC <40 × 10⁶ Mill/ejac. (Azoospermia incl.)	rFSH/ 150IU thrice weekly/ 3 months	TSC	**GG, GT, TT**: ↑ (TT most impressive)
Simoni et al. (64)	Prospective multicenter, longitudinal, open-label, two-arms	55/0	no etiology for female infertility	FSHR p.N680S (**S/S, N/N**) *FSHB* c.-211G>T (**GG, GT/TT**)	FSH <8IU/l DFI >15% (Oligo-Normo-zoospermia)	rFSH/ 150IU every 2nd day/ 3 months	DFI	FSHR p.N680S **N/N**: ↓ FSHR p.N680S **N/N** and *FSHB* c.-211G>T **GG**: ↓
Casamonti et al. (62)	Prospective, single center	40/0	/	*FSHB* c.-211G>T (**GG, GT/TT**), FSHR p.N680S (**S/S, S/N** and **N/N**) c.-29G>A (**GG, GA/AA**)	FSH <8IU/l Oligo-or Astheno- or Terato-zoospermia, or OAT	hpFSH/ 75IU every 2nd day/3 months	sperm HBA	*FSHB* c.-211 **GG, GT/TT**: ↑ FSHR p.N680S **S/S, S/N** and **N/N**: ↑ *FSHR* c.-29G>A **GG, GA/AA**: ↑

First author of the study and respective study type is listed. The study size comprises total number of treated subjects/and total number of controls. If no female factor was described, this is indicated by a slash. The SNPs are given according to their nomenclature; the bold print indicates the respective alleles coding SNPs are indicated by their corresponding amino acids. Inclusion criteria are listing specific criteria only, for more general inclusion and exclusion criteria we refer to the original manuscripts. FSH treatment is pictured by type of FSH/dosage/ and duration of treatment. Only primary endpoints are listed, and the significantly obtained pharmacogenetic results refer to this parameter. The arrows indicate an increase or decrease of the primary endpoint parameter. For further results on secondary endpoints and insignificant results see respective studies.
RCT, randomized controlled trial; TSC, total sperm count; rFSH, recombinant FSH; hpFSH, highly purified FSH; DFI, DNA fragmentation index; sperm HBA, sperm hyaluronan binding assay.

parameters between the treated—and the untreated group. The only reference to the untreated group was to show that in these subjects the parameters did not change significantly upon follow-up. Evaluating polymorphisms in the *FSHR* as putative predictive factors for response to FSH treatment, a comparison between treatment and no treatment would have revealed additional valuable information.

The group around Casamonti et al. chose the sperm-HBA binding capacity, as biomarker for fully completed spermatogenesis, as primary endpoint. As secondary objective they stratified the patients according to the SNPs in *FSHB* c.-211G<T and *FSHR* c.2039A>G and c.-29G>A in order to find predictive markers for HBA responsiveness. Over all groups (irrespective of SNP) an increase of HBA-binding capacity was observed after short-term and 3 months of treatment, this increase was also evident in secondary parameters like TSC and total motile sperm count (TMSC) (62). Substratifications of the groups for sperm parameters, baseline-HBA, clinical parameters, pharmacogenetic parameters were carried out to identify predictive factors, which contribute to responsiveness of increased HBA (see Casamonti et al. for detailed results). In terms of the stratified SNP-groups, there was no clear-cut effect of the genotype of the SNP in predicting response to treatment, neither with regard to classical semen parameters, nor to HA binding capacity. However, the patient number of the study was probably too low to make such comparisons, since

the study was statistically not powered for a pharmacogenetic approach. Additionally, the impact of sperm-HBA capacity needs to be discussed further in terms of clinical relevance for male infertility.

The pharmacogenetic approach by Ferlin was a subanalysis (n = 67) of a large population based study (n = 762) on the association of *FSHB* with FSH serum levels and sperm parameters. The 67 subjects, who were treated with FSH, showed a significant increase in sperm count, FSH and Inhibin B. T allele carriers additionally showed a significant increase in sperm concentration and total motile sperm count. The most impressive increase in sperm parameters was evident in the patients homozygous for T (compared to G allele carriers). Also the response rate in terms of doubling of sperm count was highest in the TT-group compared to GT and the wildtype GG carriers (p = 0.001). The authors point out the more severe increase in sperm count and quality in TT carriers compared to the increase seen in a general population of oligozoospermic men treated with FSH (54).

In the study by Simoni et al. the prime pharmacogenetic selection criterion was the *FSHR* p.N680S, whereby one group contained subjects homogenous for N and the other comprised homogenous S genotypes. Another inclusion criterion was a DFI>15% (**Table 2**). Total DFI decreased significantly in the homozygous N group after 3 months of treatment and in the consecutive follow-up visit after another 3 months

(57.92−43.68%, $p = 0.004$) (64). These results are in contrast to the study by Selice et al. who found the homozygous S genotype of the FSHR to be the one benefiting more from FSH treatment by improving sperm concentration and total sperm number. Simoni et al. declare study-design and inter-laboratory variability in results of semen analyses as possible reasons for these divergent results (64).

Eventually *FSHB* c.-211G>T was also evaluated in this study; comparing the brighter DFI amongst the three different genotypes for *FSHB* –c.211G>T (GG/GT/TT) there was no significant difference amongst the groups. When *FSHR* and *FSHB* genotypes were combined, a significant improvement in sperm total—and brighter DFI was observed for the homozygous *FSHR* p.N680S N and homozygous *FSHB* G genotypes ($p = 0.025$) (64). This is in contrast to the study by Ferlin and colleagues, who found the homozygous wildtype of the *FSHB* c.-211G>T to respond the least on FSH treatment. Simoni argues with the "traffic light" model by Tüttelmann et al., where the combination *FSHR* c.2039A>G AA or AG and *FSHB* c.-211G>T GG are the carriers with the best combination for FSH action (**Figure 3**) (56, 64).

Pregnancy rates were reported in the studies by Simoni and by Selice. In the latter the rate was compared amongst couples with treated males vs. males without FSH therapy, but the differences (14.8% vs. 4.6%) were not significant (63) and female factors have not been considered. In the study by Simoni, twelve pregnancies were reported during the trial, 6 in each group, both after natural conception or ART (64).

Interestingly, in all studies there were no comparisons on primary endpoints between the study arms. The statistical analyses rather focused on longitudinal effects from baseline to the end of therapy within one distinct SNP-group, rather than comparing it to the results of another SNP-group. Therefore, the predictive value of SNPs in FSHR or FSHB or the combinations thereof on putative beneficial effects of FSH on spermatogenesis are almost impossible to conclude.

Taken together, at present several pharmacogenomics studies addressed the effect of FSH treatment on spermatogenesis in idiopathic infertile men. However, due to the fact that selection criteria, treatment phase, and endpoint definitions are varying, no reliable conclusions and consequences can be drawn in terms of clinical application.

CONSIDERATIONS FOR FUTURE FSH-BASED PHARMACOGENETIC STUDIES IN INFERTILE MEN

As of today the need for treatment options for infertile men are clearly documented, warranted and should be brought to the public, the reproductive societies and the centers which daily face these patients. Besides these recipients it is also of crucial importance to convince the pharmaceutical industry that curing male infertility is a worthwhile investment. The financial support by them is a backbone to conduct proper clinical trials, but at the same time a limiting step, since study designs do not always follow the most appropriate approach, but are influenced by economic views which clearly affect the solidity of studies.

Taken into account the increasing knowledge of the importance of FSH for qualitative and quantitative normal spermatogenesis, principles of FSH-based pharmacogenetic studies emerge, which we strive to outline in the following chapter.

At the experimental side definitely more studies on the already known SNPs affecting FSH action are needed. For example it now becomes clear that some of these SNPs are displaying gender specific differences. In the case of the c.-211G>T *FSHB* SNP the genotype (GT/TT) leads to a decrease of FSH serum levels in men, presumably by affecting the transcriptional activity. In women this SNP induces an upregulation of FSH serum levels (71, 72). Keeping in mind that the majority of functional studies is being conducted in female cells or unrelated cell lines such as HEK-293 cells, it becomes very clear that human Sertoli cell systems or suitable cell lines are strongly needed.

At the genetic level it is to be assumed that the current work on SNPs from the *FSHB* and *FSHR* gene reflect only the tip of the iceberg and that there might be more upstream or downstream SNPs modulating FSH action. For example SNPs in transcription factors (e.g., SMAD, LHX3) might affect transcriptional regulation of *FSHB* or more downstream located SNPs in GDNF, or CXCL12 which impact FSHR signaling and thereby have an impact on spermatogenesis. Thus, it is crucial to decipher the FSH signaling network on spermatogenesis and to identify SNPs affecting this network. Using the potential of Genome Wide Association Studies (GWAS) this might provide novel insights into biological pathways, the discovery of novel target genes and the identification of SNPs influencing the FSH signaling network (73). It is to be envisaged that in the future a pharmacogenetic approach for identifying infertile men with a distinct set of unfavorable SNPs, will pinpoint individual patients eligible for FSH treatment and hence decrease the number of so far unexplained infertile males (idiopathic). However, the current outline of the studies is heterogeneous and shows a variety of study designs, treatments and endpoints as depicted in **Figure 4**. We therefore have made the attempt to propose an outline for FSH-based pharmacogenetic studies (**Figure 4**).

We suggest the study design to be prospective, randomized and placebo-controlled. Longitudinal evaluations within one SNP-group could reveal important information, but statistical analyses amongst the two study arms (FSH treatment vs. Placebo) are necessary, informative and can help to rule out individual variances.

For the selection of patients we suggest that two major criteria should be applied: the male and the female factor. If one wants to evaluate pregnancy rates after FSH treatment in the male, the female parameters are necessarily to be considered and mentioned. Concerning the male inclusion criteria we believe that rather commonly used sperm parameters like sperm count should be applied than functional sperm tests that reveal important additional information but are not part of a routinely used infertility workup. In terms of the pharmacogenetic selection of SNPs we strongly suggest to complement this by experimental studies (see above). By this translational approach the patient selection will be more precise, and the response to treatment putatively increased. There is no gold standard for the FSH treatment period and dosage, but a treatment for 6 months

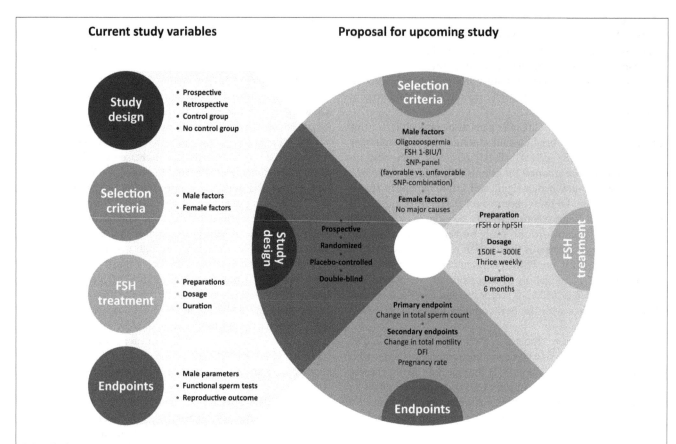

FIGURE 4 | Current study outline and proposal for upcoming study outline. The current study outlines for pharmacogenetic studies are very heterogeneous and vary in many components. With the proposal for upcoming study outline we suggest to focus on the selected parameters to generate a substantial clinical study. The colored circles indicate the major critical components of a clinical study. The circles are complemented by the respective subgroups that contribute to this parameter. In the selected parameters for proposing upcoming study outlines, the colors of the artificial pie-chart correspond to the respective parameters like study design, selection criteria, FSH treatment, and endpoints on the left side.

due to the spermatogenic cycle length of 74d, is most reasonable. From studies on patients with congenital hypogonadotropic hypogonadism we know that doses of 150 IU thrice weekly showed best treatment results, however these patients have another etiology of their impaired fertility and were treated with hCG as well (74). In a prospective, placebo-controlled clinical study in idiopathic infertile Chinese men, a FSH dose of 300 IU on alternate days for 5 months turned out to be successful (75). We therefore suggest that either dose can be applied. One of the major parameters for a successful study is the careful determination of endpoints. As suggested by the committee of the International Conference on Harmonization (ICH), on statistical principles the selection of the primary variable should reflect the accepted norms and standards in the relevant field of research (76). We therefore recommend taking the change in total sperm count as primary endpoint. Secondary endpoints may then be accomplished by further sperm parameters, functional sperm tests and pregnancy rate (after careful selection of female partners) (**Figure 4**).

Future trials could change the diagnostic and therapeutic work-up in patients with idiopathic infertility tremendously. Assessment of FSH polymorphisms and consecutive diagnose will be part of consulting and consequently will lead to FSH

treatment options for a selected group of men. A significant increase of total sperm counts by FSH treatment could improve pregnancy rates, preferentially spontaneously conceived and thereby reduce the risks for the offspring caused by ART treatment.

AUTHOR CONTRIBUTIONS

MS, LP, and JG equally compiled the available literature, designed, and wrote the manuscript, and outlined the graphics.

FUNDING

This work is supported by grants from German Research Foundation for the CRU 326 Male Germ Cells and therein GR 1547/24-1 and GR1547/25-1.

ACKNOWLEDGMENTS

The authors would like to thank all members of the Centre of Reproductive Medicine and Andrology who contributed and supported the FSH work over the last years. The graphical work was done by Kristina Selcho.

REFERENCES

1. Jungwirth A, Diemer T, Dohle GR, Giwercman A, Kopa Z, Krausz C, et al. Guidelines on male infertility. In: *European Association of Urology* (2015). p. 1–42. Available online at: https://uroweb.org/wp-content/uploads/17-Male-Infertility_LR1.pdf

2. Tüttelmann F, Ruckert C, Röpke A. Disorders of spermatogenesis: perspectives for novel genetic diagnostics after 20 years of unchanged routine. *Med Genet.* (2018) 30:12–20. doi: 10.1007/s11825-018-0181-7

3. Busch AS, Kliesch S, Tüttelmann F, Gromoll J. FSHB−211G>T stratification for follicle-stimulating hormone treatment of male infertility patients: making the case for a pharmacogenetic approach in genetic functional secondary hypogonadism. *Andrology.* (2015) 3:1050–3. doi: 10.1111/andr.12094

4. Dunnen JT, Dalgleish R, Maglott DR, Hart RK, Greenblatt MS, McGowan-Jordan J, et al. HGVS Recommendations for the description of sequence variants: 2016 update. *Hum Mutat.* (2016) 37:564–9. doi: 10.1002/humu.22981

5. Ross S, Anand SS, Joseph P, Paré G. Promises and challenges of pharmacogenetics: an overview of study design, methodological and statistical issues. *JRSM Cardiovasc Dis.* (2012) 1:1–13. doi: 10.1258/cvd.2012.012001

6. Huhtaniemi I. Hormonal regulation of spermatogenesis: mutant mice challenging old paradigms. *Eur J Endocrinol.* (2018) 179:R143–50. doi: 10.1530/EJE-18-0396

7. Attia AM, Abou-Setta AM, Al-Inany HG. Gonadotrophins for idiopathic male factor subfertility. *Cochrane Database Syst Rev.* (2013) 2013:CD005071. doi: 10.1002/14651858.CD005071.pub4

8. Santi D, Potì F, Simoni M, Casarini L. Pharmacogenetics of G-protein-coupled receptors variants: FSH receptor and infertility treatment. *Best Pract Res Clin Endocrinol Metab.* (2018) 32:189–200. doi: 10.1016/j.beem.2018.01.001

9. Colpi GM, Francavilla S, Haidl G, Link K, Behre HM, Goulis DG, et al. European academy of andrology guideline management of oligo-astheno-teratozoospermia. *Andrology.* (2018) 6:513–24. doi: 10.1111/andr.12502

10. Barbonetti A, Calogero AE, Balercia G, Garolla A, Krausz C, La Vignera S, et al. The use of follicle stimulating hormone (FSH) for the treatment of the infertile man: position statement from the Italian Society of Andrology and Sexual Medicine (SIAMS). *J Endocrinol Invest.* (2018) 41:1107–22. doi: 10.1007/s40618-018-0843-y

11. Blumenauer V, Czeromin U, Fiedler K, Gnoth C, Happel L, Krüssel JS, et al. D.I.R. Annual 2014 - The German IVF-Registry. *J Reproduktionsmed Endokrinol.* (2015) 12:509–45.

12. Esteves SC, Roque M, Bedoschi G, Haahr T, Humaidan P. Intracytoplasmic sperm injection for male infertility and consequences for offspring. *Nat Rev Urol.* (2018) 15:535–62. doi: 10.1038/s41585-018-0051-8

13. Siegel ET, Kim HG, Nishimoto HK, Layman LC. The molecular basis of impaired follicle-stimulating hormone action: evidence from human mutations and mouse models. *Reprod Sci.* (2013) 20:211–33. doi: 10.1177/1933719112461184

14. Bernard DJ, Fortin J, Wang Y, Lamba P. Mechanisms of FSH synthesis: what we know, what we don't, and why you should care. *Fertil Steril.* (2010) 93:2465–85. doi: 10.1016/j.fertnstert.2010.03.034

15. Tarulli GA, Stanton PG, Loveland KL, Rajpert-De Meyts E, McLachlan RI, Meachem SJ. A survey of Sertoli cell differentiation in men after gonadotropin suppression and in testicular cancer. *Spermatogenesis.* (2013) 3:e24014–e24014. doi: 10.4161/spmg.24014

16. França LR, Hess RA, Dufour JM, Hofmann MC, Griswold MD. The Sertoli cell: one hundred fifty years of beauty and plasticity. *Andrology.* (2016) 4:189–212. doi: 10.1111/andr.12165

17. Alves MG, Rato L, Carvalho RA, Moreira PI, Socorro S, Oliveira PF. Hormonal control of Sertoli cell metabolism regulates spermatogenesis. *Cell Mol Life Sci.* (2013) 70:777–93. doi: 10.1007/s00018-012-1079-1

18. Busch AS, Hagen CP, Main KM, Pereira A, Corvalan C, Almstrup K, et al. Genetic variation of follicle-stimulating hormone action is associated with age at testicular growth in boys. *J Clin Endocrinol Metab.* (2017) 102:1740–9. doi: 10.1210/jc.2016-4013

19. Shiraishi K, Matsuyama H. Gonadotoropin actions on spermatogenesis and hormonal therapies for spermatogenic disorders. *Endocr J.* (2017) 64:123–31. doi: 10.1507/endocrj.EJ17-0001

20. Schlatt S, Ehmcke J. Regulation of spermatogenesis: an evolutionary biologist's perspective. *Semin Cell Dev Biol.* (2014) 29:2–16. doi: 10.1016/j.semcdb.2014.03.007

21. Ding LJ, Yan GJ, Ge QY, Yu F, Zhao X, Diao ZY, et al. FSH acts on the proliferation of type a spermatogonia via Nur77 that increases GDNF expression in the Sertoli cells. *FEBS Lett.* (2011) 585:2437–44. doi: 10.1016/j.febslet.2011.06.013

22. Tadokoro Y, Yomogida K, Ohta H, Tohda A, Nishimune Y. Homeostatic regulation of germinal stem cell proliferation by the GDNF/FSH pathway. *Mech Dev.* (2002) 113:29–39. doi: 10.1016/S0925-4773(02)00004-7

23. Gloaguen P, Crépieux P, Heitzler D, Poupon A, Reiter E. Mapping the follicle-stimulating hormone-induced signaling networks. *Front Endocrinol.* (2011) 2:45. doi: 10.3389/fendo.2011.00045

24. Jiang X, Liu H, Chen X, Chen P-H, Fischer D, Sriraman V, et al. Structure of follicle-stimulating hormone in complex with the entire ectodomain of its receptor. *Proc Natl Acad Sci USA.* (2012) 109:12491–6. doi: 10.1073/pnas.1206643109

25. Huhtaniemi I, Toppari J. FSH Regulation at the molecular and cellular levels: mechanisms of action and functional effects. *Sertoli Cell Biol.* (2005) 155–69. doi: 10.1016/B978-012647751-1/50011-8

26. Walker WH, Cheng J. FSH and testosterone signaling in sertoli cells. *Reproduction.* (2005) 130:15–28. doi: 10.1530/rep.1.00358

27. Zimmermann C, Stévant I, Borel C, Conne B, Pitetti J-L, Calvel P, et al. Research resource: the dynamic transcriptional profile of sertoli cells during the progression of spermatogenesis. *Mol Endocrinol.* (2015) 29:627–42. doi: 10.1210/me.2014-1356

28. Thackray VG. Fox tales: regulation of gonadotropin gene expression by forkhead transcription factors. *Mol Cell Endocrinol.* (2014) 385:62–70. doi: 10.1016/j.mce.2013.09.034

29. Rasmussen SGF, DeVree BT, Zou Y, Kruse AC, Chung KY, Kobilka TS, et al. Crystal structure of the β2 adrenergic receptor-Gs protein complex. *Nature.* (2011) 477:549–55. doi: 10.1038/nature10361

30. Laan M, Europe PMC Funders Group. Pharmacogenetics of FSH Action. *Curr Opin Endocrinol Diabetes Obes.* (2012) 19:220–227. doi: 10.1097/MED.0b013e3283534b11

31. Zheng J, Mao J, Cui M, Liu Z, Wang X, Xiong S, et al. Novel FSHβ mutation in a male patient with isolated FSH deficiency and infertility. *Eur J Med Genet.* (2017) 60:335–9. doi: 10.1016/j.ejmg.2017.04.004

32. Consortium T 1000 GP, Auton A, Abecasis GR, Altshuler DM, Durbin RM, Abecasis GR, et al. A global reference for human genetic variation. *Nature.* (2015) 526:68. doi: 10.1038/nature15393

33. Benson CA, Kurz TL, Thackray VG. A human FSHB promoter SNP associated with low FSH levels in men impairs LHX3 binding and basal FSHB transcription. *Endocrinology.* (2013) 154:3016–21. doi: 10.1210/en.2013-1294

34. Simoni M, Gromoll J, Nieschlag E. The follicle-stimulating hormone receptor: biochemistry, molecular biology, physiology and pathophysiology. *Endocr Rev.* (1997) 18:739–73.

35. Gromoll J, Simoni M. Genetic complexity of FSH receptor function. *Trends Endocrinol Metab.* (2005) 16:368–73. doi: 10.1016/j.tem.2005.05.011

36. George JW, Dille EA, Heckert LL. Current concepts of follicle-stimulating hormone receptor gene regulation1. *Biol Reprod.* (2011) 84:7–17. doi: 10.1095/biolreprod.110.085043

37. Simoni M, Gromoll J, Höppner W, Kamischke A, Krafft T, Stähle D, et al. Mutational analysis of the follicle-stimulating hormone (FSH) receptor in normal and infertile men: identification and characterization of two discrete FSH receptor isoforms1. *J Clin Endocrinol Metab.* (1999) 84:751–5. doi: 10.1210/jcem.84.2.5500

38. Simoni M, Casarini L. Mechanisms in endocrinology: geneticsof FSH action - A 2014-and-beyond view. *Eur J Endocrinol.* (2014) 170:91–107. doi: 10.1530/EJE-13-0624

39. Wunsch A, Ahda Y, Banaz-Yaşar F, Sonntag B, Nieschlag E, Simoni M, et al. Single-nucleotide polymorphisms in the promoter region influence the expression of the human follicle-stimulating hormone receptor. *Fertil Steril.* (2005) 84:446–53. doi: 10.1016/j.fertnstert.2005.02.031

40. Strothmann K, Simoni M, Mathur P, Siakhamary S, Nieschlag E, Gromoll J. Gene expression profiling of mouse sertoli cell lines. *Cell Tissue Res.* (2004) 315:249–57. doi: 10.1007/s00441-003-0834-x

41. Wang H, Wen L, Yuan Q, Sun M, Niu M, He Z. Establishment and applications of male germ cell and Sertoli cell lines. *Reproduction.* (2016) 152:R31–40. doi: 10.1530/REP-15-0546

42. Griswold MD, Kim J-S. Site-specific methylation of the promoter alters deoxyribonucleic acid-protein interactions and prevents follicle-stimulating hormone receptor gene transcription1. *Biol Reprod.* (2001) 64:602–10. doi: 10.1095/biolreprod64.2.602

43. Nakayama T, Kuroi N, Sano M, Tabara Y, Katsuya T, Ogihara T, et al. Mutation of the follicle-stimulating hormone receptor gene 5′-untranslated region associated with female hypertension. *Hypertension.* (2006) 48:512–8. doi: 10.1161/01.HYP.0000233877.84343.d7

44. Alviggi C, Conforti A, Santi D, Esteves SC, Andersen CY, Humaidan P, et al. Clinical relevance of genetic variants of gonadotrophins and their receptors in controlled ovarian stimulation: a systematic review and meta-analysis. *Hum Reprod Update.* (2018) 24:599–614. doi: 10.1093/humupd/dmy019

45. Alviggi C, Conforti A, Caprio F, Gizzo S, Noventa M, Strina I, et al. In estimated good prognosis patients could unexpected "Hyporesponse" to controlled ovarian stimulation be related to genetic polymorphisms of FSH receptor? *Reprod Sci.* (2016) 23:1103–8. doi: 10.1177/1933719116630419

46. Mayorga MP, Gromoll J, Behre HM, Gassner C, Nieschlag E, Simoni M. Ovarian response to follicle-stimulating hormone (FSH) stimulation depends on the FSH receptor genotype*. *J Clin Endocrinol Metab.* (2000) 85:3365–9. doi: 10.1210/jcem.85.9.6789

47. Nordhoff V, Sonntag B, von Tils D, Götte M, Schüring AN, Gromoll J, et al. Effects of the FSH receptor gene polymorphism p.N680S on cAMP and steroid production in cultured primary human granulosa cells. *Reprod Biomed Online.* (2011) 23:196–203. doi: 10.1016/j.rbmo.2011.04.009

48. Gromoll J, Bröcker M, Derwahl M, Höppner W. Detection of mutations in glycoprotein hormone receptors. *Methods.* (2000) 21:83–97 doi: 10.1006/meth.2000.0977

49. Simoni M, Nieschlag E, Gromoll J. Isoforms and single nucleotide polymorphism of the FSH receptor gene: Implications for human reproduction. *Hum Reprod Update.* (2002) 8:413–21. doi: 10.1093/humupd/8.5.413

50. Kuechler A, Hauffa BP, Köninger A, Kleinau G, Albrecht B, Horsthemke B, et al. An unbalanced translocation unmasks a recessive mutation in the follicle-stimulating hormone receptor (FSHR) gene and causes FSH resistance. *Eur J Hum Genet.* (2010) 18:656–61. doi: 10.1038/ejhg.2009.244

51. Aittomäki K, Dieguez Lucena J, Pakarinen P, Sistonen P, Tapanainen J, Gromoll J, et al. Mutation in the follicle-stimulating hormone receptor gene causes hereditary hypergonadotropic ovarian failure. *Cell.* (1995) 82:959–68 doi: 10.1016/0092-8674(95)90275-9

52. Gromoll J, Simoni M, Nieschlag E. An activating mutation of the follicle-stimulating hormone receptor autonomously sustains spermatogenesis in a hypophysectomized man. *J Clin Endocrinol Metab.* (1996) 81:1367–70. doi: 10.1210/jcem.81.4.8636335

53. Desai SS, Roy BS, Mahale SD. Mutations and polymorphisms in FSH receptor: functional implications in human reproduction. *Reproduction.* (2013) 146:R235–48. doi: 10.1530/REP-13-0351

54. Ferlin A, Vinanzi C, Selice R, Garolla A, Frigo AC, Foresta C. Toward a pharmacogenetic approach to male infertility: polymorphism of follicle-stimulating hormone beta-subunit promoter. *Fertil Steril.* (2011) 96:1344–1349.e2. doi: 10.1016/j.fertnstert.2011.09.034

55. Grigorova M, Punab M, Zilaitienė B, Erenpreiss J, Ausmees K, Matulevičius V, et al. Genetically determined dosage of follicle-stimulating hormone (FSH) affects male reproductive parameters. *J Clin Endocrinol Metab.* (2011) 96:E1534–41. doi: 10.1210/jc.2011-0632

56. Tüttelmann F, Laan M, Grigorova M, Punab M, Sõber S, Gromoll J. Combined effects of the variants FSHB −211G>T and FSHR 2039A>G on male reproductive parameters. *J Clin Endocrinol Metab.* (2012) 97:3639–47. doi: 10.1210/jc.2012-1761

57. Tamburino L, La Vignera S, Tomaselli V, Condorelli RA, Mongioì LM, Calogero AE. Impact of the FSHB gene−211G/T polymorphism on male gonadal function. *J Assist Reprod Genet.* (2017) 34:671–6. doi: 10.1007/s10815-017-0896-4

58. Grigorova M, Punab M, Punab AM, Poolamets O, Vihljajev V, Žilaitiene B, et al. Reproductive physiology in young men is cumulatively affected by FSH-action modulating genetic variants: FSHR−29G/A and c.2039 A/G, FSHB−211G/T. *PLoS ONE.* (2014) 9:e94244. doi: 10.1371/journal.pone.0094244

59. Tamburino L, La Vignera S, Tomaselli V, Condorelli RA, Cannarella R, Mongioì LM, et al. The −29G/A FSH receptor gene polymorphism is associated with higher FSH and LH levels in normozoospermic men. *J Assist Reprod Genet.* (2017) 34:1289–94. doi: 10.1007/s10815-017-0970-y

60. Wu Q, Zhang J, Zhu P, Jiang W, Liu S, Ni M, et al. The susceptibility of FSHB−211G > T and FSHR G-29A, 919A > G, 2039A > G polymorphisms to men infertility: An association study and meta-analysis. *BMC Med Genet.* (2017) 18:1–15. doi: 10.1186/s12881-017-0441-4

61. Santi D, Granata AR, Simoni M. Follicle-stimulating hormone treatment of male idiopathic infertility improves pregnancy rate: a meta-analysis. *Endocr Connect.* (2015) 4: R46–58. doi: 10.1530/EC-15-0050

62. Casamonti E, Vinci S, Serra E, Fino MG, Brilli S, Lotti F, et al. Short-term FSH treatment and sperm maturation: a prospective study in idiopathic infertile men. *Andrology.* (2017) 5:414–22. doi: 10.1111/andr.12333

63. Selice R, Garolla A, Pengo M, Caretta N, Ferlin A, Foresta C. The response to fsh treatment in oligozoospermic men depends on fsh receptor gene polymorphisms. *Int J Androl.* (2011) 34(4 Part 1):306–12. doi: 10.1111/j.1365-2605.2010.01086.x

64. Simoni M, Santi D, Negri L, Hoffmann I, Muratori M, Baldi E, et al. Treatment with human, recombinant FSH improves sperm DNA fragmentation in idiopathic infertile men depending on the FSH receptor polymorphism p.N680S: a pharmacogenetic study. *Hum Reprod.* (2016) 31:1960–9. doi: 10.1093/humrep/dew167

65. Grigorova M, Punab M, Poolamets O, Sõber S, Vihljajev V, Žilaitienė B, et al. Study in 1790 Baltic men: FSHR Asn680Ser polymorphism affects total testes volume. *Andrology.* (2013) 1:293–300. doi: 10.1111/j.2047-2927.2012.00028.x

66. Nieschlag E, Simoni M, Gromoll J, Weinbauer GF. Role of FSH in the regulation of spermatogenesis: Clinical aspects. *Clin Endocrinol.* (1999) 51:139–46. doi: 10.1046/j.1365-2265.1999.00846.x

67. Ahda Y, Gromoll J, Wunsch A, Asatiani K, Zitzmann M, Nieschlag E, et al. Follicle-stimulating hormone receptor gene haplotype distribution in normozoospermic and azoospermic men. *J Androl.* (2005) 26:494–9. doi: 10.2164/jandrol.04186

68. Huszar G, Ozenci CC, Cayli S, Zavaczki Z, Hansch E, Vigue L. Hyaluronic acid binding by human sperm indicates cellular maturity, viability, and unreacted acrosomal status. *Fertil Steril.* (2003) 79 (Suppl. 3):1616–24. doi: 10.1016/S0015-0282(03)00402-3

69. Muratori M, Marchiani S, Tamburrino L, Cambi M, Lotti F, Natali I, et al. DNA fragmentation in brighter sperm predicts male fertility independently from age and semen parameters. *Fertil Steril.* (2015) 582–90.e4. doi: 10.1016/j.fertnstert.2015.06.005

70. Muratori M, Tamburrino L, Marchiani S, Cambi M, Olivito B, Azzari C, et al. Investigation on the origin of sperm DNA fragmentation: role of apoptosis, immaturity and oxidative stress monica. *Mol Med.* (2015) 21:109–122. doi: 10.2119/molmed.2014.00158

71. Schüring AN, Busch AS, Bogdanova N, Gromoll J, Tüttelmann F. Effects of the FSH-β-subunit promoter polymorphism −211G→ T on the hypothalamic-pituitary-ovarian axis in normally cycling women indicate a gender-specific regulation of gonadotropin secretion. *J Clin Endocrinol Metab.* (2013) 98:E82–6. doi: 10.1210/jc.2012-2780

72. Rull K, Grigorova M, Ehrenberg A, Vaas P, Sekavin A, Nõmmemees D, et al. FSHB −211 G>T is a major genetic modulator of reproductive physiology and health in childbearing age women. *Hum Reprod.* (2018) 33:954–66. doi: 10.1093/humrep/dey057

73. Visscher PM, Wray NR, Zhang Q, Sklar P, McCarthy MI, Brown MA, et al. 10 Years of GWAS discovery: biology, function, and translation. *Am J Hum Genet.* (2017) 101:5–22. doi: 10.1016/j.ajhg.2017. 06.005

74. Rohayem J, Hauffa BP, Zacharin M, Kliesch S, Zitzmann M. Testicular growth and spermatogenesis: new goals for pubertal hormone replacement in boys with hypogonadotropic hypogonadism?—A multicentre prospective study of hCG / rFSH treatment outcomes during adolescence. *Clin Endocrinol.* (2017) 49:75–87. doi: 10.1111/cen. 13164

75. Ding Y, Zhang X, Li J, Chen S, Zhang R, Tan W. Treatment of idiopathic oligozoospermia with recombinant human follicle-stimulating hormone: a prospective ,randomized , double-blind , placebo-controlled clinical study in Chinese population. *Clin Endocrinol.* (2015) 83:866–71. doi: 10.1111/cen.12770

76. ICH. ICH Harmonised Tripartite Guideline. *Statistical Principles for Clinical Trials. International Conference on Harmonisation E9 Expert Working Group.* (1999).

14

Role of Follicle-Stimulating Hormone in Spermatogenesis

Olayiwola O. Oduwole[1], Hellevi Peltoketo[2] and Ilpo T. Huhtaniemi[1,3]*

[1] Department of Surgery and Cancer, Institute of Reproductive and Developmental Biology, Imperial College London, London, United Kingdom, [2] Cancer and Translational Medicine Research Unit, Laboratory of Cancer Genetics and Tumor Biology, Biocenter Oulu, University of Oulu, Oulu, Finland, [3] Department of Physiology, University of Turku, Turku, Finland

*Correspondence:
Ilpo T. Huhtaniemi
ilpo.huhtaniemi@imperial.ac.uk

Spermatogenesis is a concerted sequence of events during maturation of spermatogonia into spermatozoa. The process involves differential gene-expression and cell-cell interplay regulated by the key endocrine stimuli, i.e., follicle-stimulating hormone (FSH) and luteinizing hormone (LH)-stimulated testosterone. FSH affects independently and in concert with testosterone, the proliferation, maturation and function of the supporting Sertoli cells that produce regulatory signals and nutrients for the maintenance of developing germ cells. Rodents are able to complete spermatogenesis without FSH stimulus, but its deficiency significantly decreases sperm quantity. Men carrying loss-of-function mutation in the gene encoding the ligand (FSHB) or its receptor (FSHR) present, respectively, with azoospermia or suppressed spermatogenesis. Recently, the importance of high intratesticular testosterone concentration for spermatogenesis has been questioned. It was established that it can be completed at minimal intratesticular concentration of the hormone. Furthermore, we recently demonstrated that very robust constitutive FSHR action can rescue spermatogenesis and fertility of mice even when the testosterone stimulus is completely blocked. The clinical relevance of these findings concerns a new strategy of high-dose FSH in treatment of spermatogenic failure.

Keywords: spermatogenesis, spermatogenic failure, gonadotropins, FSH, testosterone, sertoli cells, fertility

INTRODUCTION

Reproduction is controlled by the hormones functional in the hypothalamic-pituitary-gonadal (HPG) axis. In the male they concern the maintenance of testicular testosterone (T) production and spermatogenesis by the two pituitary gonadotropins, luteinizing hormone (LH) and follicle-stimulating hormone (FSH). The testicular target cells of LH are the Leydig cells present in the interstitial space, and those of FSH are the Sertoli cells present in the seminiferous tubules. LH stimulates Leydig cell T production, and FSH stimulates in Sertoli cells, in synergy with T, the production of regulatory molecules and nutrients needed for the maintenance of spermatogenesis. Hence, both T and FSH regulate spermatogenesis indirectly through Sertoli cells.

Although the principles of the hormonal regulation of spermatogenesis have been established decades ago, the recently acquired genetic information, in particular from human mutations of gonadotropin and gonadotropin receptor genes, and from genetically modified mouse models, have advanced our knowledge about the molecular events involved in the regulation of spermatogenesis. In this article, we review this information and describe some of our own studies on genetically modified mice, that reveal some new aspects of these regulatory events. Some of this information challenges the basic principles of the hormonal regulation of spermatogenesis, sheds light on its pathogenetic mechanisms, and offers new leads into its treatment.

GENERAL PRINCIPLES OF REGULATION OF SPERMATOGENESIS

Spermatogenesis is a complex and orderly sequence of events, during which diploid spermatogonia proliferate and differentiate into haploid spermatozoa in testicular seminiferous tubules (1, 2). In seminiferous tubules, the somatic Sertoli cells extend from the base of the tubule to its lumen and form a niche for germ cell maturation supporting the process qualitatively and quantitatively (1, 3–5). Sertoli cells also send signals, including paracrine factors and nutrients, to the germ cells. Starting at puberty, spermatogenesis normally continues uninterrupted throughout the lifespan (with seasonal variation in some animals) but decreasing somewhat in quantity with aging.

The spermatogenic process occurs in a stepwise fashion, and is regulated by the interplay of different autocrine, paracrine, and endocrine hormonal stimuli. The cascade involves a series of cellular mechanisms, which includes mitotic multiplication and propagation, meiotic recombination of genetic materials, and morphological maturation of spermatozoa (6, 7). The development and maintenance of spermatogenesis is dependent on the pituitary gonadotropins; FSH, and LH. Both hormones are secreted and regulated as a part of the HPG axis in response to the hypothalamic gonadotropin-releasing hormone (GnRH). GnRH stimulates the gonadotrophs in the anterior pituitary to secrete the gonadotropins in a pulsatile fashion into the systemic circulation. FSH and LH levels in turn are regulated by the negative feedback actions of gonadal sex steroids and inhibin that collectively downregulate GnRH secretion and maintain homeostasis of the HPG axis (8, 9).

FSH and LH mediate their individual actions on spermatogenesis through their cognate receptors, FSHR and LHR (LHCGR in humans). Both receptors are plasma-membrane associated G-protein coupled receptors, FSHR expressed on Sertoli cells and LHR on Leydig cells (10–13), where the latter stimulates T production (14, 15). T is considered a prerequisite for sperm production and maturation, secondary sexual characteristics and functions, and anabolic actions. T activates the androgen receptor (AR) in Sertoli cells to initiate the functional responses required for spermatogenesis (16). FSH, on the other hand, is considered to act both independently and in concert with T to stimulate Sertoli cell proliferation and to

---

Abbreviations: AR, androgen receptor; AQP8, aquaporin; CAM, constitutively activating mutation; DRD4, dopamine receptor D4; EPPIN, epididymal peptidase inhibitor; FSH, follicle-stimulating hormone; FSHβ, follicle-stimulating hormone subunit beta; FSHR, follicle-stimulating hormone receptor; GATA1, gata binding protein 1; GJA1, gap junction protein alpha 1 (Connexin43); GnRH, gonadotropin releasing hormone; GoF, gain-of-function; hpg, hypogonadal; KLF4, krüppel-like factor 4; LH, luteinizing hormone; LHβ, luteinizing hormone subunit beta; LHR/LHCGR, luteinizing hormone/choriogonadotropin receptor; LoF, loss-of-function; RHOX5, reproductive homeobox 5; T, testosterone; TJP1, tight junction protein 1; WNT3, wnt family member 3; *Fshr*-CAM, constitutively active *Fshr*; *Fshr*-KO, *fshr* knockout; LuRKO, *lhcgr* knockout.

produce signaling molecules and nutrient to support spermatid maturation (11, 17).

FSH IS AN IMPORTANT REGULATOR OF SERTOLI CELL PROLIFERATION

Sertoli cells form both structurally and biochemically a supporting environment for the maturing germ cells. Their number is determined by FSH action, in rodents during fetal and neonatal life, and in primates at neonatal and peri-pubertal age (5). In both rodents and primates, *FSHR* expression starts during the second half of gestation (18, 19), though the lack of ligand (FSH) and cAMP responsiveness imply that the receptor is initially functionally inactive (20). However, after the onset of fetal pituitary FSH production and activation of the receptor, the hormone plays a major role in Sertoli cell proliferation (21). During peri-puberty, the rising FSH concentration triggers the second phase of Sertoli cell proliferation (5, 21), and the concentration of circulating FSH correlates strongly with Sertoli cell number and testis size in adulthood (22, 23). In the absence of FSH or FSHR, the Sertoli cell number is considerably decreased, by 30–45%, in comparison to normal testicular development [**Table 1**,(5, 24, 32)]. This is of high importance, as the Sertoli cells number determines the quantity of sperm produced; a Sertoli cell is able to support a certain maximum number of germ cells (3, 5, 24, 26, 33, 34).

FSH SUPPORTS SPERMATOGENESIS QUANTITATIVELY IN RODENTS

Classical studies on animal models indicate that Sertoli cells proliferate until a finite number and differentiate toward puberty. Prepuberty, together with increasing FSH secretion, *FSHR* expression begins to fluctuate along with the stage of spermatogenesis. This is associated with maturation of the Sertoli cell population and completion of the first cycle of sperm maturation (35). In the postpubertal testis, FSH together with T evokes in Sertoli cells signals to propagate germ cell maturation (5), to provide antiapoptotic survival factors and to regulate adhesion complexes between germ cells and Sertoli cells (36).

The lack of FSH (25) or FSHR (37, 38) in mice does not lead to sterility, albeit it decreased testis size (**Figure 1**), reflecting reduced Sertoli cell number and capacity to support and nurture germ cells (24, 26). *Fshb*- and *Fshr*-knockout (-KO) mice present with complete spermatogenesis, but the amount of germ cells remained lower than in control animals. In more detail, the KO mice have <50% of spermatogonial cells and ~50% of spermatocytes in comparison to wild-type animals, and the number of germ cells is reduced further to <40% of wild-type mice at postmeiotic stages [**Table 1**, (24, 26)]. While FSH influences solely the proliferation of Sertoli cells, T and FSH impact additively on the germ cells' entry into meiosis and stimulate synergistically its completion and entry into spermiogenesis (26). Experimental data from chemically and hormonally treated rats indicate that FSH is beneficial in the early stages of spermatogenesis until round spermatids, while

TABLE 1 | Outcome of manipulation of FSH action and defects on testis mass, number of Sertoli cells, and completion of spermatogenesis.

Treatment/mouse model/human condition	Species	Testis mass or volume (%)*	Number of Sertoli cells (%)*	Number of round (r) or elongated (e) spermatids (%) or sperm count (s)*	Ratio of round spermatids to number of Sertoli cells (%)*	Reference(s)
Fshb knockout	Mouse	40	57–70	40(r), 37(e)	57	(24, 25)
Fshr knockout	Mouse	42	55**	36(r)**	69**,***	(26)
FSHR null mutation 566CT; A189V	Human	27–100	n/a	oligospermic-normospermic (s)	n/a	(27)
FSHB missense, frameshift and truncating mutations	Human	7–80	n/a or reduced number of Sertoli cells	azoospermic (s)	n/a	(28) and references therein
Acvr2a knockout (stimulation of FSH prevented)	Mouse	40–43	60–61	45(r), 41(e)	75	(24)
hpg (gonadotropin-deficient hypogonadal) + tgFSH expression	Mouse	500	162**	Increased, but low (r), hardly detectable (e)	Cannot be measured due to the absence of spermatids in *hpg* mice	(29)
(hpg + T implant) + tgFSH expression	Mouse	166	132**	161(r), 184(e)**	117**	(29)
Neonatal treatment with rhFSH	Rat	124	149	n/a	n/a	(30)
Fshr-CAM G1738C; D580H tgFSHR expression	Mouse	94	85	87(r), 87(e)	103	(31)
LuRKO; *Lhcgr* knockout	Mouse	19	29	4.8(r), 0(e)	16	(31)
Fshr-CAM/LuRKO crossbreed	Mouse	86	83	94(r), 51(e)	115	(31)

*In comparison to corresponding controls in each experiment. **Estimated from the charts presented in the article. ***All germ cells/Sertoli cells; n/a, data not available; rh, recombinant human; tg, transgenic; CAM, constitutively activating mutation.

the effect of T becomes enhanced thereafter (39–41). The germ cell to Sertoli cell ratio also decreases in the absence of FSH or FSHR [**Table 1**, (24, 26)]. Therefore, the reduction in the number of germ cells is not solely due to the decreased amount of the supporting Sertoli cells, but also because of their decreased ability to nurture germ cells.

THE CONUNDRUM OF THE ROLE OF FSH DEFICIENCY IN HUMAN SPERMATOGENESIS

To our knowledge, only one harmful (inactivating) *FSHR* mutation has been identified in men so far. In a cohort of several Finnish families of women with hypergonadotropic hypogonadism due to inactivating *FSHR*-A189V mutation, five male brothers were found to be homozygous carriers of the same mutation (27). While their homozygous female relatives had ovarian failure and infertility, the men had an unassuming phenotype which could not have been detected without the family connection. Four of the men were subfertile, phenocopying the FSH- and FSHR-deficient mice with complete but quantitatively reduced spermatogenesis, and two of them fathered two children each. In striking contrast, all men so far identified with *FSHB* mutation (*n* = 5) have been azoospermic and infertile (28). This was unanticipated, since receptor defects generally present with more severe effects in hormone action than those of ligands.

An explanation for the discrepancy between the phenotypes of men with *FSHR* and *FSHB* mutations could be the residual activity of the mutant FSHR. Indeed, when highly overexpressed *in vitro*, a small fraction of the mutant FSHR-A189V is able to reach cell membrane, where it binds FSH and activates cAMP production (42). FSHR-A189V is also able to trigger mitogen-activated protein kinase phosphorylation via β-arrestins, thus activating the signaling cascade (43).

Additional genetic and/or environmental factors besides the *FSHB* mutations may also explain the azoospermia found in the mutation carriers. The *FSHB* mutations detected, however, are independent of each other, and the men are from different ethnic backgrounds supporting the essential role of FSH in human spermatogenesis. It would be expected that men with such mutation would respond to FSH treatment. One patient was found to attain a larger testis volume after 1-year treatment, but with spermatogenesis stalled at the spermatocyte stage (28). A moderate amount of missense, frameshift, and stop-gained mutations have been identified in *FSHB* and *FSHR* genes in ExAC database of over 60,000 individuals [http://exac.broadinstitute.org/gene/ENSG00000170820; http://exac.broadinstitute.org/gene/ENSG00000131808 (44)]. The constraint metrics for the gene variations suggest that they are well tolerated, and thus more homozygous mutation carriers may be identified in the future alongside increasing exome and whole genome sequencing. For now, with few men carrying known pathogenic *FSHB* or *FSHR* mutations, and other possible related factors affecting

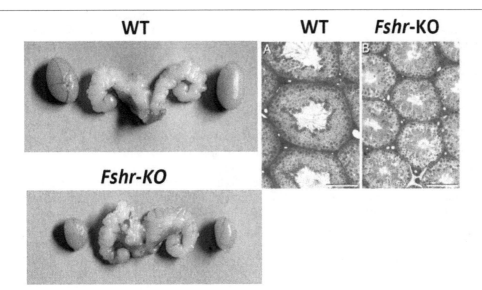

FIGURE 1 | Testes and seminal vesicles of adult wild type (WT) and *Fshr*KO) mice **(Left)**, and testicular histology of same genotypes **(Right)**. No difference is observed in seminal vesicle sizes between the two genotypes, but the size of the *Fshr*KO testes is about half that of WT. Also, while full spermatogenesis is visible in the histology of both testes, the tubular diameter is clearly narrower in the knockout testis. From (37) with permission.

spermatogenesis unrevealed, it remains unclear whether FSH action is indispensable for spermatogenesis in men or playing a supporting role. One reason for the stark contrast between the numerous mutations detected in *LHCGR* and only few in *FSHR* may be the milder "real" phenotype of *FSHB/FSHR* mutations in men (45).

EXCESSIVE FSH ACTION HAS MINOR INFLUENCE ON TESTIS DEVELOPMENT AND FUNCTION

There is a strong positive correlation between serum FSH concentration and testis development in rodents (22, 23). While the shortage of FSH or its receptor decrease spermatogenesis, neonatal administration of FSH increases to some extent the Sertoli cell number and testis size above normal in rats [**Table 1**, (30)]. Men with pituitary adenoma secreting excessive FSH appear to have normal testicular function (46, 47), suggesting that excessive FSH has no obvious effect in otherwise healthy men.

Gain-of-function (GoF) mutations of G-protein coupled receptor genes are rare. Few women with *FSHR* GoF mutations have been identified in pregnancy-associated ovarian hyperstimulation syndrome caused by constitutive activity and relaxed specificity of the receptor for hCG. However, the male relatives of the affected women did not have any reproductive or other health issues (48). A man with activating FSHR-D567G mutation has been identified to have normal spermatogenesis after hypophysectomy, even without T replacement therapy (49), suggesting that strong constitutive FSH stimulation can compensate for missing LH and reduced T action. In another case, a male carrier of an *FSHR*-N431I mutation was found to have complete spermatogenesis despite suppressed serum FSH

(50). While the FSHR-D567G mutation increased basal cAMP production 1.5-fold *in vitro*, FSHR-N431I resulted in impaired agonist-stimulated receptor desensitization and internalization, thus causing "pseudo-constitutive" receptor activation. In both cases, the enhanced receptor activity likely compensated for shortage of the ligand. With no harmful effects on male health reported, there is the possibility that normal FSH activity brings about maximal physiological response in the male.

In general, recognition of GoF mutations should be easier than loss-of-function (LoF) mutations, because the former usually alter the phenotype in heterozygous form, while the LoF mutations must be homozygous (or compound heterozygous) to be effective. The scarcity of identified *FSHR* GoF mutations implies that they may not generally be harmful for their male carriers. This is in contrast to activating *LHR* gene (*LHCGR*) mutations that cause the dramatic phenotype of early-onset precocious puberty in boys (51, 52). The transgenic mouse line expressing *FSHR*-D580H in Sertoli cells supports the benign nature of GoF *FSHR* mutations in males (31). Despite robustly induced cAMP production in the absence of ligand (53) the transgenic males present with normal testis development and function, and do not differ significantly in Sertoli or germ cell number or fertility from their wild-type littermates [**Table 1**, (31)].

FSH REGULATES GENES INVOLVED IN PROLIFERATION, STRUCTURE, AND FUNCTION OF SERTOLI CELLS

The molecular mechanisms of FSH action are discussed in other chapters of this special issue (Reiter and Casarini; Sayers and Hanyaloglu). We concentrate here on the processes and target genes of FSH action and their relationship to androgen action, to understand more precisely the role of FSH in spermatogenesis.

The regulatory system of the two gonadotropins, their feedback regulation, organization and interaction between germ and somatic cells, pose a challenge for dissecting the influence and target genes of a single factor, such as FSH. Sertoli cells present with a prominent fluctuating gene expression patterns along the seminiferous epithelial cycle (54). Therefore, their transcriptome profile analysis is highly dependent on sample source, time of collection, and culture conditions, as well as on the approach applied, *i.e.*, microarray or transcriptome sequencing.

The general phenomenon is that FSH mostly elevates the expression of a large number of Sertoli cell genes (55–57). In neonatal life, Sertoli cells proliferate extensively, and logically mainly the transcripts of genes involved in DNA replication, cell cycle and stem cell factors are enriched (54). FSH most prominently stimulates many of these genes including *Krüppel-like factor 4, Klf4* (56, 58). KLF4 is a transcription factor that can be used to reprogram Sertoli cells to pluripotent stem cells (59), but it also plays a significant role in timing and accuracy of Sertoli cell differentiation (58). In GnRH-deficient hypogonadal (*hpg*) mice the proliferation and maturation of Sertoli cells are restrained (60), but their FSH stimulation triggers, as in neonatal mice, the expression of transcripts involved in RNA and DNA binding, cell cycle and cell growth, along with signal transduction and expression of transcription factors (56). The arrest of Sertoli cell proliferation alongside cell maturation is not only due to the cessation of proliferative gene expression, but also to upregulation of genes categorized in gene ontology as negative regulators of cell proliferation (54). While FSH-stimulated *hpg* mice presented with stimulation of proliferative factors and cessation of differentiating factors (56), chronically induced cAMP production by the FSHR-D567G mutation favored in cultured Sertoli cells the expression of genes involved in cellular differentiation at the expense of proliferation (61). One possible explanation for this difference could be biased signaling upon constant FSHR activation.

The mitotic quiescence of Sertoli cells is followed by formation of tight junctions and construction of the blood-testis barrier between mature Sertoli cells, in order to separate adluminal germ cells from the circulatory and lymphatic system (1). Androgens and FSH regulate in additive and synergistic fashion the expression of several genes adjusting blood-testis barrier dynamics or its components, including tight junction proteins and junctional adhesion molecules (54). Based on current evidence, androgen action is imperative for blood-testis barrier function. FSH, instead, has a more permissive role in stimulating the organization of inter-Sertoli junction types, and junctions between Sertoli cells and germ cells such as ectoplasmic specialization and adherent junction (56, 62, 63), thereby enabling the nurturing of germ cells. The Wnt pathway is one of those activated on postnatal days 5–10 in mouse Sertoli cells (54). FSH and T target a major morphogen, Wnt3, that in turn regulates the expression of *Gja*, which encodes a gap-junction protein essential for germ cell development (64).

Alongside Sertoli cell maturation, the transcript enrichment switches from proliferative and structural genes to those more involved in metabolic and germ cell supporting processes (54). Sertoli cell-produced retinoic acids are essential for the induction of spermatogonial differentiation during the first spermatogenic wave (65). Sertoli cells present with a specific temporally regulated array of genes related to retinoic acid synthesis and action (54), and FSH may affect both ligand metabolism and receptor function (66, 67). Logically for the supportive role of FSH in spermatogenesis, it also regulates and limits the massive wave of germ cell apoptosis during the first round of spermatogenesis (68–70). This process is apparently crucial to maintain the critical cell number between some germinal cell stages and Sertoli cells, and its lack brings about sterility (70). FSH also regulates the expression of genes involved in fatty acid metabolism and mitochondrial biogenesis, which is vital for the energy metabolism of seminiferous tubules (71). Another example of FSH-induced actions of Sertoli cells on germ cells is *Aqp8*, one of the most altered genes in the absence of FSH action (57). *Aqp8* is involved in water transport through membranes (72) and is strongly down-regulated in *Fshr*-KO mice (57). Expression of *Aqp8* as well as other FSH-stimulated genes is highly dependent on the hormone action during puberty in mice, but it returns to normal in adulthood even in the absence of the receptor, suggesting that FSH action on Sertoli cell function is not equally crucial after puberty (57). Finally, the partial and global gene expression profiles earlier referred to include numerous other less well characterized FSH-dependent genes. Their in-depth characterization will further elucidate the detailed mechanisms of FSH regulation of spermatogenesis.

HIGH INTRATESTICULAR T CONCENTRATION MAY NOT BE ESSENTIAL FOR COMPLETE SPERMATOGENESIS

FSH and T regulate several aspects of spermatogenesis independently, as well as in additive and synergistic manner (26). In contrast to FSH, there has been a consensus for the absolute requirement of T for spermatogenesis in most mammalian species. An exception is the photoperiod-dependent Djungarian hamster, where the restoration of spermatogenesis is dependent on FSH (73). In other mammals, the disruption of T production through hypophysectomy, Leydig cell ablation or knockout of *Lhcgr* results in interruption of spermatogenesis (74–77). The *AR* knockout mouse acts as a conclusive proof-of-concept that spermatogenesis will not proceed beyond meiosis without the support of T (78, 79).

The site of T production is the interstitial Leydig cells, and the local intratesticular concentration of T, depending on species, is in the order of 50–100-fold higher than that in systemic circulation (80–83). Studies in rodents indicate that intratesticular T below the normal high levels can support complete spermatogenesis. Both qualitatively and quantitatively normal spermatogenesis has been reported in rats at an intratesticular T concentration 30% of control animals (84). Full spermatogenesis has also been reported in T propionate-treated and hypophysectomized rats at intratesticular T concentrations below 5% of normal (85, 86). Furthermore, treatment of *hpg* (83, 87) and *Lhcgr* knockout (LuRKO) mice (88, 89) with subcutaneous T implants restored qualitatively complete spermatogenesis in a dose-dependent manner with minimal increase in intratesticular T concentration. Similarly, human carriers of partially inactivating *LHCGR* (90) and a LoF *LHB* mutation (91) have been reported to be oligozoospermic, instead of azoospermic, at very low serum and intratesticular T concentration. The evidence together indicates that high intratesticular T concentration is not a prerequisite for complete spermatogenesis, although it apparently increases sperm production and fertility.

LH/T REGULATION OF SPERMATOGENESIS CAN BE REPLACED BY STRONG FSHR ACTIVATION

Two recently used approaches have enhanced our knowledge about the role of FSH in spermatogenesis; the serendipitous discovery of mutations in human subjects and the generation of animals lacking or overexpressing FSH or its receptor. In clinical practice, patients presenting with hypogonadotropic hypogonadism are a valuable tool to study the role of gonadotropins in spermatogenesis and subsequent fertility.

Those presenting with secondary hypogonadism consequent to idiopathic hypogonadotropic hypogonadism and Kallmann syndrome can be effectively treated with FSH and LH or with pulsatile GnRH administration (92–94).

To dissect out the effect of excessive FSH action on spermatogenesis without simultaneous LH action, we took advantage of the transgenic mice expressing constitutively active *Fshr*-D580H (*Fshr*-CAM) driven by the anti-Müllerian hormone promoter in Sertoli cells (53). *In vitro*, FSHR-D580H induced without ligand cAMP production to the same degree as the wild-type receptor at saturating FSH concentration, thereby representing a strong constitutively active receptor. Female mice carrying the mutated gene developed several abnormalities in their ovaries and other estrogen target tissues, whereas the male littermates were devoid of any discernible phenotype deviating from normal (**Figures 2A,B**).

The *Fshr*-CAM mice (53) were then crossbred into the LuRKO (77) background to generate double-mutant *Fshr*-CAM/LuRKO mice with high FSHR signaling and minimal T production [**Table 1**, (31)]. Interestingly, the mutant *Fshr*-CAM expression reversed the azoospermia and partially restored fertility of the LuRKO mice to a near-normal male phenotype (**Figures 2C,D**, **Table 1**). Despite the absence of LHR in the double-mutant mice, intratesticular and serum T concentrations increased from the

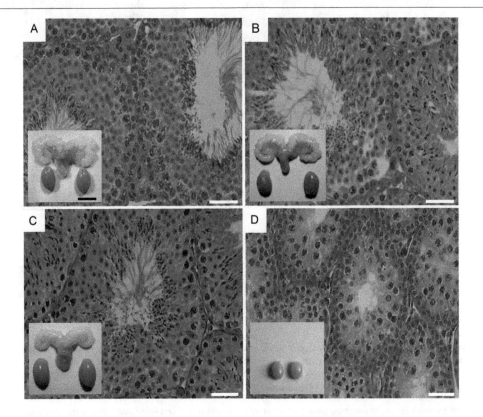

FIGURE 2 | Testicular histology and macroscopic views of testes and urogenital blocks of different mouse genotypes: **(A)** WT, **(B)** *Fshr*-CAM, **(C)** *Fshr*-CAM/LuRKO, and **(D)** LuRKO mice. **(A–C)** show normal spermatogenesis and testis and seminal vesicle (SV) sizes. In **(D)**, spermatogenesis is arrested at the round spermatid (RS) stage, with small testes and rudimentary seminal vesicle (not visible). Scale bars: 50 μm; 10 mm (insets). From (31) with permission.

very low level in LuRKO mice to ~20 and 40% of those in wild-type mice. Anatomically, testicular and reproductive accessory gland development was normal (**Figure 2C**), and the mice were fertile, but presented with delayed puberty and small litter sizes compared to wild-type mice. The surprising fertility in these mice suggested that excessive FSH action could partially substitute for missing LH. A somewhat similar observation was made with the expression of *Fshr*-D567G in *hpg* background mice (29). In this transgenic model, the presence of the mutant *FSHR* also increased, to some extent, cAMP level in Sertoli cells and T production in absence of LH but was not able to rescue mature spermatogenesis. This indicates that very robust FSH action might be needed for successful spermatogenesis in the absence of sufficient T stimulation.

To ascertain whether the observed residual Leydig cell T production was responsible for the spermatogenesis in *Fshr*-CAM/LuRKO mice, we completely blocked T action through treatment with the potent antiandrogen, flutamide.

In wild-type mice, loss of T action by flutamide treatment led, as expected, to shrunken seminal vesicles and arrest of spermatogenesis at the round spermatid stage (**Figure 3A**). Unexpectedly, identical flutamide treatment of the *Fshr*-CAM/LuRKO mice prevented only the extragonadal androgen actions but had no deleterious effect on spermatogenesis (**Figure 3B**). This suggests that the constitutively active FSHR-D580H was able to maintain spermatogenesis, even after T action was completely abolished. Hence, the constitutively active FSHR-D580H astonishingly compensated for the action of the blocked LH/T pathway. Correspondingly, expression of several androgen-dependent Sertoli cell genes including *Drd4, Rhox 5, Aqp8, Eppin,* and *Gata1,* was decreased in the flutamide-treated wild-type mice as phenocopy of the LuRKO mice (**Figure 3C**), but the treatment had no effect on expression of these androgen target genes in *Fshr*-CAM/LuRKO mice (**Figure 3D**). The azoospermic phenotype observed in wild-type mice after androgen inactivation by flutamide was similar to

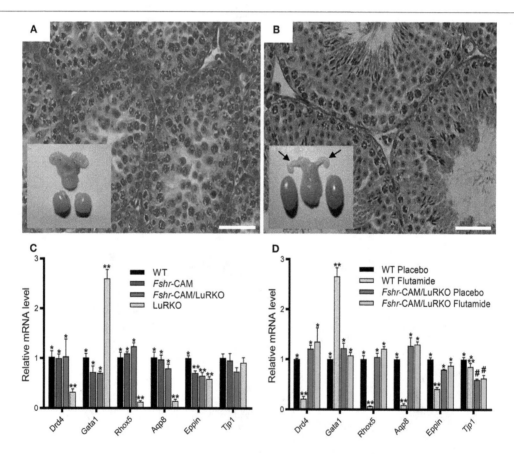

FIGURE 3 | Effect of anti-androgen flutamide treatment on wild-type (WT) and genetically modified mice. **(A,B)** Testicular histology and macroscopic views of the testes and urogenital blocks of WT and *Fshr*-CAM/LuRKO mice. **(A)** The treatment arrested spermatogenesis at round spermatid stage in WT mice and reduced their testis and seminal vesicle sizes. **(B)** Identical treatment of *Fshr*-CAM/LuRKO mice had no apparent effect on their spermatogenesis and testis size but reduced seminal vesicle size (arrows in B). **(C,D)** Expression of selected target genes in untreated **(A)** and flutamide treated **(B)** mice. **(A)** Expression of androgen-regulated (*Drd5, Rhox5, Eppin,* and *Tjp1*), postmeiotic germ cell–specific (*Aqp8*), and germ cell–regulated (*Gata1*) genes in WT, *Fshr*-CAM, *Fshr*-CAM/LuRKO, and LuRKO testes. **(B)** Effect of flutamide treatment on expression of the same androgen-regulated genes in WT and *Fshr*-CAM/LuRKO mice. Data represent mean ± SEM. $n = 3$ samples/group. Bars with different symbols differ significantly from each other ($P < 0.05$; ANOVA/Newman-Keuls). The remarkable finding is that while flutamide treatment suppressed the expression of strictly androgen-dependent genes in WT mice, the same effect was not observed in the testis of *Fshr*-CAM/LuRKO mice. Scale bars: 50 μm. From (31) with permission.

that observed in Sertoli and peritubular myoid cell-specific *AR* knockouts mice (16, 79). The *AR* knockout mice demonstrate that spermatogenesis does not proceed to completion without the indirect T effect via Sertoli cells (78, 79). Therefore, the persistent spermatogenesis observed in the double mutant mice after flutamide treatment supports the conclusion that robust and constitutive FSHR activity can compensate for missing androgen action.

FSH and T have independent mechanisms of action; FSH acting through a membrane-bound G-protein coupled receptor, and T through AR, a nuclear transcription factor. However, when scrutinized in detail, overlapping mechanisms in their mode of action exist (95, 96). Both hormones activate the mitogen-activated protein kinase and cAMP-responsive element-binding protein signaling cascades, shown to be crucial for spermatogenesis through a rapid T signaling mechanism (97), and increase of Sertoli cell intracellular Ca^{2+} (98, 99). Thus, these partly overlapping mechanisms of androgen and FSH action may explain the ability of strong FSH action to substitute for the missing T stimulus. However, the quantitatively incomplete recovery of spermatogenesis in these mice emphasizes the importance of T for qualitatively and quantitatively full spermatogenesis.

SUMMARY AND CLINICAL IMPLICATIONS

FSH function is an essential part of the complex HPG axis and its feedback control mechanisms in the regulation of testicular function. Pituitary-derived FSH provides indirect structural and metabolic support for development of spermatogonia into mature spermatids via its membrane-bound receptor in Sertoli cells. FSH also play a crucial role in determination of the number of Sertoli cells and thus their capacity to maintain spermatogenesis. In addition to proliferation and differentiation of Sertoli cells, FSH regulates the structural genes involved in the organization of cell-cell junctions as well as genes required for the metabolism and transport of regulatory and nutritive substances from Sertoli to germ cells. Although FSH is not a mandatory requirement for the completion of spermatogenesis in rodents, its deficiency, nevertheless, leads to significant reduction in sperm quantity. In humans, fertility phenotypes in carriers of inactivating *FSHB* or *FSHR* mutations varies from azoospermia to mild reduction of spermatogenesis.

In the past decades, men suffering from idiopathic hypogonadotropic hypogonadism have been treated with FSH in combination with LH to compensate for lack of endogenous gonadotropins (100). Due to the favorable influence of FSH on spermatogenesis, many studies of FSH administration have been conducted on men with idiopathic spermatogenic failure

(101–103), but with variable outcome. The general conclusion from meta-analyses is encouraging on the effect of FSH on sperm quality (103), spontaneous pregnancy rates (101, 102), and pregnancies achieved through assisted reproductive techniques (102) in several, but not in all cases. FSH-treatment has improved not only the conventional sperm parameters such as motility, number and morphology of sperm, but also the non-conventional ones such as decreased amount of DNA damage and fragmentation (104, 105).

It is presumable that certain patient groups are more responsive to FSH treatment than others, depending on their genetic background and other factors involved. For example, individuals with hetero- or homozygous polymorphisms for serine in position 680 of the FSHR are shown to respond better to FSH treatment than those with asparagine in this position (106). On the other hand, FSH administration has been shown to decrease DNA fragmentation and thus improve the quality of DNA in patients with FSHR-N680, but not with FSHR-S680 (105). The dosage and length of FSH treatment also have marked effects on the outcome. Recent studies indicate that a sufficiently long FSH treatment, preferably at least 6 months, with a high dosage of at least 150 IU per injection every other day, can improve sperm parameters significantly more than the standard FSH treatments with lower doses (103). Ding et al. (107), showed convincingly an improvement of spermatogenesis and pregnancy rates in a group of idiopathic oligozoospermic men treated with increasing doses of FSH, with the best results achieved using administration of 300 IU of recombinant human FSH every other day for 5 months. Though results from mouse experiments cannot directly be extrapolated to humans, our recent studies with *Fshr*-CAM/LuRKO mice show that robust and constant FSHR stimulation can improve spermatogenesis and fertility rate even in the absence of T. However, based on the results from meta-analyses (101–103) caution is needed with the use of FSH, especially as it relates to high dosage and long-term treatments. In addition, more carefully controlled studies should be carried out to identify individuals with possible specific genetic makeup, who would most likely benefit from FSH treatment.

AUTHOR CONTRIBUTIONS

All authors listed have made a substantial, direct and intellectual contribution to the work, and approved it for publication.

FUNDING

The original work in this review was supported by the Wellcome Trust Programme Grant (082101/Z07/Z) and the MRC Project Grant (0600002) to ITH.

REFERENCES

1. Mruk DD, Cheng CY. The mammalian blood-testis barrier: its biology and regulation. *Endocr Rev.* (2015) 36:564–91. doi: 10.1210/er.2014-1101

2. Steinberger E, Steinberger A. Spermatogenic function of the testis. In: Greep RO, Hamilton DW, editors. *Handbook of Physiology.* Washington DC: American Physiological Society (1975). p. 1–10.

3. Griswold MD. The central role of Sertoli cells in spermatogenesis. *Semin Cell Dev Biol.* (1998) 9:411–6. doi: 10.1006/scdb.1998.0203

4. Sharpe RM. Sperm counts and fertility in men: a rocky road ahead. science & Society Series on Sex and Science. *EMBO Rep.* (2012) 13:398–403. doi: 10.1038/embor.2012.50

5. Sharpe RM, McKinnell C, Kivlin C, Fisher JS. Proliferation and functional maturation of Sertoli cells, and their relevance to disorders of testis

function in adulthood. *Reproduction* (2003) 125:769–84. doi: 10.1530/rep.0.1250769

6. Ehmcke J, Hubner K, Scholer HR, Schlatt S. Spermatogonia: origin, physiology and prospects for conservation and manipulation of the male germ line. *Reprod Fertil Dev.* (2006) 18:7–12. doi: 10.1071/RD05119

7. Jan SZ, Hamer G, Repping S, de Rooij DG, van Pelt AM, Vormer TL. Molecular control of rodent spermatogenesis. *Biochim Biophys Acta* (2012) 1822:1838–50. doi: 10.1016/j.bbadis.2012.02.008

8. Hayes FJ, DeCruz S, Seminara SB, Boepple PA, Crowley WF Jr. Differential regulation of gonadotropin secretion by testosterone in the human male: absence of a negative feedback effect of testosterone on follicle-stimulating hormone secretion. *J Clin Endocrinol Metab.* (2001) 86:53–8. doi: 10.1210/jc.86.1.53

9. Manetti GJ, Honig SC. Update on male hormonal contraception: is the vasectomy in jeopardy? *Int J Impot Res.* (2010) 22:159–70. doi: 10.1038/ijir.2010.2

10. Kangasniemi M, Kaipia A, Toppari J, Perheentupa A, Huhtaniemi I, Parvinen M. Cellular regulation of follicle-stimulating hormone (FSH) binding in rat seminiferous tubules. *J Androl.* (1990) 11:336–43.

11. McLachlan RI, O'Donnell L, Meachem SJ, Stanton PG, de Kretser DM, Pratis K, et al. Identification of specific sites of hormonal regulation in spermatogenesis in rats, monkeys, and man. *Recent Prog Horm Res.* (2002) 57:149–79. doi: 10.1210/rp.57.1.149

12. Orth J, Christensen AK. Localization of 125I-labeled FSH in the testes of hypophy-sectomized rats by autoradiography at the light and electron microscope levels. *Endocrinology* (1977) 101:262–78. doi: 10.1210/endo-101-1-262

13. Simoni M, Gromoll J, Nieschlag E. The follicle-stimulating hormone receptor: biochemistry, molecular biology, physiology, and pathophysiology. *Endocr Rev.* (1997) 18:739–73. doi: 10.1210/er.18.6.739

14. McLachlan RI. The endocrine control of spermatogenesis. *Baillieres Best Pract Res Clin Endocrinol Metab.* (2000) 14:345–62. doi: 10.1053/beem.2000.0084

15. O'Shaughnessy PJ. Hormonal control of germ cell development and spermatogenesis. *Semin Cell Dev Biol.* (2014) 29:55–65. doi: 10.1016/j.semcdb.2014.02.010

16. Welsh M, Saunders PT, Atanassova N, Sharpe RM, Smith LB. Androgen action via testicular peritubular myoid cells is essential for male fertility. *FASEB J.* (2009) 23:4218–30. doi: 10.1096/fj.09-138347

17. Huhtaniemi I. A hormonal contraceptive for men: how close are we? *Prog Brain Res.* (2010) 181:273–88. doi: 10.1016/S0079-6123(08)81015-1

18. Huhtaniemi IT, Yamamoto M, Ranta T, Jalkanen J, Jaffe RB. Follicle-stimulating hormone receptors appear earlier in the primate fetal testis than in the ovary. *J Clin Endocrinol Metab.* (1987) 65:1210–4. doi: 10.1210/jcem-65-6-1210

19. Warren DW, Huhtaniemi IT, Tapanainen J, Dufau ML, Catt KJ. Ontogeny of gonadotropin receptors in the fetal and neonatal rat testis. *Endocrinology* (1984) 114:470–6. doi: 10.1210/endo-114-2-470

20. Eskola V, Nikula H, Huhtaniemi I. Age-related variation of follicle-stimulating hormone-stimulated cAMP production, protein kinase C activity and their interactions in the rat testis. *Mol Cell Endocrinol.* (1993) 93:143–8. doi: 10.1016/0303-7207(93)90117-3

21. Orth JM. The role of follicle-stimulating hormone in controlling Sertoli cell proliferation in testes of fetal rats. *Endocrinology* (1984) 115:1248–55. doi: 10.1210/endo-115-4-1248

22. Allan CM, Garcia A, Spaliviero J, Zhang FP, Jimenez M, Huhtaniemi I, et al. Complete Sertoli cell proliferation induced by follicle-stimulating hormone (FSH) independently of luteinizing hormone activity: evidence from genetic models of isolated FSH action. *Endocrinology* (2004) 145:1587–93. doi: 10.1210/en.2003-1164

23. Allan CM, Haywood M, Swaraj S, Spaliviero J, Koch A, Jimenez M, et al. A novel transgenic model to characterize the specific effects of follicle-stimulating hormone on gonadal physiology in the absence of luteinizing hormone actions. *Endocrinology* (2001) 142:2213–20. doi: 10.1210/endo.142.6.8092

24. Wreford NG, Rajendra Kumar T, Matzuk MM, de Kretser DM. Analysis of the testicular phenotype of the follicle-stimulating hormone beta-subunit knockout and the activin type II receptor knockout mice by stereological analysis. *Endocrinology* (2001) 142:2916–20. doi: 10.1210/endo.142.7.8230

25. Kumar TR, Wang Y, Lu N, Matzuk MM. Follicle stimulating hormone is required for ovarian follicle maturation but not male fertility. *Nat Genet.* (1997) 15:201–4. doi: 10.1038/ng0297-201

26. Abel MH, Baker PJ, Charlton HM, Monteiro A, Verhoeven G, De Gendt K, et al. Spermatogenesis and sertoli cell activity in mice lacking sertoli cell receptors for follicle-stimulating hormone and androgen. *Endocrinology* (2008) 149:3279–85. doi: 10.1210/en.2008-0086

27. Tapanainen JS, Aittomaki K, Min J, Vaskivuo T, Huhtaniemi IT. Men homozygous for an inactivating mutation of the follicle-stimulating hormone (FSH) receptor gene present variable suppression of spermatogenesis and fertility. *Nat Genet.* (1997) 15:205–6. doi: 10.1038/ng0297-205

28. Zheng J, Mao J, Cui M, Liu Z, Wang X, Xiong S, et al. Novel FSHβ mutation in a male patient with isolated FSH deficiency and infertility. *Eur J Med Genet.* (2017) 60:335–9. doi: 10.1016/j.ejmg.2017.04.004

29. Haywood M, Tymchenko N, Spaliviero J, Koch A, Jimenez M, Gromoll J, et al. An activated human follicle-stimulating hormone (FSH) receptor stimulates FSH-like activity in gonadotropin-deficient transgenic mice. *Mol Endocrinol.* (2002) 16:2582–91. doi: 10.1210/me.2002-0032

30. Meachem SJ, McLachlan RI, de Kretser DM, Robertson DM, Wreford NG. Neonatal exposure of rats to recombinant follicle stimulating hormone increases adult Sertoli and spermatogenic cell numbers. *Biol Reprod.* (1996) 54:36–44. doi: 10.1095/biolreprod54.1.36

31. Oduwole OO, Peltoketo H, Poliandri A, Vengadabady L, Chrusciel M, Doroszko M, et al. Constitutively active follicle-stimulating hormone receptor enables androgen-independent spermatogenesis. *J Clin Invest.* (2018) 128:1787–92. doi: 10.1172/JCI96794

32. O'Shaughnessy PJ, Monteiro A, Abel M. Testicular development in mice lacking receptors for follicle stimulating hormone and androgen. *PLoS ONE* (2012) 7:e35136. doi: 10.1371/journal.pone.0035136

33. Clermont Y, Perey B. Quantitative study of the cell population of the seminiferous tubules in immature rats. *Am J Anat.* (1957) 100:241–67. doi: 10.1002/aja.1001000205

34. Orth JM, McGuinness MP, Qiu J, Jester WF Jr, Li LH. Use of *in vitro* systems to study male germ cell development in neonatal rats. *Theriogenology* (1998) 49:431–9. doi: 10.1016/S0093-691X(97)00415-9

35. Rannikko A, Penttila TL, Zhang FP, Toppari J, Parvinen M, Huhtaniemi I. Stage-specific expression of the FSH receptor gene in the prepubertal and adult rat seminiferous epithelium. *J Endocrinol.* (1996) 151:29–35. doi: 10.1677/joe.0.1510029

36. Ruwanpura SM, McLachlan RI, Meachem SJ. Hormonal regulation of male germ cell development. *J Endocrinol.* (2010) 205:117–31. doi: 10.1677/JOE-10-0025

37. Abel MH, Wootton AN, Wilkins V, Huhtaniemi I, Knight PG, Charlton HM. The effect of a null mutation in the follicle-stimulating hormone receptor gene on mouse reproduction. *Endocrinology* (2000) 141:1795–803. doi: 10.1210/endo.141.5.7456

38. Dierich A, Sairam MR, Monaco L, Fimia GM, Gansmuller A, LeMeur M, et al. Impairing follicle-stimulating hormone (FSH) signaling *in vivo*: targeted disruption of the FSH receptor leads to aberrant gametogenesis and hormonal imbalance. *Proc Natl Acad Sci USA.* (1998) 95:13612–7. doi: 10.1073/pnas.95.23.13612

39. McLachlan RI, Wreford NG, Meachem SJ, De Kretser DM, Robertson DM. Effects of testosterone on spermatogenic cell populations in the adult rat. *Biol Reprod.* (1994) 51:945–55. doi: 10.1095/biolreprod51.5.945

40. McLachlan RI, Wreford NG, Tsonis C, De Kretser DM, Robertson DM. Testosterone effects on spermatogenesis in the gonadotropin-releasing hormone-immunized rat. *Biol Reprod.* (1994) 50:271–80. doi: 10.1095/biolreprod50.2.271

41. Meachem SJ, McLachlan RI, Stanton PG, Robertson DM, Wreford NG. FSH immunoneutralization acutely impairs spermatogonial development in normal adult rats. *J Androl.* (1999) 20:756–62.

42. Rannikko A, Pakarinen P, Manna PR, Beau I, Misrahi M, Aittomaki K, et al. Functional characterization of the human FSH receptor with an inactivating Ala189Val mutation. *Mol Hum Reprod.* (2002) 8:311–7. doi: 10.1093/molehr/8.4.311

43. Tranchant T, Durand G, Gauthier C, Crepieux P, Ulloa-Aguirre A, Royere D, et al. Preferential beta-arrestin signalling at low receptor density revealed by functional characterization of the human FSH receptor A189 V mutation. *Mol Cell Endocrinol.* (2011) 331:109–18. doi: 10.1016/j.mce.2010.08.016

44. Lek M, Karczewski KJ, Minikel EV, Samocha KE, Banks E, Fennell T, et al. Analysis of protein-coding genetic variation in 60,706 humans. *Nature* (2016) 536:285–91. doi: 10.1038/nature19057

45. Huhtaniemi I. Male hypogonadism resulting from mutations in the genes for gonadotropin subunits and their receptors. In: Winters S, Huhtaniemi I, editors. *Male Hypogonadism* New York, NY: Humana Press (2017). p. 127–52. doi: 10.1007/978-3-319-53298-1_6

46. Galway AB, Hsueh AJ, Daneshdoost L, Zhou MH, Pavlou SN, Snyder PJ. Gonadotroph adenomas in men produce biologically active follicle-stimulating hormone. *J Clin Endocrinol Metab.* (1990) 71:907–12. doi: 10.1210/jcem-71-4-907

47. Snyder PJ. Gonadotroph cell pituitary adenomas. *Endocrinol Metab Clin North Am.* (1987) 16:755–64. doi: 10.1016/S0889-8529(18)30472-9

48. Lussiana C, Guani B, Mari C, Restagno G, Massobrio M, Revelli A. Mutations and polymorphisms of the FSH receptor (FSHR) gene: clinical implications in female fecundity and molecular biology of FSHR protein and gene. *Obstet Gynecol Surv.* (2008) 63:785–95. doi: 10.1097/OGX.0b013e31818957eb

49. Gromoll J, Simoni M, Nieschlag E. An activating mutation of the follicle-stimulating hormone receptor autonomously sustains spermatogenesis in a hypophysectomized man. *J Clin Endocrinol Metab.* (1996) 81:1367–70.

50. Casas-Gonzalez P, Scaglia HE, Perez-Solis MA, Durand G, Scaglia J, Zarinan T, et al. Normal testicular function without detectable follicle-stimulating hormone. a novel mutation in the follicle-stimulating hormone receptor gene leading to apparent constitutive activity and impaired agonist-induced desensitization and internalization. *Mol Cell Endocrinol.* (2012) 364:71–82. doi: 10.1016/j.mce.2012.08.011

51. Jeha GS, Lowenthal ED, Chan WY, Wu SM, Karaviti LP. Variable presentation of precocious puberty associated with the D564G mutation of the LHCGR gene in children with testotoxicosis. *J Pediatr.* (2006) 149:271–4. doi: 10.1016/j.jpeds.2006.03.017

52. Macedo DB, Silveira LF, Bessa DS, Brito VN, Latronico AC. Sexual precocity-genetic bases of central precocious puberty and autonomous gonadal activation. *Endocr Dev.* (2016) 29:50–71. doi: 10.1159/000438874

53. Peltoketo H, Strauss L, Karjalainen R, Zhang M, Stamp GW, Segaloff DL, et al. Female mice expressing constitutively active mutants of FSH receptor present with a phenotype of premature follicle depletion and estrogen excess. *Endocrinology* (2010) 151:1872–83. doi: 10.1210/en.2009-0966

54. Zimmermann C, Stevant I, Borel C, Conne B, Pitetti JL, Calvel P, et al. Research resource: the dynamic transcriptional profile of sertoli cells during the progression of spermatogenesis. *Mol Endocrinol.* (2015) 29:627–42. doi: 10.1210/me.2014-1356

55. McLean DJ, Friel PJ, Pouchnik D, Griswold MD. Oligonucleotide microarray analysis of gene expression in follicle-stimulating hormone-treated rat Sertoli cells. *Mol Endocrinol.* (2002) 16:2780–92. doi: 10.1210/me.2002-0059

56. Sadate-Ngatchou PI, Pouchnik DJ, Griswold MD. Follicle-stimulating hormone induced changes in gene expression of murine testis. *Mol Endocrinol.* (2004) 18:2805–16. doi: 10.1210/me.2003-0203

57. Soffientini U, Rebourcet D, Abel MH, Lee S, Hamilton K, Fowler PA, et al. Identification of Sertoli cell-specific transcripts in the mouse testis and the role of FSH and androgen in the control of Sertoli cell activity. *BMC Genomics* (2017) 18:972. doi: 10.1186/s12864-017-4357-3

58. Godmann M, Katz JP, Guillou F, Simoni M, Kaestner KH, Behr R. Kruppel-like factor 4 is involved in functional differentiation of testicular Sertoli cells. *Dev Biol.* (2008) 315:552–66. doi: 10.1016/j.ydbio.2007.12.018

59. Sun H, Zhang G, Dong F, Wang F, Cao W. Reprogramming sertoli cells into pluripotent stem cells. *Cell Reprogram* (2014) 16:196–205. doi: 10.1089/cell.2013.0083

60. Myers M, Ebling FJ, Nwagwu M, Boulton R, Wadhwa K, Stewart J, et al. Atypical development of Sertoli cells and impairment of spermatogenesis in the hypogonadal (hpg) mouse. *J Anat.* (2005) 207:797–811. doi: 10.1111/j.1469-7580.2005.00493.x

61. Strothmann K, Simoni M, Mathur P, Siakhamary S, Nieschlag E, Gromoll J. Gene expression profiling of mouse Sertoli cell lines. *Cell Tissue Res.* (2004) 315:249–57. doi: 10.1007/s00441-003-0834-x

62. Sluka P, O'Donnell L, Bartles JR, Stanton PG. FSH regulates the formation of adherens junctions and ectoplasmic specialisations between rat Sertoli cells *in vitro* and *in vivo*. *J Endocrinol.* (2006) 189:381–95. doi: 10.1677/joe.1.06634

63. Stanton PG. Regulation of the blood-testis barrier. *Semin Cell Dev Biol.* (2016) 59:166–73. doi: 10.1016/j.semcdb.2016.06.018

64. Basu S, Arya SP, Usmani A, Pradhan BS, Sarkar RK, Ganguli N, et al. Defective Wnt3 expression by testicular Sertoli cells compromise male fertility. *Cell Tissue Res.* (2018) 371:351–63. doi: 10.1007/s00441-017-2698-5

65. Raverdeau M, Gely-Pernot A, Feret B, Dennefeld C, Benoit G, Davidson I, et al. Retinoic acid induces Sertoli cell paracrine signals for spermatogonia differentiation but cell autonomously drives spermatocyte meiosis. *Proc Natl Acad Sci USA.* (2012) 109:16582–7. doi: 10.1073/pnas.1214936109

66. Guo X, Morris P, Gudas L. Follicle-stimulating hormone and leukemia inhibitory factor regulate Sertoli cell retinol metabolism. *Endocrinology* (2001) 142:1024–32. doi: 10.1210/endo.142.3.7996

67. Santos NC, Kim KH. Activity of retinoic acid receptor-alpha is directly regulated at its protein kinase A sites in response to follicle-stimulating hormone signaling. *Endocrinology* (2010) 151:2361–72. doi: 10.1210/en.2009-1338

68. Billig H, Furuta I, Rivier C, Tapanainen J, Parvinen M, Hsueh AJ. Apoptosis in testis germ cells: developmental changes in gonadotropin dependence and localization to selective tubule stages. *Endocrinology* (1995) 136:5–12. doi: 10.1210/endo.136.1.7828558

69. Meachem SJ, Ruwanpura SM, Ziolkowski J, Ague JM, Skinner MK, Loveland KL. Developmentally distinct *in vivo* effects of FSH on proliferation and apoptosis during testis maturation. *J Endocrinol.* (2005) 186:429–46. doi: 10.1677/joe.1.06121

70. Rodriguez I, Ody C, Araki K, Garcia I, Vassalli P. An early and massive wave of germinal cell apoptosis is required for the development of functional spermatogenesis. *EMBO J.* (1997) 16:2262–70. doi: 10.1093/emboj/16.9.2262

71. Regueira M, Riera MF, Galardo MN, Camberos Mdel C, Pellizzari EH, Cigorraga SB, et al. FSH and bFGF regulate the expression of genes involved in Sertoli cell energetic metabolism. *Gen Comp Endocrinol.* (2015) 222:124–33. doi: 10.1016/j.ygcen.2015.08.011

72. Yeung CH, Callies C, Tuttelmann F, Kliesch S, Cooper TG. Aquaporins in the human testis and spermatozoa - identification, involvement in sperm volume regulation and clinical relevance. *Int J Androl.* (2010) 33:629–41. doi: 10.1111/j.1365-2605.2009.00998.x

73. Huhtaniemi I. A short evolutionary history of FSH-stimulated spermatogenesis. *Hormones* (2015) 14:468–78. doi: 10.14310/horm.2002.1632

74. Bartlett JM, Kerr JB, Sharpe RM. The effect of selective destruction and regeneration of rat Leydig cells on the intratesticular distribution of testosterone and morphology of the seminiferous epithelium. *J Androl.* (1986) 7:240–53. doi: 10.1002/j.1939-4640.1986.tb00924.x

75. Lei ZM, Mishra S, Zou W, Xu B, Foltz M, Li X, et al. Targeted disruption of luteinizing hormone/human chorionic gonadotropin receptor gene. *Mol Endocrinol.* (2001) 15:184–200. doi: 10.1210/mend.15.1.0586

76. Russell LD, Clermont Y. Degeneration of germ cells in normal, hypophysectomized and hormone treated hypophysectomized rats. *Anat Rec.* (1977) 187:347–66. doi: 10.1002/ar.1091870307

77. Zhang FP, Poutanen M, Wilbertz J, Huhtaniemi I. Normal prenatal but arrested postnatal sexual development of luteinizing hormone receptor knockout (LuRKO) mice. *Mol Endocrinol.* (2001) 15:172–83. doi: 10.1210/mend.15.1.0582

78. Chang C, Chen YT, Yeh SD, Xu Q, Wang RS, Guillou F, et al. Infertility with defective spermatogenesis and hypotestosteronemia in male mice lacking the androgen receptor in Sertoli cells. *Proc Natl Acad Sci USA.* (2004) 101:6876–81. doi: 10.1073/pnas.0307306101

79. De Gendt K, Swinnen JV, Saunders PT, Schoonjans L, Dewerchin M, Devos A, et al. A Sertoli cell-selective knockout of the androgen receptor causes spermatogenic arrest in meiosis. *Proc Natl Acad Sci USA.* (2004) 101:1327–32. doi: 10.1073/pnas.0308114100

80. Huhtaniemi I, Nikula H, Rannikko S. Pituitary-testicular function of prostatic cancer patients during treatment with a gonadotropin-releasing hormone agonist analog. I. Circulating hormone levels. *J Androl.* (1987) 8:355–62. doi: 10.1002/j.1939-4640.1987.tb00975.x

81. Jarow JP, Chen H, Rosner TW, Trentacoste S, Zirkin BR. Assessment of the androgen environment within the human testis: minimally invasive method to obtain intratesticular fluid. *J Androl*. (2001) 22:640–5. doi: 10.1002/j.1939-4640.2001.tb02224.x

82. Roth MY, Lin K, Amory JK, Matsumoto AM, Anawalt BD, Snyder CN, et al. Serum LH correlates highly with intratesticular steroid levels in normal men. *J Androl*. (2010) 31:138–45. doi: 10.2164/jandrol.109.008391

83. Singh J, O'Neill C, Handelsman DJ. Induction of spermatogenesis by androgens in gonadotropin-deficient (hpg) mice. *Endocrinology* (1995) 136:5311–21. doi: 10.1210/endo.136.12.7588276

84. Cunningham GR, Huckins C. Persistence of complete spermatogenesis in the presence of low intratesticular concentrations of testosterone. *Endocrinology* (1979) 105:177–86. doi: 10.1210/endo-105-1-177

85. Santulli R, Sprando RL, Awoniyi CA, Ewing LL, Zirkin BR. To what extent can spermatogenesis be maintained in the hypophysectomized adult rat testis with exogenously administered testosterone? *Endocrinology* (1990) 126:95–101. doi: 10.1210/endo-126-1-95

86. Sun YT, Irby DC, Robertson DM, de Kretser DM. The effects of exogenously administered testosterone on spermatogenesis in intact and hypophysectomized rats. *Endocrinology* (1989) 125:1000–10. doi: 10.1210/endo-125-2-1000

87. Spaliviero JA, Jimenez M, Allan CM, Handelsman DJ. Luteinizing hormone receptor-mediated effects on initiation of spermatogenesis in gonadotropin-deficient (hpg) mice are replicated by testosterone. *Biol Reprod*. (2004) 70:32–8. doi: 10.1095/biolreprod.103.019398

88. Oduwole OO, Vydra N, Wood NE, Samanta L, Owen L, Keevil B, et al. Overlapping dose responses of spermatogenic and extragonadal testosterone actions jeopardize the principle of hormonal male contraception. *FASEB J*. (2014) 28:2566–76. doi: 10.1096/fj.13-249219

89. Pakarainen T, Zhang FP, Makela S, Poutanen M, Huhtaniemi I. Testosterone replacement therapy induces spermatogenesis and partially restores fertility in luteinizing hormone receptor knockout mice. *Endocrinology* (2005) 146:596–606. doi: 10.1210/en.2004-0913

90. Bruysters M, Christin-Maitre S, Verhoef-Post M, Sultan C, Auger J, Faugeron I, et al. A new LH receptor splice mutation responsible for male hypogonadism with subnormal sperm production in the propositus, and infertility with regular cycles in an affected sister. *Hum Reprod*. (2008) 23:1917–23. doi: 10.1093/humrep/den180

91. Achard C, Courtillot C, Lahuna O, Meduri G, Soufir JC, Liere P, et al. Normal spermatogenesis in a man with mutant luteinizing hormone. *N Engl J Med*. (2009) 361:1856–63. doi: 10.1056/NEJMoa0805792

92. Buchter D, Behre HM, Kliesch S, Nieschlag E. Pulsatile GnRH or human chorionic gonadotropin/human menopausal gonadotropin as effective treatment for men with hypogonadotropic hypogonadism: a review of 42 cases. *Eur J Endocrinol*. (1998) 139:298–303. doi: 10.1530/eje.0.1390298

93. Burgues S, Calderon MD. Subcutaneous self-administration of highly purified follicle stimulating hormone and human chorionic gonadotrophin for the treatment of male hypogonadotrophic hypogonadism. Spanish collaborative group on male hypogonadotropic hypogonadism. *Hum Reprod*. (1997) 12:980–6. doi: 10.1093/humrep/12.5.980

94. Nieschlag E, Buchter D, Von Eckardstein S, Abshagen K, Simoni M, Behre HM. Repeated intramuscular injections of testosterone undecanoate for substitution therapy in hypogonadal men. *Clin Endocrinol*. (1999) 51:757–63. doi: 10.1046/j.1365-2265.1999.00881.x

95. Plant TM, Marshall GR. The functional significance of FSH in spermatogenesis and the control of its secretion in male primates. *Endocr Rev*. (2001) 22:764–86. doi: 10.1210/edrv.22.6.0446

96. Walker WH, Cheng J. FSH and testosterone signaling in Sertoli cells. *Reproduction* (2005) 130:15–28. doi: 10.1530/rep.1.00358

97. Toocheck C, Clister T, Shupe J, Crum C, Ravindranathan P, Lee TK, et al. Mouse spermatogenesis requires classical and nonclassical testosterone signaling. *Biol Reprod*. (2016) 94:11. doi: 10.1095/biolreprod.115.132068

98. Gorczynska E, Handelsman DJ. Androgens rapidly increase the cytosolic calcium concentration in Sertoli cells. *Endocrinology* (1995) 136:2052–9. doi: 10.1210/endo.136.5.7720654

99. Lyng FM, Jones GR, Rommerts FF. Rapid androgen actions on calcium signaling in rat sertoli cells and two human prostatic cell lines: similar biphasic responses between 1 picomolar and 100 nanomolar concentrations. *Biol Reprod*. (2000) 63:736–47. doi: 10.1095/biolreprod63.3.736

100. Rastrelli G, Corona G, Mannucci E, Maggi M. Factors affecting spermatogenesis upon gonadotropin-replacement therapy: a meta-analytic study. *Andrology* (2014) 2:794–808. doi: 10.1111/andr.262

101. Attia AM, Abou-Setta AM, Al-Inany HG. Gonadotrophins for idiopathic male factor subfertility. *Cochrane Database Syst Rev*. (2013) 8:CD005071. doi: 10.1002/14651858.CD005071.pub4

102. Santi D, Granata AR, Simoni M. FSH treatment of male idiopathic infertility improves pregnancy rate: a meta-analysis. *Endocr Connect*. (2015) 4:R46–58. doi: 10.1530/EC-15-0050

103. Valenti D, La Vignera S, Condorelli RA, Rago R, Barone N, Vicari E, et al. Follicle-stimulating hormone treatment in normogonadotropic infertile men. *Nat Rev Urol*. (2013) 10:55–62. doi: 10.1038/nrurol.2012.234

104. Colacurci N, De Leo V, Ruvolo G, Piomboni P, Caprio F, Pivonello R, et al. Recombinant FSH improves sperm DNA damage in male infertility: a phase II clinical trial. *Front Endocrinol*. (2018) 9:383. doi: 10.3389/fendo.2018.00383

105. Simoni M, Santi D, Negri L, Hoffmann I, Muratori M, Baldi E, et al. Treatment with human, recombinant FSH improves sperm DNA fragmentation in idiopathic infertile men depending on the FSH receptor polymorphism p.N680S: a pharmacogenetic study. *Hum Reprod*. (2016) 31:1960–9. doi: 10.1093/humrep/dew167

106. Selice R, Garolla A, Pengo M, Caretta N, Ferlin A, Foresta C. The response to FSH treatment in oligozoospermic men depends on FSH receptor gene polymorphisms. *Int J Androl*. (2011) 34:306–12. doi: 10.1111/j.1365-2605.2010.01086.x

107. Ding YM, Zhang XJ, Li JP, Chen SS, Zhang RT, Tan WL, et al. Treatment of idiopathic oligozoospermia with recombinant human follicle-stimulating hormone: a prospective, randomized, double-blind, placebo-controlled clinical study in Chinese population. *Clin Endocrinol*. (2015) 83:866–71. doi: 10.1111/cen.12770

15

In Vivo and In Vitro Impact of Carbohydrate Variation on Human Follicle-Stimulating Hormone Function

George R. Bousfield[1]*, Jeffrey V. May[1], John S. Davis[2,3,4], James A. Dias[5]
and T. Rajendra Kumar[6]

[1] Department of Biological Sciences, Wichita State University, Wichita, KS, United States, [2] Department of Obstetrics and Gynecology, University of Nebraska Medical Center, Omaha, NE, United States, [3] Department of Biochemistry and Molecular Biology, University of Nebraska Medical Center, Omaha, NE, United States, [4] Nebraska-Western Iowa Health Care System, Omaha, NE, United States, [5] Department of Biomedical Sciences, School of Public Health, University at Albany, Albany, NY, United States, [6] Department of Obstetrics and Gynecology, University of Colorado Anschutz Medical Campus, Aurora, CO, United States

*Correspondence:
George R. Bousfield
george.bousfield@wichita.edu

Human follicle-stimulating hormone (FSH) exhibits both macro- and microheterogeneity in its carbohydrate moieties. Macroheterogeneity results in three physiologically relevant FSHβ subunit variants, two that possess a single N-linked glycan at either one of the two βL1 loop glycosylation sites or one with both glycans. Microheterogeneity is characterized by 80 to over 100 unique oligosaccharide structures attached to each of the 3 to 4 occupied N-glycosylation sites. With respect to its receptor, partially glycosylated (hypoglycosylated) FSH variants exhibit higher association rates, greater apparent affinity, and greater occupancy than fully glycosylated FSH. Higher receptor binding-activity is reflected by greater *in vitro* bioactivity and, in some cases, greater *in vivo* bioactivity. Partially glycosylated pituitary FSH shows an age-related decline in abundance that may be associated with decreased fertility. In this review, we describe an integrated approach involving genetic models, *in vitro* signaling studies, FSH biochemistry, relevance of physiological changes in FSH glycoform abundance, and characterize the impact of FSH macroheterogeneity on fertility and reproductive aging. We will also address the controversy with regard to claims of a direct action of FSH in mediating bone loss especially at the peri- and postmenopausal stages.

Keywords: pituitary, N-glycosylation, follicle-stimulating hormone, bone, female Infertility

STRUCTURAL ATTRIBUTES OF FOLLICLE-STIMULATING HORMONE (FSH) AND ITS SUBUNITS

Follicle-stimulating hormone is one of three gonadotropins in the human glycoprotein hormone family. This hormone family is part of the cystine knot growth factor superfamily, a large group of homo- and heterodimeric signaling molecules (1). FSH plays a central role in reproduction, particularly in females. In the ovary, FSH stimulates follicle development and estrogen synthesis. In the testis, FSH maintains Sertoli cell function, which supports spermatogenesis. Although currently controversial (2, 3), FSH has been claimed to play a direct role in osteoporosis by stimulating differentiation of osteoclasts, which are responsible for removing bone (4). The idea put forth is that in the postmenopausal period when FSH levels rise, activation of osteoclasts results in bone loss. Reports of non-gonadal actions of FSH have recently been summarized (5).

Follicle-stimulating hormone is composed of two dissimilar, cystine knot motif glycoprotein subunits: a common α-subunit and hormone-specific β-subunit (**Figure 1**) (6). The FSHα subunit amino-acid sequence and disulfide bond organization, including a cystine knot motif, are identical to those in the other glycoprotein hormones, luteinizing hormone (LH), thyroid-stimulating hormone (TSH), and chorionic gonadotropin (CG) (7). However, the N-glycan populations at both glycosylated residues, Asn^{52} and Asn^{78}, differ from those of the other glycoprotein hormone α-subunits such that these otherwise identical subunits can be distinguished from each other and from free α-subunit by their oligosaccharide populations (8–10). The hormone-specific FSHβ subunit shares 34–40% sequence homology, six conserved disulfide bonds, cystine knot motif, and seatbelt loop with the other human glycoprotein hormone β-subunits (7, 11, 12). While there are two potential N-glycosylation sites in FSHβ, partially glycosylated variants exist that are missing either one of these oligosaccharides (13). These contribute to an unknown degree of charge variation in FSH preparations and result in the classic FSH isoforms (14, 15). The classic interpretation of FSH isoforms was based solely on the notion that variant patterns of negatively charged sialic acid or, to a much lesser extent, sulfate residues terminated oligosaccharide branches, which gave rise to differentially charged isoforms. The observation of hypo-glycosylation further refines our understanding of isoforms, in that net charge may vary, due to presence or absence of entire glycans.

FSH GLYCOSYLATION HETEROGENEITY

Follicle-stimulating hormone glycosylation exhibits both macro- and microheterogeneity (**Table 1**). Macroheterogeneity herein refers to the presence or absence of glycosylation at any one potential glycosylation site. Examples of FSH macroheterogeneity involve the absence of either FSHβ Asn^7 or Asn^{24} oligosaccharides in a population of fully processed and secreted FSH. Microheterogeneity herein refers to as many as 80 to over 100 unique oligosaccharide structures, which can be detected once released from each of the 3–4 glycan-occupied Asn residues in FSH.

Differences in electrophoretic mobility of FSH subunits, revealed by subunit-specific Western blots, provide a convenient means to distinguish four FSH variants resulting from macroheterogeneity. Fully glycosylated hFSHβ migrates as a 24-kDa band (hereinafter, 24k-FSHβ), $desN^{24}$glycan-FSHβ migrates as a 21-kDa band (21k-FSHβ), and $desN^7$glycan-FSHβ migrates as an 18-kDa band (18k-FSHβ). The FSH heterodimers that incorporate these β-subunit variants are designated, FSH^{24}, FSH^{21}, and FSH^{18}, respectively (19), and are shown in **Figure 2**. Pituitary extracts also possess a non-glycosylated, 15-kDa FSHβ variant (20). However, the corresponding FSH^{15} does not appear to be physiologically relevant, because subunit association is extremely inefficient when both FSHβ glycans are missing, and little, if any, FSH heterodimer is secreted (21). FSH^{24} and FSH^{21} are detected in FSH derived from human pituitary extracts, as well as from urinary protein preparations (**Table 1**). When FSH is separated into fully- and hypo-glycosylated fractions, the latter often include FSH^{18}, which can constitute as much as 40% of the hypo-glycosylated FSH preparation (13). As most $hFSH^{21}$ preparations also possess $hFSH^{18}$, and are not easily separated, it has become a convention to abbreviate the mixture of physiologically relevant hypo-glycosylated FSH preparations as $hFSH^{21/18}$.

Follicle-stimulating hormone microheterogeneity results from a structurally heterogeneous population of oligosaccharides attached to each glycosylated Asn residue of the four glycosylation sequons in FSH. Microheterogeneity in this hormone has largely been evaluated at the whole hormone level in studies of pituitary and urinary FSH preparations (16, 22–25). Human pituitary FSH oligosaccharides are 85–98% complex-type, 88–99% are sialylated, 36–46% are biantennary, 30–49% are triantennary, 5–15% are tetra-antennary, while only 4–7% are sulfated (**Table 1**). The low extent of oligosaccharide sulfation appears to be a human-specific characteristic (no data exist for nonhuman primate FSH glycans), as FSH preparations from cattle, pigs, sheep, and horses possess higher levels of sulfated oligosaccharides, ranging from 13 to 58% (23, 26). Accordingly, a major factor in determining hFSH clearance rates is the extent of sialic acid termination at the non-reducing ends of oligosaccharide branches. As compared with naturally occurring hFSH preparations, recombinant hFSH preparation oligosaccharides exhibit a reduced degree of branching, consisting of largely (55%) biantennary glycans. However, the degree of sialylation in these preparations lags that of urinary hFSH to a lesser extent, because the most abundant urinary FSH triantennary and tetra-antennary glycans are one sialic acid residue short of a full complement (16, 25, 27).

As mentioned above, microheterogeneity contributes to charge variation in FSH, and this has been reported to alter FSH biological activity (14, 28, 29). Comparisons of microheterogeneity in early studies were challenged not only by the large number of oligosaccharide structures encountered, but also by the different

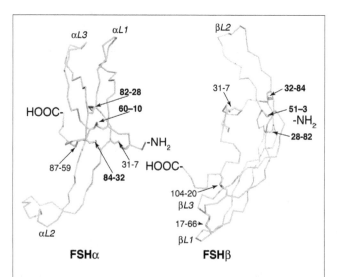

FIGURE 1 | Follicle-stimulating hormone (FSH) subunit peptide moieties. Wire-frame models of FSH subunits extracted from pdb 1FL7 using MacPyMOL v1.8.2.3. FSHα backbone is green and FSHβ backbone is cyan. Disulfide bonds are indicated as yellow sticks. Cystine knot loops are designated by subunit (α or β) and number (1–3). Pairs of numbers refer to Cys residues involved in a disulfide bond. Bold numbers indicate Cys Knot disulfide bonds.

TABLE 1 | Macro- and microheterogeneity of hFSH preparations.

FSH preparation	Macroheterogeneity (% relative abundance)						
	Pituitary hFSH	Urinary hFSH	Pituitary hFSH[24]	Pituitary hFSH[21]	Pituitary hFSH[21/18]	Recombinant GH$_3$ hFSH[24]	Recombinant GH$_3$ hFSH[21]
FSH[24]	77	86	100	–	–	89	–
FSH[21]	23	14	–	100	60	11	54
FSH[18]	–[a]	–	–	–	40	–	46
FSH[15]	–	–	–	–	–	–	–

Oligosaccharide type	Types of oligosaccharides (% relative abundance)					
						Recombinant GH$_3$-hFSH[b]
Biantennary	38.2	37.2	47.1	51.2	28.6	55.5
Triantennary(3)[c]	41.0	44.0	30.7	35.9	2.5	0
Triantennary(6)[d]	0	0	0	0	0	29.7
Tetra-antennary	15.0	14.8	10.6	6.0	0.01	0
Neutral	0.3	2.2	9.9	4.5	74.2	12.3
Sialylated	99.1	97.5	75.4	78.8	20.7	87.7
Sulfated	6.5	4.2	39.3	35.0	9.6	0
Sial/sulfat	5.9	3.9	24.0	18.3	4.5	0
Core fucose	43.0	23.9	45.1	47.8	23.0	50.6
Antenna-fucose	0.3	0	3.6	0.8	0.4	19.9
Bisect GlcNAc	32.6	23.9	17.9	23.2	7.9	47.0
GalNAc	2.8	1.7	20.3	13.8	14.1	10.5

Relative abundance determined by Western blot and mass spectrometry, respectively. Data are limited to those preparations for which both glycoform abundance and glycan microheterogeneity exist.
[a]– = not detected.
[b] = glycoforms not separated.
[c]Triantennary(3) = third branch attached to Man(α1–3) branch.
[d]Triantennary(6) = third branch attached to Man(α1–6) branch.
Data derived from Ref. (16–18). FSH, follicle-stimulating hormone.

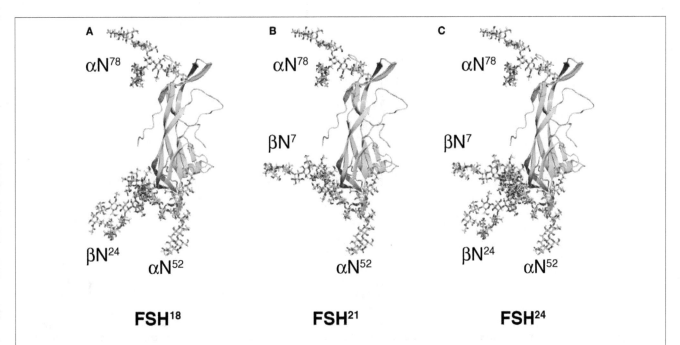

FIGURE 2 | Follicle-stimulating hormone (FSH) glycoform models. Models of FSH heterodimers extracted from pdb 4AY9 decorated with the most abundant glycan observed at each N-glycosylation site by nano-ESI-ion mobility-MS (Bousfield, G. R. and Harvey, D. J., unpublished). Subunits are shown as cartoons rendered by MacPyMOL with subunits and their oligosaccharides colored as in **Figure 1**; FSHα green and FSHβ cyan. Oligosaccharides shown as sticks were created and attached to the FSH model using GLYCAM [Woods Group. (2005–2017) GLYCAM Web. Complex Carbohydrate Research Center, University of Georgia, Athens, GA, USA. (http://glycam.org)]. **(A)** FSH[18], which lacks Asn[24] glycan. **(B)** FSH[21], which lacks Asn[7] glycan. **(C)** FSH[24], which possesses all four N-glycans.

analytical methods each group employed, as each of these exhibited bias toward or against specific families of oligosaccharides. We recently characterized microheterogeneity in three purified human pituitary FSH glycoform preparations, as well as highly purified pituitary, urinary, and recombinant hFSH preparations using nano-electrospray mass spectrometry (13, 16–18). Because over 33–109 structures were detected in each sample, comparing oligosaccharide populations derived from different FSH preparations proved challenging.

The oligosaccharide structures shown in **Figure 3** represent those present in at least 1% relative abundance in at least FSH preparation. Using this criterion, a total of 54 glycans were selected for comparison. The glycans are organized by position in the N-glycan biosynthetic pathway or by the number of complex branches. Within each antennary group, 2-, 3-, or 4-branch glycans, monosaccharide composition is the basis of organization. Structures 1–7 are oligomannose glycan intermediates found in ER and *cis*Golgi-derived glycoprotein precursors (**Figure 3A**). In multi-glycosylation site glycoproteins, these can be found in glycoproteins possessing mature glycans at other sites, when glycan processing at individual sites differs (30). Structures 8 and 9 exhibit the beginnings of complex oligosaccharide synthesis (**Figure 3A**), structures 10–34 are biantennary glycans (**Figures 3A–C**), structures 35–48 are triantennary glycans (**Figures 3C,D**), and structures 49–54 are tetra-antennary glycans (**Figure 3D**). The oligosaccharide populations of fully

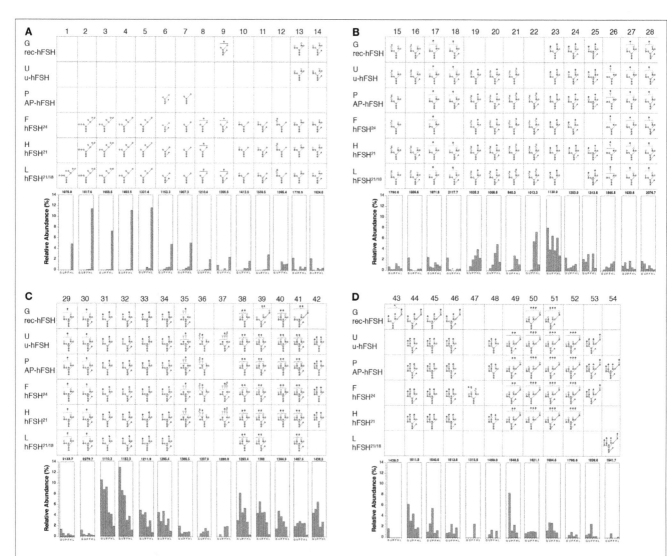

FIGURE 3 | Human follicle-stimulating hormone (FSH) oligosaccharide microheterogeneity. Summary of results of nano-ESI mass spectrometry studies showing only those oligosaccharides present at >1% relative abundance in at least one hFSH preparation. The glycan diagram indicates it was detected in the preparation. The Consortium for Functional Glycomics monosaccharide symbols are used in conjunction with Oxford Glycobiology Institute linkage indicators (1–2, −; 1–3, \; 1–4, |; 1–6,/; solid lines indicate β-linkage and dashed lines indicate α-linkage). The bar graphs at the bottom of each panel indicate the relative abundance of the structure in each preparation. The preparations are indicated by single letters as follows: G is GH₃-recombinant hFSH; U is urinary hFSH; P is pituitary hFSH; F is fully glycosylated pituitary hFSH²⁴; H is hypo-glycosylated pituitary hFSH²¹/¹⁸; and L is hFSH²¹/¹⁸ isolated from hLH preparations. The structures are distributed across four panels beginning with the high mannose precursors and ending with tetra-antennary oligosaccharides, the largest found in hFSH. **(A)** Structures 1–14. **(B)** Structures 15–28. **(C)** Structures 29–42. **(D)** Structures 43–54.

glycosylated FSH[24] and hypo-glycosylated FSH[21] preparations, F and D, respectively, possessed 51 of the 54 major glycans identified in these studies, and 45 of these, representing 88% of these more abundant glycans, were detected in both preparations. Pituitary and urinary FSH preparations P and U, respectively, both possessed 38 glycans (75%) in common with glycoforms F and D, while the hypo-glycosylated hFSH[21/18] preparation L, possessed 35 glycans (68%) found in glycoform preparations F and D. Recombinant hFSH preparation G, expressed by stably transfected GH₃ cells, displayed the lowest qualitative similarity to FSH[24] and FSH[21], possessing only 28 (55%) of the glycans found in glycoforms F and D. Moreover, the triantennary recombinant hFSH oligosaccharides displayed a different branching pattern.

Raising the cutoff to 4% relative abundance identified four groups of highly abundant glycans. The first group revealed a unique pattern of glycosylation for hFSH[21/18] preparation L, consisting of a series of high mannose oligosaccharide intermediates possessing 9, 8, 7, 6, 5, and 3 mannose residues (structures 1–7, **Figure 3A**). Taken in isolation, this observation suggests that these glycoforms may not have exited the biosynthetic pathway. However, complex oligosaccharides, identical to those found in all other FSH preparations examined in this study, were also present in hFSH-L, suggesting oligosaccharide processing occurred at least at one glycosylation site in the Golgi. Glycosylation site-specific glycan analysis, when sufficient samples are available, or top–down proteomics for limited samples, have the potential to demonstrate the presence of both oligomannose and complex glycans in the same hypo-glycosylated hFSH molecule to support this hypothesis. Oligosaccharide structures 2–7 were also found in two pituitary glycoform preparations, hFSH[24] and hFSH[21]. However, in both cases, these glycans were present in very low abundance, consistent with their being N-glycan biosynthetic intermediates. Moreover, both secreted hFSH preparations, urinary hFSH and recombinant hFSH, were devoid of oligomannose structures 1–7. In the case of urinary hFSH, this could have

resulted either from rapid clearance of oligomannose-containing hFSH from the circulation or bias during purification.

As only secreted recombinant hFSH was recovered from conditioned medium, the absence of oligomannose glycans indicated that mature hFSH secreted by the GH₃ cell line possessed only complex N-glycans. Moreover, the antibody used to capture recombinant hFSH appeared to capture all FSH forms, reducing the likelihood of purification biasing the oligosaccharide population (13). The high abundance of biosynthetic intermediate and low abundance of complex glycans in hFSH[21/18] preparation L was notable because it exhibited the highest receptor binding-activity of any hFSH preparation we have studied. This led to the concern that we were studying a physiologically irrelevant glycoform. However, subsequent demonstration of significant biological activity differences between other pituitary and recombinant FSH glycoform preparations eliminated this concern (18, 31, 32).

Three clusters of high-abundance, complex glycans were noted in the other five hFSH preparations comprising oligosaccharide structures 22–23, 31–34, and 38–42. Group 2 structure 23, a disialylated, biantennary glycan possessing one GalNAc substituted for Gal, was highly abundant in all five preparations. This was notable, because the absence of sulfated GalNAc from hFSH N-glycans has been attributed to impaired recognition of a Pro-Leu-Arg motif in the common α-subunit of hFSH by β1, 4-N-acetylgalactosaminyltransferase-T3 and -T4 (βGalNAct-T3 and βGalNAc-T4, respectively), as compared with hCG and hLH. The resulting reduction in FSH oligosaccharide sulfation was proposed as a consequence of altered motif access in this hormone, probably due to conformational change (33).

Comparison of Pro-Leu-Arg motifs in both hCG crystal structures, 1hcn (12) and 1hrp (11), with those in the two hFSH structures found in 1fl7 (6) showed positions of the Pro⁴⁰ and Leu⁴¹ residue side chains were very similar in all six possible alignments (**Figure 4**). The Arg⁴² side chains were closely aligned in only one comparison, u-hCGα2:r-hFSHα1 (**Figure 4D**),

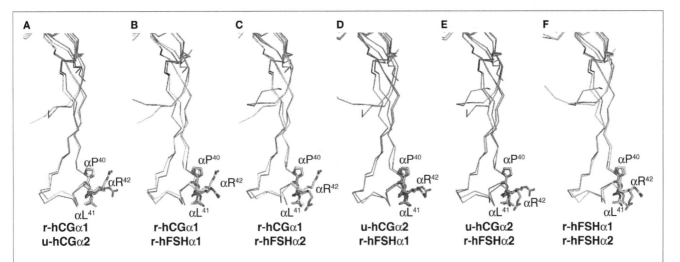

FIGURE 4 | Comparison of Pro-Leu-Arg motif in hCG and follicle-stimulating hormone (FSH) crystal structures. Cystine knot loop αL2 in the common α-subunits from each hormone structure were aligned using MacPyMOL. The backbone traces are shown and the side chains for Pro⁴⁰, Leu⁴¹, and Arg⁴² shown as sticks. The residues are labeled because the flattening effect of printing appears to invert the order of Leu⁴¹ and Arg⁴². Chemically deglycosylated recombinant selenomethionine hCGα is r-hCGα1 (1hcn), chemically deglycosylated urinary hCGα is u-hCGα2 (1hrp), recombinant insect cell hFSH (1fl7) resulted in two models identified as r-hFSHα1 and r-hFSHα2, respectively. **(A–F)** α-subunit models aligned as indicated.

suggesting flexibility in that region of the subunit (6, 34). Indeed, molecular dynamics simulations of FSH bound and unbound to the FSH receptor (FSHR) high-affinity binding site support flexibility in residue 40–47 region as unbound FSH exhibits root mean square fluctuations >1 Å (35). Unbound FSH is the form of the heterodimer recognized by β4GalNAc transferases. When FSH is bound to FSHR, this region loses flexibility, indicating it can achieve a stable conformation when bound to another protein. Thus, pituitary βGalNAc transferases are likely to bind this motif in both hLH and hFSH, consistent with the widespread distribution of GalNAc in hFSH oligosaccharides. The frequent appearance of GalNAc in sulfate-deficient glycans suggests an alternative hypothesis to explain reduced sulfation; human sialyltransferases compete more effectively with sulfotransferase in the human pituitary, leading to preferential addition of Neu5Ac to GalNAc. As N-glycan branches terminated with Neu5Ac-GalNAc were first reported for hLH oligosaccharides, finding this type of glycan is not unprecedented (36).

In fact, hLH possesses the greatest abundance of sialic acid of all characterized mammalian LH preparations (23, 36, 37). Moreover, structure 23 is part of a series of 15 GalNAc-containing, biantennary glycans observed in at least one of the six hFSH preparations (structures 10–25, **Figures 3A,B**). While two other structures are possible for the *m/z* 1130.9 ion associated with structure 23 (17), they do not permit addition of the two sialic acid residues associated with this oligosaccharide because the 5th hexosamine in the alternative structures is a bisecting GlcNAc residue and the single antenna possessing a Gal residue provides attachment for only one Neu5Ac residue. Group 3 glycan structures 31–34, are conventional, disialylated, biantennary oligosaccharides in which Neu5Ac residues are attached to Gal residues (**Figure 3C**). Structures 31 and 32 were the most abundant oligosaccharides derived from recombinant, urinary, and pituitary hFSH (**Figure 3C**). As 85–100% core-fucosylated glycans are found on the other human pituitary hormone LHβ and TSHβ subunits, structure

31 most likely reflects FSHα subunit glycosylation, while structure 32 reflects FSHβ subunit glycosylation (36, 38). The 4th high abundance glycan cluster, comprising structures 38–42, includes triantennary oligosaccharides possessing only two sialic acid residues. For this group of oligosaccharides, recombinant hFSH differed in the location of the two branch-mannose residues. In pituitary hFSH, GlcNAc transferase IV initiated a third glycan branch on Man (α1–3), while in recombinant hFSH GlcNAc transferase V initiated a third branch on Man (α1–6) (**Figure 3C**, compare row G with the other five rows). This suggested a difference in the relative activities of GlcNAc transferases IV and V between pituitary gonadotropes and somatotrope-derived GH₃ cells, despite the expression of both transferase genes in GH₃ cells (18). Another feature of recombinant hFSH glycans was antenna-linked fucose residues, such as observed in structure 43, one of the >1% abundance class of oligosaccharides (18).

IMPACT OF FSH GLYCOSYLATION HETEROGENEITY ON COGNATE RECEPTOR BINDING

The FSHR is a G-protein-coupled receptor (GPCR) with a leucine-rich repeat extracellular domain comprising 358 amino-acid residues. This ligand binding domain is connected to a 337-residue, hepta-helical transmembrane domain (39, 40). Crystal structures of the high-affinity FSH binding domain in complex with FSH revealed that the interface of the complex involves contacts exclusively *via* protein–protein interactions (41, 42). FSH oligosaccharides added by modeling do not appear to interact with the extracellular domain engaged with FSH, as they are located on a face of the hormone, which is oriented away from the hormone receptor interface (**Figure 5**). Since it is well established that FSH carbohydrate is necessary for full FSHR activation (43–46), it seems reasonable to assume that

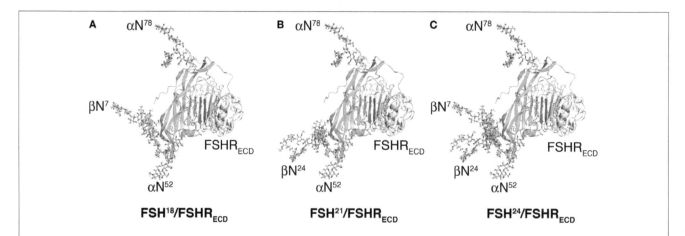

FIGURE 5 | Follicle-stimulating hormone (FSH) glycoform models bound to monomeric FSH receptor (FSHR) extracelluar domain model (FSHR_ECD). FSH glycoform models are oriented as in **Figure 2**. The FSHR_ECD model was extracted from pdb 4AY9 and rendered as cartoon using MacPyMOL. The FSH glycoform models were aligned to the FSH model extracted from the pdb file along with the FSHR_ECD to illustrate the positions of oligosaccharides relative to the high-affinity binding site in the FSHR. **(A)** Glycosylated model of FSH¹⁸ and FSHR extracellular domain. **(B)** Glycosylated model of FSH²¹ and FSHR extracellular domain. **(C)** Glycosylated model of FSH²⁴ and FSHR extracellular domain.

the carbohydrate affects hormone conformation, which in turn modulates activity. The structure of the entire FSHR (extracellular domain and transmembrane domains) in complex with FSH has yet to be determined, and until then, carbohydrate interaction with the transmembrane domain cannot be ruled out. Alternatively, carbohydrate modulation of FSH conformation may affect the final disposition of FSHR extracellular domain (FSHR$_{ECD}$) hinge region putative interactions with extracellular loops of the transmembrane domains (34, 47). Consistent with the absence of FSH carbohydrate interaction with FSHR$_{ECD}$, isolated hybrid-type oligosaccharides related to structure 12 in **Figure 3** have no effect on FSHR binding (48). Nevertheless, these oligosaccharides significantly inhibit both basal granulosa cell steroidogenesis, as well as FSH-stimulated steroidogenesis (48). The low affinity of carbohydrate–protein interactions requires sufficiently high oligosaccharide concentrations in inhibition studies that hormone contamination can inhibit binding assays. In our hands, a minimum of two purification steps is necessary to eliminate residual hormone assay interference (48). Accordingly, we attributed hormone contamination in the oligosaccharide preparation as the reason for a report that hCG-derived oligosaccharides inhibited both receptor binding and cellular activation (49).

Loss of a single FSHβ oligosaccharide has three effects on FSH binding to its receptor. First, hypo-glycosylated hFSH immediately engages FSHR preparations, whereas fully glycosylated hFSH^{24} exhibits about a 30-min lag before FSHR binding begins in earnest (13). Second, hypo-glycosylated hFSH$^{21/18}$ exhibits a 2.8- to over 14-fold higher apparent affinity for the FSHR as compared with hFSH^{24} (**Table 2**). Third, hypo-glycosylated hFSH$^{21/18}$ occupies 2- to threefold more FSHRs than FSH^{24} (13, 18). A glance at the structures of FSH glycoforms bound to the FSHR$_{ECD}$ immediately raises the question of how loss of either FSHβ N-glycan facilitates FSH association with the receptor, as neither glycan is close to the binding site (**Figure 5**). This leaves yet to be defined hindrance by the FSHR transmembrane domain or FSHR oligomerization as potential mechanisms.

The crystal structure of the high-affinity binding site of the FSHR$_{ECD}$ comprised two FSHR domains associated back to back, sandwiched by FSH ligands (41). There was no indication of FSH oligosaccharide interaction with the receptor. The crystal structure of the entire FSHR$_{ECD}$ with FSH bound revealed a strikingly different FSHR$_{ECD}$ conformation as trimeric FSHR–FSH complexes (42). To obtain diffractable crystals in both studies, endoglycosidase-F digestion reduced FSH and FSHR$_{ECD}$ N-glycans to single GlcNAc residues, which eliminated oligosaccharide influence on hormone-receptor binding. The trimeric

FSHR crystal structure suggested FSH αAsn^{52} oligosaccharide, when present, would restrict ligand binding to one glycosylated FSH ligand per FSHR trimer as a biantennary glycan attached to this Asn residue would occupy the center of the trimeric complex (47). While no subsequent studies supporting the dimeric FSHR model have been reported, several lines of evidence appear to support the trimeric FSHR$_{ECD}$ model. Biochemical data in support of the trimeric FSHR model were provided when recombinant-mutant des-αN^{52}-hFSH exhibited threefold greater binding to CHO cells expressing hFSHRs as compared with recombinant wt-hFSH (47). Small molecule allosteric FSHR modulators were reported to increase FSH binding ~threefold, suggesting trimeric FSHR complexes dissociating to form FSHR monomers (50–52). Incorporating a transmembrane domain model to the FSHR$_{ECD}$ trimer model predicted that only a single β-arrestin could bind to the trimeric FSHR. Addition of an allosteric modulator to β-arrestin binding assays produced a threefold increase in β-arrestin binding, supporting a model that allosteric small molecule FSHR modulators dissociate FSHR trimers into monomers, thereby increasing FSH access (47). However, a superresolution microscopic technique, dual-color photoactivatable dyes, and localization microscopy (PD-PALM) revealed the closely related LHR existed as a variety of oligomeric forms as well as monomers in the cell membrane (53). Docking of complete LHR models in this study provided a variety of conformations of LHR oligomers, including trimeric LHRs. Similar studies with FSHRs would help clarify the relationship of FSHRs.

As greater FSHR occupancy is directly proportional to FSH-stimulated cAMP production by target cells, increased hypo-glycosylated hFSH binding to FSHR is expected to provide a correspondingly greater cellular activation than fully glycosylated hFSH (54). However, since the model of an FSHR trimer can only accommodate one G protein, it is unlikely that the increase in cAMP is due to occupancy alone. Another possibility is that occupancy by hypo-glycosylated FSH fails to engage the GRK/arrestin pathway which would otherwise attenuate the reengagement of G protein subsequent to activation of adenyl cyclase. Another possibility is that hypo-glycosylated FSH creates a more stable complex with FSHR such that during intracellular trafficking, cAMP- and arrestin-mediated persistent signaling (55) is enhanced. Finally, one may also suggest that since the FSH/FSHR complex appears to recycle to the cell surface (56, 57), the high-affinity binding of hypo-glycosylated FSH may have a proclivity for FSHR, thus failing to dissociate upon relocation to the plasma membrane and perhaps reformation of the putative trimeric structures. This could affect the dynamic stoichiometry of the cell surface unoccupied receptor cohort whose ontogeny resets not only with

TABLE 2 | Follicle-stimulating hormone (FSH) receptor-binding activities of pituitary and recombinant hFSH glycoform preparations.

FSH preparation	Pituitary hFSH	Urinary hFSH	Pituitary hFSH^{24}	Pituitary hFSH$^{21/18}$	Recombinant GH$_3$ hFSH^{24}	Recombinant GH$_3$ hFSH^{21}
FSH RLA potency (IU/mg)	8,560	10,000	18,737	269,445	20,844	57,942
FSH^{21}/FSH^{24} ratio				14.4		2.8

The radioiodinated tracer was 2.5 ng/tube ^{125}I-hFSH and the receptor preparation was 250,000 FSHR-expressing CHO cells/tube.
Data derived from Ref. (16, 18).

new FSHR synthesis but also by occupancy/recycling engaged by other members of the orchestra[1] of glycoforms.

FSHR-MEDIATED SIGNALING *IN VITRO* AND *IN VIVO*

Biased signaling has underpinned GPCR drug development for years but only recently has the mechanism of this phenomenon been revealed in the GPCR field, including the FSHR (51, 58–60). The realization that one GPCR can activate several effector proteins to activate different pathways has prompted the challenging of previously accepted dogma and may help to explain previously unexplained observations. An example of such dogma is that both FSHR and LH/CGR primarily signal *via* Gαs leading to the activation of the cAMP/protein kinase A (PKA) pathway and subsequently leading to steroidogenesis (51, 61–64). Alternative pathways, such as phospholipase C/inositol trisphosphate metabolism were first recognized over 25 years ago (65, 66); however, most studies examining the actions of gonadotropin glycosylation variants remain fixed on the primary pathway. The concept of biased signaling predicts that the specificity of signal transduction depends on, at least in part, the structure of the ligand [reviewed in Ref. (58, 59)]. In support of this idea, a partially deglycosylated eLH variant (67) (eLHdg) was found to exhibit biased signaling through the FSHR (68). While incapable of activating the cAMP/PKA pathway and eliciting steroidogenesis in granulosa cells, binding of eLHdg to FSHR recruited β-arrestins and activated ERK MAPK signaling *via* a cAMP-independent pathway (68).

Another recent study showed that the oligosaccharide complexity of recombinant hFSH preparations differentially affected gene expression and steroidogenesis in human granulosa cells (69). Our own studies with hFSH glycoforms have found evidence for biased signaling, albeit in different cell types. The hFSH[21/18] glycoforms were more active than hFSH[24] in activating the cAMP/PKA pathway and phosphorylation of PKA substrates *via* Gαs in human KGN granulosa cells (31). The actions of FSH[21/18] were 10-fold greater than FSH[24] on induction of CYP19A1 and estrogen (31). The obvious next step is to determine if this biased signaling by hFSH[24] occurs in gonadal cells, which is an active area of pursuit using both *in vitro* and *in vivo* genetic approaches.

GENETIC MODELS TO STUDY THE PHYSIOLOGY OF FSH GLYCOFORMS

Fshb Knockout Mice

As mentioned above, hypo-glycosylated FSH[21/18] has been shown to be more avid compared with fully glycosylated FSH[24] in several receptor binding assays (13, 18), and more potent when tested

using primary granulosa cell- or immortalized granulosa cell-based *in vitro* assays (31). Translation of these *in vitro* observations from biochemistry to physiology required the development of new models as well as implementation of existing mouse models. Accordingly, *in vivo* effects of FSH glycoforms FSH[21/18] and FSH[24] were evaluated using the experimental design of an *in vivo* pharmacological rescue approach. In this experimental paradigm, first, immature *Fshb* null female mice (at 21 days of age) were injected i.p. with different doses of FSH glycoforms separately and at different times postinjection, ovaries were collected for subsequent selected gene expression analysis by quantitative real-time PCR. In these studies, hypo-glycosylated FSH[21/18] elicited *in vivo* bioactivity comparable to that of FSH[24]; however, these analyses also indicated that differences exist between FSH[21/18] and FSH[24] glycoforms in inducing a unique subset of FSH-responsive genes (32). Second, to assess the upstream signaling pathways which control FSH-induced gene expression, immunofluorescence analysis was performed on ovarian sections obtained from *Fshb* null female mice injected with FSH[21/18] and FSH[24] glycoforms using p-CREB and p-PKA substrate antibodies. At three different time points tested (0.5, 1, and 2 h), both glycoforms were equally effective and significantly upregulated p-PKA and p-PKA substrates (nuclear accumulation in granulosa cells) over PBS-injected controls, with maximal induction observed at the 1-h time point (32).

In a third set of experiments, ovarian protein extracts were obtained from *Fshb* null female mice at different time points after injecting with FSH glycoforms separately. These extracts were subjected to Western blot analysis followed by densitometry quantification. When induction of p-CREB, p-PKA substrate and p-p38, p-p44/42, and p-AKT was compared, FSH[21/18] hypo-glycosylated FSH, similar to the above assays, was as active as that of FSH[24], the fully glycosylated FSH (32). Finally, in ovarian weight gain response assays, FSH[21/18] was equally potent as that of the FSH[24], although FSH[21/18] elicited better estradiol induction compared with that by FSH[24] (32). Thus, the *in vivo* pharmacological rescue experiments suggest biased agonism exhibited by different FSH glycoforms and, as would be expected, these are nuanced. In addition to determining if this phenomenon occurs *in vivo* as a function of age (particularly in regard to bone density given the correlation of age with changing FSH glycoform abundance), it will also be critical to determine if these nuances correlate with fertility or embryo quality, having great potential impact on therapeutic use.

In vivo pharmacological rescue of *Fshb* null male mice was also performed using recombinant human FSH glycoforms and measurement of testicular weight gain between postnatal day 5 and 10 in *Fshb* null male mice (32). When injected separately into *Fshb* null male mice at postnatal day 5, both FSH glycoforms significantly induced testicular weight gain by day 10 compared with that in PBS-injected controls (32). Testis weight correlated well with testis tubule size, as well as number of germ cells per tubule. Hypo-glycosylated FSH[21/18] was more active than FSH[24] (32). Similarly, a subset of FSH-responsive genes in mouse Sertoli cells responded much better to hypo-glycosylated FSH[21/18] than fully glycosylated FSH[24]. Furthermore, the number of BrdU+ Sox9+ proliferating Sertoli cells was also found significantly higher in testes of mice injected with FSH[21/18] compared with FSH[24] (32).

---

[1]Each of the FSH molecules is analogous to a member of the orchestra. Their seat is the receptor and their glycoforms are the instruments which they bring to play. The role of each molecule in the orchestra performance will be dependent on the glycoform instrument they bring with them. Like an orchestral performance, one must envision FSH signaling as a complex symphony which may be deconstructed but with loss to the nuance and impact of the full symphony.

It is likely that different human FSH glycoforms act *via* different FSHR-mediated downstream signaling pathways in mouse Sertoli cells, similar to granulosa cells, and elicit distinct gene/protein expression changes. These observations suggest there may be a therapeutic potential advantage of using glycoform-specific hFSH preparations for treatment of male factor fertility, such as marginal sperm counts.

Evaluation of FSH[15] in *Fshb* Null Mice

In vitro expression, purification and characterization of recombinant human FSH glycoforms in somatotrope-derived GH$_3$ cells often results in FSH[21/18] and FSH[24] as the most abundant FSH glycoforms identified by mass spectrometry (18). However, according to the all or none FSHβ glycosylation concept, FSH dimers containing non-glycosylated FSHβ (expected to be 15 kDa in denaturing gels) could also exist in pituitaries (20). To test the biological significance of non-glycosylated FSHβ, separate lines of transgenic mice were first generated that expressed, either a human *FSHB*-mutant transgene (*HFSHB*[7Δ24Δ]) encoding a glycosylation defective 15k-FSHβ subunit or a human *FSHB* WT transgene (*HFSHB*[WT])-encoding wild-type (WT) FSHβ subunit, specifically in gonadotropes. The transgenes were subsequently introduced onto an *Fshb* null genetic background by intercrossing using a genetic rescue strategy (70).

Real-time qPCR assays, immuno co-localization, and Western blot analyses under denaturing conditions confirmed that the transgene encoded mRNA and the corresponding subunits were abundantly expressed in pituitaries (21). While WT human FSHβ subunit-containing, inter-species hybrid FSH was readily detectable by Western blot analysis under non-denaturing conditions of *HFSHB* [WT] mouse pituitaries, FSH dimer containing double N-glycosylation-mutant human FSHβ subunit was barely detectable in pituitaries of *HFSHB*[WT] mice on an *Fshb* null genetic background (21). Consistent with these expression data, mutant FSHβ subunit-containing FSH dimer was not detectable in either short-term pituitary organ culture media or serum samples by specific RIAs (21). Furthermore, gonad histology, gonad gene expression, and fertility assays all indicated that the double N-glycosylation-mutant *HFSHB* transgene failed to rescue *Fshb* null mice (21). Taken together, these genetic experiments confirmed that the double N-glycosylation-mutant human FSHβ subunit-containing FSH dimer is unstable *in vivo*. Such a dimer is also secretion incompetent and even when secreted in low amounts, it fails to rescue mice lacking FSH. Thus, at least one N-glycosylation site on human FSHβ subunit is essential for efficient FSH dimer assembly, secretion, and biological activity *in vivo*.

SUMMARY OF INTEGRATED RESULTS

Implementation of Glycoforms in ART/IVF

Fundamental and heretofore unrecognized differences in human FSH relating to the number and location of FSH glycans resulting in FSH glycoforms, FSH[24], FSH[21], and FSH[18] (16, 19) have been summarized. Moreover, the seminal observation from analysis of individual human pituitaries was that the abundance of FSH[21]

declines with age in women [**Table 3** and (16)] raises the question whether this had implications for therapeutic intervention. FSH[21] is elevated in young women of reproductive age, but declines thereafter leading to a condition of FSH[24] dominance. Thus, the active reproductive period is characterized by the presence of FSH[21], while the period of declining fertility and reproductive senescence is characterized by significantly diminished FSH[21] along with FSH[24] dominance.

In this regard, it is noteworthy that current hFSH products available commercially for clinical use, whether they are of menopausal or recombinant origin, consist overwhelmingly of FSH[24] (18). Thus, despite the general success of IVF, there has not been a systematic clinical trial which considers that a form of the hormone associated physiologically with a period of decreased reproductive function rather than the form of the hormone present during the reproductive period may be compromising both yield and quality of embryos. It is believed that the clinical utilization of hypo-glycosylated FSH[21/18] preparations for IVF would represent a paradigm shift in the treatment of infertility. The use of something truly different, an apparently more active and more physiologically relevant FSH, might provide the basis for improved ovarian stimulation and overall pregnancy outcome. Thus, an emerging question is whether the shift from FSH[21] to FSH[24] dominance occurs as a result of normal aging or a premature change and represents an underlying cause of subfertility/infertility. To place this in context, a brief overview of controlled ovarian stimulation (COS) is warranted.

The use of COS began in the 1980s as a means to enhance/improve the chances of generating a pregnancy *via* the combination of procedures involved in *in vitro* fertilization (IVF). Prior to this, "natural cycle" IVF was utilized, which generated on average, a single utilizable oocyte (71). Not surprisingly, success *via* this method was severely limited. COS was developed as a means to generate multiple oocytes, which would increase the chances for successful fertilization, enhance embryo development, and coupled with multiple embryo transfer to the uterus, increase pregnancy rates. Indeed, COS proved invaluable as the preferred mechanism underlying IVF (72, 73). In parallel to COS, increased focus on IVF Laboratory practice coupled with IVF Laboratory Certification greatly moved IVF from "experimental procedure" status to that of standard of care (74). At the core of COS is the utilization of hFSH, the fundamental endocrine driver of ovarian follicle development (72).

The history of COS has witnessed a number of modifications aimed at increasing IVF success. Among these are: the utilization of GnRH agonist or antagonists to block endogenous gonadotropin production; utilization of urinary-derived human menopausal gonadotropin or well-controlled recombinant cDNA-driven expression of hFSH produced primarily using cells

---

TABLE 3 | Relative abundance of FSH[21] in individual human pituitaries.

No. of pituitaries	2	4	4
Age range (years)	21–24	39–43	58–71
FSH[21]	62 ± 10.5	41 ± 8.2	17 ± 3.7

Based on band density in Western blots using anti-FSHβ monoclonal antibody RFSH20 (16).

of Chinese hamster ovary origin; the use of FSH alone or the combined use of FSH coupled with LH; variable gonadotropin dosage and administration regimens; and utilization of supplemental progesterone to offset or oppose estradiol levels (72, 73, 75). Often, modifications have been undertaken to treat women with special conditions that impact success including women with PCOS, older women, and women with cancer (76). Indeed, a women's age is one of the most predictive factors underlying success with IVF due in large part to the diminishing pool of primordial follicles. The common and overriding feature of the above modifications is the utilization of FSH.

The mechanistic functions and potential differences among FSH glycoforms remain largely unknown. As noted above, differences in receptor binding and the subsequent impact upon certain intracellular signaling systems and cell function can and have been demonstrated (77, 78). The fundamental mechanisms underlying female fertility in terms of producing a viable oocyte still remain largely unknown. However, there are clearly defined stages, which offer targets for differential regulation. These stages include primordial follicle activation, preantral follicle growth, antral follicle growth, and dominant follicle selection. An intriguing hypothesis is that hFSH glycoforms function during different stages of follicle development. This might explain in part, the reported differences in glycoform stimulation of ovarian gene expression and cellular signaling pathways observed in the immature *Fshb* null mice (32).

Follicle development up to the antral stage is not dependent upon FSH in the mouse (79, 80). Nevertheless, preantral follicles are responsive to FSH (81, 82). Owing to the recently reported *in vivo* activities of the glycoforms, could FSH$^{21/18}$ preparations function to drive preantral follicle development to provide follicles appropriately responsive to FSH^{24}? Might supplementation with FSH$^{21/18}$ for one or two cycles prior to COS overcome what appears to be a natural decline in fertility with age concomitant with a decline in the levels of hFSH$^{21/18}$? One proposes supplementation in the event that FSH$^{21/18}$ drives preantral follicle development, so that replacement of FSH^{24} by FSH$^{21/18}$ under standard COS strategies may not provide for improved results if FSH$^{21/18}$ is needed during the earlier stages of follicle development and ineffective in later stages. Furthermore, such treatment paradigms might serve to ameliorate the decreased responsiveness of older women to COS with commercially available FSH, which is essentially FSH^{24}. There is, for example, some evidence that microheterogeneity differences affect estradiol production (78).

FSH$^{21/18}$ supplementation over an extended period to promote preantral follicle development, which would serve to provide appropriately developed follicles for continued development, perhaps with either glycoform. Owing to potential differences in uptake and circulating half-life, and whether the glycoforms are under episodic as opposed to a more tonic secretion, differences in hFSH glycoform dose and administration regimen may be needed to provide for a more physiological representation. Clearly, the discovery of FSH$^{21/18}$ and the initial characterization of its activity provide the basis for new ideas concerning COS and IVF. These data indicate that FSH$^{21/18}$ and FSH^{24} exist, and they exhibit differences in both *in vitro* and *in vivo* activities, and their relative abundance changes with age. These data provide

a compelling basis for continued investigation. Central to the improvement of IVF outcomes will be the understanding of how and when these two glycoforms function to promote the proper developmental program of the follicle.

Implementation of FSH Glycoforms to Preserve Bone

Follicle-stimulating hormone has been reported to have direct effects on bone, attributed to FSH-driven (83–85) osteoclast development and activity (86–89). During the premenopausal period, when ovarian reserve is waning and FSH levels are rising because of the lack of negative feedback by ovarian estrogen (90), the abundance of fully glycosylated hFSH^{24} in the pituitary also rises. It is well established that declining levels of estradiol during the menopausal transition affects bone mineral density, and other metabolic parameters (91). Since the 1940s it has been assumed that reduced bone mineral density was due to a simple sex steroid deficiency (92). Previous reports, largely from one laboratory, have challenged this view by providing evidence that elevated FSH during menopause or ovarian deficiency might explain the bone loss (86, 93). A number of observations highlight the potential importance of FSH in mediating, at least in part, bone loss in humans (94) not associated with changes in steroid hormones (84). A recent study found that FSH, but not estrogen, was strongly associated with bone loss in postmenopausal women treated for breast cancer (95). Furthermore, polymorphisms in the *FSHR* are associated with accelerated bone loss in women (96). As such, the levels of estrogen and FSH may contribute in multiple ways to bone mineral density during aging.

It should be appreciated that the extra-gonadal actions of FSH have only been recently identified and the actions of FSH on bone have been controversial [reviewed in Ref. (97)]. Allan et al. (98) reported that FSH produced anabolic effects on bone that correlated with inhibin and testosterone levels. Ritter et al. (99) found that treatment of mice with FSH had no effect on bone loss or gain and did not increase osteoclast formation. Two other groups found little correlation of FSH levels and bone mineral density (2, 100). In contrast, other studies provide evidence that FSH can promote the development of human osteoclast precursor cells (89) and induce the production of bone-resorbing cytokines (87, 88, 93). These are relevant observations since the immune system plays a role in a variety of disease states linking inflammatory responses and bone loss (101). Furthermore, several lines of evidence support the initial observations that loss of either *Fshb* or *Fshr* confers protection from bone loss in mice (86).

Geng et al. (102) showed that exogenous FSH enhanced osteoclast differentiation and treatment with neutralizing antibodies to FSH or a GST–FSHβ fusion protein prevented bone loss in ovariectomized rats. Likewise, Zhu et al. (103) reported that treatment of ovariectomized mice with an FSH antibody prevented bone loss. Our data show that treatment of murine and human osteoclast precursor cells with FSH^{24}, but not FSH^{21}, increases the formation of multi-nucleated, TRAP (tartrate-resistant acid phosphatase-5b, a bone resorption marker) positive osteoclasts (Davis et al., unpublished). FSH also works together with receptor activator of nuclear factor-κB (NFκB) ligand (RANKL) to induce expression of MMP9 and cathepsin-k (CTSK) in osteoclasts. These data are in agreement with our own and indicate that FSH[24] increases *TNFα and IRAK* mRNA in human CD14[+] osteoclast precursors. TNFα is important for osteoclast formation (93, 104, 105). These findings indicate that the age-related increase in hFSH[24] may regulate bone, a nontraditional FSH target. Evidence points to the ability of FSH to activate Gα[i] in bone cells, resulting in a reduction in cAMP levels (86), which contrasts to the activation of Gα[s] and increase in cAMP in granulosa cells. In bone, FSH stimulates MAPK and NFκB osteoclastogenic intracellular signaling pathways (86). Our data indicate that FSH[24] is responsible for activating these signaling pathways and formation of osteoclasts. Hence, there is a critical need to settle the controversy regarding a role for FSH in targeting osteoclasts in women.

AUTHOR CONTRIBUTIONS

GB, JM, JSD, JD, and TK authored individual sections of the review. GB, JM, JD, JD, and TK reviewed the entire manuscript.

FUNDING

This work was supported by the National Institute on Aging (grant number AG029531 to GB, JM, JD, and TK) and The Edgar L. & Patricia M. Makowski Endowment (to TK). This work was supported in part by a Senior Career Scientist Award (to JSD) from the United States (US) Department of Veterans Affairs Biomedical Laboratory Research and Development Service.

REFERENCES

1. Hearn MTW, Gomme PT. Molecular architecture and biorecognition processes of the cystine knot protein superfamily: part I. The glycoprotein hormones. *J Mol Recognit* (2000) 13:223–78. doi:10.1002/1099-1352(200009/10)13:5<223::AID-JMR501>3.0.CO;2-L

2. Gao J, Tiwari-Pandey R, Samadfam R, Yang Y, Miao D, Karaplis AC, et al. Altered ovarian function affects skeletal homeostasis independent of the action of follicle-stimulating hormone. *Endocrinology* (2007) 148(6):2613–21. doi:10.1210/en.2006-1404

3. Williams GR. Hypogonadal bone loss: sex steroids or gonadotropins? *Endocrinology* (2007) 148(6):2610–2. doi:10.1210/en.2007-0337

4. Agrawal M, Zhu G, Sun L, Zaidi M, Iqbal J. The role of FSH and TSH in bone loss and its clinical relevance. *Curr Osteoporos Rep* (2010) 8(4):205–11. doi:10.1007/s11914-010-0028-x

5. Kumar TR. Extragonadal actions of FSH: a critical need for novel genetic models. *Endocrinology* (2018) 159(1):2–8. doi:10.1210/en.2017-03118

6. Fox KM, Dias JA, Van Roey P. Three-dimensional structure of human follicle-stimulating hormone. *Mol Endocrinol* (2001) 15:378–89. doi:10.1210/mend.15.3.0603

7. Bousfield GR, Jia L, Ward DN. Gonadotropins: chemistry and biosynthesis. 3rd ed. In: Neill JD, editor. *Knobil and Neill: Physiology of Reproduction*. San Diego: Elsevier (2006). p. 1581–634.

8. Maghnin-Rogister G, Closset J, Hennen G. Differences in the carbohydrate portion of the α subunit of porcine lutropin (LH), follitropin (FSH) and thyrotropin (TSH). *FEBS Lett* (1975) 60(2):263–6. doi:10.1016/0014-5793(75)80727-7

9. Nilsson B, Rosen SW, Weintraub BD, Zopf DA. Differences in the carbohydrate moieties of the common α-subunits of human chorionic gonadotropin, luteinizing hormone, follicle-stimulating hormone, and thyrotropin: preliminary structural inferences from direct methylation analysis. *Endocrinology* (1986) 119:2737–43. doi:10.1210/endo-119-6-2737

10. Gotschall RR, Bousfield GR. Oligosaccharide mapping reveals hormone-specific glycosylation patterns on equine gonadotropin α-subunit Asn[56]. *Endocrinology* (1996) 137(6):2543–57. doi:10.1210/endo.137.6.8641208

11. Lapthorn AJ, Harris DC, Littlejohn A, Lustbader JW, Canfield RE, Machin KJ, et al. Crystal structure of human chorionic gonadotropin. *Nature* (1994) 369:455–61. doi:10.1038/369455a0

12. Wu H, Lustbader JW, Liu Y, Canfield RE, Hendrickson WA. Structure of human chorionic gonadotropin at 2.6 Å resolution from MAD analysis of the selenomethionyl protein. *Structure* (1994) 2:545–58. doi:10.1016/S0969-2126(00)00054-X

13. Bousfield GR, Butnev VY, Butnev VY, Hiromasa Y, Harvey DJ, May JV. Hypo-glycosylated human follicle-stimulating hormone (hFSH21/18) is much more active in vitro than fully-glycosylated hFSH (hFSH24). *Mol Cell Endocrinol* (2014) 382:989–97. doi:10.1016/j.mce.2013.11.008

14. Ulloa-Aguirre A, Midgley AR Jr, Beitins IZ, Padmanbhan V. Follicle-stimulating isohormones: characterization and physiological relevance. *Endocr Rev* (1995) 16(6):765–87. doi:10.1210/edrv-16-6-765

15. Bousfield GR, Butnev VY, Bidart JM, Dalpathado D, Irungu J, Desaire H. Chromatofocusing fails to separate hFSH isoforms on the basis of glycan structure. *Biochemistry* (2008) 47(6):1708–20. doi:10.1021/bi701764w

16. Bousfield GR, Butnev VY, Rueda-Santos MA, Brown A, Smalter Hall A, Harvey DJ. Macro and micro heterogeneity in pituitary and urinary follicle-stimulating hormone glycosylation. *J Glycomics Lipidomics* (2014) 4:125. doi:10.4172/2153-0637.1000125

17. Bousfield GR, Butnev VY, White WK, Smalter Hall A, Harvey DJ. Comparison of follicle-stimulating hormone glycosylation microheterogeneity by quantitative negative mode nano-electrospray mass spectrometry of peptide-N-glycanase-released oligosaccharides. *J Glycomics Lipidomics* (2015) 5(1):129. doi:10.4172/2153-0637.1000129

18. Butnev VY, Butnev VY, May JV, Shuai B, Tran P, White WK, et al. Production, purification, and characterization of recombinant hFSH glycoforms for functional studies. *Mol Cell Endocrinol* (2015) 405:41–52. doi:10.1016/j.mce.2015.01.026

19. Davis JS, Kumar TR, May JV, Bousfield GR. Naturally occurring follicle-stimulating hormone glycosylation variants. *J Glycomics Lipidomics* (2014) 4:e117. doi:10.4172/2153-0637.1000e117

20. Walton WJ, Nguyen VT, Butnev VY, Singh V, Moore WT, Bousfield GR. Characterization of human follicle-stimulating hormone isoforms reveals a non-glycosylated β-subunit in addition to the conventional glycosylated β-subunit. *J Clin Endocrinol Metab* (2001) 86:3675–85. doi:10.1210/jcem.86.8.7712

21. Wang H, Butnev VY, Bousfield GR, Kumar TR. A human FSHB transgene encoding the double N-glycosylation mutant (Asn7Δ Asn25Δ) FSHβ fails to rescue Fshb null mice. *Mol Cell Endocrinol* (2016) 426:113–24. doi:10.1016/j.mce.2016.02.015

22. Renwick AGC, Mizuochi T, Kochibe N, Kobata A. The asparagine-linked sugar chains of human follicle-stimulating hormone. *J Biochem* (1987) 101:1209–21. doi:10.1093/oxfordjournals.jbchem.a121985

23. Green ED, Baenziger JU. Asparagine-linked oligosaccharides on lutropin, follitropin, and thyrotropin II. Distributions of sulfated and sialylated oligosaccharides on bovine, ovine, and human pituitary glycoprotein hormones. *J Biol Chem* (1988) 263(1):36–44.

24. Wolfenson C, Groisman J, Couto AS, Hedenfalk M, Cortvrindt RG, Smitz JE, et al. Batch-to-batch consistency of human-derived gonadotrophin preparations compared with recombinant preparations. *Reprod Biomed Online* (2005) 10(4):442–54. doi:10.1016/S1472-6483(10)60819-X

25. Lombardi A, Andreozzi C, Pavone V, Triglione V, Angiolini L, Caccia P. Evaluation of the oligosaccharide composition of commercial follicle stimulating hormone preparations. *Electrophoresis* (2013) 34(16):23–94–2406. doi:10.1002/elps.201300045

26. Dalpathado DS, Irungu JA, Go EP, Butnev VY, Norton K, Bousfield GR, et al. Comparative glycomics of the glycoprotein hormone follicle-stimulating hormone (FSH): glycopeptide analysis of isolates from two mammalian species. *Biochemistry* (2006) 45(28):8665–73. doi:10.1021/bi060435k

27. Gervais A, Hammel Y-A, Pelloux S, Lepage P, Baer G, Carte N, et al. Glycosylation of human recombinant gonadotrophins: characterization and

batch-to-batch consistency. *Glycobiology* (2003) 13(3):179–89. doi:10.1093/glycob/cwg020

28. Ulloa-Aguirre A, Timossi C, Damian-Matsumura P, Dias JA. Role of glycosylation in function of follicle-stimulating hormone. *Endocrine* (1999) 11(3):205–15. doi:10.1385/ENDO:11:3:205

29. Ulloa-Aguirre A, Dias JA, Bousfield GR. Gonadotropins. In: Simoni M, Huhtaniemi I, editors. *Endocrinology of the Testis and Male Reproduction.* Cham: Springer (2017). p. 1–52.

30. Bousfield GR, Butnev VY, Butnev VY, Nguyen VT, Gray CM, Dias JA, et al. Differential effects of a asparagine⁵⁶ oligosaccharide structure on equine lutropin and follitropin hybrid conformation and receptor-binding activity. *Biochemistry* (2004) 43:10817–33. doi:10.1021/bi049857p

31. Jiang C, Hou X, Wang C, May JF, Butnev VY, Bousfield GR, et al. Hypoglycosylated hFSH has greater bioactivity than fully-glycosylated recombinant hFSH in human granulosa cells. *J Clin Endocrinol Metab* (2015) 100(6):E852–60. doi:10.1210/jc.2015-1317

32. Wang H, May J, Shuai B, May JV, Bousfield GR, Kumar TR. Evaluation of *in vivo* bioactivities of recombiant hypo-(FSH²¹/¹⁸) and fully-(FSH²⁴) glycosylated human FSH glycoforms in *Fshb* null mice. *Mol Cell Endocrinol* (2016) 437:224–36. doi:10.1016/j.mce.2016.08.031

33. Mengeling BJ, Manzella SM, Baenziger JU. A cluster of basic amino acids within an α-helix is essential for α-subunit recognition by the glycoprotein hormone N-acetylgalactosaminyltransferase. *Proc Natl Acad Sci U S A* (1995) 92:502–6. doi:10.1073/pnas.92.2.502

34. Jiang X, Dias JA, He X. Structural biology of glycoprotein hormones and their receptors: insights to signaling. *Mol Cell Endocrinol* (2014) 384(1):424–51. doi:10.1016/j.mce.2013.08.021

35. Meher BR, Dixit A, Bousfield GR, Lushington GH. Glycosylation effects on FSH-FSHR interaction dynamics: a case study of different FSH glycoforms by molecular dynamics simulations. *PLoS One* (2015) 10(9):e0137897. doi:10.1371/journal.pone.0137897

36. Weisshaar G, Hiyama J, Renwick AGC, Nimtz M. NMR investigations of the N-linked oligosaccharides at individual glycosylation sites of human lutropin. *Eur J Biochem* (1991) 195:257–68. doi:10.1111/j.1432-1033.1991.tb15702.x

37. Weisshaar G, Hiyama J, Renwick AGC. Site-specific N-glycosylation of ovine lutropin: structural analysis by one- and two-dimensional 1H-NMR spectroscopy. *Eur J Biochem* (1990) 192:741–51. doi:10.1111/j.1432-1033.1990.tb19285.x

38. Hiyama J, Weisshaar G, Renwick AGC. The asparagine-linked oligosaccharides at individual glycosylation sites in human thyrotropin. *Glycobiology* (1992) 2(5):401–9. doi:10.1093/glycob/2.5.401

39. Sprengel R, Braun T, Nikolics K, Segaloff DL, Seeburg PH. The testicular receptor for follicle stimulating hormone: structure and functional expression of cloned cDNA. *Mol Endocrinol* (1990) 4:525–30. doi:10.1210/mend-4-4-525

40. Minegishi T, Nakamura K, Takakura Y, Ibuki Y, Igarashi M. Cloning and sequencing of human FSH receptor cDNA. *Biochem Biophys Res Commun* (1991) 175(3):1125–30. doi:10.1016/0006-291X(91)91682-3

41. Fan QR, Hendrickson WA. Structure of human follicle-stimulating hormone in complex with its receptor. *Nature* (2005) 433:269–77. doi:10.1038/nature03206

42. Jiang X, Liu H, Chen X, Chen PH, Fischer D, Sriraman V, et al. Structure of follicle-stimulating hormone in complex with the entire ectodomain of its receptor. *Proc Natl Acad Sci U S A* (2012) 109(31):12491–6. doi:10.1073/pnas.1206643109

43. Manjunath P, Sairam MR, Sairam J. Studies on pituitary follitropin. X. Biochemical, receptor binding and immunological properties of deglycosylated ovine hormone. *Mol Cell Endocrinol* (1982) 28:125–38. doi:10.1016/0303-7207(82)90026-0

44. Calvo FO, Keutmann HT, Bergert ER, Ryan RJ. Deglycosylated human follitropin: characterization and effects on adenosine cyclic 3′,5′-phosphate production in porcine granulosa cells. *Biochemistry* (1986) 25:3938–43. doi:10.1021/bi00361a030

45. Bishop LA, Robertson DM, Cahir N, Schofield PR. Specific roles for the asparagine-linked carbohydrate residues of recombinant human follicle stimulating hormone in receptor binding and signal transduction. *J Mol Endocrinol* (1994) 8(6):722–31. doi:10.1210/me.8.6.722

46. Flack MR, Froehlich J, Bennet AP, Anasti J, Nisula BC. Site-directed mutagenesis defines the individual roles of the glycosylation sites on follicle-stimulating hormone. *J Biol Chem* (1994) 269(19):14015–20.

47. Jiang X, Fischer D, Chen X, McKenna SD, Liu H, Sriraman V, et al. Evidence for follicle-stimulating hormone receptor as a functional trimer. *J Biol Chem* (2014) 289(20):14273–82. doi:10.1074/jbc.M114.549592

48. Nguyen VT, Singh V, Butnev VY, Gray CM, Westfall S, Davis JS, et al. Inositol phosphate stimulation by LH requires the entire α Asn⁵⁶ oligosaccharide. *Mol Cell Endocrinol* (2003) 199(1–2):73–86. doi:10.1016/S0303-7207(02)00297-6

49. Thotakura NR, Weintraub BD, Bahl OP. The role of carbohydrate in human choriogonadotropin (hCG) action. Effects of N-linked carbohydrate chains from hCG and other glycoproteins on hormonal activity. *Mol Cell Endocrinol* (1990) 70(3):263–72. doi:10.1016/0303-7207(90)90217-V

50. Janovick JA, Maya-Nunez G, Ulloa-Aguirre A, Huhtaniemi IT, Dias JA, Verbost PM, et al. Increased plasma membrane expression of human follicle-stimulating hormone receptor by a small molecule thienopyr(im)idine. *Mol Cell Endocrinol* (2009) 298(1–2):84–8. doi:10.1016/j.mce.2008.09.015

51. Dias JA, Bonnet B, Weaver BA, Watts J, Kuuetzman K, Thomas RM, et al. A negative allosteric modulator demonstrates biased antagonism of the follicle stimulating hormone receptor. *Mol Cell Endocrinol* (2011) 333(2):143–50. doi:10.1016/j.mce.2010.12.023

52. van Koppen CJ, Verbost PM, van de Lagemaat R, Karsents WJ, Loozen HJ, vn Acterberg TA, et al. Signaling of an allosteric, nanomolar potent, low molecular weight agonist for the follicle-stimulating hormone receptor. *Biochem Pharmacol* (2013) 85(8):1162–70. doi:10.1016/j.bcp.2013.02.001

53. Jonas KC, Fanelli F, Huhtaniemi IT, Hanyaloglu AC. Single molecule analysis of functionally asymmetric G protein-coupled receptor (GPCR) oligomers reveals diverse spatial and structural assemblies. *J Biol Chem* (2015) 290:3875–92. doi:10.1074/jbc.M114.622498

54. Bhaskaran RS, Ascoli M. The post-endocytotic fate of the gonadotropin receptors is an important determinant of the desensitization of gonadotropin responses. *J Mol Endocrinol* (2005) 34(2):447–57. doi:10.1677/jme.1.01745

55. Calebiro D, Nikolaev VO, Gagliani MC, de Filippis T, Dees C, Tacchetti C, et al. Persistent cAMP-signals triggered by internalized G-protein-coupled receptors. *PLoS Biol* (2009) 7(8):e1000172. doi:10.1371/journal.pbio.1000172

56. Krishnamurthy H, Kishi H, Shi M, Galet C, Bhaskaran RS, Hirakawa T, et al. Postendocytotic trafficking of the follicle-stimulating hormone (FSH)-FSH receptor complex. *Mol Endocrinol* (2003) 17(11):2162–76. doi:10.1210/me.2003-0118

57. Kluetzman KS, Thomas RM, Nechamen CA, Dias JA. Decreased degradation of internalized follicle-stimulating hormone caused by mutation of aspartic acid 6.30(550) in a protein kinase-CK2 consensus sequence in the third intracellular loop of human follicle-stimulating hormone receptor. *Biol Reprod* (2011) 84:1154–63. doi:10.1095/biolreprod.110.087965

58. Landomiel F, Gallay N, Jégot G, Tranchant T, Durand G, Bourquard T, et al. Biased signalling in follicle stimulating hormone action. *Mol Cell Endocrinol* (2014) 382(1):452–9. doi:10.1016/j.mce.2013.09.035

59. Luttrell LM. Minireview: more than just a hammer: ligand 'bias' and pharmaceutical discovery. *Mol Endocrinol* (2014) 28(3):281–94. doi:10.1210/me.2013-1314

60. Shukla AK. Biasing GPCR signaling from inside. *Sci Signal* (2014) 7:e3. doi:10.1126/scisignal.2005021

61. Means AR, MacDonald E, Soderling TR, Corbin JD. Testicular adenosine 3′:5′-monophosphate-dependent protein kinase. Regulation by follicle-stimulating hormone. *J Biol Chem* (1974) 249(4):1131–8.

62. Marsh JM. The role of cyclic AMP in gonadal steroidogenesis. *Biol Reprod* (1976) 14(1):30–53. doi:10.1095/biolreprod14.1.30

63. Dattatreyamurty B, Figgs LW, Reichert LE Jr. Physical and functional association of follitropin receptors with cholera toxin-sensitive guanine nucleotide-binding protein. *J Biol Chem* (1987) 262(24):11737–45.

64. Hunzicker-Dunn M, Maizels ET. FSH signaling pathways in immature granulosa cells that regulate target gene expression: branching out from protein kinase A. *Cell Signal* (2006) 18(9):1351–9. doi:10.1016/j.cellsig.2006.02.011

65. Davis JS, Weakland LL, West LA, Farese RV. Luteinizing hormone stimulates the formation of inositol trisphosphate and cyclic AMP in rat granulosa cells. *Biochem J* (1986) 238:597–604. doi:10.1042/bj2380597

66. Davis JS, Weakland LL, Farese RV, West LA. Luteinizing hormone increases inositol trisphosphate and cytosolic Ca^{2+} in isolated bovine luteal cells. *J Biol Chem* (1987) 262(18):8515–21.

67. Butnev VY, Singh V, Nguyen VT, Bousfield GR. Truncated eLHβ and asparagine[56]-deglycosylated eLHα combine to produce a potent follicle-stimulating hormone antagonist. *J Endocrinol* (2002) 172(3):545–55. doi:10.1677/joe.0.1720545

68. Wehbi V, Tranchant T, Durand G, Musnier A, Decourtye G, Piketty V, et al. Partially deglycosylated equine LH preferentially activates beta-arrestin-dependent signaling at the follicle-stimulating hormon receptor. *Mol Endocrinol* (2010) 24(3):561–73. doi:10.1210/me.2009-0347

69. Loreti N, Fresno C, Barrera D, Andreone L, Albarran SL, Fernandez EA, et al. The glycan structure in recombinant human FSH affects endocrine activity and global gene expression in human granulosa cells. *Mol Cell Endocrinol* (2013) 366(1):68–80. doi:10.1016/j.mce.2012.11.021

70. Kumar TR, Low MJ, Matzuk MM. Genetic rescue of follicle-stimulating hormone beta-deficient mice. *Endocrinology* (1998) 139(7):3289–95. doi:10.1210/endo.139.7.6111

71. Zech NH, Zech M, Baldauf S, Comploj G, Murtinger M, Spitzer D, et al. Ovarian stimulation in ART--Unwinding pressing issues. *Minerva Ginecol* (2015) 67(2):127–47.

72. Grainger DA, Tjaden BL, Ttpati LL. Assisted reproductive technologies. 2nd ed. In: Goldman MB, Troisi R, Rexfode KM, editors. *Women & Health.* Waltham, MA: Academic Press (2013). p. 307–20.

73. Jungheim ES, Meyer M, Broughton DE. Best practices for controlled ovarian stimulation in IVF. *Semin Reprod Med* (2015) 33:77–82. doi:10.1055/s-0035-1546424

74. May JV. Ovarian hyperstimulation: effects on oocyte quality and communication between physician and embryologist to optimize oocyte quality. In: May JV, editor. *Infertility and Reproductive Medicine Clinics of North America: Assisted Reproduction, Laboratory Considerations.* Philadelphia, PA: W.B Saunders Co (1998):163–79.

75. Vuong TNL, Phung HT, Ho MT. Recombinant follicle-stimulating hormone and recombinant luteinizing hormone versus recombinant follicle-stimulating hormone alone during GnRH antagonist ovarian stimulation in patients aged >= 35 years: a randomized controlled trial. *Hum Reprod* (2015) 30:1188–95. doi:10.1093/humrep/dev038

76. Cakmak H, Rosen MP. Ovarian stimulation in cancer patients. *Fert Seril* (2013) 99:1476–84. doi:10.1016/j.fertnstert.2013.03.029

77. Williams RS, Vensel T, Sistrom CL, Kipersztok S, Rhoton-Vlasak A, Drury K. Pregnancy rates in varying age groups after in vitro fertilization: a comparison of follitropin alfa (Gonal F) and follitropin beta (Follistim). *Am J Obstet Gynecol* (2003) 189(2):342–6; discussion 346–7. doi:10.1067/S0002-9378(03)00728-2

78. Orvieto R, Nahum R, Rabinson J, Ashkenazi J, Anteby EY, Meltcer S. Follitropin-alpha (Gonal-F) versus follitropin-beta (Puregon) in controlled ovarian hyperstimulation for in vitro fertilization: is there any difference? *Fertil Steril* (2009) 91(4 Suppl):1522–5. doi:10.1016/j.fertnstert.2008.08.112

79. Kumar TR, Wang Y, Lu N, Matzuk MM. Follicle stimulating hormone is required for ovarian follicle maturation but not male fertility. *Nat Genet* (1997) 15(2):201–4. doi:10.1038/ng0297-201

80. Kumar TR. Mouse models for gonadotropins: a 15-year saga. *Mol Cell Endocrinol* (2007) 260-262:249–54. doi:10.1016/j.mce.2006.09.002

81. McGee EA, Perlas E, LaPolt PS, Tsafriri A, Hsueh AJ. Follicle-stimulating hormone enhances the development of preantral follicles in juvenile rats. *Biol Reprod* (1997) 57(5):990–8. doi:10.1095/biolreprod57.5.990

82. Abel MH, Wootton AN, Wilkins V, Huhtaniemi I, Kinight PG, Charlton HM. The effect of a null mutation in the follicle-stimulating hormone receptor gene on mouse reproduction. *Endocrinology* (2000) 141(5):1795–803. doi:10.1210/endo.141.5.7456

83. Ebeling PR, Atley LM, Guthrie JR, Burger HG, Dennerstein L, Hopper JL, et al. Bone turnover markers and bone density across the menopausal transition. *J Clin Endocrinol Metab* (1996) 81(9):3366–71. doi:10.1210/jc.81.9.3366

84. Sowers MR, Jannausch M, McConnell D, Little R, Greendale GA, Finkelstein JS, et al. Hormone predictors of bone mineral density changes during the menopausal transition. *J Clin Endocrinol Metab* (2006) 91(4):1261–7. doi:10.1210/jc.2005-1836

85. Lo JC, Burnett-Bowie SAM, Finkelstein JS. Bone and the perimenopause. *Obstet Gynecol Clin North Am* (2011) 38(3):503–17. doi:10.1016/j.ogc.2011.07.001

86. Sun L, Peng Y, Sharrow AC, Iqbal J, Zhang Z, Papachristou DJ, et al. FSH directly regulates bone mass. *Cell* (2006) 125(2):247–60. doi:10.1016/j.cell.2006.01.051

87. Cannon JG, Cortez-Cooper M, Meaders E, Stallings J, Haddow S, Kraj B, et al. Follicle-stimulating hormone, interleukin-1, and bone density in adult women. *Am J Physiol Regul Integr Comp Physiol* (2010) 298(3):R790–8. doi:10.1152/ajpregu.00728.2009

88. Sun L, Zhang Z, Zhu LL, Peng Y, Liu X, Li J, et al. Further evidence for direct pro-resorptive actions of FSH. *Biochem Biophys Res Commun* (2010) 394(1):6–11. doi:10.1016/j.bbrc.2010.02.113

89. Cannon JG, Kraj B, Sloan G. Follicle-stimulating hormone promotes RANK expression on human monocytes. *Cytokine* (2011) 53(2):141–4. doi:10.1016/j.cyto.2010.11.011

90. Crandall CJ, Tseng CH, Karlamangla AS, Finkelstein JS, Randolph JF Jr, Thurston RC, et al. Serum sex steroid levels and longitudinal changes in bone density in relation to the final menstrual period. *J Clin Endocrinol Metab* (2013) 98(4):E654–63. doi:10.1210/jc.2012-3651

91. Dennerstein L, Lehert P, Guthrie JR, Burger HG. Modeling women's health during the menopausal transition: a longitudinal analysis. *Menopause* (2007) 14(1):53–62. doi:10.1097/01.gme.0000229574.67376.ba

92. Riggs BL, Khosla S, Melton LJ III. Sex steroids and the construction and conservation of the adult skeleton. *Endocr Rev* (2002) 23(3):279–302. doi:10.1210/edrv.23.3.0465

93. Iqbal J, Sun L, Kumar TR, Blair HC, Zaidi M. Follicle-stimulating hormone stimulates TNF production from immune cells to enhance osteoblast and osteoclast formation. *Proc Natl Acad Sci U S A* (2006) 103(40):14925–30. doi:10.1073/pnas.0606805103

94. Devleta B, Adem B, Senada S. Hypergonadotropic amenorrhea and bone density: new approach to an old problem. *J Bone Miner Metab* (2004) 22(4):360–4. doi:10.1007/s00774-004-0495-1

95. Tabatabai LS, Bloom J, Stewart S, Sellmeyer DE. FSH levels predict bone loss in premenopausal women treated for breast cancer more than one year after treatment. *J Clin Endocrinol Metab* (2016) 101(3):1257–62. doi:10.1210/jc.2015-3149

96. Rendina D, Gianfrancesco F, De Filippo G, Merlotti D, Esposito T, Mingione A, et al. FSHR gene polymorphisms influence bone mineral density and bone turnover in postmenopausal women. *Eur J Endocrinol* (2010) 163(1):165–72. doi:10.1530/eje-10-0043

97. Colaianni G, Cuscito C, Colucci S. FSH and TSH in the regulation of bone mass: the pituitary/immune/bone axis. *Clin Dev Immunol* (2013) 2013:382698. doi:10.1155/2013/382698

98. Allan CM, Kalak R, Dunstan CR, McTavish KJ, Zhou H, Handelsman DJ, et al. Follicle-stimulating hormone increases bone mass in female mice. *Proc Natl Acad Sci U S A* (2010) 107(52):22629–34. doi:10.1073/pnas.1012141108

99. Ritter V, Thuering B, Saint Mezard P, Luong-Nguyen NH, Seltenmeyer Y, Junker U, et al. Follicle-stimulating hormone does not impact male bone mass in vivo or human male osteoclasts in vitro. *Calcif Tissue Int* (2008) 82(5):383–91. doi:10.1007/s00223-008-9134-5

100. Gourlay ML, Specker BL, Li C, Hammett-Stabler CA, Renner JB, Rubin JE. Follicle-stimulating hormone is independently associated with lean mass but not BMD in younger postmenopausal women. *Bone* (2012) 50(1):311–6. doi:10.1016/j.bone.2011.11.001

101. Faienza MF, Ventura A, Marzano F, Cavallo L. Postmenopausal osteoporosis: the role of immune system cells. *Clin Dev Immunol* (2013) 2013:575936. doi:10.1155/2013/575936

102. Geng W, Yan X, Du H, Cui J, Li L, Chen F. Immunization with FSHbeta fusion protein antigen prevents bone loss in a rat ovariectomy-induced osteoporosis model. *Biochem Biophys Res Commun* (2013) 434(2):280–6. doi:10.1016/j.bbrc.2013.02.116

103. Zhu LL, Blair H, Cao J, Yuen T, Latif R, Guo L, et al. Blocking antibody to the beta-subunit of FSH prevents bone loss by inhibiting bone resorption and stimulating bone synthesis. *Proc Natl Acad Sci U S A* (2012) 109(36):14574–9. doi:10.1073/pnas.1212806109

104. Ralston SH, Russell RG, Gowen M. Estrogen inhibits release of tumor necrosis factor from peripheral blood mononuclear cells in postmenopausal women. *J Bone Miner Res* (1990) 5(9):983–8. doi:10.1002/jbmr.5650050912

16

Glycosylation Pattern and *in vitro* Bioactivity of Reference Follitropin alfa and Biosimilars

Laura Riccetti[1], Samantha Sperduti[1], Clara Lazzaretti[1,2], Danièle Klett[3],
Francesco De Pascali[3], Elia Paradiso[1,2], Silvia Limoncella[1], Francesco Potì[4],
Simonetta Tagliavini[5], Tommaso Trenti[5], Eugenio Galano[6], Angelo Palmese[6],
Abhijeet Satwekar[6], Jessica Daolio[7], Alessia Nicoli[7], Maria Teresa Villani[7],
Lorenzo Aguzzoli[7], Eric Reiter[3], Manuela Simoni[1,3,8,9] and Livio Casarini[1,8*]

[1] Unit of Endocrinology, Department of Biomedical, Metabolic and Neural Sciences, University of Modena and Reggio Emilia, Modena, Italy, [2] International PhD School in Clinical and Experimental Medicine, University of Modena and Reggio Emilia, Modena, Italy, [3] PRC, INRA, CNRS, IFCE, Université de Tours, Nouzilly, France, [4] Unit of Neurosciences, Department of Medicine and Surgery, University of Parma, Parma, Italy, [5] Department of Laboratory Medicine and Pathological Anatomy, Azienda USL, NOCSAE, Modena, Italy, [6] Analytical Development Biotech Products, Merck Serono S.p.A. (an affiliate of Merck KGaA, Darmstadt, Germany), Rome, Italy, [7] Azienda Unità Sanitaria Locale—IRCCS di Reggio Emilia, Department of Obstetrics and Gynaecology, Fertility Center, ASMN, Reggio Emilia, Italy, [8] Center for Genomic Research, University of Modena and Reggio Emilia, Modena, Italy, [9] Unit of Endocrinology, Department of Medical Specialties, Azienda Ospedaliero-Universitaria, Modena, Italy

Correspondence:
Livio Casarini
livio.casarini@unimore.it

Recombinant follicle-stimulating hormone (FSH) (follitropin alfa) and biosimilar preparations are available for clinical use. They have specific FSH activity and a unique glycosylation profile dependent on source cells. The aim of the study is to compare the originator (reference) follitropin alfa (Gonal-f®)- with biosimilar preparations (Bemfola® and Ovaleap®)-induced cellular responses *in vitro*. Gonadotropin N-glycosylation profiles were analyzed by ELISA lectin assay, revealing preparation specific-patterns of glycan species (Kruskal-Wallis test; $p < 0.05$, $n = 6$) and by glycotope mapping. Increasing concentrations of Gonal-f® or biosimilar (1×10^{-3}-1×10^{3} ng/ml) were used for treating human primary granulosa lutein cells (hGLC) and FSH receptor (FSHR)-transfected HEK293 cells *in vitro*. Intracellular cAMP production, Ca^{2+} increase and β-arrestin 2 recruitment were evaluated by BRET, CREB, and ERK1/2 phosphorylation by Western blotting. 12-h gene expression, and 8- and 24-h progesterone and estradiol synthesis were measured by real-time PCR and immunoassay, respectively. We found preparation-specific glycosylation patterns by lectin assay (Kruskal-Wallis test; $p < 0.001$; $n = 6$), and similar cAMP production and β-arrestin 2 recruitment in FSHR-transfected HEK293 cells (cAMP EC_{50} range = 12 ± 0.9-24 ± 1.7 ng/ml; β-arrestin 2 EC_{50} range = 140 ± 14.1-313 ± 18.7 ng/ml; Kruskal-Wallis test; $p \geq 0.05$; $n = 4$). Kinetics analysis revealed that intracellular Ca^{2+} increased upon cell treatment by 4 μg/ml Gonal-f®, while equal concentrations of biosimilars failed to induced a response (Kruskal-Wallis test; $p < 0.05$; $n = 3$). All preparations induced both 8 and 24 h-progesterone and estradiol synthesis in hGLC, while no different EC_{50}s were demonstrated (Kruskal-Wallis test; $p > 0.05$; $n = 5$). Apart from preparation-specific intracellular Ca^{2+} increases achieved at supra-physiological hormone doses, all compounds induced similar intracellular responses and steroidogenesis, reflecting similar bioactivity, and overall structural homogeneity.

Keywords: FSH, biosimilar, gonal-F, bemfola, ovaleap, glycosylation, assisted reproduction (ART)

INTRODUCTION

Follicle-stimulating hormone (FSH) is a heterodimeric glycoprotein hormone produced by the pituitary and acting on the gonads (1). In fertile women, FSH controls reproduction supporting ovarian granulosa cell proliferation and follicular growth by binding to its G protein-coupled receptor (FSHR) (2).

FSH shares a 92-amino acid residue α subunit with other glycoprotein hormones and has a 111-amino acid residue, hormone-specific β subunit (3). Two N-linked heterogeneous oligosaccharide populations are bound to each protein backbone subunit and are involved in hormone folding and half-life, receptor binding, and activation (4, 5). After gonadotropin binding, FSHR conformation rearrangements occur, triggering intracellular signal transduction. Gαs protein signaling leads to adenylyl cyclase stimulation and cyclic-AMP (cAMP)/protein kinase A (PKA)-pathway activation (6, 7), resulting in cAMP-response element binding protein (CREB) (8, 9) and extracellular-regulated kinase 1/2 (ERK1/2) (10) phosphorylation. These phospho-proteins are key players modulating steroidogenesis, proliferation and survival/apoptosis (8, 11), all molecular events underlying reproductive functions (12). Upon ligand binding, FSHR recruits other heterotrimeric Gα proteins, including Gαq and Gαi (13–16), as well as other interactors (17), linking FSH action to multiple intracellular signaling pathways, such as the rapidly-activated, phospholipase C-dependent (18), cytosolic calcium cation (Ca^{2+}) release (19). FSHR internalization and recycling is mediated by β-arrestin 1 and 2, which triggers G protein-independent ERK1/2 signaling (20, 21).

FSH exists in a number of isoforms differing in content and composition of oligosaccharides attached to the protein backbone (22). FSH glycoforms were proposed as biased receptor ligands (5, 23, 24) due to isoform-specific contact with FSHR (25) and intracellular signaling (26). Glycosylation is a post-translational process influencing the isoelectric point (pI) and half-life of the gonadotropin (27). In women, more glycosylated and acidic FSH isoforms, mainly due to sialylation, exhibit a prolonged in vivo half-life due to reduced kidney clearance and are secreted mostly during the early and mid-follicular phase, compared to FSH basic glycoforms, which are predominant before ovulation (28, 29). Highly acidic FSH isoforms are produced more after the menopause than during the fertile lifespan (30), suggesting that glycoform composition of circulating hormones is dynamic and might have a physiological role.

Several formulations of exogenous FSH may be used in assisted reproductive technologies (ART) to induce multiple follicle development. Both urinary and recombinant FSH and other gonadotropin preparations are commercially available, as well as follitropin alfa biosimilar drugs, which are recombinant compounds similar to the originator (31–33). Previous studies attempted to address effects of these preparations on ART outcomes, given their different glycosylation states featured as post-translational modifications by the cellular source and/or purification processes (31, 34, 35). In fact, previous analyses by mass spectrometry found preparation-specific pattern of glycans bound to the FSH β-subunits (36, 37).

In this study, the biochemical composition and hormone-induced cell response of the originator follitropin alfa and two biosimilar preparations were analyzed in vitro. Glycosylation pattern was assessed in regard to cAMP production, Ca^{2+} release, β-arrestin 2 recruitment, CREB, and ERK1/2 phosphorylation and steroid (i.e., progesterone and estradiol) synthesis, which were analyzed in human primary granulosa-lutein cells (hGLC) and HEK293 cells transiently transfected with the human FSHR cDNA.

MATERIALS AND METHODS

Follitropin Alfa Reference Preparation (Gonal-f®) and Biosimilars

The reference follitropin alfa and two biosimilar preparations were analyzed: Gonal-f® provided by Merck KGaA (Darmstadt, Germany), Ovaleap® purchased from Teva Pharmaceutical Industries (Tel Aviv, Israel) and Bemfola® from Finox Biotech (Kirchberg, Switzerland). Different batches of each preparation were tested by performing both biochemical and functional evaluations, as follows: two batches of Gonal-f® (AU016646, BA045956), two batches of Ovaleap® (S27266, R38915), and three batches of Bemfola® (PPS30400, PNS30388, PNS30230). Additional Gonal-f® (199F005, 199F049, 199F051) and Ovaleap® (S06622) batches were used for glycopeptide mapping. Comparison of hormone induced-signaling in vitro were performed by stimulating cells with gonadotropins concentrations expressed by mass rather than International Units (IU), since the latter depends of the in vivo activity in rats (38). Gonal-f® and biosimilar dosages were determined starting by the batch concentration declared by providers, consisting of 44 μg/ml for Gonal-f®, Ovaleap® and Bemfola®. Recombinant human choriogonadotropin (hCG; Ovitrelle®, Merck KGaA) was used as a negative control where indicated.

Silver Staining and Western Blotting Analysis

According to gonadotropin quantification provided by the producers, 300 ng of each compound were subjected to 12% SDS-PAGE. Gel electrophoresis was performed under denaturing-reducing or *non*-denaturing-*non* reducing conditions, followed by silver staining and Western blotting. Denaturing conditions consisted of boiling samples 5 min at 100°C, while reducing conditions were obtained by adding 2-mercaptoethanol (Sigma-Aldrich, St. Louis, MO, USA), disrupting disulfide bonds (39). Silver staining was performed after acrylamide gel electrophoresis, as previously described (40, 41). Briefly, fixation was performed by incubating gels 1 h in 50% ethanol buffer, in the presence of 12% acetic acid and $5 \times 10{-4}\%$ formalin (all from Sigma-Aldrich). After washes, gels were stained with 0.2% $AgNO_3$ buffer 30 min-treatment and signals were developed by 3% Na_2CO_3 buffer, 0.0005% formalin and $4 \times 10{-4}\%$ $Na_2S_2O_3$ before to be stopped. Originator follitropin alpha and biosimilars were evaluated by Western blotting using a rabbit anti-human polyclonal primary antibody against FSHβ/FSH (SAB1304978; Sigma-Aldrich), while the secondary antibody was anti-rabbit human horseradish peroxidase (HRP)-conjugated (#NA9340V; GE HealthCare, Little Chalfont, UK). Recombinant hCG (Ovitrelle; Merck KGaA) was used as a negative control. Signals were developed with ECL (GE HealthCare) and acquired using the VersaDoc Imaging System (Bio-Rad Laboratories Inc., Hercules, CA, USA).

Lectin ELISA Assay and Glycopeptide Mapping

The technique was described previously (41, 42) and adapted to preparations used in this study. A 96-well-microtiter plate was coated overnight at 4°C with the anti-human gonadotropin α subunit monoclonal antibody HT13.3 (43), which recognizes all human glycoprotein hormone α subunits, in 0.1 M sodium carbonate/hydrogen carbonate buffer (pH = 9.6). Plates were washed with a saline buffer (TBS-T; 25 mM Tris, 140 mM NaCl, 3 mM KCl, 0.05%, Tween 20; pH = 7.4) and *non*-specific sites were saturated by 1 h-treatment at room temperature (RT) using TBS-T containing 2% polyvinylpyrrolidone K30 (Fluka, Sigma-Aldrich). Duplicate 5 ng samples of each hormone preparation were then incubated over-night, in 100 μl/well of the saturation buffer. After washing, biotinylated lectins (Vector laboratories Ltd, AbCys Biologie, Paris, France) were placed into wells and incubated for 2 h at RT. Lectins used were: *Sambucus nigra* agglutinin (SNA), *Maackia amurensis* agglutinin (MAA), *Artocarpus Polyphemus* lectin (jacalin), *Ricinus communis* agglutinin (RCA-1, ricin), *Datura stramonium* agglutinin (DSA), wheat germ agglutinin (WGA), *Phaseolus vulgaris* agglutinin (PHA-E) (**Supplemental Table 1**). They were diluted in saturation buffer containing 1 mM $CaCl_2$, 1 mM $MgCl_2$, and 1 mM $MnCl_2$. Plates were washed and peroxidase labeled NeutrAvidin^{TM} (Pierce, Interchim, Montluçon, France) was added in each well (100 μl in TBS-T), for 1 h at RT. After incubation with TMB ELISA peroxidase substrate standard solution (UP664781; Interchim, Montluçon, France) 20 min at RT, reactions were stopped by adding 50 μl/well of 2 N H_2SO_4, and absorbance measured at 450 nm wavelength using a spectrophotometer. Blank values, consisting of samples

maintained in the absence of hormones, were subtracted to obtain ELISA data.

Additional information about reagents, glycopeptide mapping, hydrophilic interaction chromatography, and mass spectrometry analysis is provided in the supplemental section (**Supplemental Material and Methods**).

Cell Culture and Transfection

HEK293 cells were cultured in Dulbecco's Modified Eagle Medium (DMEM) supplemented with 10% FBS, 4.5 g/l glucose, 100 IU/ml penicillin, 0.1 mg/ml streptomycin, and 1 mM glutamine (all from Sigma-Aldrich). Transient transfections were performed in 96-well plates using Metafectene PRO (Biontex Laboratories GmbH, München, Germany), in order to obtain exogenous FSHR and cAMP CAMYEL-, β-arrestin 2- or aequorin Ca^{2+}-BRET biosensor protein expression (15), as previously described (41). For cAMP evaluation, 50 ng/well of FSHR-expressing plasmid were mixed together with 0.5 μl/well of Metafectene PRO in serum-free medium and incubated 20 min. A 50 μl aliquot of cAMP CAMYEL biosensor-expressing plasmid-Metafectene PRO mix was added to each well-containing 1×10^5 cells, in a total volume of 200 μl/well, and incubated 2-days before stimulation with gonadotropins. One hundred ng/well of FSHR-Rluc8- and 100 ng/well of β-arrestin 2 biosensor-expressing plasmids were used for evaluating β-arrestin 2 recruitment. One hundred ng/well of FSHR- and 100 ng/well of aequorin biosensor-expressing plasmids were used to prepare cells for measure changes in intracellular Ca^{2+}. All samples were prepared in duplicate and BRET measurements were performed using 2-day transfected cells, in 40 μl/well PBS and 1 mM Hepes.

Human primary granulosa lutein cells (hGLC) were isolated from ovarian follicles of about twenty donor women undergoing oocyte retrieval for ART, following written consent and with local Ethics Committee permission (Nr. 796 19th June 2014, Reggio Emilia, Italy). Patients had to match these criteria: absence of endocrine abnormalities and viral/bacterial infections, age between 25 and 45 years. Cells were recovered from the follicular washing fluid using a 50% Percoll density gradient (GE Healthcare, Little Chalfont, UK), following a protocol previously described (7, 44, 45). In order to restore expression of gonadotropin receptors (46), hGLC were cultured 6 days, then serum-starved over-night before use in experiments. Cells were cultured at 37°C and 5% CO_2 in McCoy's 5A medium, supplemented with 10% FBS, 2 mM L-glutamine, 100 IU/ml penicillin, 100 μg/ml streptomycin and 250 ng/ml Fungizone (Sigma-Aldrich).

BRET Measurement of cAMP Production, and β-arrestin Recruitment and Intracellular Ca^{2+} Increase

Intracellular cAMP and Ca^{2+} increase, and β-arrestin 2 recruitment were evaluated following a previously described procedure (15, 41, 47). Cyclic-AMP production and Ca^{2+} increase were evaluated in transiently transfected HEK293 cells using the *FSHR*-expressing plasmid, together with the BRET-based cAMP biosensor CAMYEL (48), or the aequorin Ca^{2+}-biosensor expression vector (49), respectively, while BRET experiments cannot be performed in hGLC due to sub-optimal transfection efficiency and the high mortality rate in this cell model. Recruitment of β-arrestin 2 was assessed after transient transfection of HEK293 cells with the C-terminal, *Rluc*-tagged *FSHR* cDNA plasmid (provided by Dr. Aylin C. Hanyaloglu, Imperial College, London, UK) and N-terminal, yPET-tagged β-arrestin 2 (provided by Dr. Mark G. Scott, Cochin Institute, Paris, France). Cells were incubated 30 min in 40 μl/well PBS and 1 mM Hepes, in the presence or in the absence of increasing concentrations of Gonal-f® or biosimilars (1×10^{-3}-1×10^3 ng/ml range), and intracellular cAMP increase and β-arrestin 2 recruitment were measured upon addition of 10 μl/well of 5 μM Coelenterzine h (Interchim). A 4×10^3 ng/ml hormone concentration-induced intracellular Ca^{2+} increase was evaluated over 100 s in transfected cells. Recombinant follitropin alfa or biosimilar addition occurred at the 25 s time-point. Light emissions were detected at 475 ± 30 and 530 ± 30 nm wavelengths using the CLARIOstar plate reader equipped with a monocromator (BMG Labtech, Ortenberg, Germany).

Evaluation of ERK1/2 and CREB Phosphorylation

Hormone-induced ERK1/2 and CREB phosphorylation was analyzed by Western blotting following a protocol previously described (50). Human GLCs were seeded in 24-well plates (1×10^5 cells/well) and treated for 15 min with increasing concentrations of gonadotropin (1×10^1-1×10^3 ng/ml range). Cells were immediately lysed for protein extraction in ice-cold RIPA buffer along with PhosStop phosphatase inhibitor and a protease inhibitor cocktail (Roche, Basel, Switzerland). Cell lysates were subjected to 12% SDS-PAGE and Western blotting, while pERK1/2 and pCREB activation were evaluated using specific rabbit antibodies (#9101 and #9198, respectively; Cell Signaling Technology Inc., Danvers, MA, USA). Sample loads were normalized to total ERK1/2 (#4695; Cell Signaling Technology Inc.). Membranes were treated with secondary anti-rabbit HRP-conjugated antibody (#NA9340V; GE HealthCare) and signals developed with ECL (GE HealthCare). Signal detection employed the VersaDoc system using the QuantityOne analysis software (Bio-Rad Laboratories Inc.). Protein density volumes were semi-quantitatively evaluated by the ImageJ software (U. S. National Institutes of Health, Bethesda, MD, USA) (51).

Gene Expression Analysis

Hormone 50% effective concentrations (EC_{50}s) were calculated from the cAMP dose-response curves and used for hGLC treatments before FSH-target gene expression analysis. Cells were seeded at 5×10^4 cells/well in 24-well plates and exposed to gonadotropins for 8 h, and RNA was then extracted using the automated workstation EZ1 Advanced XL (Qiagen, Hilden, Germany). Equal amounts of total RNA were retrotranscribed by iScript reverse transcriptase (Bio-Rad Laboratories Inc.), according to a previously validated protocol

(52). The expression of *STARD1* and *CYP19A1* genes encoding steroid-acute regulatory protein (StAR) and aromatase enzymes, respectively, was evaluated by real time PCR (7, 44) using specific primer sequences and protocols previously validated (7). Target gene expression was normalized to *ribosomal protein subunit 7* (*RPS7*) gene expression using the $2^{-\Delta\Delta Ct}$ method (53). Experiments were recorded as the mean value of duplicates.

Steroid Hormone Stimulation Protocol and Measurement

Human GLCs were seeded in 24-well plates (4×10^4 cells/well) and treated 8 or 24 h with increasing hormone concentrations (1×10^{-3}-1×10^3 ng/ml). Where appropriate, 1 μM 4-androstene-3,17-dione (androstenedione; #A9630; Sigma-Aldrich) was added, as a substrate to be converted to estrogen by the aromatase enzyme. Stimulations were terminated by freezing samples and total progesterone or estradiol was measured in the cell media by an immunoassay analyzer (ARCHITECT second Generation system; Abbot Diagnostics, Chicago, IL, USA).

Statistical Analysis

Data were graphically represented using box and whiskers plots, histograms, X-Y graphs and tables, and indicated as means ± standard error of means (SEM). Western blotting results were normalized to total ERK signals. Intracellular Ca^{2+} increase was represented as kinetics of acceptor emissions measured at 525 ± 30 nm, and area under the curve (AUC) values were extrapolated for comparisons between preparations. Dose-response curves for cAMP and β-arrestin 2 were obtained by data interpolation using *non*-linear regression. BRET data were represented as induced BRET changes by subtracting the ratio of donor/acceptor biosensor emissions of the untreated cells from the values of the stimulated cells. Data distributions were analyzed by D'Agostino and Pearson normality test, while differences were evaluated by Kruskal-Wallis or Friedman test with Dunn's multiple comparison *post-test* and considered significant when $p < 0.05$. Statistics were performed using the GraphPad Prism 6.01 software (GraphPad Software Inc., San Diego, CA, USA).

RESULTS

Western Blotting and Silver Staining Analysis

Samples comprising 300 ng/well of *non*-denatured and denatured Gonal-f® and biosimilar preparations were loaded onto a 12% acrylamide gel and separated by SDS gel electrophoresis under denaturing-reducing and *non*-denaturing-*non* reducing conditions. Denaturing conditions refer to 100°C-boiled samples, while reducing conditions were obtained by adding 2-mercaptoethanol. While no signals were detected under *non* denaturing-*non* reducing conditions by Western blotting (data not shown), two bands corresponding to the reference follitropin alfa and biosimilar preparations were revealed under denaturing-reducing conditions (**Figure 1A**). Ovaleap® and Gonal-f® preparations featured an ~20 KDa band, while a band corresponding to about 23 KDa molecular weight characterized

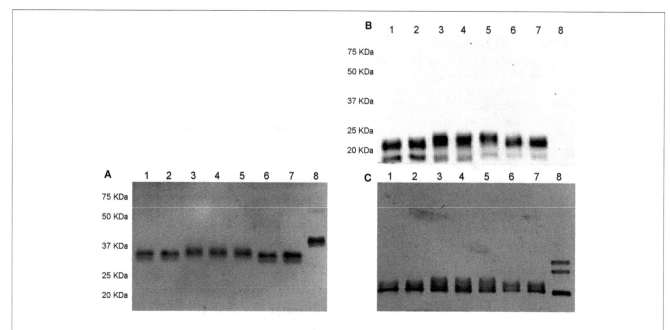

FIGURE 1 | Western blotting **(A)** and silver staining analysis **(B,C)** of Gonal-f® and biosimilars under *non*-denaturing-*non* reducing and denaturing-reducing conditions. Samples comprising 300 ng of each preparation, according to the quantification provided by the manufacturer, were loaded. FSH presence was detected by rabbit anti-human polyclonal primary antibody against FSHβ/FSH. Recombinant hCG was used as negative control. Samples were loaded as follows: (1) Ovaleap® batch R38915, (2) Ovaleap® batch S27266, (3) Bemfola® batch PPS30400, (4) Bemfola® batch PNS30388, (5) Bemfola® batch PNS30230, (6) Gonal-f® batch AU016646, (7) Gonal-f® batch BA045956, (8) recombinant hCG. **(A)** Evaluation of FSH preparations under denaturing-reducing conditions, by Western blotting, using anti-FSHβ antibody. **(B)** Silver staining analysis of FSH preparations under *non-denaturing-non reducing* conditions. **(C)** Analysis of FSH preparations under denaturing-reducing conditions, by silver staining.

Bemfola®. All preparations displayed a 15 KDa band of varying intensity. Recombinant hCG served as a negative control, providing no signal using the anti-FSH antibody.

Analysis by silver staining under *non* denaturing-*non* reducing conditions revealed that all preparations shared an overall similar protein pattern characterized by a single band at about 37 KDa molecular weight (**Figure 1B**). hCG resulted in a 40 KDa band. All samples displayed signals at about 20 KDa molecular weight (**Figure 1C**). Interestingly, no 15-KDa signals were detected, oppositely to that demonstrated by Western blotting, likely to be attributed to the low amount of FSHβ bound by the antibody and undetectable using silver staining due to sub-optimal sensitivity of this method (54). Three 35–20 KDa bands corresponding to recombinant hCG Ovitrelle® were detected, as previously described (41).

Reference Follitropin Alfa and Biosimilar Reactivity to Lectins

The carbohydrate structure of follitropin alfa and biosimilars was investigated by ELISA, using a panel consisting of seven lectins characterized by specific recognition of different glycan features (**Supplemental Table 1**). Batches of each hormone were considered as experimental replicates and absorbance values measured at 450 nm were compared (**Table 1**).

Bemfola® displayed structural peculiarities and variability, emerging by lectin analysis (**Supplemental Table 2**), due to significantly higher reactivity against ricin than other preparations (Kruskal-Wallis test; $p < 0.05$; $n = 16$; **Table 1**). Moreover, lectin assay revealed higher affinity of Bemfola® to DSA than Gonal-f® (Kruskal Wallis test; $p < 0.05$; $n = 6$). Ricin recognizes Galβ(1,4)GlcNAc monomers with higher affinity in the absence of sialylation in the terminal galactose, while DSA lectin binds Galβ(1,4) linked N-acetylglucosamine oligomers and a branched pentasaccharide sequence, including two N-acetyl lactosamine repeats linked to a mannose (55). No signal was detected with SNA lectin regardless of the hormone tested, indicating that sialic acid of the α(2,6) type is absent (56), likely due to the absence of galactoside α(2,6) sialyltransferase enzyme expression by CHO-K1 cells (57). Sialic acid of α(2,3) type is detected by MAA lectin in all samples (58), without any significant preparation-specific pattern. Jacalin failed to produce any signal, demonstrating the absence of O-glycans of the Galβ1-3GalNac or GalNac type (59). PHA-E lectin recognizes bi-antennary complex-type N-glycan with outer Gal and bisecting GlcNAc sequences (60), while WGA lectin reacts with GlcNAc sequences and sialic acid (61). Antennarity (**Table 2**), sialylation (**Table 3**), and sialic acid (**Table 4**) distribution were analyzed by glycopeptide mapping of Gonal-f® and Ovaleap® batches.

These features were similarly represented among preparations (Kruskal-Wallis test; $p \geq 0.05$; $n = 6$), as well as among batches (**Supplemental Results**), at least in Gonal-f® and Bemfola® (Chi-square test; $p \geq 0.05$), which appeared to be homogeneous, overall (**Supplemental Tables 3–5**).

TABLE 1 | ELISA lectin analysis of reference and biosimilar follitropin alfa preparations.

Lectins	Gonal-f® Absorbance (nm; means ± SEM*10³)	Ovaleap® Absorbance (nm; means ± SEM*10³)	Bemfola® Absorbance (nm; means ± SEM*10³)	p^a
MAA	74 ± 10	56 ± 1	60 ± 6	0.236
SNA	−2 ± 1	−35 ± 1	−40 ± 1	0.236
Jacalin	−1 ± 8	−9 ± 4	−17 ± 2	0.749
Ricin	120 ± 3	70 ± 2	180 ± 2	<0.0001
DSA	250 ± 8	370 ± 13	460 ± 8	0.001
PHA–E	1300 ± 30	1350 ± 40	1300 ± 30	0.814
WGA	100 ± 7	50 ± 5	80 ± 3	0.809

[a] Kruskal Wallis test and Dunn's post-test.

TABLE 2 | Antennarity of reference and biosimilar follitropin alfa preparations.

Glycosylation site	Antennarity distribution	Gonal-f® (means ± SEM)	Ovaleap® (means ± SEM)	p^a
Asn52	Di-antennary	88.5 ± 0.5	90.6 ± 0.9	>0.999
	Tri-antennary	11.0 ± 0.6	9.1 ± 0.7	
	Tetra-antennary	0.4 ± 0.1	0.5 ± 0.2	
	A-Index	2.1 ± 0.0	2.1 ± 0.0	
Asn78	Di-antennary	91.5 ± 0.4	93.0 ± 0.5	>0.999
	Tri-antennary	8.3 ± 0.4	6.9 ± 0.2	
	Tetra-antennary	0.2 ± 0.1	0.2 ± 0.1	
	A-Index	2.1 ± 0.0	2.1 ± 0.0	
Asn7	Di-antennary	10.7 ± 0.4	6.0 ± 0.6	>0.999
	Tri-antennary	66.5 ± 1.1	73.2 ± 1.7	
	Tetra-antennary	19.3 ± 0.9	17.3 ± 1.7	
	One Repeat containing	3.3 ± 0.4	3.4 ± 0.5	
	A-Index	3.2 ± 0.0	3.2 ± 0.0	
Asn24	Mono-antennary	0.4 ± 0.1	0.3 ± 0.0	>0.999
	Di-antennary	87.5 ± 0.7	83.0 ± 1.2	
	Tri-antennary	7.7 ± 0.4	10.5 ± 0.3	
	Tetra-antennary	4.5 ± 0.3	6.1 ± 1.2	
	One Repeat containing	0.1 ± 0.0	0.3 ± 0.0	
	A-Index	2.2 ± 0.0	2.2 ± 0.0	

[a] Kolmogorov-Smirnov test.

TABLE 3 | Sialylation distribution in reference and biosimilar follitropin alfa preparations.

Glycosylation site	Sialylation indexes	Gonal-f® (means ± SEM)	Ovaleap® (means ± SEM)	p^a
Asn52	S-extent (%)	96.0 ± 0.1	97.5 ± 0.2	>0.999
	S-index	2.0 ± 0.0	2.0 ± 0.0	
Asn78	S-extent (%)	85.0 ± 0.3	90.1 ± 0.2	0.400
	S-index	1.8 ± 0.0	1.9 ± 0.0	
Asn7	S-extent (%)	91.3 ± 0.2	95.4 ± 0.4	0.100
	S-index	2.9 ± 0.0	3.0 ± 0.0	
Asn24	S-extent (%)	88.0 ± 0.2	92.3 ± 0.7	0.100
	S-index	1.9 ± 0.0	2.0 ± 0.0	

[a] Mann-Whitney's U-test.

TABLE 4 | Sialic acid distribution in reference and biosimilar follitropin alfa preparations.

Glycosylation site	Sialic acid	Gonal-f® (means ± SEM)	Ovaleap® (means ± SEM)	p^a
Asn52	NANA	97.3 ± 0.1	94.0 ± 0.1	>0.999
	NGNA	0.2 ± 0.1	4.2 ± 0.3	
	O-Acetylated NANA	2.5 ± 0.1	1.8 ± 0.3	
Asn78	NANA	95.0 ± 0.3	89.9 ± 0.2	>0.999
	NGNA	0.0 ± 0.0	4.4 ± 0.2	
	O-Acetylated NANA	5.0 ± 0.3	5.8 ± 0.4	
Asn7	NANA	97.5 ± 0.4	95.4 ± 0.5	>0.999
	NGNA	0.0 ± 0.0	2.9 ± 0.2	
	O-Acetylated NANA	2.5 ± 0.4	1.7 ± 0.6	
Asn24	NANA	92.8 ± 0.3	90.2 ± 0.5	>0.999
	NGNA	0.2 ± 0.1	3.6 ± 0.1	
	O-Acetylated NANA	7.0 ± 0.4	6.2 ± 0.4	

[a] Kolmogorov-Smirnov test.

Evaluation of Intracellular cAMP Increase and β-Arrestin 2 Recruitment

Transfected, FSHR-expressing HEK293 cells were used to compare intracellular cAMP increases and β-arrestin 2 recruitment induced by 30-min treatment with increasing doses of reference follitropin alfa and biosimilars. Different batches of each preparation were tested and dose-response curves obtained by plotting cAMP and β-arrestin 2 levels in a semi-log X-Y graph (**Supplemental Figure 1**), in order to calculate and compare EC_{50} values obtained from the individual dose-response-curves (**Figure 2**).

Although preparation-specific carbohydrate structures were detected (**Table 1**), no significant differences were found between Gonal-f® and biosimilars' EC_{50} required for activating cAMP (**Table 5**; 12.9 ± 2.5–24.2 ± 6.0 ng/ml range; Kruskal-Wallis test, $p \geq 0.05$; $n = 4$; **Figure 2A**) and β-arrestin 2

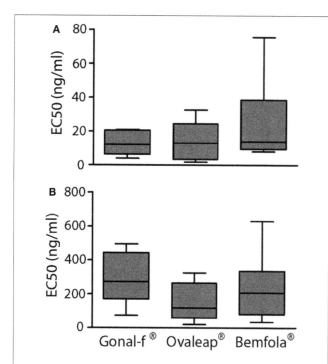

FIGURE 2 | EC$_{50}$ of cAMP response and β-arrestin 2 recruitment induced by Gonal-f® and biosimilars in transfected HEK293 cells. **(A)** Cells were transiently co-transfected with FSHR and CAMYEL sensor. cAMP was measured by BRET after 30 min stimulation with increasing doses of Gonal-f®, Ovaleap®, and Bemfola®. **(B)** Cells were transiently co-transfected with FSHR-Rluc8 and β-arrestin 2 –YPET sensors. β-arrestin 2 recruitment was measured by BRET after 30 min stimulation with increasing doses of hormones. EC$_{50}$ values were extrapolated by non-linear regression. Data are represented as box and whiskers graphs (Kruskal Wallis test, $p \geq 0.05$; $n = 4$).

TABLE 5 | Efficiency (EC$_{50}$) of 30 min-cAMP and β-arrestin 2 production induced by reference and biosimilar follitropin alfa preparations in transfected, FSHR-expressing HEK293 cells.

Preparation	EC$_{50}$ cAMP (ng/ml; means ± SEM; $n = 4$)	p^a	EC$_{50}$ β-arrestin 2 (ng/ml; means ± SEM; $n = 4$)	p^a
Gonal-f®	12.9 ± 2.5	0.561	278.6 ± 56.9	0.223
Ovaleap®	14.7 ± 3.9		140.7 ± 42.6	
Bemfola®	24.2 ± 6.0		234.9 ± 57.2	

^{a} Kruskal-Wallis test.

Gonal-f® and biosimilars' patterns of ERK1/2 phosphorylation were detected, pCREB activation occurred upon cell treatment by 0.5 ng/ml Gonal-f, differently to that obtained using both biosimilars (Friedman test, $p < 0.05$; $n = 4$). Interestingly, cell treatment by Gonal-f® and Bemfola® maximal concentrations (15 ng/ml) resulted in slightly decreased levels of CREB phosphorylation, not differing, however, significantly from the *plateau* levels of pCREB activation.

STARD1 and CYP19A1 Gene Expression Analysis

Expression of FSH target genes was analyzed by real time PCR in hGLC. For this purpose, cells were stimulated 12 h by Gonal-f®, Ovaleap® or Bemfola®. Hormones were administered at the EC$_{50}$ calculated from cAMP data (12 ng/ml Gonal-f® and Ovaleap®, 24 ng/ml Bemfola®). Total RNA was reverse-transcribed to cDNA and used for *STARD1* and *CYP19A1* gene expression analysis by real-time PCR. Data were normalized over the *RPS7* gene expression and represented as fold-increase over unstimulated cells in a bar-graph as means ± SEM (**Figure 4**).

Gonal-f®, Ovaleap®, and Bemfola® resulted in about 15-fold *STARD1* and 3-fold *CYP19A1* increase compared to the basal level (Kruskal-Wallis test, $p < 0.05$; $n = 4$). In particular, Ovaleap®-induced *CYP19A1* expression level lower than what was obtained by Bemfola® treatment (Kruskal-Wallis test, $p < 0.05$; $n = 4$). Treatment using different batches did not to affect *STARD1* and *CYP19A1* expression levels, since no significant differences between lots of any preparation occurred (Kruskal-Wallis test, $p \geq 0.05$; $n = 4$; data not shown).

Steroid Synthesis Analysis

Progesterone production and androgen-to-estrogen conversion were evaluated in hGLC treated for 8 or 24 h with hormones. For this purpose, cells were maintained under continuous stimulation by increasing gonadotropin concentrations (1×10^{-3}-1×10^{3} ng/ml range) until reactions were stopped by freezing cell plates. To evaluate estradiol synthesis, androstenedione was added into wells as a substrate for the aromatase enzyme. Eight- and Twenty-four hours progesterone and estradiol dose-response curves were obtained and evaluated by *non*-linear regression, EC$_{50}$ values calculated, and compared (**Table 6**).

Reflecting cAMP accumulation, cell stimulation with Gonal-f®, Ovaleap®, and Bemfola® resulted in similar 8- and 24-h

(**Table 5**; 140.7 ± 42.6–278.6 ± 56.9 ng/ml range; Kruskal-Wallis test, $p \geq 0.05$; $n = 4$; **Figure 2B**), consistent between batches (cAMP: 10 ± 0.0–28 ± 0.0 ng/ml range; β-arrestin 2: 64 ± 0.0–610 ± 0.2 ng/ml range; Kruskal-Wallis test, $p \geq 0.05$; $n = 4$; **Supplemental Figure 1**) and confirming similar potencies *in vitro*.

Analysis of pERK1/2 and pCREB Activation

The phosphorylation of ERK1/2 and CREB was evaluated in hGLC, which naturally express endogenous FSHR. Cells were treated for 15 min with increasing hormone concentrations, and phospho-protein activation was evaluated by Western blotting and semi-quantitatively measured (**Figure 3**). Total ERK served as a normalizer.

Similar ERK1/2 and CREB phosphorylation patterns were observed after stimulating cells with increasing doses of different batches of each preparation (**Supplemental Figure 2**). Mean results from batches of Gonal-f®, Ovaleap®, and Bemfola® were calculated and average hormone-specific pERK1/2 and pCREB activation results were reported (**Figure 3**). All preparations induced protein phosphorylation within the 1.5–15 ng/ml range (Kruskal-Wallis test, $p < 0.05$; $n = 4$), consistently between different batches of each preparation (Friedman test, $p \geq 0.05$; $n = 4$). While no statistically significant differences between

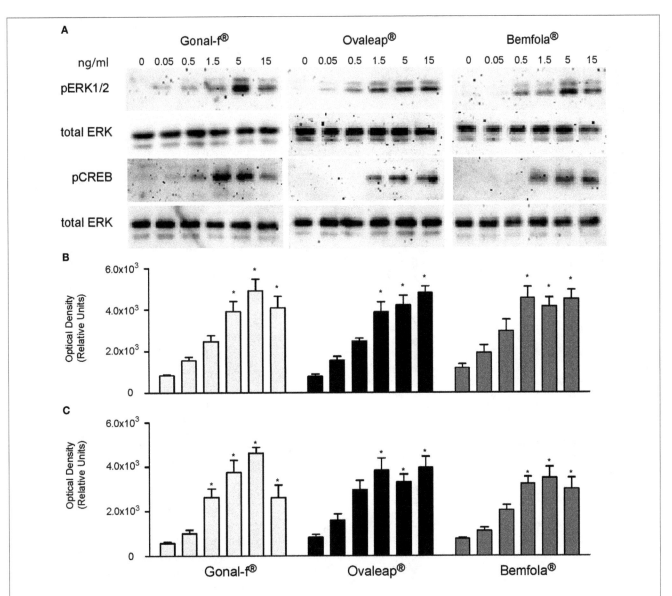

FIGURE 3 | Evaluation of pERK1/2 and pCREB activation after Gonal-f® and biosimilars treatment of hGLC. Cells were stimulated by increasing doses of preparations. ERK1/2 and CREB phosphorylation were evaluated after 15 min by Western blotting (images representative of four independent experiments) **(A)**. **(B,C)** Densitometric analysis of pERK1/2 **(B)** and pCREB **(C)** signals. The values were normalized to total ERK and represented as means ± SEM, then statistically evaluated (* = significant vs. control (0 dose); Kruskal Wallis test; $p < 0.05$; $n = 4$).

progesterone and estradiol production curves (Kruskal-Wallis test; $p \geq 0.05$; $n = 5$), confirmed using different batches (Kruskal-Wallis test; $p \geq 0.05$; $n = 5$; data not shown), as well as in similar progesterone and estradiol *plateau* levels (Kruskal-Wallis test; $p \geq 0.05$; $n = 5$; **Supplemental Table 6**).

Intracellular Ca²⁺ Increase

Kinetics of intracellular Ca^{2+} increase was evaluated in a transiently transfected HEK293 cell line that co-expressed both FSHR- and Ca^{2+}-biosensors, by BRET. Cells were monitored for over 100 s and 4×10^3 ng/ml hormone addition occurred at the 25 s time-point (**Figure 5**). A 10–20-fold supra-physiological FSH concentration was used, compared to FSH serum levels described in cycling women (62), due to the lack of an

intracellular Ca^{2+} signal at lower hormone concentrations (data not shown). Thapsigargin and vehicle treatment were used as positive and negative controls, respectively. Data were represented as means ± SEM. AUC values were calculated to compare preparation-specific intracellular Ca^{2+} increase.

Addition of vehicle failed to induce any intracellular Ca^{2+} increase, confirming the lack of activity exerted by the solvent used for hormone dilution on calcium response. After confirming the absence of batch-specific results (Kruskal-Wallis test; $p \geq 0.05$; $n = 3$; data not shown), cell treatment by Gonal-f® induced rapid intracellular Ca^{2+} increase, which was about 230-fold higher than vehicle (Kruskal-Wallis test; $p < 0.05$; $n = 3$) and occurred within 1–2 s after hormone addition. Bemfola® and Ovaleap® induced only a minimal, not significant intracellular

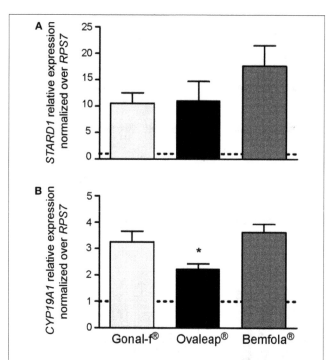

FIGURE 4 | *STARD1* and *CYPA19A1* gene expression analysis. The expression of *STARD1* **(A)** and *CYPA19A1* **(B)** gene was evaluated in hGLC stimulated for 12 h with the EC$_{50}$ of Gonal-f® or biosimilars (12 ng/ml Gonal-f® and Ovaleap®, 24 ng/ml Bemfola®) by real-time PCR. Each value was normalized over the *RPS7* gene expression (means ± SEM; $n = 4$). Unstimulated cells served as control and are indicated as a dotted line. (*= significant vs. Bemfola®, Kruskal Wallis test; $p < 0.05$).

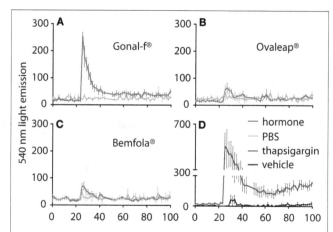

FIGURE 5 | Calcium response kinetics in transfected HEK293 cells treated with Gonal-f® or biosimilars. Cells were transiently co-transfected with FSHR and aequorin sensors, then stimulated in duplicates with a fixed dose (4 × 10^3 ng/ml) of **(A)** Gonal-f®, **(B)** Ovaleap®, **(C)** Bemfola®. **(D)** Thapsigargin, PBS and hormone diluent were used as positive and negative controls, respectively. BRET signal was measured for 100 s. Data are represented as means ± SEM ($n = 3$). Area under the curve (AUC) values were calculated and differences were considered for $p < 0.05$ (Kruskal Wallis test).

TABLE 6 | FSH EC$_{50}$ values (ng/ml) in inducing 8 h- and 24 h-progesterone and estradiol production induced by reference and biosimilar follitropin alfa preparations (means±SEM; $n = 5$) in human primary granulosa cells.

Preparation	Progesterone	p^a	Estradiol	p^a
8 h				
Gonal-f®	1.5 ± 0.3		10.3 ± 4.4	
Ovaleap®	10.9 ± 3.7	0.285	5.6 ± 1.9	0.899
Bemfola®	4.4 ± 1.5		7.1 ± 2.6	
24 h				
Gonal-f®	15.4 ± 5.5		3.3 ± 1.0	
Ovaleap®	5.7 ± 1.2	0.799	2.5 ± 0.8	0.803
Bemfola®	7.3 ± 2.0		3.4 ± 1.0	

^{a} Kruskal-Wallis test.

Ca^{2+} increase (Kruskal-Wallis test; $p \geq 0.05$; $n = 3$). Maximal levels of intracellular Ca^{2+} were achieved under thapsigargin treatment, which served as a positive control and induced an about 600-fold greater increase compared to the basal level (Kruskal-Wallis test; $p < 0.05$; $n = 3$).

DISCUSSION

We compared the biochemical profiles and hormone-induced cell responses of the reference follitropin alfa (Gonal-f®) and two biosimilars, Ovaleap® and Bemfola®, *in vitro*, revealing

overall comparable hormone-induced intracellular signaling and steroidogenesis. Only the originator follitropin alfa induced hormone-specific pattern of CREB phosphorylation and, at supra-physiological concentrations (62), intracellular Ca^{2+} increase to transfected, FSHR-expressing cell lines.

Several gonadotropin formulations are commercially available, differing by source, purification process, and purity. Clinicians choose freely what preparation or combination of preparations will be administered to women undergoing ART (35). These preparations may differ in oligosaccharide content and number of branches attached to the protein backbone (63), depending on the glycosyltransferases equipment of the source cell. Gonal-f® is expressed by Chinese hamster ovary (CHO) cell lines (64), ensuring high bioactivity and batch-to-batch consistency (65, 66). Bemfola® is produced by a pre-adapted dihydrofolate reductase deficient CHO (CHO DHFR-) host cell line (67) and has demonstrated similar efficacy and safety *in vivo* as compared to the reference follitropin alfa, in a multi-center phase 3 study (68). Ovaleap® is also produced by a CHO-derived cell line after adaptation to serum free conditions (69) and has been demonstrated to be similar to follitropin alfa *in vivo* in a phase 3 clinical study (70).

Gonal-f® and Ovaleap® share two similar Western blotting patterns under denaturing and reducing conditions, likely due to specifically glycosylated FSH β-subunits (36, 37), while Bemfola® featured a ~23 instead of 20 KDa band according to its specific glycosylation pattern detected by mass spectrometry (36). Most of these signals were confirmed by silver staining, except for the absence of the 15 KDa band, likely due to sub-optimal sensitivity of the method (54). Analysis of native proteins contained in Gonal-f® and Ovaleap® batches, which were obtained by omitting treatment of samples by 100°C-heating and 2-mercaptoethanol reduction, revealed a single 37

KDa band consistent with the FSH heterodimer (71), while Bemfola® resulted in slightly higher apparent molecular weight. On the other hand, lectin assay revealed higher DSA signal in Bemfola® than Gonal-f®, likely due to different multiantennary complex structures on N-glycans demonstrated by glycopeptide mapping (36), and suggesting Bemfola®-specific glycosylation patterns. Lower ricin binding to Ovaleap® than to Bemfola® and Gonal-f® indicated a different content of Galβ1-4GlcNAc molecules (72).

Naturally occurring variations in carbohydrate structures were characterized during the follicular phase of the cycle (22) and might affect FSH bioactivity in vivo (73). Highly glycosylated FSH isoforms prevail at the early stages, while serum levels of less-acidic (sialylated) glycoforms increase at the mid-cycle until ovulation (29), suggesting a functional role of glycosylation and sialylated structures in modulating FSH bioactivity (26). However, crystallographic structures of FSH in complex with the receptor ectodomain suggested that carbohydrates are not located in the binding interface between the hormone and FSHR (74, 75), making unclear the physiological role of FSH sugar residues in hormone activity. In fact, analysis of signaling cascades revealed that cell treatment by Gonal-f® and biosimilars resulted in similar dose-response curves for both cAMP and β-arrestin 2, as well as ERK1/2 phosphorylation pattern. These results were replicated using different batches and are strengthened by similar ratios between EC_{50}s observed for cAMP and β-arrestin 2 recruitment, confirming previously reported results obtained with follitropin alfa (15). On the other hand, the crystallographic structure of the human FSH bound to the extracellular binding domain of FSHR was obtained using partially deglycosylated hormone-receptor complexes (74). Therefore, it might be not fully descriptive of the role of sugar chains linked to the hormone in binding the receptor, providing a basis for explaining preparation-specific features, such as the higher potency of Gonal-f® in inducing CREB activation. These characteristics are likely linked to a relatively wide FSH EC_{50} range of progesterone response (**Table 6**; from 1.5 ± 0.3 to 10.9 ± 3.7 ng/ml), although not significantly different, presumably due to biased signaling (76, 77) of preparations.

Preparation-specific glycosylation patterns may be reflected by cellular response to supra-physiological doses of FSH in vitro. Biosimilar compounds induce barely detectable Ca^{2+} increases in FSHR-expressing HEK293 cells, which differed to that of Gonal-f® as previously reported using human pituitary FSH (78). FSHR is known to modulate intracellular Ca^{2+} increase via a molecular mechanism involving the phospholipase C (19). However, Gonal-f®-induced Ca^{2+} increase was obtained by hormone concentrations usually not achieved in vivo (62), while cAMP activation, and ERK1/2 CREB phosphorylation occurs at FSH doses achievable in serum, suggesting a supraphysiological shift from Gαs to Gαq protein-mediated activation of intracellular signaling cascades (8, 79). These data should be confirmed in other cell models, such as hGLC, since the pattern of intracellular signaling pathways is cell-specific and depends on the number and variety of GPCRs located at the cell surface (12, 79–81). Most importantly, preparation-specific activation of cAMP/β-arrestin 2 and intracellular Ca^{2+} increase indicated that these hormones might act as biased ligands under particular conditions, as well as the high sensitivity of the cAMP response detectable in vitro.

Confirming similar, FSH-induced STARD1 expression in hGLC, no differences in 8 and 24 h-progesterone and estradiol production between hormones was found, despite their structural peculiarities and lower Ovaleap®-induced CYP19A1 expression levels. Previous studies reported preparation-specific intracellular signaling resulting in similar long-term effects, measurable as 24-h steroid production (41, 45). These data are reminiscent of the earlier debate about recombinant and urinary FSH preparations, which provided similar pregnancy rate per fresh transfer (35, 68), as well as similar pharmacokinetic profiles (82). However, the matter is still debated. Different ART outcomes, depending on the use of Bemfola® vs. Gonal-f®, were postulated, possibly explained by different glycosylation, especially sialylation patterns between the two preparations and/or higher batch-to-batch variability (36) and estradiol production (82), observed with Bemfola®. Further in vivo investigations and extensive clinical experience are necessary to characterize the possible occurrence of biosimilar preparation-specific effects (31).

CONCLUSIONS

Different glycosylation profiles are characteristic of the follitropin alfa and subsequent biosimilar preparations, likely due to the specific enzymatic equipment of the source cell lines. These molecular peculiarities do not result in major preparation-specific signals mediated at the intracellular level and steroid synthesis, which were found to be overall similar when follitropin alfa and biosimilars are used at concentrations resembling those obtained under physiological conditions. In light of the specific molecular features of these commercial compounds and of the slight differences demonstrated by the present study, and considering the relevance of their use for clinical purposes, the comparison between the reference follitropin alfa and biosimilar preparations merits further investigations in a variety of experimental settings.

AUTHOR CONTRIBUTIONS

LR wrote a manuscript draft, performed experiments, and data analysis. SS, CL, DK, FD, EP, SL, ST, EG, AP, and AS contributed to experiments and edited the manuscript. FP and TT provided scientific and methodological assistance and edited the manuscript. JD, AN, MV, and LA provided assistance to experimental procedures and manuscript editing. ER and MS provided scientific support, data interpretation, and manuscript drafting. LC provided experiment management, data analysis and interpretation, and manuscript editing.

FUNDING

This study was supported by the Departments of Excellence Programme of the Italian Ministry of University and Research to the Department of Biomedical, Metabolic and Neural Sciences, University of Modena and Reggio Emilia (Italy) and by the French National Research Agency (ANR) under the program Investissements d'Avenir Grant Agreement (LabEx MabImprove: ANR-10-LABX-53), and ARD 2020 Biomédicaments grant from Région Center Val de Loire. MS is a LE STUDIUM RESEARCH FELLOW, Loire Valley Institute for Advanced Studies, Orléans & Tours, France,—INRA—Center Val de Loire, 37380 Nouzilly, France, receiving funding from the European Union's Horizon 2020 research and innovation programme under the Marie Skłodowska-Curie grant agreement No. 665790.

SUPPLEMENTARY MATERIAL

Supplemental Figure 1 | Cyclic-AMP response and β-arrestin 2 recruitment induced by different batches of Gonal-f® and biosimilars in trasfected HEK293 cells. **(A–C)** Cells were transiently co-transfected with FSHR and the CAMYEL sensor. Cyclic-AMP was measured by BRET after 30 min stimulation with increasing doses of **(A)** Gonal-f®, **(B)** Ovaleap®, and **(C)** Bemfola® batches. **(D–F)** Recruitment of β-arrestin 2 was measured in FSHR-Rluc8 and β-arrestin 2-YPET biosensor-expressing cells by BRET, after 30-min treatment of with increasing doses of **(D)** Gonal-f®, **(E)** Ovaleap®, and **(F)** Bemfola®. Data were represented as means ± SEM. No significant differences between EC_{50} values were found (Kruskal Wallis test, $p \geq 0.05$; $n = 4$).

Supplemental Figure 2 | Densitometric analysis of pERK1/2 and pCREB activation induced by different batches of Gonal-f® and biosimilars in hGLC. Cells were stimulated with increasing doses of FSH preparations and 15 min- ERK1/2 **(A)** and CREB **(B)** phosphorylation evaluated by semi-quantitative Western blotting. Values were normalized to total ERK and represented as means ± SEM. Differences between batches of each preparation was statistically evaluated (Kruskal Wallis test; $p \geq 0.05$; $n = 4$).

Supplemental Table 1 | Lectin specific binding sites.

Supplemental Table 2 | ELISA lectin analysis of different batches of originator and biosimilar follitropin alfa. Lectins were used as follows: MAA ($n = 20$), SNA ($n = 14$), Jacalin ($n = 6$), ricin ($n = 16$), DSA ($n = 6$), PHA-E ($n = 8$), WGA ($n = 8$). Hormone reactivity to lectins was represented as absorbance measured at 450 nm (means ± SEM)*10^3, after subtracting values obtained in the absence of gonadotropin. Data were analyzed by Kruskal-Wallis test, taking $p < 0.05$ as significant.

Supplemental Table 3 | Antennarity distribution of Gonal-f® and Ovaleap® batches.

Supplemental Table 4 | Sialylation distribution of follitropin alfa and Ovaleap® batches. Asn^7, Asn^{24}, Asn^{52}, and Asn^{78} were analyzed in terms of percentage.

Supplemental Table 5 | Sialic acids distribution of follitropin alfa originator and Ovaleap® batches.

Supplemental Table 6 | Eight h- and twenty four hours-progesterone and estradiol *plateau* levels induced by Gonal-f® and biosimilar stimulation of human primary granulosa cells. Data are represented as means ± SEM (Kruskal-Wallis test, $p \geq 0.05$; $n = 5$).

Supplemental Data Sheet 1 | Glycopeptide mapping.

Supplemental Data Sheet 2 | Supplemental Results.

REFERENCES

1. Themmen APN, Huhtaniemi IT. Mutations of gonadotropins and gonadotropin receptors: elucidating the physiology and pathophysiology of pituitary-gonadal function. *Endocr Rev.* (2000) 21:551–83. doi: 10.1210/edrv.21.5.0409

2. Simoni M, Gromoll J, Nieschlag E. The follicle-stimulating hormone receptor: biochemistry, molecular biology, physiology, and pathophysiology. *Endocr Rev.* (1997) 18:739–73. doi: 10.1210/er.18.6.739

3. Lamminen T, Jokinen P, Jiang M, Pakarinen P, Simonsen H, Huhtaniemi I. Human FSHβ subunit gene is highly conserved. *Mol Hum Reprod.* (2005) 11:601–5. doi: 10.1093/molehr/gah198

4. Bishop LA, Robertson DM, Cahir N, Schofield PR. Specific roles for the asparagine-linked carbohydrate residues of recombinant human follicle stimulating hormone in receptor binding and signal transduction. *Mol Endocrinol.* (1994) 8:722–31. doi: 10.1210/me.8.6.722

5. Ulloa-Aguirre A, Timossi C, Damián-Matsumura P, Dias JA. Role of glycosylation in function of follicle-stimulating hormone. *Endocrine.* (1999) 11:205–16. doi: 10.1385/ENDO:11:3:205

6. Gloaguen P, Crépieux P, Heitzler D, Poupon A, Reiter E. Mapping the follicle-stimulating hormone-induced signaling networks. *Front Endocrinol.* (2011) 2:45. doi: 10.3389/fendo.2011.00045

7. Casarini L, Moriondo V, Marino M, Adversi F, Capodanno F, Grisolia C, et al. FSHR polymorphism p.N680S mediates different responses to FSH *in vitro*. *Mol Cell Endocrinol.* (2014) 393:83–91. doi: 10.1016/j.mce.2014.06.013

8. Conti M. Specificity of the cyclic adenosine 3′,5′-monophosphate signal in granulosa cell function. *Biol Reprod.* (2002) 67:1653–61. doi: 10.1095/biolreprod.102.004952

9. Hunzicker-Dunn M, Maizels ET. FSH signaling pathways in immature granulosa cells that regulate target gene expression: branching out from protein kinase A. *Cell Signal.* (2006) 18:1351–9. doi: 10.1016/j.cellsig.2006.02.011

10. Seger R, Hanoch T, Rosenberg R, Dantes A, Merz WE, Strauss JF, et al. The ERK signaling cascade inhibits gonadotropin-stimulated steroidogenesis. *J Biol Chem.* (2017) 292:8847. doi: 10.1074/jbc.A117.006852

11. Ulloa-Aguirre A, Reiter E, Crépieux P. FSH receptor signaling: complexity of interactions and signal diversity. *Endocrinology.* (2018) 159:3020–35. doi: 10.1210/en.2018-00452

12. Casarini L, Santi D, Simoni M, Potì F. "Spare" luteinizing hormone receptors: facts and fiction. *Trends Endocrinol Metab.* (2018) 29:208–17. doi: 10.1016/j.tem.2018.01.007

13. Quintana J, Hipkin RW, Sánchez-Yagüe J, Ascoli M. Follitropin (FSH) and a phorbol ester stimulate the phosphorylation of the FSH receptor in intact cells. *J Biol Chem.* (1994) 269:8772–9.

14. Saltarelli D. Heterotrimeric Gi/o proteins control cyclic AMP oscillations and cytoskeletal structure assembly in primary human granulosa-lutein cells. *Cell Signal.* (1999) 11:415–33. doi: 10.1016/S0898-6568(99)00012-1

15. Ayoub MA, Landomiel F, Gallay N, Jégot G, Poupon A, Crépieux P, et al. Assessing gonadotropin receptor function by resonance energy transfer-based assays. *Front Endocrinol.* (2015) 6:130. doi: 10.3389/fendo.2015.00130

16. Escamilla-Hernandez R, Little-Ihrig L, Zeleznik AJ. Inhibition of rat granulosa cell differentiation by overexpression of Gαq. *Endocrine.* (2008) 33:21–31. doi: 10.1007/s12020-008-9064-z

17. Nechamen CA, Thomas RM, Dias JA. APPL1, APPL2, Akt2 and FOXO1a interact with FSHR in a potential signaling complex. *Mol Cell Endocrinol.* (2007) 260-2:93–9. doi: 10.1016/j.mce.2006.08.014

18. Lin YF, Tseng MJ, Hsu HL, Wu YW, Lee YH, Tsai YH. A novel follicle-stimulating hormone-induced G alpha h/phospholipase C-delta1 signaling pathway mediating rat sertoli cell Ca2+-influx. *Mol Endocrinol.* (2006) 20:2514–27. doi: 10.1210/me.2005-0347

19. Minegishi T, Tano M, Shinozaki H, Nakamura K, Abe Y, Ibuki Y, et al. Dual coupling and down regulation of human FSH receptor in CHO cells. *Life Sci.* (1997) 60:2043–50. doi: 10.1016/S0024-3205(97)00191-4

20. Kara E, Crépieux P, Gauthier C, Martinat N, Piketty V, Guillou F, et al. A phosphorylation cluster of five serine and threonine residues in the C-terminus of the follicle-stimulating hormone receptor is important for desensitization but not for beta-arrestin-mediated ERK activation. *Mol Endocrinol.* (2006) 20:3014–26. doi: 10.1210/me.2006-0098

21. Reiter E, Ahn S, Shukla AK, Lefkowitz RJ. Molecular mechanism of β-arrestin-biased agonism at seven-transmembrane receptors. *Annu Rev Pharmacol Toxicol.* (2012) 52:179–97. doi: 10.1146/annurev.pharmtox.010909. 105800

22. Wide L, Eriksson K. Dynamic changes in glycosylation and glycan composition of serum FSH and LH during natural ovarian stimulation. *Ups J Med Sci.* (2013) 118:153–64. doi: 10.3109/03009734.2013. 782081

23. Davis JS, Kumar TR, May JV, Bousfield GR. Naturally occurring follicle-stimulating hormone glycosylation variants. *J Glycomics Lipidom.* (2014) 04:e117. doi: 10.4172/2153-0637.1000e117

24. Ulloa-Aguirre A, Zarinan T. The follitropin receptor: matching structure and function. *Mol Pharmacol.* (2016) 90:596–608. doi: 10.1124/mol. 116.104398

25. Meher BR, Dixit A, Bousfield GR, Lushington GH. Glycosylation effects on FSH-FSHR interaction dynamics: a case study of different FSH glycoforms by molecular dynamics simulations. *PLoS ONE.* (2015) 10:e0137897. doi: 10.1371/journal.pone.0137897

26. Jiang C, Hou X, Wang C, May JV, Butnev VY, Bousfield GR, et al. Hypoglycosylated hFSH has greater bioactivity than fully glycosylated recombinant hFSH in human granulosa cells. *J Clin Endocrinol Metab.* (2015) 100:E852–60. doi: 10.1210/jc.2015-1317

27. Helenius A, Aebi M. Intracellular functions of N-linked glycans. *Science.* (2001) 291:2364–9. doi: 10.1126/science.291.5512.2364

28. Ulloa-Aguirre A, Timossi C, Barrios-de-Tomasi J, Maldonado A, Nayudu P. Impact of carbohydrate heterogeneity in function of follicle-stimulating hormone: studies derived from *in vitro* and *in vivo* models. *Biol Reprod.* (2003) 69:379–89. doi: 10.1095/biolreprod.103.016915

29. Anobile CJ, Talbot JA, McCann SJ, Padmanabhan V, Robertson WR. Glycoform composition of serum gonadotrophins through the normal menstrual cycle and in the post-menopausal state. *Mol Hum Reprod.* (1998) 4:631–9. doi: 10.1093/molehr/4.7.631

30. Wide L, Hobson BM. Qualitative difference in follicle-stimulating hormone activity in the pituitaries of young women compared to that of men and elderly women. *J Clin Endocrinol Metab.* (1983) 56:371–5. doi: 10.1210/jcem-56-2-371

31. Orvieto R, Seifer DB. Biosimilar FSH preparations- are they identical twins or just siblings? *Reprod Biol Endocrinol.* (2016) 14:32. doi: 10.1186/s12958-016-0167-8

32. Roger SD, Mikhail A. Biosimilars: opportunity or cause for concern? *J Pharm Pharm Sci.* (2007) 10:405–10. Available online at: https://sites.ualberta.ca/~csps/JPPS10_3/ReviewArticle_1308/R_1380.html

33. Santi D, Simoni M. Biosimilar recombinant follicle stimulating hormones in infertility treatment. *Expert Opin Biol Ther.* (2014) 14:1399–409. doi: 10.1517/14712598.2014.925872

34. Brinsden P, Akagbosu F, Gibbons LM, Lancaster S, Gourdon D, Engrand P, et al. A comparison of the efficacy and tolerability of two recombinant human follicle-stimulating hormone preparations in patients undergoing *in vitro* fertilization-embryo transfer. *Fertil Steril.* (2000) 73:114–6. doi: 10.1016/S0015-0282(99)00450-1

35. Casarini L, Brigante G, Simoni M, Santi D. Clinical applications of gonadotropins in the female: assisted reproduction and beyond. *Prog Mol Biol Transl Sci.* (2016) 143:85–119. doi: 10.1016/bs.pmbts.2016. 08.002

36. Mastrangeli R, Satwekar A, Cutillo F, Ciampolillo C, Palinsky W, Longobardi S. *In-vivo* biological activity and glycosylation analysis of a biosimilar recombinant human follicle-stimulating hormone product (Bemfola) compared with its reference medicinal product (GONAL-f). *PLoS ONE.* (2017) 12:e0184139. doi: 10.1371/journal.pone.0184139

37. Walton WJ, Nguyen VT, Butnev VY, Singh V, Moore WT, Bousfield GR. Characterization of human FSH isoforms reveals a nonglycosylated β-subunit in addition to the conventional glycosylated β-subunit. *J Clin Endocrinol Metab.* (2001) 86:3675–85. doi: 10.1210/jc.86.8.3675

38. Steelman SL, Pohley FM. Assay of the follicle stimulating hormone based on the augmentation with human chorionic gonadotropin. *Endocrinology.* (1953) 53:604–16. doi: 10.1210/endo-53-6-604

39. Smithies O. Disulfide-bond cleavage and formation in proteins. *Science.* (1965) 150:1595–8. doi: 10.1126/science.150.3703.1595

40. Chevallet M, Luche S, Rabilloud T. Silver staining of proteins in polyacrylamide gels. *Nat Protoc.* (2006) 1:1852–8. doi: 10.1038/nprot.2006.288

41. Riccetti L, Klett D, Ayoub MA, Boulo T, Pignatti E, Tagliavini S, et al. Heterogeneous hCG and hMG commercial preparations result in different intracellular signalling but induce a similar long-term progesterone response *in vitro. Mol Hum Reprod.* (2017) 23:685–97. doi: 10.1093/molehr/gax047

42. Legardinier S, Klett D, Poirier JC, Combarnous Y, Cahoreau C. Mammalian-like nonsialyl complex-type N-glycosylation of equine gonadotropins in Mimic™ insect cells. *Glycobiology.* (2005) 15:776–90. doi: 10.1093/glycob/cwi060

43. Bidart JM, Troalen F, Bousfield GR, Birken S, Bellet DH. Antigenic determinants on human choriogonadotropin alpha-subunit. I. Characterization of topographic sites recognized by monoclonal antibodies. *J Biol Chem.* (1988) 263:10364–9.

44. Casarini L, Lispi M, Longobardi S, Milosa F, La Marca A, Tagliasacchi D, et al. LH and hCG action on the same receptor results in quantitatively and qualitatively different intracellular signalling. *PLoS ONE.* (2012) 7:e46682. doi: 10.1371/journal.pone.0046682

45. Casarini L, Riccetti L, De Pascali F, Nicoli A, Tagliavini S, Trenti T, et al. Follicle-stimulating hormone potentiates the steroidogenic activity of chorionic gonadotropin and the anti-apoptotic activity of luteinizing hormone in human granulosa-lutein cells *in vitro. Mol Cell Endocrinol.* (2016) 422:103–14. doi: 10.1016/j.mce.2015.12.008

46. Nordhoff V, Sonntag B, von Tils D, Götte M, Schüring AN, Gromoll J, et al. Effects of the FSH receptor gene polymorphism p.N680S on cAMP and steroid production in cultured primary human granulosa cells. *Reprod Biomed Online.* (2011) 23:196–203. doi: 10.1016/j.rbmo.2011.04.009

47. Riccetti L, Yvinec R, Klett D, Gallay N, Combarnous Y, Reiter E, et al. Human luteinizing hormone and chorionic gonadotropin display biased agonism at the LH and LH/CG receptors. *Sci Rep.* (2017) 7:940. doi: 10.1038/s41598-017-01078-8

48. Jiang LI, Collins J, Davis R, Lin KM, DeCamp D, Roach T, et al. Use of a cAMP BRET sensor to characterize a novel regulation of cAMP by the sphingosine 1-phosphate/G13 pathway. *J Biol Chem.* (2007) 282:10576–84. doi: 10.1074/jbc.M609695200

49. Tricoire L, Tsuzuki K, Courjean O, Gibelin N, Bourout G, Rossier J, et al. Calcium dependence of aequorin bioluminescence dissected by random mutagenesis. *Proc Natl Acad Sci USA.* (2006) 103:9500–5. doi: 10.1073/pnas.0603176103

50. Casarini L, Riccetti L, De Pascali F, Gilioli L, Marino M, Vecchi E, et al. Estrogen modulates specific life and death signals induced by LH and hCG in human primary granulosa cells *in vitro. Int J Mol Sci.* (2017) 18:926. doi: 10.3390/ijms18050926

51. Schneider CA, Rasband WS, Eliceiri KW. NIH Image to ImageJ: 25 years of image analysis. *Nat Methods.* (2012) 9:671–5. doi: 10.1038/nmeth.2089

52. Riccetti L, De Pascali F, Gilioli L, Poti F, Giva LB, Marino M, et al. Human LH and hCG stimulate differently the early signalling pathways but result in equal testosterone synthesis in mouse Leydig cells *in vitro. Reprod Biol Endocrinol.* (2017) 15:2. doi: 10.1186/s12958-016-0224-3

53. Livak KJ, Schmittgen TD. Analysis of relative gene expression data using real-time quantitative PCR and the 2−ΔΔCT method. *Methods.* (2001) 25:402–8. doi: 10.1006/meth.2001.1262

54. Kavran JM, Leahy DJ. Silver staining of SDS-polyacrylamide Gel. *Methods Enzymol.* 541:169–76. doi: 10.1016/B978-0-12-420119-4.00014-8

55. Yamashita K, Totani K, Ohkura T, Takasaki S, Goldstein IJ, Kobata A. Carbohydrate binding properties of complex-type oligosaccharides on immobilized Datura stramonium lectin. *J Biol Chem.* (1987) 262:1602–7.

56. Shibuya N, Goldstein IJ, Broekaert WF, Nsimba-Lubaki M, Peeters B, Peumans WJ. The elderberry (Sambucus nigra L.) bark lectin recognizes the Neu5Ac(alpha 2-6)Gal/GalNAc sequence. *J Biol Chem.* (1987) 262:1596–601.

57. Xu X, Nagarajan H, Lewis NE, Pan S, Cai Z, Liu X, et al. The genomic sequence of the Chinese hamster ovary (CHO)-K1 cell line. *Nat Biotechnol.* (2011) 29:735–41. doi: 10.1038/nbt.1932

58. Wang WC, Cummings RD. The immobilized leukoagglutinin from the seeds of Maackia amurensis binds with high affinity to complex-type Asn-

linked oligosaccharides containing terminal sialic acid-linked alpha-2,3 to penultimate galactose residues. *J Biol Chem.* (1988) 263:4576–85.

59. Kabir S. Jacalin: a jackfruit (Artocarpus heterophyllus) seed-derived lectin of versatile applications in immunobiological research. *J Immunol Methods.* (1998) 212:193–211. doi: 10.1016/S0022-1759(98)00021-0

60. Narasimhan S, Freed JC, Schachter H. The effect of a "bisecting" N-acetylglucosaminyl group on the binding of biantennary, complex oligosaccharides to concanavalin A, Phaseolus vulgaris erythroagglutinin (E-PHA), and Ricinus communis agglutinin (RCA-120) immobilized on agarose. *Carbohydr Res.* (1986) 149:65–83. doi: 10.1016/S0008-6215(00)90370-7

61. Monsigny M, Roche AC, Sene C, Maget-Dana R, Delmotte F. Sugar-lectin interactions: how does wheat-germ agglutinin bind sialoglycoconjugates? *Eur J Biochem.* (1980) 104:147–53. doi: 10.1111/j.1432-1033.1980.tb04410.x

62. Sherman BM, Korenman SG. Hormonal characteristics of the human menstrual cycle throughout reproductive life. *J Clin Invest.* (1975) 55:699–706. doi: 10.1172/JCI107979

63. Grass J, Pabst M, Chang M, Wozny M, Altmann F. Analysis of recombinant human follicle-stimulating hormone (FSH) by mass spectrometric approaches. *Anal Bioanal Chem.* (2011) 400:2427–38. doi: 10.1007/s00216-011-4923-5

64. Howles CM. Genetic engineering of human FSH (Gonal-F). *Hum Reprod Update.* (1996) 2:172–91. doi: 10.1093/humupd/2.2.172

65. Bassett RM, Driebergen R. Continued improvements in the quality and consistency of follitropin alfa, recombinant human FSH. *Reprod Biomed Online.* (2005) 10:169–77. doi: 10.1016/S1472-6483(10)60937-6

66. Wolfenson C, Groisman J, Couto AS, Hedenfalk M, Cortvrindt RG, Smitz JE, et al. Batch-to-batch consistency of human-derived gonadotrophin preparations compared with recombinant preparations. *Reprod Biomed Online.* (2005) 10:442–54. doi: 10.1016/S1472-6483(10)60819-X

67. EMA/65507/2013 rev.1. *Assessment Report.* Bemfola International non-Proprietary Name: Follitropin Alfa (2014). p. 1–76.

68. Rettenbacher M, Andersen AN, Garcia-Velasco JA, Sator M, Barri P, Lindenberg S, et al. A multi-centre phase 3 study comparing efficacy and safety of Bemfola(Ⓡ) versus Gonal-f(Ⓡ) in women undergoing ovarian stimulation for IVF. *Reprod Biomed Online.* (2015) 30:504–13. doi: 10.1016/j.rbmo.2015.01.005

69. EMA/CHMP/41467/2013. *Ovaleap International Non-Proprietary Name: Follitropin Alfa.* (2013). p. 1–72.

70. Strowitzki T, Kuczynski W, Mueller A, Bias P. Randomized, active-controlled, comparative phase 3 efficacy and safety equivalence trial of Ovaleap(Ⓡ) (recombinant human follicle-stimulating hormone) in infertile women using assisted reproduction technology (ART). *Reprod Biol Endocrinol.* (2016) 14:1. doi: 10.1186/s12958-015-0135-8

71. Fox KM, Dias JA, Van Roey P. Three-dimensional structure of human follicle-stimulating hormone. *Mol Endocrinol.* (2001) 15:378–89. doi: 10.1210/mend.15.3.0603

72. Green ED, Brodbeck RM, Baenziger JU. Lectin affinity high-performance liquid chromatography. Interactions of N-glycanase-released oligosaccharides with Ricinus communis agglutinin I and Ricinus communis agglutinin II. *J Biol Chem.* (1987) 262:12030–9.

73. Campo S, Andreone L, Ambao V, Urrutia M, Calandra RS, Rulli SB. Hormonal regulation of follicle-stimulating hormone glycosylation in males. *Front Endocrinol.* (2019) 10:17. doi: 10.3389/fendo.2019.00017

74. Fan QR, Hendrickson WA. Structure of human follicle-stimulating hormone in complex with its receptor. *Nature.* (2005) 433:269–277. doi: 10.1038/nature03206

75. Jiang X, Liu H, Chen X, Chen PH, Fischer D, Sriraman V, et al. Structure of follicle-stimulating hormone in complex with the entire ectodomain of its receptor. *Proc Natl Acad Sci USA.* (2012) 109:12491–6. doi: 10.1073/pnas.1206643109

76. Ayoub MA, Yvinec R, Jégot G, Dias JA, Poli S-M, Poupon A, et al. Profiling of FSHR negative allosteric modulators on LH/CGR reveals biased antagonism with implications in steroidogenesis. *Mol Cell Endocrinol.* (2016) 436:10–22. doi: 10.1016/j.mce.2016.07.013

77. Klein Herenbrink C, Sykes DA, Donthamsetti P, Canals M, Coudrat T, Shonberg J, et al. The role of kinetic context in apparent biased agonism at GPCRs. *Nat Commun.* (2016) 7:10842. doi: 10.1038/ncomms10842

78. Younglai EV, Kwan TK, Kwan CY, Lobb DK, Foster WG. Dichlorodiphenylchloroethylene elevates cytosolic calcium concentrations and oscillations in primary cultures of human granulosa-lutein cells. *Biol Reprod.* (2004) 70:1693–700. doi: 10.1095/biolreprod.103.026187

79. Jonas KC, Chen S, Virta M, Mora J, Franks S, Huhtaniemi I, et al. Temporal reprogramming of calcium signalling via crosstalk of gonadotrophin receptors that associate as functionally asymmetric heteromers. *Sci Rep.* (2018) 8:2239. doi: 10.1038/s41598-018-20722-5

80. Tranchant T, Durand G, Gauthier C, Crépieux P, Ulloa-Aguirre A, Royère D, et al. Preferential β-arrestin signalling at low receptor density revealed by functional characterization of the human FSH receptor A189 V mutation. *Mol Cell Endocrinol.* (2011) 331:109–18. doi: 10.1016/j.mce.2010.08.016

81. Zhu X, Gilbert S, Birnbaumer M, Birnbauer L. Dual signaling potential is common among Gs-coupled receptors and dependent on receptor density. *Mol Pharmacol.* (1994) 46:460–9.

82. Wolzt M, Gouya G, Sator M, Hemetsberger T, Irps C, Rettenbacher M, et al. Comparison of pharmacokinetic and safety profiles between Bemfola(Ⓡ) and Gonal-f(Ⓡ) after subcutaneous application. *Eur J Drug Metab Pharmacokinet.* (2016) 41:259–65. doi: 10.1007/s13318-015-0257-6

17

Biased Signaling and Allosteric Modulation at the FSHR

Flavie Landomiel, Francesco De Pascali, Pauline Raynaud, Frédéric Jean-Alphonse,
Romain Yvinec, Lucie P. Pellissier, Véronique Bozon, Gilles Bruneau, Pascale Crépieux,
Anne Poupon and Eric Reiter*

PRC, INRA, CNRS, IFCE, Université de Tours, Nouzilly, France

*Correspondence:
Eric Reiter
eric.reiter@inra.fr

Knowledge on G protein-coupled receptor (GPCRs) structure and mechanism of activation has profoundly evolved over the past years. The way drugs targeting this family of receptors are discovered and used has also changed. Ligands appear to bind a growing number of GPCRs in a competitive or allosteric manner to elicit balanced signaling or biased signaling (i.e., differential efficacy in activating or inhibiting selective signaling pathway(s) compared to the reference ligand). These novel concepts and developments transform our understanding of the follicle-stimulating hormone (FSH) receptor (FSHR) biology and the way it could be pharmacologically modulated in the future. The FSHR is expressed in somatic cells of the gonads and plays a major role in reproduction. When compared to classical GPCRs, the FSHR exhibits intrinsic peculiarities, such as a very large NH2-terminal extracellular domain that binds a naturally heterogeneous, large heterodimeric glycoprotein, namely FSH. Once activated, the FSHR couples to Gαs and, in some instances, to other Gα subunits. G protein-coupled receptor kinases and β-arrestins are also recruited to this receptor and account for its desensitization, trafficking, and intracellular signaling. Different classes of pharmacological tools capable of biasing FSHR signaling have been reported and open promising prospects both in basic research and for therapeutic applications. Here we provide an updated review of the most salient peculiarities of FSHR signaling and its selective modulation.

Keywords: GPCR, reproduction, follicle-stimulating hormone, β-arrestin, G protein, signaling, bias, trafficking

INTRODUCTION

Follicle stimulating hormone (FSH) plays a crucial role in the control of male and female reproduction. FSH is a heterodimeric glycoprotein consisting of an α-subunit non-covalently associated with a β-subunit. The α-subunit is shared with luteinizing hormone (LH), chorionic gonadotropin (CG) and thyroid-stimulating hormone (TSH), whereas the β chain is specific of each glycoprotein hormone (1). FSH is synthesized and secreted by the pituitary and binds to a plasma membrane receptor (FSHR) that belongs to the class A of the G protein-coupled receptor (GPCR) superfamily. The FSHR displays a high degree of tissue specificity as it is expressed in Sertoli and granulosa cells located in the male and female gonads, respectively (2). FSH is required for normal growth and maturation of ovarian follicles in women and for normal spermatogenesis in men (3). Female mice with FSHβ or FSHR gene knockout present an incomplete follicle development leading to infertility, whereas males display oligozoospermia and subfertility (4, 5).

Consistently, women expressing non-functional variants of the FSHR are infertile while men are oligozoospermic, yet fertile (6). To date, only native forms of FSH, either purified from urine or by using recombinant technology, are being used in reproductive medicine with no other pharmacological agents being currently available in clinic (7–9). Novel classes of FSHR agonists with varying pharmacological profiles could potentially help improving the overall efficiency of assisted reproductive technology. On the other hand, FSHR antagonists could represent an avenue for non-steroidal approach to contraception (10). This paper offers an updated overview of the way FSHR signals and of how selective modulation of its signaling can be achieved.

STRUCTURE OF THE FSHR

For the vast majority of GPCRs, the orthosteric site (i.e., the region that binds the natural ligand), is located in a cavity defined by the transmembrane helices. This is not the case for the FSHR, which binds its natural ligand, FSH, through its characteristic large horse-shoe-shaped extracellular domain (ECD). Consequently, the orthosteric site spans over the nine leucine rich repeats (LRRs) of the ECD (**Figure 1**). The first crystal structure of FSH bound to part of the ECD came out in 2005 and led to a detailed understanding of the molecular basis leading to the specificity of hormone binding (11). The ECD of the receptor contains 12 LRRs linked to three disulfide bonds and two unstructured sequence motifs that define the hinge region connecting the ECD to transmembrane domains (TMD). However, the recombinant protein used for crystallization did not include amino acid residues in the hinge region. Therefore, the receptor activation mechanism remained poorly understood, until recently, when another crystal structure including the hinge region was reported (12). Interestingly, it revealed a two-step activation mechanism of the receptor: interaction of FSH with LRR1-9 reshapes hormone conformation, so that exposed residues located at the interface of the hormone α- and β-subunits form a binding pocket for sulfated Tyr335 of the hinge region, resulting in a conformational change of the latter (13, 14). This two-step interaction process not only stabilizes the FSH/FSHR interaction but also relieves the tethered inverse agonistic activity previously mapped within the hinge region (15). Since no structural data of gonadotropin receptor TMD are currently available, homology modeling with other GPCRs is necessary. The structure of human neuropeptide Y1 receptor that recently came out (PDB:5BZQ) displays the highest identity with FSHR (25%) and LHR (24%) TM domains. Prior to that, gonadotropin receptor TM domains have been successfully modeled using adenosine receptor crystal structure (16). This revealed the existence of two adjacent pockets that could accommodate small ligands. These sites have been assigned P1 and P2 (major and minor site, respectively). The P1 site is located between TMs III, IV, V, and VI, and P2 between TMs I, II, III, and VII (**Figure 1A**) (17). These putative TM domain allosteric sites have been confirmed in studies utilizing chimeric receptors and

mutagenesis. Interestingly, it was found that a FSHR small-molecule agonist at high concentration specifically displaced the binding of radiolabelled adenosine A3 receptor (A3R) agonist on A3R (18). This suggests a similarity between glycoprotein receptor and A3R in the TMD region for the allosteric binding pocket (19). As suggested from studies on other GPCRs, allosteric sites distinct from P1 and P2 may also exist and affect FSHR activity (20).

FSHR COUPLING TO G PROTEINS

By analogy with other GPCRs, it is reasonable to posit that FSH binding leads to conformational rearrangements within the transmembrane regions, thereby causing the recruitment and coupling of signal transducers (G proteins, β-arrestins) that ultimately trigger a complex intracellular signaling network (21, 22). The primary transduction effector described for the FSHR is Gαs that triggers the canonical adenylyl cyclase/cAMP/protein kinase A (PKA) signaling cascade. Once activated, PKA phosphorylates many proteins such as transcription factors of the cAMP response element-binding protein (CREB) family (23–31). cAMP action is also mediated by the Exchange Proteins directly Activated by cAMP (EPACs) (32–34). Upon cAMP binding, EPAC1/2 stimulate Ras-related protein (RAP1/2), small GTPases that lead to protein kinase B phosphorylation (PKB) (35, 36). In addition, the FSHR has been reported to interact with Gαi and Gαq. Gαi inhibits adenylate cyclase, blocking Gαs-induced cAMP production (37). The stimulation of Gαq requires in vitro stimulation with high FSH concentrations (>50 nM) (22, 38–40). This coupling leads to the production of inositol 1,4,5 triphosphate (IP3) and diacylglycerol (DAG), increased intracellular calcium concentration and activation of protein kinase C (PKC). Pleiotropic coupling of FSHR to various heterotrimeric proteins suggests the co-existence of multiple active conformations of the receptor in the plasma membrane (41, 42).

FSHR COUPLING TO β-ARRESTIN

Similarly to most GPCRs, the FSHR interacts with β-arrestins, scaffolding proteins that control receptor desensitization, internalization and recycling (24, 43–46). Classically, β-arrestins are recruited following (i) receptor activation and (ii) receptor phosphorylation by G protein-coupled receptor kinases (GRK). Due to steric hindrance, FSHR coupling to Gαs is impaired once β-arrestins are recruited (47, 48). In a model of rat primary Sertoli cells that express the FSHR endogenously, it has been demonstrated that agonist-induced cAMP levels decreased upon β-arrestin overexpression, consistently with its role in FSHR desensitization (49). In heterologous cells, the carboxyl tail of FSHR has been reported to be phosphorylated on several serine and threonine residues (43). In addition to these classical functions, it has become increasingly clear that β-arrestins can also initiate specific, G protein-independent signaling events leading to the activation of many pathways,

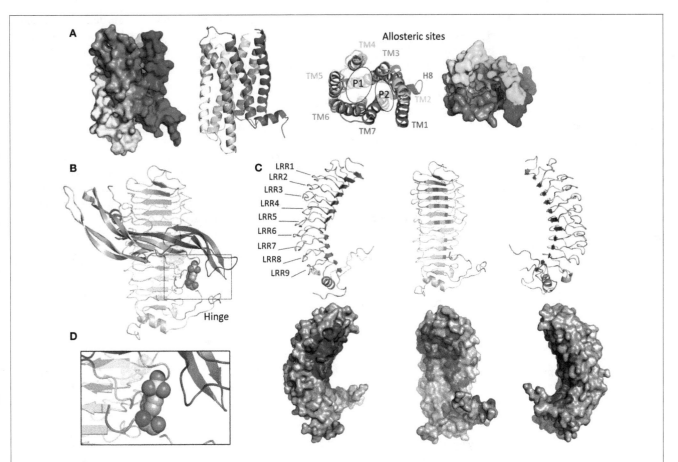

FIGURE 1 | Orthosteric and allosteric sites in the FSHR. **(A)** Cartoon and surface view of the transmembrane regions of the FSHR showing P1 and P2 allosteric sites. **(B)** Complex between the ectodomain of the FSHR (gray) and FSH (violet: alpha chain, pink: beta chain). The colored spheres represent sulphated Tyr355. **(C)** Residues involved in FSH binding are shown in red. **(D)** Close-up on the interaction between sulphated Tyr335 (colored spheres) and FSH.

amongst which the ERK (Extracellular signal-Regulated Kinase) MAP (Mitogen-Activated Protein) kinase pathway has been the most studied (50). Of note, ERK activation kinetics at the FSHR has been reported to vary in heterologous cells as a function of the upstream transduction mechanism involved: β-arrestin-mediated ERK activation is delayed but more sustained compared to Gαs-dependent ERK activation, which occurs early but is transient (43). Consistent with the concept of "phosphorylation barcode" which links particular GRK-mediated phosphorylation signatures at the receptor level to the activation of distinct β-arrestin-dependent functions (51, 52), a relationship has been found between the subtype of GRK involved in FSHR phosphorylation and the nature of β-arrestin-mediated actions. In particular, β-arrestins recruited to GRK2 or GRK3-phosphorylated FSHR favor receptor desensitization whereas GRK5 or GRK6-mediated phosphorylation of FSHR were involved in β-arrestin-dependent ERK activation (43, 53, 54). Recently, phosphorylation of Tyrosine383 in β-arrestin 2 has proved to be crucial for β-arrestin-mediated ERK activation by the FSHR and other GPCRs. More precisely, ligand-induced receptor activation provokes MEK (Mitogen-activated protein kinase kinase)-mediated phosphorylation of Tyr^{383}, necessary

for β-arrestin 2-mediated ERK recruitment and activation (55). β-arrestins also play a role in FSHR-induced translation, mediated by a β-arrestin/p70S6K/ribosomal S6 complex that assembles in heterologous and in primary Sertoli cells. Upon FSH stimulation, activation of G protein-dependent signaling enhances p70S6K activity within the β-arrestin/p70S6K/rpS6 preassembled complex, leading to the fast and robust translation of 5′ oligopyrimidine track (5′TOP) mRNA (56). In addition, the balance between FSHR-mediated proliferation vs apoptosis seems to be regulated by β-arrestins. In hGL5 human granulosa cells, silencing of β-arrestins leads to an increase in cAMP/PKA and a decrease in β-arrestin-mediated proliferative pathway, resulting in cell death (57). Evidence reported for other GPCRs demonstrated that the internalized receptor can form molecular complexes involving simultaneous interactions with Gαs to the core domain and β-arrestin to the C-tail of the receptor (58). These complexes, named "megaplexes," are able to signal from the endosome by inducing a second wave of cAMP (58, 59). Based on structural evidence, a two-step mechanism for β-arrestin recruitment has been proposed (60). First, β-arrestins are recruited to the phosphorylated C-tail, resulting in a so-called "partially engaged" complex which the authors reported to be sufficient for ERK signaling and internalization. Interestingly, this conformation allows the receptor to simultaneously couple to G protein α subunit. Second, a conformational rearrangement of β-arrestins allows them to interact with the receptor core domain, forming a "fully engaged complex" incompatible with further G protein coupling (58, 60–62). More recently, a separate study uncovered another mechanism of β-arrestin activation that the authors called "catalytic activation." Upon ligand-induced recruitment of inactivated β-arrestin to the receptor core domain, a conformational change in β-arrestin occurs that exposes a PIP2-binding motif and allows β-arrestin to bind membrane lipid rafts independently of the receptor. Interestingly, the authors noticed an accumulation of active β-arrestin in clathrin-coated endocytic structures in the absence of the receptor, revealing the existence of a receptor C-tail-independent β-arrestin activation mechanism (63). No evidence currently exist that the aforementioned mechanisms also apply to the FSHR. Further studies will be necessary to clarify the molecular mechanisms involved in β-arrestin recruitment and activation at the FSHR and to determine their possible peculiarities.

FSHR INTERACTION WITH OTHER PARTNERS

Beside G proteins, GRKs and β-arrestins, the signal is also transduced at the FSHR by other direct binding partners (44). For example, adaptor protein, phosphotyrosine interacting with the Adapter protein with PH domain, PTB domain, and leucine zipper 1 (APPL1) binds intracellular loop 1 of the FSHR (64). This protein has lately retained the greatest attention in the gonadotropin community for two main reasons. The first one is that this adapter protein links the FSHR directly to inositide phosphate metabolism and Ca^{2+} release in granulosa cells (65), hence it induces cAMP-independent signaling; the second is that, like β-arrestins, APPL1 recruitment plays a role in the subcellular routing of FSHR. This discovery had been heralded by the previously identified interaction between GAIP-interacting protein C-tail (GIPC) adaptor and the FSHR (or the LHR), presumably requiring the carboxyterminal end of the receptor. Interestingly, GIPC reroutes the internalized FSHR from Early Endosomes (EE) to recycling Very Early Endosomes (VEE), and by these means, enables sustained ERK phosphorylation (66). Likewise, in HEK293 cells, APPL1 has been shown to convey internalized FSHR, as well as LHR, to VEE for recycling, and PKA-dependent phosphorylation of APPL1 leads to endosomal cAMP signaling (67). These two sets of observations on ERK MAP kinases and cAMP suggest that spatially restricted FSH signaling may be generalized to several of its components. In addition, 14-3-3τ has been shown to interact directly with the second intracellular loop of the receptor FSHR (68, 69). The 14-3-3τ interaction site on the FSHR encompasses the ERW motif involved in G protein association (70), that is consistent with the observation that 14-3-3τ overexpression in HEK293 cells reduces FSH-induced cAMP response (68). The co-occurrence of these direct binding partners as well as G protein, GRK and β-arrestins, raises fundamental questions about their

sequence/dynamics of interaction on a single FSHR or about the possibility that FSHR oligomers might cluster transduction assembly of variable composition at the plasma membrane and in intracellular compartments.

TRAFFICKING AND ENDOSOMAL SIGNALING

Compartmentalization of signaling is now viewed as an important feature for many signaling proteins and plays key roles in cellular responses. This is particularly the case for membrane receptors such as GPCRs since, in the past years, several examples have revealed connections between membrane compartmentalization, endocytic trafficking and signaling patterns. Originally thought to function solely at the plasma membrane, the multifunctional protein β-arrestin assemble signaling molecules (e.g., MAPK, Src, etc) that direct GPCRs to the endocytic pathway and regulate their post-endocytic fate, as mentioned above. For some GPCRs forming a stable interaction with β-arrestin, β-arrestin/receptor/signaling molecule complexes are found in endosomes, allowing prolonged signaling from these intracellular structures (71–73). The nature of the β-arrestin binding motifs, in particular serine/threonine clusters in the C-tail of the receptor, regulates the stability of this interaction. GPCRs that display high affinity binding to β-arrestin, are classified as class B (74, 75). In the FSHR, a cluster of 5 serines/threonines is involved in both internalization and binding of β-arrestin to the receptor and is consistent with the class B definition. Such interaction was confirmed by bioluminescence energy transfer experiments (BRET) and co-immunoprecipitation experiments, however no imaging data have confirmed the existence of a functional complex in endosomes (24, 43). In addition, it is unclear whether β-arrestin-mediated ERK signaling by FSHR requires β-arrestin localization in endosomes. Recently, both the FSHR and LHR were reported to predominantly localize to an atypical endosome denoted as VEE (**Figure 2**). Alteration of this endosomal trafficking by blocking internalization inhibits activation of ERK through the LHR, suggesting that VEE are a location for signaling (66). These particular endosomes are upstream of the classical endosomes and are devoid of typical early endosomes markers such as the Rab5 GTPase or the phosphatidylinositol-3-phosphate (PI(3)P) or the PI(3)P-bound EEA1 proteins. Morphologically, they are smaller (<400 nm) than conventional sorting EE but their exact nature remains to be defined. Interestingly, gonadotropin receptor localization in VEE requires an intact receptor C-tail and the GIPC PDZ-domain protein (66). PDZ motifs are found in several GPCRs to regulate their spatial localization or trafficking (76). The PDZ motif of the LHR directly binds GIPC that sequesters the receptor into VEE following agonist-induced internalization. In fact, in cells depleted in GIPC or expressing LHR lacking the distal PDZ motif in its C-tail, the receptors are rerouted and accumulated into the classical EE where they fail to recycle back to the plasma membrane. In addition, they were not able to signal to ERK MAP kinases (66), suggesting that endosomal ERK activity occurs from this specific compartment.

It is worth noting that the FSHR does not display a known PDZ ligand in its C-tail and the exact mechanism on how GIPC controls FSHR fate remains to be determined. However, APPL1, a known FSHR binding partner, localizes to a subset of VEE and displays a PDZ motif previously shown to interact with GIPC (64, 65, 77). A possible scenario would be that FSHR, *via* its interaction with APPL1, connects with GIPC and is targeted to VEE where it activates ERK (78). Earlier work supports the idea that endosomal APPL1 defines a signaling platform upstream of the Rab5/PI(3)P endosomes. Disruption of EE leads to the accumulation of the EGFR Tyrosine kinase receptor in APPL1 vesicles, leading to a sustained activation of ERK from this compartment (79, 80). As shown for the LHR, the endosomal cAMP/PKA dependent phosphorylation of APPL1 on Ser410 is necessary for the recycling of the receptor (67).

This concept of endosomal signaling compartmentalization was further supported by the findings that GPCR can induce a second phase of G protein activation following their internalization (81–83). This allowed the advent of a new paradigm where some GPCRs do not only transduce and activate G proteins from the plasma membrane but also from endocytic compartments (the so-called "megaplex" mentioned above). Interestingly, the two other members of the glycoprotein hormone receptor family, TSHR and LHR, were both shown to transduce *via* Gαs and promote sustained cAMP production from endocytic compartments (59, 67, 84, 85). While the TSHR acts from EE and *trans*-Golgi compartments, the LHR signaling is restricted to the VEE. It has yet to be shown whether the FSHR also activates G proteins from the VEE but the fact that it shares several features with GPCRs known to signal from endosomes, including LHR, V2R or PTHR, supports this possibility. FSHR trafficking mimics the LHR as discussed above and it displays a phosphorylation code similar to those found in the C-tail of V2R and PTHR. More precisely, the formation of a "megaplex" has been shown to induce cAMP from the EE in response to PTHR activation (86, 87). That the FSHR could signal in endocytic compartments through G proteins in a similar way as the PTHR, but from VEE, is conceivable, but further studies are needed to demonstrate this possibility. Despite the identification of structural determinants in the FSHR C-tail that regulate its trafficking (88), very little is known about the mechanisms involved in the post-endocytic trafficking of this receptor.

BIASED SIGNALING AND ITS QUANTIFICATION

The action of a given ligand on its cognate receptor has classically been characterized by its effect on downstream effectors (second messengers). Compared to the reference ligand (generally, the physiological ligand), a pharmacological agent can be either an agonist (it produces a biological response similar to that of the reference ligand), an antagonist (it blocks the biological response elicited by the reference ligand) or an inverse agonist (it produces an opposite biological response that leads to a decrease in the receptor basal activity). Importantly, it has long been thought that these characteristics hold irrespectively of effector

measured (89). However, some ligands did not match with one of these categories, because they displayed both agonist and antagonist (or inverse agonist) activities at the same receptor, depending on the downstream pathway measured. For instance, carvedilol, a clinically used β-blocker, has a clear inverse agonist profile on Gαs-dependent activity at the β2 adrenergic receptor while being a weak partial agonist for β-arrestin-dependent ERK activation (90). To deal with these discrepancies, the concept of biased signaling or functional selectivity, recently came to the fore (89, 91, 92). According to this concept, a ligand is biased when it triggers imbalanced responses, compared to a reference ligand acting on the same receptor (classically the endogenous ligand). Importantly, a biased ligand can selectively activate only a subset of the biological responses or activate all of them but with different efficacies compared to the reference ligand. As these ideas hold profound implications and potential for the design of new therapeutics, biased signaling is a very active area of research in pharmacology (93, 94). Over the last decade, biased signaling has been evidenced in many different receptors, including gonadotropin receptors, as will be discussed in a forthcoming section. By analogy with a ligand bias, the notion of receptor bias has been proposed (95). Two receptors, diverging only by a mutation or a polymorphism, once activated by the same ligand may induce two signaling pathways with different relative efficacies. Importantly, biased signaling has been extended to allosteric ligands, which can modulate not only the efficacy of a given ligand-induced receptor signal but also select and bias the activation of the receptor toward a subset of the biological responses (93). Ligand bias and receptor bias must be set apart from system bias or observational bias (95). System bias refers to bias that are due to the particular biological system used (some transducer molecules, such as G proteins, may be expressed differentially in different cell types for instance). Observational bias refers to the modification or amplification of the signals inherent to the specific assays used for the measurements. Besides being supported by numerous experimental evidences, biased signaling is consistent with the receptor conformation theory, which views a receptor population as an ensemble of conformations that evolve dynamically, according to some energy landscape and subjected to external perturbations (96). In such theory, ligand-induced receptor activation is concomitant with a stabilization of some receptor conformations and a modification of the receptor conformation energy landscape, resulting from the interaction of the ligand with its receptor. Several studies have thus shown that receptor conformational equilibrium models, such as the extended ternary complex model, can satisfactorily explain ligand bias (97, 98). Several groups have attempted to address the problem of bias quantification. Considering a given receptor and two signaling pathways (A and B), the objective is to be able to classify ligand bias, as having for instance a low, a moderate or a high bias toward pathway A vs pathway B, when compared to a reference ligand. The most popular method to quantify ligand bias uses dose-response data and the so-called operational model (99, 100). The latter is widely used to perform regression on dose-response data, which have in many cases a sigmoid shape. The parameters of the operational model are derived from a

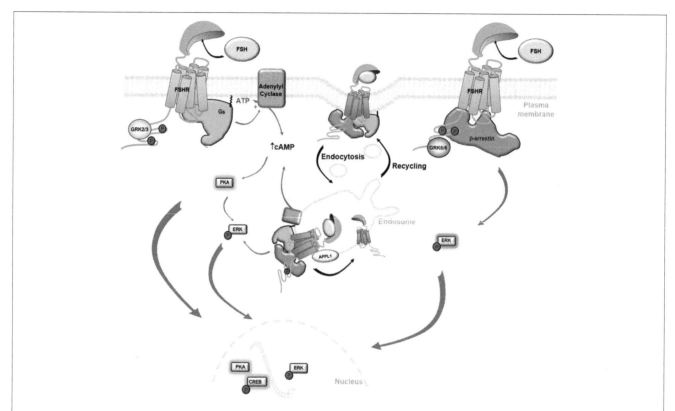

FIGURE 2 | FSHR signaling and trafficking. Upon FSH binding, the FSHR mainly activates Gαs protein, leading to conversion of ATP to cAMP by adenylyl cyclases and activation of intracellular effector kinases, including PKA. After stimulation, GRK phosphorylates and desensitizes the FSHR. Phosphorylated FSHR recruits β-arrestin, which in turn induces its own signaling, including ERK activation, as well as receptor internalization in the endosomes. FSHR potentially activates G protein-dependent and -independent signaling from the endosomal compartment, before quickly recycling back to the plasma membrane. Effector proteins drive the cellular responses, including gene transcription, cell proliferation and differentiation. APPL1, Adaptor protein, phosphotyrosine interacting with PH domain and leucine zipper 1; CREB, cAMP response element binding protein; ERK, extracellular signal-regulated kinase; FSH, Follicle-stimulating hormone; GRK, G protein-coupled receptor kinase; PKA, protein Kinase A.

simple chemical reaction scheme that takes into account ligand receptor association/dissociation reactions and that links the ligand-receptor concentration to the biological response thanks to a logistic function (similar to enzymatic reaction models). The usefulness of this model for the quantification of ligand bias is associated with the interpretation of its parameters. In particular, the two main parameters of the operational model are the ligand-receptor dissociation constant K_a and the intrinsic efficacy τ (which describes the ability of the ligand-receptor association to be converted into a response). With these two coefficients, a single transduction coefficient, given by $\log(\tau/K_a)$, has been proposed to characterize the agonism of a ligand for a given signaling pathway (100). This coefficient can then be compared between two pathways and between two ligands, to ensure normalization. Hence

$$\Delta\log(\tau/K_a) = \log(\tau/K_a)_{\text{ligand A}} - \log(\tau/K_a)_{\text{ligand B}}$$

quantifies the activation of a pathway by ligand A, compared to ligand B. In addition,

$$\Delta\Delta\log(\tau/K_a) = \Delta\log(\tau/K_a)_{\text{pathway 1}} - \Delta\log(\tau/K_a)_{\text{pathway 2}}$$

evaluates the differences of activation between the two pathways. Finally, the bias is defined as

$$\text{bias} = 10^{\Delta\Delta\log(\tau/Ka)}$$

This procedure for bias quantification, together with its statistical significance, has been detailed as a step-by-step protocol using Prism (v6.0; GraphPad Software) (101–103). Other logistic regressions that lead to different quantifications and parameter interpretations have been proposed and compared (104). A notion of dose-dependent ligand bias, which may reveal subtle nonlinear effects of the ligand, has also been defined using logistic function (105). Overall, the statistical regression of dose-response data (sigmoid curves) can be ambiguous and lead to a misinterpretation of the results. Moreover, it has been shown experimentally that different procedures may exhibit discrepancies between each other, and may fail to detect ligand bias or lead to false positives, probably due to the presence of system or observational bias (104). A semi-quantitative method to classify ligand bias that would be more robust than quantitative methods has been proposed, based on logistic regression (104). However, the major concern of the operational approach to quantify ligand bias is that it disregards an important aspect of signaling pathways, namely the temporal activation of the different signaling processes (106). This has been revealed by the relatively simple observation that the bias value, as calculated with the operational model, could change as a function of the kinetics of response (107). Actually, the apparent bias can even be in an opposite direction for two different time points when the biological responses are measured. While part of the explanation of this phenomena resides in the different time scales at stake within a signal transduction pathway (binding kinetics, second messenger and effector kinetics), it also reveals the whole complexity of a receptor trafficking system (108), that can certainly not be condensed into a single number. Thus, methodological developments such as dynamical versions of the operational model and/or the extended ternary complex model (109, 110) must be developed to address this complexity and allow better characterization of the effect of a ligand on its cognate receptor.

BIASED SIGNALING AT THE FSHR

To date, different classes of biases have been reported to elicit selective modulation at the FSHR (**Figure 3**). Ligand bias can be provoked by small molecule ligands, glycosylation variants of FSH or by antibodies acting at FSH or FSHR. Receptor bias due to mutations or single nucleotide polymorphisms (SNP) at the FSHR have also been reported.

Small Molecule Ligands
Several classes of chemical compounds exhibiting the ability to modulate FSHR-mediated signaling upon binding have been identified to date. Readers interested in the chemical diversity of currently known FSHR small molecules classes can refer to **Figure 2** of Anderson et al. in the same special issue of Frontiers in Endocrinology (19). According to their mode of action and effect on the receptor, they can be divided in four classes: allosteric agonists, positive allosteric modulators (PAMs), negative allosteric modulators (NAMs) and neutral allosteric ligands (NALs) (111). While PAMs or NAMs need the presence of FSH to detect the enhancement or the decrease of FSHR activation, respectively, agonists have the capacity to activate it on their own. Even though NALs do not influence signaling, they can potentially prevent other allosteric modulators from binding (112). Thiazolidinones, identified by screening combinatorial chemical scaffolds, were the first class of FSHR allosteric agonists to be reported (113). The allosteric nature of thiazolidinone derivatives was confirmed thanks to experiments involving FSHR/TSHR chimeras, which showed that their binding site was localized in the TMD (114). A nanomolar potent thiazolidinone FSHR agonist was reported to trigger signaling pathways similar to FSH, both *in vitro* and *in vivo* (115). Interestingly, some thiazolidinone analogs demonstrated biased agonism by mobilizing the Gαi protein instead of Gαs or both as observed for other thiazolidinone analogs or FSH preparations (116). Besides, high throughput screening on substituted benzamides allowed the identification of a series of FSHR PAMs that showed improved selectivity

against LHR and TSHR. Interesting pharmacokinetic properties were also described for two selected compounds (117). A dihydropyridine compound, Org 24444-0, is another PAM, which displayed a good selectivity toward FSHR and induced cAMP production in presence of FSH (118). The compound was also able to reproduce the effects of FSH on the follicle phase maturation in mature female rats. Among the currently known NAMs, tetrahydroquinolines constitute a good example of biased signaling. It was indeed established that the compounds inhibited FSHR-induced cAMP production, without inhibiting FSH binding (119). Unfortunately, the tetrahydroquinolines did not display any *in vivo* activity. Three other NAMs have been characterized by Dias et al. (120, 121). The first one, ADX61623, was reported to inhibit cAMP and progesterone but not estradiol production in rat granulosa primary cells. Using ^{125}I-hFSH, it was established that ADX61623 did not compete with FSH, but rather increased FSH binding, suggesting that it does not bind the extracellular domain of FSHR. When tested *in vivo*, the compound was not able to decrease FSH-induced preovulatory follicle development (120). Two similar compounds were described later: ADX68692 and ADX68693. Both were reported to inhibit cAMP and progesterone production in rat granulosa primary cells, but while ADX68692 also affected estradiol and decreased the number of oocytes recovered in mature female rat, ADX68693 had no effect on estradiol, nor on the number of retrieved oocytes (121). Interestingly, ADX68692 and ADX68693 were also reported to exert similar actions on the LHR (122). The first FSHR competitive antagonist described in scientific literature, suramin, was reported to inhibit testosterone production and FSHR signaling, by competing with FSH binding (123). Another non-competitive antagonist of human and rat FSHR showing the same behavior was later identified (124).

Glycosylation Variants
Gonadotropins present natural heterogeneity in their glycan moieties that contribute up to nearly 30% of the hormone's mass (125–128). The presence of glycans has important outcomes on the *in vivo* half-life of the hormone because, by doubling its diameter, it limits its glomerular filtration. FSH contains two potential N-linked oligosaccharides on each subunit that are sources of heterogeneities. Importantly, these glycan chains are involved in FSH folding, assembly, stability, quality control, secretion, transport as well as the biological activity and potency (15, 129–138). The α chain is glycosylated at asparagine 52 (Asn52) and Asn78, while the FSH β subunit can be glycosylated at Asn7 and Asn24. Partially glycosylated variants that are missing either one or both of these oligosaccharides on FSHβ have been reported in equine FSHβ, human FSHβ (hFSH β), rhesus FSHβ and Japanese macaque FSHβ (139–142). Glycosylation profile of each subunit plays a critical role in the activity and clearance of FSH (131, 143, 144). Interestingly, while FSHα subunit amino-acid sequences are identical to LH, TSH and CG α-subunits, the N-glycan populations at Asn52 and Asn78 differ from those of the other hormones (145–147). FSHβ subunit shares 34–40% of sequence homology with the other human glycoprotein hormone β-subunits, yet the main structural hallmarks (i.e., six disulfide bonds, cystine

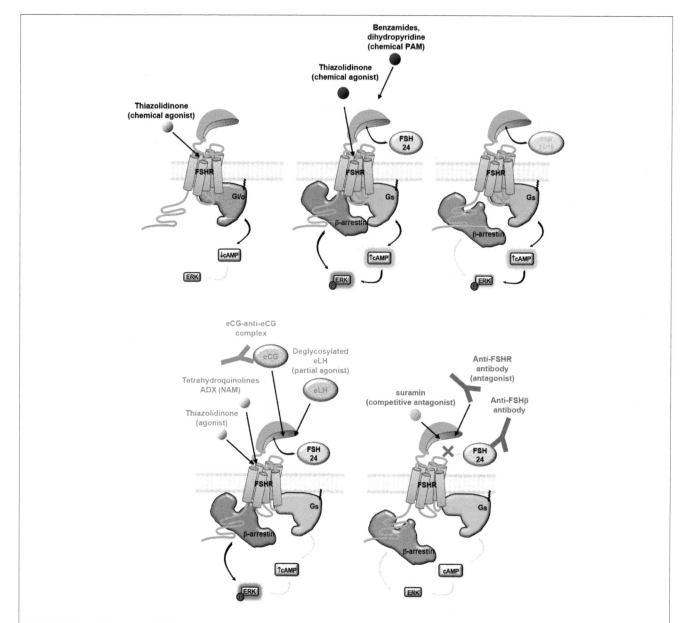

FIGURE 3 | Ligand bias at the FSHR. Balanced agonists or PAM at the FSHR induce both G protein and β-arrestin recruitment. FSH binding to the FSHR can be prevented using small competitive ligands, antibodies directed against the binding pocket of the FSHR or directly against FSH. Biased signaling toward Gαi, Gαs, or β-arrestin recruitment can result from glycosylation forms of FSH (fully glycosylated FSH24 vs partially glycosylated FSH21-18), antibody or small chemical compounds.

knot motif and seatbelt loop) are conserved (148, 149). Interestingly, the abundance of the glycosylated variants in FSHβ subunit appears to be physiologically regulated (141). Although glycosylations are involved in the FSH bioactivity, they are not directly interacting with the receptor binding site (11, 12, 15, 150). Removal of the carbohydrate residue at position 78 from α-subunit significantly increases receptor binding affinity of human FSH. Likewise, carbohydrate at position 52 of the α-subunit was found to be essential for bioactivity since its removal resulted in significant decrease in potency. Furthermore, β-subunit carbohydrates are essential for FSHβ/FSHα heterodimerization (138, 151). In binding assays,

hypoglycosylated FSH (triglycosylated FSH21/18, missing either Asn7 or Asn24-linked oligosaccharide on the β chain) was 9–26-fold more active than fully glycosylated FSH (tetraglycosylated FSH24) (139). Likewise, a deglycosylated FSH variant, which possesses only α-subunit oligosaccharides, is significantly more bioactive *in vitro* and more efficient in receptor binding than the tetraglycosylated form of the hormone (141, 142, 152). However, this hypoglycosylated FSH is not physiologically relevant because subunit heterodimerization is extremely inefficient when both FSHβ glycans are missing, precluding secretion of enough active forms (151). In contrast, ovulated eggs and subsequent *in vitro* embryo development was increased by hyperglycosylated

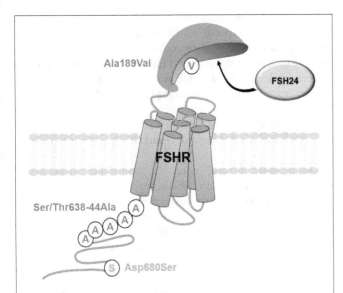

FIGURE 4 | Mutation-induced receptor bias at the FSHR. Mutations can lead to biased signal transduction at the FSHR upon exposure to fully glycosylated FSH (FSH24). Green, Gs-biased mutants; purple, β-arrestin-biased mutant.

FSH (153). FSH variant abundance is tightly correlated with fertility: FSH24 predominates in men and post-menopausal women whereas FSH21/18 is more abundant in younger females. This observation suggests that hypoglycosylated FSH may play a preferential role in efficient stimulation of ovarian follicle development (154). Noteworthy, FSH variants have been reported to exhibit biased signaling: FSH21/18 is better to activate the cAMP/PKA pathway and is 10-fold more potent in inducing CYP19A1 and estrogen than fully glycosylated FSH24 (155). Bias at the FSHR has also been reported with partially deglycosylated eLH (eLHdg) preparation. β-arrestin depletion revealed that eLHdg induced β-arrestin recruitment to the FSHR and activated both ERK and PI3K pathways in a β-arrestin-dependent and Gαs/cAMP-independent manner (156). Altogether, these data suggest that FSH glycoforms may act as physiological bias (157). A recent study revealing signaling bias between human LH and hCG is consistent with this hypothesis (158).

Antibody

Particular antibodies have been shown to selectively modulate FSHR activation, likely eliciting structural constraints and stabilizing distinct conformations of FSH and/or its receptor (21). Monoclonal antibodies against bovine FSHβ and anti-peptide antibodies targeting ovine FSHβ both significantly enhanced biological activity in mice (159, 160). Interestingly, in non-equine species, equine CG (eCG) binds to both FSHR and LHR and elicits their activation (161–164). Studies have evaluated the impact on gonadotropin bioactivities of different eCG/anti-eCG antibody complexes generated using individual sera from a large number of eCG-treated goats. Interestingly, both inhibition and hyperstimulation of LH and FSH bioactivity were recorded (165). In a follow-up study, Wehbi et al. investigated the effects of these complexes on FSH signaling in more details (166). Three

stimulatory complexes were tested, displaying modulatory effect on cAMP production but all exhibited increased β-arrestin-dependent ERK response, suggesting biased properties. Recently, Ji et al. developed two anti-FSHβ monoclonal antibodies using synthetic peptides located at the binding interface of FSHR (167). Strikingly, this study demonstrated that blocking FSH action using antibodies against FSHβ protects ovariectomized mice against bone loss, by stimulating new bone formation and reducing bone removal besides inhibiting fat accumulation. Direct targeting of GPCR with antibody or antibody fragments in order to modulate their signaling is increasingly viewed as a viable approach that even led to therapeutic applications in the last few years (168). The FSHR has been targeted by antibodies in different studies. Recombinant filamentous phages displaying at their surface three overlapping N-terminal decapeptides of the FSHR, A18–27, B25–34, and C29–38 peptides were used for immunizing ewes and female mice. When tested in vitro, antiA and antiB immunoglobulins behaved as antagonists for FSH binding and for cAMP production, whereas antiC immunoglobulins did not compete for hormone binding but displayed agonist activity on FSHR-mediated cAMP response (169). Studies using polyclonal and monoclonal antibodies or scFv fragments specific of the hinge region of FSHR, LHR, or TSHR, while not affecting hormone binding, all revealed agonistic activities, unequivocally establishing the role of the hinge region in the activation of these receptors (170–172). More recently, recombinant nanobodies capable of specifically recognizing FSHR and of inhibiting cAMP accumulation have been identified (173). Even though the biased nature of the above-discussed anti-FSHR antibodies have not been assessed in the original studies, it is tempting to speculate that antibodies and antibody fragments hold a lot of promises as research tools and as therapeutic agents capable of eliciting functional selectivity at the FSHR.

Single Nucleotide Polymorphisms and Mutations

Induced or natural mutations have been shown to elicit biased signaling in various GPCRs (174–176). In the FSHR, active and inactive mutations and SNP have been reported (177) but most of them are insufficiently documented to suggest they could induce a receptor bias. However, some studies suggested that a mutation or a SNP at the FSHR can modify the balance between different signaling pathways (**Figure 4**). The Ala189Val inactive mutation, leading to subfertility in men and infertility in women, impairs the G protein pathway but not β-arrestin-dependent ERK activation (6, 178). However, this Ala189Val mutation provokes intracellular retention of the FSHR, hence decreases its plasma membrane expression level (179). Tranchant et al. demonstrated that the FSHR also elicits preferential β-arrestin-dependent signaling when its plasma membrane density is similar to that of the Ala189Val mutant. Therefore, the Ala189Val mutation could very well represent a case of system bias rather than of receptor bias. Uchida et al. described an inactivating mutation (Met512Ile) in the FSHR of a woman with ovarian hyperstimulation syndrome (OHSS) but probably not related with this pathology (179). The mutant receptor led to decreased cAMP and PI3K responses whereas ERK activation remained unchanged compared to wild-type FSHR. Further investigations are required to ascertain whether the imbalance between the different signaling pathways is caused by a true receptor bias or whether it also results from affected cell surface expression of the receptor. Another case is the Asp431Ile mutation in the extracellular loop 1 (EL1) that has been found in a man with undetectable circulating FSH but normal spermatogenesis (180). This mutation leads to a marked decrease in FSH-induced desensitization and internalization compared to the wild-type receptor.

The FSHR gene carries about 2,000 SNPs, among which the SNP p.N680S (c.2039A>G) is a discrete marker of ovarian response. Women bearing the serine variant display resistance to FSH compared with those bearing the asparagine variant. p.N680S S homozygous FSHR differently stimulates intracellular cAMP and leads to different kinetics of ERK and CREB phosphorylation (181). Kara et al. have shown that site-directed mutagenesis of all the five ser/thr residues located in the C-tail at position 638–644 of the rat FSHR reduced its ability to interact with β-arrestins upon FSH stimulation (43). Interestingly, the internalization of the mutant receptor was reduced while its ability to activate ERK via the β-arrestin-dependent pathway was increased, indicating receptor bias.

CONCLUSIONS

The observation that FSHR transduction can be finely tuned by a variety of biased ligands, mutations or polymorphisms, further emphasizes the importance to better understand the complex signaling networks that are modulated (i.e., activated or inhibited) downstream of the FSHR. These novel biased ligands and receptor variants are great research tools that should really help us deciphering the molecular mechanisms involved in FSHR-associated physiopathology. In addition, a number of existing ligands and mutants have been characterized solely by measuring plasma membrane expression and/or cAMP response. Further characterization is required and may generate insightful findings. Biased ligands also open intriguing prospects in drug discovery. In particular, low molecular weight agonists of the FSHR could lead to the development of orally-active treatments.

Such administration route would bypass the multiple injections of gonadotropin preparations that remain needed in the current protocols used in assisted reproduction. Moreover, it becomes possible to sort out the pathways leading to ovulation and those responsible for OHSS, and the availability of pathway-selective low molecular weight agonists at the FSHR could pave the way for the development of safer treatments, presenting reducing risks of OHSS. Modulation of relative FSH and LH activities could also open new avenues in the treatment of polycystic ovarian syndrome (PCOS).

On a more general note, the availability of allosteric compounds active at the FSHR, opens the unprecedented opportunity to enhance or dampen the transduction activities of the FSHR *in vivo*, while conserving the rhythmicity and biochemical diversity of endogenous FSH, a property that no orthosteric compound can match. The conditions of application of such treatments will obviously require extensive pre-clinical and clinical studies. Despite of these limitations, hampering any hope for short-term clinical use, the advent of biased and allosteric compounds certainly represents an important juncture in a field that has uniquely relied for so long on natural and recombinant gonadotropins to treat infertility. Finally, orally active low molecular weight FSHR antagonists may also lead to novel classes of oral contraceptives devoid of the side effects associated with current sex steroid-based contraceptives.

AUTHOR CONTRIBUTIONS

Each author wrote a section of the review. AP and LPP designed **Figures 1–4** respectively. ER integrated all the contributions into the final manuscript. All authors edited the complete paper.

FUNDING

This publication was funded with support from the French National Research Agency under the program Investissements d'avenir Grant Agreement LabEx MabImprove: ANR-10-LABX-53 and ARD2020 Biomédicaments grant from Région Centre. FDP is recipient of a doctoral fellowship from INRA and Région Centre. FJ-A is recipient of a Le Studium fellowship.

REFERENCES

1. Pierce JG, Parsons TF. Glycoprotein hormones: structure and function. *Ann Rev Biochem.* (1981) 50:465–95. doi: 10.1146/annurev.bi.50.070181.002341
2. Simoni M, Gromoll J, Nieschlag E. The follicle-stimulating hormone receptor: biochemistry, molecular biology, physiology, and pathophysiology. *Endocr Rev.* (1997) 18:739–73. doi: 10.1210/er.18.6.739
3. Themmen APN, Huhtaniemi IT. Mutations of gonadotropins and gonadotropin receptors: elucidating the physiology and pathophysiology of pituitary-gonadal function. *Endocr Rev.* (2000) 21:551–83. doi: 10.1210/edrv.21.5.0409
4. Dierich A, Sairam MR, Monaco L, Fimia GM, Gansmuller A, Lemeur M, et al. Impairing follicle-stimulating hormone (FSH) signaling *in vivo*: targeted disruption of the FSH receptor leads to aberrant gametogenesis and hormonal imbalance. *Cell Biol.* (1998) 95:13612–7.
5. Kumar TR, Wang Y, Lu N, Matzuk MM. Follicle stimulating hormone is required for ovarian follicle maturation but not male fertility. *Nat Genet.* (1997) 15:201–4. doi: 10.1038/ng0297-201
6. Aittomäki K, Lucena JL, Pakarinen P, Sistonen P, Tapanainen J, Gromoll J, et al. Mutation in the follicle-stimulating hormone receptor gene causes hereditary hypergonadotropic ovarian failure. *Cell.* (1995) 82:959–68.
7. Lunenfeld B. Historical perspectives in gonadotrophin therapy. *Hum Reprod Update.* (2004) 10:453–67. doi: 10.1093/humupd/dmh044
8. Macklon NS, Stouffer RL, Giudice LC, Fauser BC. The science behind 25 years of ovarian stimulation for *in vitro* fertilization. *Endocr Rev.* (2006) 27:170–207. doi: 10.1210/er.2005-0015

9. Croxtall JD, McKeage K. Corifollitropin alfa: a review of its use in controlled ovarian stimulation for assisted reproduction. *BioDrugs.* (2011) 25:243–54. doi: 10.2165/11206890-000000000-00000

10. Naz RK, Gupta SK, Gupta JC, Vyas HK, Talwar AG. Recent advances in contraceptive vaccine development: a mini-review. *Hum Reprod.* (2005) 20:3271–83. doi: 10.1093/humrep/dei256

11. Fan QR, Hendrickson WA. Structural bology of glycoprotein hormones and their receptors. *Endocrine.* (2005) 26:179–88. doi: 10.1385/ENDO:26:3:179

12. Jiang X, Liu H, Chen X, Chen PH, Fischer D, Sriraman V, et al. Structure of follicle-stimulating hormone in complex with the entire ectodomain of its receptor. *Proc Natl Acad Sci USA.* (2012) 109:12491–6. doi: 10.1073/pnas.1206643109

13. Ahn S, Shenoy SK, Wei H, Lefkowitz RJ. Differential kinetic and spatial patterns of beta-arrestin and G protein-mediated ERK activation by the angiotensin II receptor. *J Biol Chem.* (2004) 279:35518–25. doi: 10.1074/jbc.M405878200

14. Costagliola S, Panneels V, Bonomi M, Koch J, Many MC, Smits G, et al. Tyrosine sulfation is required for agonist recognition by glycoprotein hormone receptors. *EMBO J.* (2002) 21:504–13. doi: 10.1093/emboj/21.4.504

15. Jiang X, Dias JA, He X. Structural biology of glycoprotein hormones and their receptors: Insights to signaling. *Mol Cell Endocrinol.* (2014) 382:424–51. doi: 10.1016/j.mce.2013.08.021

16. Heitman LH, Kleinau G, Brussee J, Krause G, Ijzerman AP. Determination of different putative allosteric binding pockets at the lutropin receptor by using diverse drug-like low molecular weight ligands. *Mol Cell Endocrinol.* (2012) 351:326–36. doi: 10.1016/j.mce.2012.01.010

17. Arey BJ. Allosteric modulators of glycoprotein hormone receptors: discovery and therapeutic potential. *Endocrine.* (2008) 34:1–10. doi: 10.1007/s12020-008-9098-2

18. Nataraja S, Sriraman V, Palmer S. Allosteric regulation of the follicle-stimulating hormone receptor. *Endocrinology.* (2018) 159:2704–16. doi: 10.1210/en.2018-00317

19. Anderson RC, Newton CL, Millar RP. Small molecule follicle-stimulating hormone receptor agonists and antagonists. *Front Endocrinol.* (2018) 9:757. doi: 10.3389/fendo.2018.00757

20. Gentry PR, Sexton PM, Christopoulos A. Novel allosteric modulators of G protein-coupled receptors. *J Biol Chem.* (2015) 290:19478–88. doi: 10.1074/jbc.R115.662759

21. Ulloa-Aguirre A, Crépieux P, Poupon A, Maurel MC, Reiter E. Novel pathways in gonadotropin receptor signaling and biased agonism. *Rev Endocr Metab Disord.* (2011) 12:259–74. doi: 10.1007/s11154-011-9176-2

22. Gloaguen P, Crepieux P, Heitzler D, Poupon A, Reiter E. Mapping the follicle-stimulating hormone-induced signaling networks. *Front Endocrinol.* (2011) 2:45. doi: 10.3389/fendo.2011.00045

23. Abou-Issa H, Reichert LE Jr. Modulation of follicle-stimulating hormone-sensitive rat testicular adenylate cyclase activity by guanyl nucleotides. *Endocrinology.* (1979) 104:189–93.

24. Ayoub MA, Landomiel F, Gallay N, Jegot G, Poupon A, Crepieux P, et al. Assessing Gonadotropin receptor function by resonance energy transfer-based assays. *Front Endocrinol.* (2015) 6:130. doi: 10.3389/fendo.2015.00130

25. Dattatreyamurty B, Figgs LW, Reichert LE. Physical and functional association of follitropin receptors with cholera toxin-sensitive guanine nucleotide-binding protein. *J Biol Chem.* (1987) 262:11737–45.

26. Gershengorn MC, Osman R. Minireview: insights into G protein-coupled receptor function using molecular models. *Endocrinology.* (2001) 142:2–10. doi: 10.1210/endo.142.1.7919

27. Hansson VV, Skalhegg BS, Tasken K. Cyclic-AMP-dependent protein kinase (PKA) in testicular cells. Cell specific expression, differential regulation and targeting of subunits of PKA. *J Steroid Biochem Mol Biol.* (2000) 73:81–92. doi: 10.1016/S0960-0760(00)00057-1

28. Hunzicker-Dunn M, Maizels ET. FSH signaling pathways in immature granulosa cells that regulate target gene expression: branching out from protein kinase A. *Cell Signal.* (2006) 18:1351–9. doi: 10.1016/j.cellsig.2006.02.011

29. Musnier A, Heitzler D, Boulo T, Tesseraud S, Durand G, Lécureuil C, et al. Developmental regulation of p70 S6 kinase by a G protein-coupled receptor dynamically modeled in primary cells. *Cell Mol Life Sci.* (2009) 66:3487–503. doi: 10.1007/s00018-009-0134-z

30. Remy JJ, Lahbib-Mansais Y, Yerle M, Bozon V, Couture L, Pajot E, et al. The porcine follitropin receptor: cDNA cloning, functional expression and chromosomal localization of the gene. *Gene.* (1995) 163:257–61. doi: 10.1016/0378-1119(95)00385-J

31. Ulloa-Aguirre A, Lira-Albarrán S. Clinical applications of gonadotropins in the male. *Prog Mol Biol Transl Sci.* (2016) 143:121–74. doi: 10.1016/bs.pmbts.2016.08.003

32. de Rooij J, Zwartkruis FJ, Verheijen MH, Cool RH, Nijman SM, Wittinghofer A, et al. Epac is a Rap1 guanine-nucleotide-exchange factor directly activated by cyclic AMP. *Nature.* (1998) 396:474–7. doi: 10.1038/24884

33. Kawasaki H, Springett GM, Toki S, Canales JJ, Harlan P, Blumenstiel JP, et al. A Rap guanine nucleotide exchange factor enriched highly in the basal ganglia. *Proc Natl Acad Sci USA.* (1998) 95:13278–83. doi: 10.1073/pnas.95.22.13278

34. Wayne CM, Fan H-Y, Cheng X, Richards JS. Follicle-stimulating hormone induces multiple signaling cascades: evidence that activation of Rous sarcoma oncogene, RAS, and the epidermal growth factor receptor are critical for granulosa cell differentiation. *Mol Endocrinol.* (2007) 21:1940–57. doi: 10.1210/me.2007-0020

35. Gonzalez-Robayna IJ, Falender AE, Ochsner S, Firestone GL, Richards JS. Follicle-Stimulating hormone (FSH) stimulates phosphorylation and activation of protein kinase B (PKB/Akt) and serum and glucocorticoid-lnduced kinase (Sgk): evidence for A kinase-independent signaling by FSH in granulosa cells. *Mol Endocrinol.* (2000) 14:1283–300. doi: 10.1210/mend.14.8.0500

36. Meroni SB, Riera MF, Pellizzari EH, Galardo MN, Cigorraga SB. FSH activates phosphatidylinositol 3-kinase/protein kinase B signaling pathway in 20-day-old Sertoli cells independently of IGF-I. *J Endocrinol.* (2004) 180:257–65. doi: 10.1677/joe.0.1800257

37. Gorczynska E, Spaliviero J, Handelsman DJ. The relationship between 3′,5′-cyclic adenosine monophosphate and calcium in mediating follicle-stimulating hormone signal transduction in Sertoli cells. *Endocrinology.* (1994) 134:293–300. doi: 10.1210/endo.134.1.8275946

38. Conti M. Specificity of the cyclic adenosine 3′,5′-monophosphate signal in granulosa cell function. *Biol Reprod.* (2002) 67:1653–61. doi: 10.1095/biolreprod.102.004952

39. Ito J, Shimada M, Terada T. Effect of protein kinase C activator on mitogen-activated protein kinase and p34(cdc2) kinase activity during parthenogenetic activation of porcine oocytes by calcium ionophore. *Biol Reprod.* (2003) 69:1675–82. doi: 10.1095/biolreprod.103.018036

40. Quintana J, Hipkin RW, Sanchez-Yague J, Ascoli M. Follitropin (FSH) and a phorbol ester stimulate the phosphorylation of the FSH receptor in intact cells. *J Biol Chem.* (1994) 269:8772–9.

41. Swaminath G, Xiang Y, Lee TW, Steenhuis J, Parnot C, Kobilka BK. Sequential binding of agonists to the beta2 adrenoceptor. Kinetic evidence for intermediate conformational states. *J Biol Chem.* (2004) 279:686–91. doi: 10.1074/jbc.M310888200

42. Zürn A, Zabel U, Vilardaga J-P, Schindelin H, Lohse MJ, Hoffmann C. Fluorescence resonance energy transfer analysis of alpha 2a-adrenergic receptor activation reveals distinct agonist-specific conformational changes. *Mol Pharmacol.* (2009) 75:534–41. doi: 10.1124/mol.108.052399

43. Kara E, Crepieux P, Gauthier C, Martinat N, Piketty V, Guillou F, et al. A phosphorylation cluster of five serine and threonine residues in the C-terminus of the follicle-stimulating hormone receptor is important for desensitization but not for beta-arrestin-mediated ERK activation. *Mol Endocrinol.* (2006) 20:3014–26. doi: 10.1210/me.2006-0098

44. Ulloa-Aguirre A, Reiter E, Crepieux P. FSH receptor signaling: complexity of interactions and signal diversity. *Endocrinology.* (2018) 159:3020–35. doi: 10.1210/en.2018-00452

45. De Pascali F, Reiter E. β-arrestins and biased signaling in gonadotropin receptors. *Minerva Ginecol.* (2018) 70:525–38. doi: 10.23736/S0026-4784.18.04272-7

46. Reiter E, Lefkowitz RJ. GRKs and beta-arrestins: roles in receptor silencing, trafficking and signaling. *Trends Endocrinol Metab.* (2006) 17:159–65. doi: 10.1016/j.tem.2006.03.008

47. Nakamura K, Krupnick JG, Benovic JL, Ascoli M. Signaling and phosphorylation-impaired mutants of the rat follitropin receptor

reveal an activation- and phosphorylation-independent but arrestin-dependent pathway for internalization. *J Biol Chem.* (1998) 273:24346–54. doi: 10.1074/jbc.273.38.24346

48. Troispoux C, Guillou F, Elalouf JM, Firsov D, Iacovelli L, De Blasi A, et al. Involvement of G protein-coupled receptor kinases and arrestins in desensitization to follicle-stimulating hormone action. *Mol Endocrinol.* (1999) 13:1599–614. doi: 10.1210/mend.13.9.0342

49. Marion S, Robert F, Crepieux P, Martinat N, Troispoux C, Guillou F, et al. G protein-coupled receptor kinases and beta arrestins are relocalized and attenuate cyclic 3',5'-adenosine monophosphate response to follicle-stimulating hormone in rat primary Sertoli cells. *Biol Reprod.* (2002) 66:70–6. doi: 10.1095/biolreprod66.1.70

50. Lefkowitz RJ, Shenoy SK. Transduction of receptor signals by beta-arrestins. *Science.* (2005) 308:512–7. doi: 10.1126/science.1109237

51. Butcher AJ, Prihandoko R, Kong KC, McWilliams P, Edwards JM, Bottrill A, et al. Differential G-protein-coupled receptor phosphorylation provides evidence for a signaling bar code. *J Biol Chem.* (2011) 286:11506–18. doi: 10.1074/jbc.M110.154526

52. Nobles KN, Xiao K, Ahn S, Shukla AK, Lam CM, Rajagopal S, et al. Distinct phosphorylation sites on the beta(2)-adrenergic receptor establish a barcode that encodes differential functions of beta-arrestin. *Sci Signal.* (2011) 4:ra51. doi: 10.1126/scisignal.2001707

53. Heitzler D, Durand G, Gallay N, Rizk A, Ahn S, Kim J, et al. Competing G protein-coupled receptor kinases balance G protein and beta-arrestin signaling. *Mol Syst Biol.* (2012) 8:590. doi: 10.1038/msb.2012.22

54. Reiter E, Ayoub MA, Pellissier LP, Landomiel F, Musnier A, Tréfier A, et al. β-arrestin signalling and bias in hormone-responsive GPCRs. *Mol Cell Endocrinol.* (2017) 449:28–41. doi: 10.1016/j.mce.2017.01.052

55. Cassier E, Gallay N, Bourquard T, Claeysen S, Bockaert J, Crépieux P, et al. Phosphorylation of β-arrestin2 at Thr383 by MEK underlies β-arrestin-dependent activation of Erk1/2 by GPCRs. *eLife.* (2017) 6:e23777. doi: 10.7554/eLife.23777

56. Tréfier A, Musnier A, Landomiel F, Bourquard T, Boulo T, Ayoub MA, et al. G protein-dependent signaling triggers a β-arrestin-scaffolded p70S6K/rpS6 module that controls 5'TOP mRNA translation. *FASEB J.* (2018) 32:1154–69. doi: 10.1096/fj.201700763R

57. Casarini L, Reiter E, Simoni M. beta-arrestins regulate gonadotropin receptor-mediated cell proliferation and apoptosis by controlling different FSHR or LHCGR intracellular signaling in the hGL5 cell line. *Mol Cell Endocrinol.* (2016) 437:11–21. doi: 10.1016/j.mce.2016.08.005

58. Thomsen ARB, Plouffe B, Cahill TJ, Shukla AK, Tarrasch JT, Dosey AM, et al. GPCR-G protein-β-arrestin super-complex mediates sustained G protein signaling. *Cell.* (2016) 166:907–19. doi: 10.1016/j.cell.2016.07.004

59. Calebiro D, Nikolaev VO, Gagliani MC, de Filippis T, Dees C, Tacchetti C, et al. Persistent cAMP-signals triggered by internalized G-protein-coupled receptors. *PLoS Biol.* (2009) 7:e1000172. doi: 10.1371/journal.pbio.1000172

60. Shukla AK, Westfield GH, Xiao K, Reis RI, Huang LY, Tripathi-Shukla P, et al. Visualization of arrestin recruitment by a G-protein-coupled receptor. *Nature.* (2014) 512:218–22. doi: 10.1038/nature13430

61. Kumari P, Srivastava A, Banerjee R, Ghosh E, Gupta P, Ranjan R, et al. Functional competence of a partially engaged GPCR-beta-arrestin complex. *Nat Commun.* (2016) 7:13416. doi: 10.1038/ncomms13416

62. Cahill TJ III, Thomsen AR, Tarrasch JT, Plouffe B, Nguyen AH, Yang F, et al. Distinct conformations of GPCR-beta-arrestin complexes mediate desensitization, signaling, and endocytosis. *Proc Natl Acad Sci USA.* (2017) 114:2562–7. doi: 10.1073/pnas.1701529114

63. Eichel K, Jullié D, Barsi-Rhyne B, Latorraca NR, Masureel M, Sibarita J-B, et al. Catalytic activation of β-arrestin by GPCRs. *Nature.* (2018) 557:381–6. doi: 10.1038/s41586-018-0079-1

64. Nechamen CA, Thomas RM, Cohen BD, Acevedo G, Poulikakos PI, Testa JR, et al. Human follicle-stimulating hormone (FSH) receptor interacts with the adaptor protein APPL1 in HEK 293 cells: potential involvement of the PI3K pathway in FSH signaling. *Biol Reprod.* (2004) 71:629–36. doi: 10.1095/biolreprod.103.025833

65. Thomas RM, Nechamen CA, Mazurkiewicz JE, Ulloa-Aguirre A, Dias JA. The adapter protein APPL1 links FSH receptor to inositol 1,4,5-trisphosphate production and is implicated in

intracellular Ca(2+) mobilization. *Endocrinology.* (2011) 152:1691–701. doi: 10.1210/en.2010-1353

66. Jean-Alphonse F, Bowersox S, Chen S, Beard G, Puthenveedu MA, Hanyaloglu AC. Spatially restricted G protein-coupled receptor activity via divergent endocytic compartments. *J Biol Chem.* (2014) 289:3960–77. doi: 10.1074/jbc.M113.526350

67. Sposini S, Jean-Alphonse FG, Ayoub MA, Oqua A, West C, Lavery S, et al. Integration of GPCR signaling and sorting from very early endosomes via opposing APPL1 mechanisms. *Cell Rep.* (2017) 21:2855–67. doi: 10.1016/j.celrep.2017.11.023

68. Cohen BD, Nechamen CA, Dias JA. Human follitropin receptor (FSHR) interacts with the adapter protein 14-3-3tau. *Mol Cell Endocrinol.* (2004) 220:1–7. doi: 10.1016/j.mce.2004.04.012

69. Dias JA, Mahale SD, Nechamen CA, Davydenko O, Thomas RM, Ulloa-Aguirre A. Emerging roles for the FSH receptor adapter protein APPL1 and overlap of a putative 14-3-3τ interaction domain with a canonical G-protein interaction site. *Mol Cell Endocrinol.* (2010) 329:17–25. doi: 10.1016/j.mce.2010.05.009

70. Timossi C, Maldonado D, Vizcaíno A, Lindau-Shepard B, Conn PM, Ulloa-Aguirre A. Structural determinants in the second intracellular loop of the human follicle-stimulating hormone receptor are involved in G(s) protein activation. *Mol Cell Endocrinol.* (2002) 189:157–68. doi: 10.1016/S0303-7207(01)00720-1

71. Lohse MJ, Hoffmann C. Arrestin interactions with G protein-coupled receptors. *Handb Exp Pharmacol.* (2014) 219:15–56. doi: 10.1007/978-3-642-41199-1_2

72. Oakley RH, Laporte SA, Holt JA, Barak LS, Caron MG. Molecular determinants underlying the formation of stable intracellular G protein-coupled receptor-β-arrestin complexes after receptor endocytosis. *J Biol Chem.* (2001) 276:19452–60. doi: 10.1074/jbc.M101450200

73. Peterson YK, Luttrell LM. The diverse roles of arrestin scaffolds in G protein-coupled receptor signaling. *Pharmacol Rev.* (2017) 69:256–97. doi: 10.1124/pr.116.013367

74. Luttrell LM, Lefkowitz RJ. The role of beta-arrestins in the termination and transduction of G-protein-coupled receptor signals. *J Cell Sci.* (2002) 115(Pt 3):455–65.

75. Zhou XE, He Y, de Waal PW, Gao X, Kang Y, Van Eps N, et al. Identification of phosphorylation codes for arrestin recruitment by G protein-coupled receptors. *Cell.* (2017) 170:457–69.e13. doi: 10.1016/j.cell.2017.07.002

76. Romero G, von Zastrow M, Friedman PA. Role of PDZ proteins in regulating trafficking, signaling, and function of GPCRs: means, motif, and opportunity. *Adv Pharmacol.* (2011) 62:279–314. doi: 10.1016/B978-0-12-385952-5.00003-8

77. Nechamen CA, Thomas RM, Dias JA. APPL1, APPL2, Akt2 and FOXO1a interact with FSHR in a potential signaling complex. *Mol Cell Endocrinol.* (2007) 260-2:93–9. doi: 10.1016/j.mce.2006.08.014

78. Lin DC, Quevedo C, Brewer NE, Bell A, Testa JR, Grimes ML, et al. APPL1 associates with TrkA and GIPC1 and is required for nerve growth factor-mediated signal transduction. *Mol Cell Biol.* (2006) 26:8928–41. doi: 10.1128/MCB.00228-06

79. Kalaidzidis I, Miaczynska M, Brewinska-Olchowik M, Hupalowska A, Ferguson C, Parton RG, et al. APPL endosomes are not obligatory endocytic intermediates but act as stable cargo-sorting compartments. *J Cell Biol.* (2015) 211:123–44. doi: 10.1083/jcb.201311117

80. Zoncu R, Perera RM, Balkin DM, Pirruccello M, Toomre D, De Camilli P. A phosphoinositide switch controls the maturation and signaling properties of APPL endosomes. *Cell.* (2009) 136:1110–21. doi: 10.1016/j.cell.2009.01.032

81. Thomsen ARB, Jensen DD, Hicks GA, Bunnett NW. Therapeutic targeting of endosomal G-protein-coupled receptors. *Trends Pharmacol Sci.* (2018) 39:879–91. doi: 10.1016/j.tips.2018.08.003

82. Tsvetanova NG, Irannejad R, von Zastrow M. G protein-coupled receptor (GPCR) signaling via heterotrimeric G proteins from endosomes. *J Biol Chem.* (2015) 290:6689–96. doi: 10.1074/jbc.R114.617951

83. Vilardaga JP, Jean-Alphonse FG, Gardella TJ. Endosomal generation of cAMP in GPCR signaling. *Nat Chem Biol.* (2014) 10:700–6. doi: 10.1038/nchembio.1611

84. Godbole A, Lyga S, Lohse MJ, Calebiro D. Internalized TSH receptors en route to the TGN induce local Gs-protein signaling and gene transcription. *Nat Commun.* (2017) 8:443. doi: 10.1038/s41467-017-00357-2

85. Lyga S, Volpe S, Werthmann RC, Gotz K, Sungkaworn T, Lohse MJ, et al. Persistent cAMP signaling by internalized LH receptors in ovarian follicles. *Endocrinology.* (2016) 157:1613–21. doi: 10.1210/en.2015-1945

86. Wehbi VL, Stevenson HP, Feinstein TN, Calero G, Romero G, Vilardaga JP. Noncanonical GPCR signaling arising from a PTH receptor-arrestin-Gbetagamma complex. *Proc Natl Acad Sci USA.* (2013) 110:1530–5. doi: 10.1073/pnas.1205756110

87. Jean-Alphonse FG, Wehbi VL, Chen J, Noda M, Taboas JM, Xiao K, et al. beta2-adrenergic receptor control of endosomal PTH receptor signaling via Gbetagamma. *Nat Chem Biol.* (2017) 13:259–61. doi: 10.1038/nchembio.2267

88. Krishnamurthy H, Kishi H, Shi M, Galet C, Bhaskaran RS, Hirakawa T, et al. Postendocytotic trafficking of the follicle-stimulating hormone (FSH)-FSH receptor complex. *Mol Endocrinol.* (2003) 17:2162–76. doi: 10.1210/me.2003-0118

89. Urban JD, Clarke WP, von Zastrow M, Nichols DE, Kobilka B, Weinstein H, et al. Functional selectivity and classical concepts of quantitative pharmacology. *J Pharmacol Exp Ther.* (2006) 320:1–13. doi: 10.1124/jpet.106.104463

90. Wisler JW, DeWire SM, Whalen EJ, Violin JD, Drake MT, Ahn S, et al. A unique mechanism of beta-blocker action: carvedilol stimulates beta-arrestin signaling. *Proc Natl Acad Sci USA.* (2007) 104:16657–62. doi: 10.1073/pnas.0707936104

91. Evans BA, Sato M, Sarwar M, Hutchinson DS, Summers RJ. Ligand-directed signalling at β-adrenoceptors. *Br J Pharmacol.* (2010) 159:1022–38. doi: 10.1111/j.1476-5381.2009.00602.x

92. Kenakin T. Functional selectivity and biased receptor signaling. *J Pharmacol Exp Ther.* (2011) 336:296–302. doi: 10.1124/jpet.110.173948

93. Kenakin T, Christopoulos A. Signalling bias in new drug discovery: detection, quantification and therapeutic impact. *Nat Rev Drug Discov.* (2013) 12:205–16. doi: 10.1038/nrd3954

94. Michel MC, Charlton SJ. Biased agonism in drug discovery - is it too soon to choose a path? *Mol Pharmacol.* (2018) 93:259–65. doi: 10.1124/mol.117.110890

95. Smith JS, Lefkowitz RJ, Rajagopal S. Biased signalling: from simple switches to allosteric microprocessors. *Nat Rev Drug Discov.* (2018) 17:243–60. doi: 10.1038/nrd.2017.229

96. Kenakin T. Theoretical aspects of GPCR–ligand complex pharmacology. *Chem Rev.* (2017) 117:4–20. doi: 10.1021/acs.chemrev.5b00561

97. Edelstein SJ, Changeux J-P. Biased allostery. *Biophys J.* (2016) 111:902–8. doi: 10.1016/j.bpj.2016.07.044

98. Roth S, Bruggeman FJ. A conformation-equilibrium model captures ligand–ligand interactions and ligand-biased signalling by G-protein coupled receptors. *FEBS J.* (2014) 281:4659–71. doi: 10.1111/febs.12970

99. Black JW, Leff P. Operational models of pharmacological agonism. *Proc R Soc Lond Series B Biol Sci.* (1983) 220:141–62. doi: 10.1098/rspb.1983.0093

100. Kenakin T, Watson C, Muniz-Medina V, Christopoulos A, Novick S. A simple method for quantifying functional selectivity and agonist bias. *ACS Chem Neurosci.* (2012) 3:193–203. doi: 10.1021/cn200111m

101. van der Westhuizen ET, Breton B, Christopoulos A, Bouvier M. Quantification of ligand bias for clinically relevant 2-adrenergic receptor ligands: implications for drug taxonomy. *Mol Pharmacol.* (2014) 85:492–509. doi: 10.1124/mol.113.088880

102. Namkung Y, Le Gouill C, Lukashova V, Kobayashi H, Hogue M, Khoury E, et al. Monitoring G protein-coupled receptor and beta-arrestin trafficking in live cells using enhanced bystander BRET. *Nat Commun.* (2016) 7:12178. doi: 10.1038/ncomms12178

103. Rajagopal S, Ahn S, Rominger DH, Gowen-MacDonald W, Lam CM, DeWire SM, et al. Quantifying ligand bias at seven-transmembrane receptors. *Mol Pharmacol.* (2011) 80:367–77. doi: 10.1124/mol.111.072801

104. Onaran HO, Ambrosio C, Ugur Ö, Koncz EM, Grò MC, Vezzi V, et al. Systematic errors in detecting biased agonism: analysis of current methods and development of a new model-free approach. *Sci Rep.* (2017) 7:44247. doi: 10.1038/srep44247

105. Barak LS, Peterson S. Modeling of bias for the analysis of receptor signaling in biochemical systems. *Biochemistry.* (2012) 51:1114–25. doi: 10.1021/bi201308s

106. Grundmann M, Kostenis E. Temporal bias: time-encoded dynamic GPCR signaling. *Trends Pharmacol Sci.* (2017) 38:1110–24. doi: 10.1016/j.tips.2017.09.004

107. Klein Herenbrink C, Sykes DA, Donthamsetti P, Canals M, Coudrat T, Shonberg J, et al. The role of kinetic context in apparent biased agonism at GPCRs. *Nat Commun.* (2016) 7:10842. doi: 10.1038/ncomms10842

108. Lane JR, May LT, Parton RG, Sexton PM, Christopoulos A. A kinetic view of GPCR allostery and biased agonism. *Nat Chem Biol.* (2017) 13:929–37. doi: 10.1038/nchembio.2431

109. Bridge LJ, Mead J, Frattini E, Winfield I, Ladds G. Modelling and simulation of biased agonism dynamics at a G protein-coupled receptor. *J Theor Biol.* (2018) 442:44–65. doi: 10.1016/j.jtbi.2018.01.010

110. Hoare SRJ, Pierre N, Moya AG, Larson B. Kinetic operational models of agonism for G-protein-coupled receptors. *J Theor Biol.* (2018) 446:168–204. doi: 10.1016/j.jtbi.2018.02.014

111. Christopoulos A, Changeux JP, Catterall WA, Fabbro D, Burris TP, Cidlowski JA, et al. International Union of Basic and Clinical Pharmacology. XC. multisite pharmacology: recommendations for the nomenclature of receptor allosterism and allosteric ligands. *Pharmacol Rev.* (2014) 66:918–47. doi: 10.1124/pr.114.008862

112. Burford NT, Watson J, Bertekap R, Alt A. Strategies for the identification of allosteric modulators of G-protein-coupled receptors. *Biochem Pharmacol.* (2011) 81:691–702. doi: 10.1016/j.bcp.2010.12.012

113. Maclean D, Holden F, Davis AM, Scheuerman RA, Yanofsky S, Holmes CP, et al. Agonists of the follicle stimulating hormone receptor from an encoded thiazolidinone library. *J Combin Chem.* (2004) 6:196–206. doi: 10.1021/cc0300154

114. Yanofsky SD, Shen ES, Holden F, Whitehorn E, Aguilar B, Tate E, et al. Allosteric activation of the Follicle-stimulating Hormone (FSH) receptor by selective, nonpeptide agonists. *J Biol Chem.* (2006) 281:13226–33. doi: 10.1074/jbc.M600601200

115. Sriraman V, Denis D, de Matos D, Yu H, Palmer S, Nataraja S. Investigation of a thiazolidinone derivative as an allosteric modulator of follicle stimulating hormone receptor: evidence for its ability to support follicular development and ovulation. *Biochem Pharmacol.* (2014) 89:266–75. doi: 10.1016/j.bcp.2014.02.023

116. Arey BJ, Yanofsky SD, Claudia Pérez M, Holmes CP, Wrobel J, Gopalsamy A, et al. Differing pharmacological activities of thiazolidinone analogs at the FSH receptor. *Biochem Biophys Res Commun.* (2008) 368:723–8. doi: 10.1016/j.bbrc.2008.01.119

117. Yu HN, Richardson TE, Nataraja S, Fischer DJ, Sriraman V, Jiang X, et al. Discovery of substituted benzamides as follicle stimulating hormone receptor allosteric modulators. *Bioorgan Med Chem Lett.* (2014) 24:2168–72. doi: 10.1016/j.bmcl.2014.03.018

118. van Koppen CJ, Verbost PM, van de Lagemaat R, Karstens W-JF, Loozen HJJ, van Achterberg TAE, et al. Signaling of an allosteric, nanomolar potent, low molecular weight agonist for the follicle-stimulating hormone receptor. *Biochem Pharmacol.* (2013) 85:1162–70. doi: 10.1016/j.bcp.2013.02.001

119. van Straten NCR, van Berkel THJ, Demont DR, Karstens W-JF, Merkx R, Oosterom J, et al. Identification of substituted 6-amino-4-phenyltetrahydroquinoline derivatives: potent antagonists for the follicle-stimulating hormone receptor. *J Med Chem.* (2005) 48:1697–700. doi: 10.1021/jm049676l

120. Dias JA, Bonnet B, Weaver BA, Watts J, Kluetzman K, Thomas RM, et al. A negative allosteric modulator demonstrates biased antagonism of the follicle stimulating hormone receptor. *Mol Cell Endocrinol.* (2011) 333:143–50. doi: 10.1016/j.mce.2010.12.023

121. Dias JA, Campo B, Weaver BA, Watts J, Kluetzman K, Thomas RM, et al. Inhibition of follicle-stimulating hormone-induced preovulatory follicles in rats treated with a nonsteroidal negative allosteric modulator of follicle-stimulating hormone receptor1. *Biol Reprod.* (2014) 90:19. doi: 10.1095/biolreprod.113.109397

122. Ayoub MA, Yvinec R, Jegot G, Dias JA, Poli SM, Poupon A, et al. Profiling of FSHR negative allosteric modulators on LH/CGR reveals biased antagonism

with implications in steroidogenesis. *Mol Cell Endocrinol.* (2016) 436:10–22. doi: 10.1016/j.mce.2016.07.013

123. Danesi R, La Rocca RV, Cooper MR, Ricciardi MP, Pellegrini A, Soldani P, et al. Clinical and experimental evidence of inhibition of testosterone production by suramin. *J Clin Endocrinol Metab.* (1996) 81:2238–46.

124. Arey BJ, Deecher DC, Shen ES, Stevis PE, Meade EH, Wrobel J, et al. Identification and characterization of a selective, nonpeptide follicle-stimulating hormone receptor antagonist. *Endocrinology.* (2002) 143:3822–9. doi: 10.1210/en.2002-220372

125. Bousfield GR, Butnev VY, White WK, Hall AS, Harvey DJ. Comparison of follicle-stimulating hormone glycosylation microheterogenity by quantitative negative mode nano- electrospray mass spectrometry of peptide-N glycanase- released oligosaccharides. *J Glycomics Lipidomics.* (2015) 311:587–96. doi: 10.4172/2153-0637.1000129

126. Fox KM, Dias JA, Roey PV. Three-dimensional structure of human follicle-stimulating hormone. *Mol Endocrinol.* (2001) 15:378–89. doi: 10.1210/mend.15.3.0603

127. Rapoport B, McLachlan SM, Kakinuma A, Chazenbalk GD. Critical relationship between autoantibody recognition and thyrotropin receptor maturation as reflected in the acquisition of complex carbohydrate. *J Clin Endocrinol Metab.* (1996) 81:2525–33. doi: 10.1210/jcem.81.7.8675572

128. Dias JA, Van Roey P. Structural biology of human follitropin and its receptor. *Arch Med Res.* (2001) 32:510–9. doi: 10.1016/S0188-4409(01)00333-2

129. Baenziger JU, Green ED. Pituitary glycoprotein hormone oligosaccharides: structure, synthesis and function of the asparagine-linked oligosaccharides on lutropin, follitropin and thyrotropin. *Biochim Biophys Acta.* (1988) 947:287–306.

130. Bishop LA, Nguyen TV, Schofield PR. Both of the β-subunit carbohydrate residues of follicle-stimulating hormone determine the metabolic clearance rate and *in vivo* potency. *Endocrinology.* (1995) 136:2635–40. doi: 10.1210/endo.136.6.7750487

131. Dalpathado DS, Irungu J, Go EP, Butnev VY, Norton K, Bousfield GR, et al. Comparative glycomics of the glycoprotein follicle stimulating hormone: glycopeptide analysis of isolates from two mammalian species. *Biochemistry.* (2006) 45:8665–73. doi: 10.1021/bi060435k

132. Grass J, Pabst M, Chang M, Wozny M, Altmann F. Analysis of recombinant human follicle-stimulating hormone (FSH) by mass spectrometric approaches. *Anal Bioanal Chem.* (2011) 400:2427–38. doi: 10.1007/s00216-011-4923-5

133. Grossmann M, Weintraub BD, Szkudlinski MW. Novel insights into the molecular mechanisms of human thyrotropin action: structural, physiological, and therapeutic implications for the glycoprotein hormone family. *Endocr Rev.* (1997) 18:476–501. doi: 10.1210/edrv.18.4.0305

134. Jiang X, Fischer D, Chen X, McKenna SD, Liu H, Sriraman V, et al. Evidence for follicle-stimulating hormone receptor as a functional trimer. *J Biol Chem.* (2014) 289:14273–82. doi: 10.1074/jbc.M114.549592

135. Lambert A, Rodgers M, Mitchell R, Wood AM, Wardle C, Hilton B, et al. *In-vitro* biopotency and glycoform distribution of recombinant human follicle stimulating hormone (Org 32489), Metrodin and Metrodin-HP. *Mol Hum Reprod.* (1995) 1:270–7. doi: 10.1093/molehr/1.5.270

136. Sairam MR, Bhargavi GN. A role for glycosylation of the alpha subunit in transduction of biological signal in glycoprotein hormones. *Science.* (1985) 229:65–7. doi: 10.1126/science.2990039

137. Ulloa-Aguirre A, Midgley AR, Beitins IZ, Padmanabhan V. Follicle-stimulating isohormones: characterization and physiological relevance. *Endocr Rev.* (1995) 16:765–87. doi: 10.1210/edrv-16-6-765

138. Ulloa-Aguirre A, Timossi C, Barrios-de-Tomasi J, Maldonado A, Nayudu P. Impact of carbohydrate heterogeneity in function of follicle-stimulating hormone: studies derived from *in vitro* and *in vivo* models1. *Biol Reprod.* (2003) 69:379–89. doi: 10.1095/biolreprod.103.016915

139. Bousfield GR, Butnev VY, Butnev VY, Hiromasa Y, Harvey DJ, May JV. Hypo-glycosylated Human Follicle-Stimulating Hormone (hFSH 21/18) is much more active *in vitro* than Fully-glycosylated hFSH (hFSH 24). *Mol Cell Endocrinol.* (2014) 382:989–97. doi: 10.1016/j.mce.2013.11.008

140. Bousfield GR, Butnev VY, Gotschall RR, Baker VL, Mooreb WT. Structural features of mammalian gonadotropins. *Mol Cell Endocrinol.* (1996) 125:3–19. doi: 10.1016/S0303-7207(96)03945-7

141. Bousfield GR, Butnev VY, Walton WJ, Nguyen VT, Huneidi J, Singh V, et al. All-or-none N-glycosylation in primate follicle-stimulating hormone β-subunits. *Mol Cell Endocrinol.* (2007) 260–2:40–8. doi: 10.1016/j.mce.2006.02.017

142. Walton WJ, Nguyen VT, Butnev VY, Singh V, Moore WT, Bousfield GR. Characterization of human FSH isoforms reveals a nonglycosylated β-subunit in addition to the conventional glycosylated β-subunit. *J Clin Endocrinol Metab.* (2001) 86:3675–85. doi: 10.1210/jc.86.8.3675

143. Dias JA, Lindau-Shepard B, Hauer C, Auger I. Human follicle-stimulating hormone structure-activity relationships. *Biol Reprod.* (1998) 58:1331–6. doi: 10.1095/biolreprod58.6.1331

144. Ulloa-Aguirre A, Timossi C, Damian-Matsumura P, Dias JA. Role of glycosylation in function of follicle-stimulating hormone. *Endocrine.* (1999) 11:205–15. doi: 10.1385/ENDO:11:3:205

145. Gotschall RR, Bousfield GR. Oligosaccharide mapping reveals hormone-specific glycosylation patterns on equine gonadotropin α-subunit Asn56. *Endocrinology.* (1996) 137:2543–57. doi: 10.1210/endo.137.6.8641208

146. Maghuin-Rogister G, Closset J, Hennen G. Differences in the carbohydrate portion of the α subunit of porcine lutropin (LH), follitropin (FSH) and thyrotropin (TSH). *FEBS Lett.* (1975) 60:263–6. doi: 10.1016/0014-5793(75)80727-7

147. Nilsson B, Rosen SW, Weintraub BD, Zopf DA. Differences in the carbohydrate moieties of the common α-subunits of human chorionic gonadotropin, luteinizing hormone, follicle-stimulating hormone, and thyrotropin: preliminary structural inferences from direct methylation analysis. *Endocrinology.* (1986) 119:2737–43.

148. Lapthorn AJ, Harris DC, Littlejohn A, Lustbader JW, Canfield RE, Machin KJ, et al. Crystal structure of human chorionic gonadotropin. *Nature.* (1994) 369:455–61. doi: 10.1038/369455a0

149. Wu H, Lustbader JW, Liu Y, Canfield RE, Hendrickson WA. Structure of human chorionic gonadotropin at 2.6 å resolution from MAD analysis of the selenomethionyl protein. *Structure.* (1994) 2:545–58.

150. Miguel RN, Sanders J, Furmaniak J, Smith BR. Glycosylation pattern analysis of glycoprotein hormones and their receptors. *J Mol Endocrinol.* (2017) 58:25–41. doi: 10.1530/JME-16-0169

151. Wang H, Butnev V, Bousfield GR, Rajendra Kumar T. A human FSHB transgene encoding the double N-glycosylation mutant [Asn (7Δ) Asn (24Δ)] FSHβ subunit fails to rescue Fshb null mice. *Mol Cell Endocrinol.* (2016) 426:113–24. doi: 10.1016/j.mce.2016.02.015

152. Meher BR, Dixit A, Bousfield GR, Lushington GH. Glycosylation effects on FSH-FSHR interaction dynamics: a case study of different fsh glycoforms by molecular dynamics simulations. *PLoS ONE.* (2015) 10:1–23. doi: 10.1371/journal.pone.0137897

153. Trousdale RK, Yu B, Pollak SV, Husami N, Vidali A, Lustbader JW. Efficacy of native and hyperglycosylated follicle-stimulating hormone analogs for promoting fertility in female mice. *Fertil Steril.* (2009) 91:265–70. doi: 10.1016/j.fertnstert.2007.11.013

154. Andersen CY, Leonardsen L, Ulloa-Aguirre A, Barrios-De-Tomasi J, Moore L, Byskov AG. FSH-induced resumption of meiosis in mouse oocytes: effect of different isoforms. *Mol Hum Reprod.* (1999) 5:726–31. doi: 10.1093/molehr/5.8.726

155. Jiang C, Hou X, Wang C, May JV, Butnev VY, Bousfield GR, et al. Hypoglycosylated hFSH has greater bioactivity than fully glycosylated recombinant hFSH in human granulosa cells. *J Clin Endocrinol Metab.* (2015) 100:E852–60. doi: 10.1210/jc.2015-1317

156. Wehbi V, Tranchant T, Durand G, Musnier A, Decourtye J, Piketty V, et al. Partially deglycosylated equine LH preferentially activates beta-arrestin-dependent signaling at the follicle-stimulating hormone receptor. *Mol Endocrinol.* (2010) 24:561–73. doi: 10.1210/me.2009-0347

157. Timossi CM, Barrios-de-Tomasi J, González-Suárez R, Arranz MC, Padmanabhan V, Conn PM, et al. Differential effects of the charge variants of human follicle-stimulating hormone. *J Endocrinol.* (2000) 165:193–205. doi: 10.1677/joe.0.1650193

158. Riccetti L, Yvinec R, Klett D, Gallay N, Combarnous Y, Reiter E, et al. Human luteinizing hormone and chorionic gonadotropin display biased agonism at the LH and LH/CG receptors. *Sci Rep.* (2017) 7:940. doi: 10.1038/s41598-017-01078-8

159. Ferasin L, Gabai G, Beattie J, Bono G, Holder AT. Enhancement of FSH bioactivity *in vivo* using site-specific antisera. *J Endocrinol.* (1997) 152:355–63. doi: 10.1677/joe.0.1520355

160. Glencross RG, Lovell RD, Holder AT. Monoclonal antibody enhancement of fsh-induced uterine growth in snell dwarf mice. *J Endocrinol.* (1993) 136:R5–7. doi: 10.1677/joe.0.136R005

161. Combarnous Y, Guillou F, Martinat N. Comparison of *in vitro* Follicle-Stimulating Hormone (FSH) activity of equine gonadotropins (Luteinizing Hormone, FSH, and Chorionic Gonadotropin) in male and female rats. *Endocrinology.* (1984) 115:1821–7. doi: 10.1210/endo-115-5-1821

162. Guillou F, Combarnous Y. Purification of equine gonadotropins and comparative study of their acid-dissociation and receptor-binding specificity. *Biochim Biophys Acta.* (1983) 755:229–36.

163. Combarnous Y, Hennen G, Ketelslegers M. Pregnant mare serum gonadotropin exhibits higher affinity for lutropin than for follitropin receptors of porcine testis. *FEBS Lett.* (1978) 90:65–8. doi: 10.1016/0014-5793(78)80299-3

164. Licht P, Gallo AB, Aggarwal BB, Farmer SW, Castelino JB, Papkoff H. Biological and binding activities of equine pituitary gonadotrophins and pregnant mare serum gonadotrophin. *J Endocrinol.* (1979) 83:311–22. doi: 10.1677/joe.0.0830311

165. Hervé V, Roy F, Bertin J, Guillou F, Maurel M-C. Antiequine chorionic gonadotropin (eCG) antibodies generated in goats treated with eCG for the induction of ovulation modulate the luteinizing hormone and follicle-stimulating hormone bioactivities of eCG differently. *Endocrinology.* (2004) 145:294–303. doi: 10.1210/en.2003-0595

166. Wehbi V, Decourtye J, Piketty V, Durand G, Reiter E, Maurel M-C. Selective modulation of follicle-stimulating hormone signaling pathways with enhancing equine chorionic gonadotropin/antibody immune complexes. *Endocrinology.* (2010) 151:2788–99. doi: 10.1210/en.2009-0892

167. Ji Y, Liu P, Yuen T, Haider S, He J, Romero R, et al. Epitope-specific monoclonal antibodies to FSHβ increase bone mass. *Proc Natl Acad Sci USA.* (2018) 115:2192–7. doi: 10.1073/pnas.1718144115

168. Hutchings CJ, Koglin M, Olson WC, Marshall FH. Opportunities for therapeutic antibodies directed at G-protein-coupled receptors. *Nat Rev Drug Discov.* (2017) 16:787–810. doi: 10.1038/nrd.2017.91

169. Abdennebi L, Couture L, Grebert D, Pajot E, Salesse R, Remy JJ. Generating FSH antagonists and agonists through immunization against FSH receptor N-terminal decapeptides. *J Mol Endocrinol.* (1999) 22:151–9. doi: 10.1677/jme.0.0220151

170. Agrawal G, Dighe RR. Critical Involvement of the Hinge region of the follicle-stimulating hormone receptor in the activation of the receptor. *J Biol Chem.* (2009) 284:2636–47. doi: 10.1074/jbc.M808199200

171. Dhar N, Mohan A, Thakur C, Chandra NR, Dighe RR. Dissecting the structural and functional features of the Luteinizing hormone receptor using

receptor specific single chain fragment variables. *Mol Cell Endocrinol.* (2016) 427:1–12. doi: 10.1016/j.mce.2016.02.022

172. Majumdar R, Railkar R, Dighe RR. Insights into differential modulation of receptor function by hinge region using novel agonistic lutropin receptor and inverse agonistic thyrotropin receptor antibodies. *FEBS Lett.* (2012) 586:810–7. doi: 10.1016/j.febslet.2012.01.052

173. Crepin R, Veggiani G, Djender S, Beugnet A, Planeix F, Pichon C, et al. Whole-cell biopanning with a synthetic phage display library of nanobodies enabled the recovery of follicle-stimulating hormone receptor inhibitors. *Biochem Biophys Res Commun.* (2017) 493:1567–72. doi: 10.1016/j.bbrc.2017.10.036

174. Chen X, Bai B, Tian Y, Du H, Chen J. Identification of serine 348 on the apelin receptor as a novel regulatory phosphorylation site in apelin-13-induced G protein-independent biased signaling. *J Biol Chem.* (2014) 289:31173–87. doi: 10.1074/jbc.M114.574020

175. Gorvin CM, Babinsky VN, Malinauskas T, Nissen PH, Schou AJ, Hannyaloglu AC, et al. A calcium-sensing receptor mutation causing hypocalcemia disrupts a transmembrane salt bridge to activate beta-arrestin-biased signaling. *Sci Signal.* (2018) 11:518. doi: 10.1126/scisignal.aan3714

176. Woo AY, Jozwiak K, Toll L, Tanga MJ, Kozocas JA, Jimenez L, et al. Tyrosine 308 is necessary for ligand-directed Gs protein-biased signaling of beta2-adrenoceptor. *J Biol Chem.* (2014) 289:19351–63. doi: 10.1074/jbc.M114.558882

177. Desai SS, Roy BS, Mahale SD. Mutations and polymorphisms in FSH receptor: functional implications in human reproduction. *Reproduction.* (2013) 146:R235–48. doi: 10.1530/REP-13-0351

178. Tranchant T, Durand G, Gauthier C, Crepieux P, Ulloa-Aguirre A, Royere D, et al. Preferential beta-arrestin signalling at low receptor density revealed by functional characterization of the human FSH receptor A189 V mutation. *Mol Cell Endocrinol.* (2011) 331:109–18. doi: 10.1016/j.mce.2010.08.016

179. Uchida S, Uchida H, Maruyama T, Kajitani T, Oda H, Miyazaki K, et al. Molecular analysis of a mutated FSH receptor detected in a patient with spontaneous ovarian hyperstimulation syndrome. *PLoS ONE.* (2013) 8:e75478. doi: 10.1371/journal.pone.0075478

180. Casas-Gonzalez P, Scaglia HE, Perez-Solis MA, Durand G, Scaglia J, Zarinan T, et al. Normal testicular function without detectable follicle-stimulating hormone. A novel mutation in the follicle-stimulating hormone receptor gene leading to apparent constitutive activity and impaired agonist-induced desensitization and internalization. *Mol Cell Endocrinol.* (2012) 364:71–82. doi: 10.1016/j.mce.2012.08.011

181. Casarini L, Moriondo V, Marino M, Adversi F, Capodanno F, Grisolia C, et al. FSHR polymorphism p.N680S mediates different responses to FSH *in vitro*. *Mol Cell Endocrinol.* (2014) 393:83–91. doi: 10.1016/j.mce.2014.06.013

18

Structure-Function Relationships of the Follicle-Stimulating Hormone Receptor

Alfredo Ulloa-Aguirre[1]*, Teresa Zariñán[1], Eduardo Jardón-Valadez[2],
Rubén Gutiérrez-Sagal[1] and James A. Dias[3]

[1] Red de Apoyo a la Investigación, Universidad Nacional Autónoma de México and Instituto Nacional de Ciencias Médicas y Nutrición Salvador Zubirán, Mexico City, Mexico, [2] Departamento de Ciencias Ambientales, Universidad Autónoma Metropolitana Unidad Lerma, Lerma, Mexico, [3] Department of Biomedical Sciences, School of Public Health, University at Albany, Albany, NY, United States

*Correspondence:
Alfredo Ulloa-Aguirre
aulloaa@unam.mx

The follicle-stimulating hormone receptor (FSHR) plays a crucial role in reproduction. This structurally complex receptor is a member of the G-protein coupled receptor (GPCR) superfamily of membrane receptors. As with the other structurally similar glycoprotein hormone receptors (the thyroid-stimulating hormone and luteinizing hormone-chorionic gonadotropin hormone receptors), the FSHR is characterized by an extensive extracellular domain, where binding to FSH occurs, linked to the signal specificity subdomain or hinge region. This region is involved in ligand-stimulated receptor activation whereas the seven transmembrane domain is associated with receptor activation and transmission of the activation process to the intracellular loops comprised of amino acid sequences, which predicate coupling to effectors, interaction with adapter proteins, and triggering of downstream intracellular signaling. In this review, we describe the most important structural features of the FSHR intimately involved in regulation of FSHR function, including trafficking, dimerization, and oligomerization, ligand binding, agonist-stimulated activation, and signal transduction.

Keywords: follicle-stimulating hormone receptor (FSHR), follitropin receptor, structure, G protein-coupled receptor (GPCR), glycoprotein hormone receptors

INTRODUCTION

The glycoprotein hormone (GPH) receptors (GPHR), are members of the highly conserved Class A subfamily (or rhodopsin-like family) of the G protein-coupled receptor (GPCR) superfamily (1–5). GPCRs are 7-transmembrane-helix protein molecules that transmit intracellular effects through activating intracellular signaling mediated by members of the guanine-nucleotide-binding signal-transducing proteins (G proteins); they are characterized by a single polypeptide chain that traverses the lipid bilayer of the plasma membrane seven times, forming characteristic transmembrane α-helices linked by alternating extracellular and intracellular sequences or loops, with an extracellular amino-terminus end and an intracellular carboxyl-terminal tail (C-tail) of variable lengths. In the case of GPHRs, common features include a large amino-terminal extracellular domain (ECD), where recognition and binding of their cognate ligands, follicle-stimulating hormone or follitropin (FSH), luteinizing hormone (LH), and thyroid-stimulating hormone (TSH) occur (6). This domain contains a central structural motif of imperfect leucine-rich repeats [12 in the FSH receptor (FSHR), 9 in the luteinizing hormone/chorionic gonadotropin receptor (LHCGR) and 11 in the TSH receptor (TSHR) (7–9)] that is shared with several cell surface plasma membrane receptors. The leucine-rich repeats motif comprises a surface that is involved in selectivity for ligands and specific protein-protein interactions, and is formed by successive repeating units (β-strand and α-helix) that collectively predispose the ECD to adopt a horse shoe-shaped tertiary structure (see **Figure 1A** in the schematic representation of the FSHR, a prototypical member of the GPHR family) (7, 10). At the COOH-terminal end of the large ECD resides the "hinge" region, which links the leucine-rich repeat (LRR) ECD with the serpentine, seven-transmembrane α-helical domains (7TMD) and that plays a critical role of signaling functionality of the receptor (7) (**Figure 1B**). The hinge region of all GPHRs is involved not only in high affinity binding of the ligand but in also receptor activation, intramolecular signal transduction and silencing of basal activity in the absence of ligand (9).

The *FSHR* is about 190 Kb long and is located on chromosome 2p21–p16 (11); its coding region comprises 10 exons, each varying in size from 69 to 1,234 bp, and 9 introns with sizes 108 to 15 kb. Exons 1–9 of the receptor gene encode the large ECD, including the hinge region, whereas exon 10 encodes the COOH-terminal end of the hinge region, the 7TMD (which contains 3 extracellular loops and 3 intracellular loops) and the intracellular C-tail (3, 11). The human FSHR (hereafter abbreviated as only FSHR) protein is composed of 695 amino acid residues; the first set of 17 amino acids encodes the signal sequence, which after cleavage results in a predicted cell surface plasma membrane (PM)-expressed, mature FSHR of 678 amino acid residues exhibiting an approximate molecular weight of 75 kDa as predicted from its cDNA sequence (12). However, further cleavage of the FSHR occurs at the C-tail, but the exact location of this cleavage has yet to be determined (13). Three of four potential N-linked glycosylation sites yields receptor forms with molecular weights (as determined by gel electrophoresis) of ~80 to ~87 kDa for the mature receptor (14). A high degree sequence homology is present in both the FSHR and its closely related LHCGR. In fact, their sequence homology is ~46% in the ECD and ~72% in the 7TMD (12, 15). Of the three domains of the gonadotropin receptors, the intracellular sequences, which include the intervening loops and the C-tail, present the lowest sequence homology (~27% identity), except the NH_2-ends of the carboxyl-termini, which have cysteine residues for palmitoylation and the primary sequence motif $[F(X)_6LL]$ that is involved in intracellular trafficking from the endoplasmic reticulum to the PM (16–18). Both of these structural features are quite common in the rhodopsin-like GPCR Class and likely play a role in signaling specificity particularly when two members of the same family (FSHR and LHR) are coexpressed in the same cell (granulosa cell).

Gonadotropins and their receptors play an essential role in reproduction. In the ovary, FSHR is predominantly expressed in granulosa cells of developing follicles, where the FSH-activated receptor triggers activation of a complex signaling network that promotes follicle growth and maturation, and induces in the granulosa cells the necessary enzymes for converting the androgens provided by the theca cells under the LH stimulus

to estrogens (19). In the testis, the Sertoli cells lining the seminiferous tubules are the targets of FSH action, where the gonadotropin promotes their growth and maturation and, together with testosterone produced by LH-stimulated Leydig cells, initiates, and supports high quality spermatogenesis (20, 21). Interestingly, a recent study in transgenic mice showed that a constitutively active mutant (CAM) FSHR may support normal spermatogenesis alone in the absence of androgens (22). Whether this finding in mice is relevant in humans remains an open question.

In recent years there have been reports of FSHR detected in other than the canonical gonadal tissues. Extragonadal FSHRs, which include bone (23, 24), monocytes (25, 26), different sites of the female reproductive tract and the developing placenta (27), endothelial cells from umbilical vein (28) and blood vessels from malignant tumors and metastases (29–31), and the liver (32), have been identified employing different detection approaches, mainly immunohistochemistry and more recently *in vitro* and *in vivo* imaging of FSH-conjugated NIRII-fluorophore (33). It has been proposed that these extragonadal FSHRs might play a role in diverse physiological processes, mainly related with osteoclast-mediated bone resorption and angiogenesis (34–40). However, expression of FSHRs in some extragonadal tissues has been recently questioned (41). Regarding their structure-function relationship, it is interesting to note that the FSHRs mRNA transcripts identified in human monocytes and osteoclasts apparently correspond to receptor isoforms or variants resulting from differential splicing that do not transduce signals in response to FSH *via* the canonical G_s protein pathway (26) but rather, probably, through G_{i2} which in turn triggers MEK/Erk, NF-kB, and Akt activation leading to increased osteoclast formation (23).

More recently, Liu and colleagues (42) showed that immunoneutralization of circulating FSH levels via administration of either a polyclonal or monoclonal anti-FSHβ antibody to mice, not only led to attenuation in bone loss in ovariectomized animals but also prevented adipose tissue accumulation and parallely enhanced brown adipose tissue and thermogenesis, probably by blocking the inhibition promoted by FSH on uncoupling protein 1 (Ucp1) expression, a regulator of white fat beiging and thermogenesis (43). Given the physiological and therapeutic implications of extragonadal FSHRs, more studies, particularly in humans, are warranted to confirm that extragonadal FSHRs are expressed at sufficient densities to evoke significant biological effects particularly when exposed to increased FSH levels, as those present during the peri- and postmenopause.

The FSHR protein includes a number of specific primary sequences involved in many of the functions of the receptor. These sequences are involved in outward trafficking from its site of synthesis (the endoplasmic reticulum; ER) to the PM (upward trafficking), agonist binding and activation, signal transduction, desensitization and internalization, and degradation or recycling (downward trafficking). Alterations in any of these primary sequences by gene mutations or due to single nucleotide polymorphisms (SNPs), may potentially result in abnormal function of the receptor protein and eventually to disease.

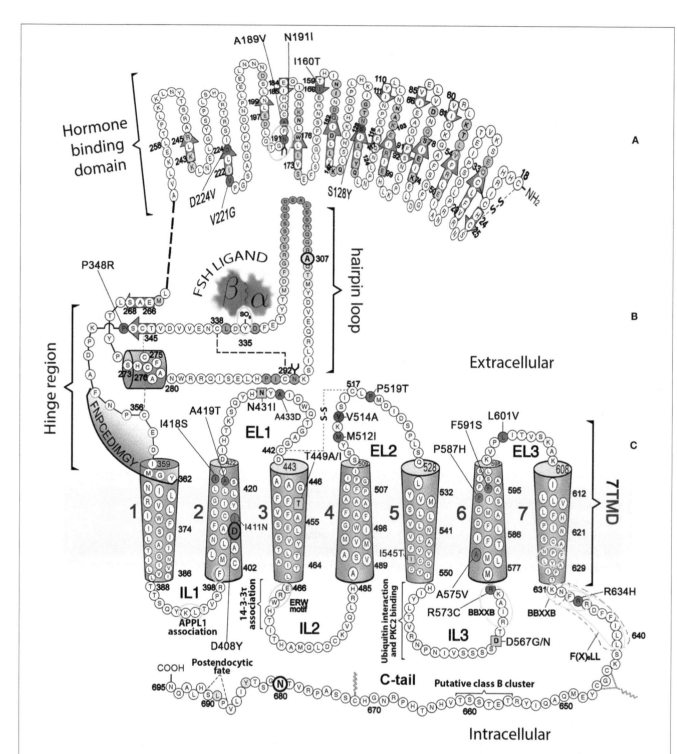

FIGURE 1 | Schematic representation of the FSHR, showing its amino acid sequence and domains involved in different receptor functions, including binding to agonist, activation, and signal transduction. **(A)** Hormone specific binding domain. Residues buried in the FSH/FSHR interface and located in the high affinity-binding site are colored circles (green, binding to FSH α-subunit only; blue, binding to FSH β-subunit only; orange, residues that interact with both FSH subunits). Beta strands located in the concave (corresponding to the leucine-rich repeats) or convex surface of ECD are indicated by the colorless arrows. Mutations in this domain leading to promiscuous ligand binding are depicted in magenta (S128Y), whereas mutations in residues leading to loss-of-function are colored in red. The majority of these mutations provoke defects in receptor trafficking. **(B)** Hinge region with the sulfated tyrosine (in position 335) involved in ligand-provoked binding to the FSH subunits is indicated by the green oval. **(C)** 7TMD with the α helices represented as cylinders. The location of naturally occurring loss-of-function mutations are shown as red-colored circles, while the gain-of-function mutations are represented by green squares. The mutation at V514 (magenta circle at the EL2), led to increased plasma membrane expression of the receptor and OHSS at low FSH doses [reviewed in (4)]. Also indicated are sequences and residues located in the cytoplasmic side involved in association of the receptor with interacting proteins, receptor activation, upward trafficking, internalization, and post-endocytic fate. For details, see the text.

DOMAINS AND MOTIFS INVOLVED IN FSHR UPWARD TRAFFICKING

The endoplasmic reticulum (ER) is the cell organelle where the life cycle of GPCRs begins; here, the newly synthesized peptide sequence is translocated, folded into secondary and tertiary structures via disulfide bonds formation and assembled into quaternary complexes. Properly folded receptors are then exported to the ER-Golgi intermediate complex and then to the Golgi apparatus and trans-Golgi network; here, processing is completed, and the receptor proteins are ready to complete their outward trafficking to the PM and become exposed to cognate ligands (44, 45). Similar to other GPCRs, if the FSHR is not correctly folded the quality control surveillance of the proteosome removes the misfolded receptor. If properly folded, in the ER FSHR continues its transit to the Golgi and the PM (46). N-linked glycosylation (as well as disulfide bond formation) is a frequent feature of GPCRs that occurs during biosynthesis and facilitates folding of protein precursors by increasing their solubility, protecting from detrimental non-productive protein-protein interactions and stabilizing protein conformation (47). Glycosylation plays a crucial role in folding, maturation, and intracellular trafficking of the receptors from the ER to the PM (48). As mentioned above, the ECD of the FSHR contains four potential N-linked glycosylation sites (sequence NXS/T, where X is any amino acid except proline) at positions 191, 199, 293, and 318 (12). However, the crystal structure of the FSHR ECD at residues 25 to 250 in complex with FSH (7, 49) (see below) has provided positive evidence for glycosylation at only one of these sites. That structure revealed that carbohydrate is attached at residue N191, which protrudes into solvent, while no incorporation of carbohydrate complex occurs at residue N199, which projects from the flat β-sheet into the hormone-receptor binding interface and if present would prevent hormone binding, as might be predicted by the FSH-FSHR ECD crystal structure (14). Information is lacking on FSHR glycosylation at residues 293 and 318, albeit some studies suggest that it might occur at two of the three (at positions 191, 199, 293) N-linked glycosylation consensus sequences (50) (**Figure 1A**). Naturally occurring mutations at the ECD of the FSHR (51, 52) near or at putative glycosylation sites are deleterious, emphasizing the important role of glycosylation on receptor targeting to the cell surface and insertion into the PM. In fact, the A189V, and N191I naturally occurring FSHR mutations lead to a profound defect in targeting the receptor protein to the PM, confirming the role of the conserved 189AFNGT193 motif (which hosts one glycosylation site) in FSHR trafficking. Nevertheless, it is not known whether the A189V mutant FSHR is glycosylated at position N191, given that V189 as well as I191 may potentially impair proper receptor LRR formation, particularly its α-helical portion, and hence receptor trafficking.

On the other hand, mutagenesis, and biochemical studies suggest that in the rat FSHR glycosylation is present at two glycosylation consensus sequences and that disruption of either of these two glycosylation sites (N191 or N293) does not apparently affect receptor folding and trafficking to the PM (50). The authors interpretation of this finding is that in this rodent

species, at least one glycosylation site at the ECD is needed for FSHR folding and efficient trafficking to the PM (50). Absence of glycosylation of the mature rat FSHR does not impact on binding or affinity, albeit glycans appear to be important structures for the maturation of the newly synthesized receptor helping on folding, conformational stability, and correct routing to the plasma membrane.

Mutations at the amino-terminal end of the ECD also affects cell surface residency of the FSHR. In this region, alanine scanning mutagenesis identified two regions comprising amino acid residues V9-L31 and E39-N47 which are apparently important for receptor trafficking (53, 54). Mutations in several amino acid residues, specifically at F30, I40, D43, L44, R46, and N47 significantly decreased cell surface PM expression due to failure for proper trafficking (54). Although mutations at these sites might impair glycosylation of the receptor, the abnormal trafficking was more likely due to abnormal NH_2-terminal folding and trapping FSHR intermediates by surveillance mechanisms that incidentally may interfere with appropriate glycosylation processing in the ER-Golgi.

In addition to the above described 189AFNGT193 motif in the FSHR, where mutations influence upward trafficking of gonadotropin receptors, other sequence motifs located in intracellular domains seem to be involved in the exit of these and other GPCRs from the ER and the Golgi. Among these export motifs is the $F(X)_6LL$ (where X is any amino acid) sequence described by Duvernay and colleagues (16, 55) located between residues 633 and 641 in the FSHR (**Figure 1C**). The C-tail sequence of the FSHR also contains the minimal BBXXB motif reversed (BXXBB, where B represents a basic amino acid and X any other amino acid) in its juxtamembrane region (residues 631KNFRR635) (56); the last arginine residues of this latter motif (at positions 634 and 635) and the preceding F633 also are included within the NH_2-terminal end of the $F(X)_6LL$ sequence, and hence substitutions in these residues impaired trafficking and PM expression of the receptor (56, 57). The intracellular loop (IL) 3 of the FSHR also contains this BXXBB motif (residues 569RIAKR573) and either deletion or replacement of its basic residues with alanine also impairs PM expression of the receptor (56, 58).

There are other naturally-occurring mutations that affect trafficking of the FSHR besides those at exon 7 already described, as well as those that impact on ECD glycosylation. These have been identified by virtue of their causal relationship to intracellular retention of FSHR and include the I160T and D224V mutations (at exons 6 and 9, respectively) at the ECD (59, 60), D408Y at the TMD2 (61), and P519T at the extracelullar loop (EL) 2 (62) (**Figure 1** red-filled circles). There have been few studies of the molecular physiopathogenesis leading to impaired upward trafficking of these FSHR mutants. The Pro519Thr mutation in the middle of the EL2 results in complete failure of FSHR to bind FSH and incompetence for triggering intracellular signaling. The loss of a proline residue at this position may potentially provoke a severe conformational flexibility that leads to misfolding and intracellular trapping of the mutant receptor. The peptide backbone of proline, which is constrained in a ring structure, is associated with a forced turn in the protein sequence, which is lost when the less constraining threonine is present instead. Thus, it is possible that the abrupt turn at the middle of the EL2 [where the highly conserved motif KVSIC*X*PMDV/T/I (residues 513–522 in the FSHR) present in all three glycoprotein hormone receptors is located], may be an obligatory requisite for both signal transduction activity and proper routing of the receptor to the PM membrane (62). The remaining mutations (at positions 160, 224, and 408) also occur at highly conserved residues or sequences across species (12), supporting their importance on FSHR function, at least on its proper intracellular routing to the PM.

The above mentioned FSHR D408Y mutation represents an interesting paradigm to explore the molecular mechanisms subserving misfolding and impaired intracellular trafficking of mutant FSHR to the PM. Potential alterations in the secondary structure of the D408Y mutant receptor have been proposed using template-based modeling techniques. Bramble et al. (61) compared a model of the WT FSHR to a model of FSHR containing the D408Y mutation using the RaptorX software (63). The exercise detected a distorted helical structure upstream at the site of the mutation at the 7TMD helix 2; this observation was corroborated by a calculated decreased in the helicity score of the 400 to 410 region using ExPASy secondary structure predictor (61). A caveat should be noted, however, that template-based-modeling relies on known structures of proteins (templates) that display sequence homology with the unknown protein [by homology modeling or fold recognition of individual amino acids in the context of all known structures (protein threading)]. Therefore, the accuracy of prediction of protein structure using template-based modeling of membrane proteins will be limited by the fact that there are not many solved structures of GPCR TM domains. This will likely resolve in the near future as the use of cryo-electron microscopy becomes more accessible to scientists studying GPCRs (64), which undoubtedly will transform further understanding of how GPCRs function. In the absence of such advances and complementary to this new resource, alternative approaches, such as molecular dynamics (MD) simulations, had emerged (65). All-atom MD simulations provides atomistic grounds for understanding membrane folding processes, protein-lipid affinity, and protein conformational changes, among other important phenomena for studying membrane proteins physiology in an aqueous environment. For example, in the case of the D408Y FSHR mutant, all atom MD simulations performed for a period of 20 ns within a lipid bilater environment of polyunsaturated lipids predicted that mutations at residue 408 would only affect *very slightly* the secondary structure. This is because the H-bonds stabilizing the helical domains are located in the hydrophobic core of the bilayer, where electrostatic interactions are enhanced due to the non-polar environment of the lipid hydrocarbon tails. However, contacts between TMD2 and TMD7 are indeed disrupted upon replacement of aspartic acid with tyrosine at position 408 (**Figure 2**). Here Y408 made contacts (with S456 at TMD3, C584 at TMD6, and H615 at TM7) not observed in the WT receptor (**Figure 3**). This indicated that replacements at position 408 may severely impact on the conformational dynamics of the receptor and thereby promote distinct fluctuations throughout to the

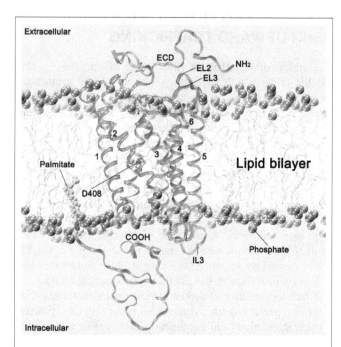

FIGURE 2 | Follicle stimulating hormone receptor (magenta ribbons) in a lipid membrane bilayer (violet spheres and sticks). The 7TMD domains are identified with numbers 1–7. Extracellular loops 2 and 3, and the intracellular loop 3, are labeled as EL2, EL3 and IL3, respectively. The NH$_2$ terminus with a fragment of the ectodomain (ECD) (starting at residue 317) is depicted in the extracellular side. Palmitoylated cysteine residues anchored in the membrane are depicted in cyan spheres. The lipid heads are represented by the phosphorous atoms, which are depicted as violet spheres, and the lipid tails are represented as free-drawn vertical lines in the background. Water molecules at the intra- and extraccelular sides are depicted as a continum solvent in violent.

whole receptor structure (**Figure 4**), which may potentially lead to *misfolding* and *retention* of the mutant receptor within the cell by the quality control system of the cell.

Dimerization and Upward Trafficking

Association between GPCRs, either in the form of dimers or oligomers, plays a pivotal role in GPCR function, influencing intracellular trafficking, ligand binding, and signaling regulation (66–68). In the case of the FSHR, the receptor self-associates early during receptor biosynthesis, and using both biochemical and super-resolution imaging approaches evidence supports the quaternary association at the PM as both monomers and higher order structures (dimers and oligomers) (13, 69, 70). Nevertheless, whether association of FSHRs in the ER is an *obligatory* pre-requisite for trafficking to the PM, as with other GPCRs (71–77), is an open question. Although biochemical studies have found that both the ECD and TMD contribute to early FSHR association, the sites of interaction(s) remain to be identified. In fact, in one study (69), mutations in TMD helix 1 and/or 4, which have previously been suggested to be involved in dimerization of the α1β-adrenergic receptor, dopamine D2 receptor, and CCR5 (78–80), failed to alter the propensity of the FSHR to associate. Nevertheless, some domains potentially involved in intracellular FSHR-FSHR interactions have been

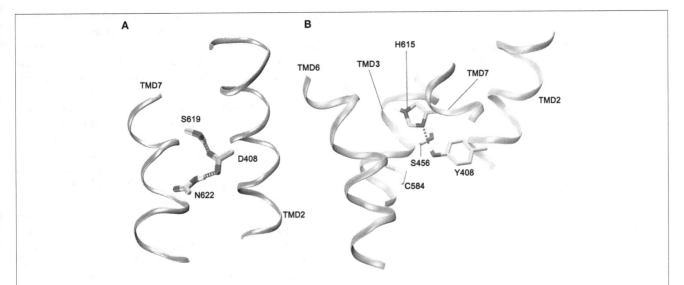

FIGURE 3 | Contacts between side chain atoms of residues at helix 2 (TMD2) and residues at helices 3 (TMD3), 6 (TMD6), and 7 (TMD7). **(A)** Side chain interactions in the WT FSHR with the carboxyl group of D408 forming hydrogen bonds with S619 and N622. **(B)** Side chain interactions of Y408 at TMD helix 2 and residues at TMD helix 3, helix 6, and helix 7. A hydrogen bond between Y408 and H615 is shown; C584 is depicted since it is close neighbor of Y408 within a 3.5 Å cut-off. Side chains are depicted as sticks, and the color code is: carbon,cyan; oxigen,red; hydrogen, white; sulfur,yellow; and nitrogen, blue. Only small fragments of the helical regions are depicted (green or cyan ribbons for the WT and 408 mutant receptors, respectively).

identified employing short interfering sequences specific for particular TMDs and the C-tail (57). That study suggested that association of FSHRs may occur via multiple contact sites at the 7TMD, including helices 5, 6, and 7, and the C-tail. Although in how this FSHR-FSHR interaction might influence upward traffic of the FSHR to the PM has not yet been particularly addressed, the same study also demonstrated that heterozygous mutations causing misrouting of the receptor led to defective upward intracellular trafficking and interfered with proper maturation of the WT, functional FSHR (57). The more recent crystal structure of the FSHR ECD, which included the entire 350 amino acid of the ECD, demonstrated an additional mode of association of hormone with the ECD that includes the hinge region of the receptor (**Figure 1B**) and represented a trimeric receptor structure (14, 81). This latter observation will be an important platform for defining the number of FSH molecules hosted by the receptor but whose formation during the biosynthetic process and role in receptor trafficking has not been yet documented. In this vein it is possible that association of FSHR receptors as dimers or trimers may facilitate coupling the receptor to several and distinct G proteins and adaptors. In fact, a recent study has shown that heteromers of adenosine A2A receptor and dopamine D2 receptor homodimers associated to distinct G proteins, may modulate signal transduction selectivity through different molecular interactions with effectors (82).

Heterodimerization of FSHR with the closely related LHCGR, has been studied employing different experimental approaches (57, 70, 83, 84). However, it is not yet known whether such hetero-association also occurs early during biosynthesis, as demonstrated for FSHR homodimers, or later, when the individual receptors are already at the cell surface PM. In any case, the presence of FSHR-LHCGR heterodimers appears to

convey important physiological implications, particularly during follicular maturation, as it may prevent premature luteinization of the follicle or ovarian hyperstimulation, according with the level of expression of each receptor (83). As in the case of association between FSHRs, it is still unknown which are the potential contact sites of interaction between these receptors, although experiments using mutant FSHRs coexpressed with the WT LHCGR suggest that this hetero-association may also occur via multiple inter-TMD contacts (57).

FSHR DOMAINS INVOLVED IN LIGAND BINDING AND RECEPTOR ACTIVATION

The Extracellular Domain (ECD) and Ligand Binding

As described above and shown in **Figure 1A**, the mature, PM expressed FSHR exhibits a large ectodomain, where recognition and binding of its cognate ligand occurs (14). The current dogma is that in the FSHR ECD resides both the binding site for agonist and the region essential for ligand-provoked triggering of receptor activation. The first reported structure of the FSH complexed with the extracellular-hormone binding domain of the FSHR (FSHR_HB) (49) documented the important structural relationship between FSH and FSHR. However, the expressed protein used for crystalization did not include the signal specificity subdomain or hinge region, which had been considered as a separate structure participating on FSHR activation (85–87). This groundbreaking structure showed for the first time that FSH binds to FSHR_HB like a "handclasp" and that most β-strands in the inner surface are involved in ligand binding (**Figure 1A**). Moreover, extensive previous mutagenesis

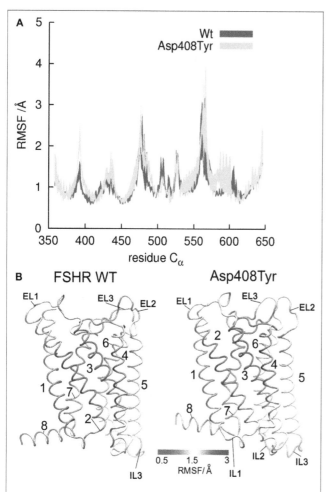

FIGURE 4 | Root mean square fluctiations (RMSF) for α-carbon atoms of the WT FSHR and the mutant D408Y. **(A)** Fluctuations calculated for residues in the tansmembrane domain from Y362 to C646. Helical regions display lower RMSF values since they are rather rigid within the bilayer hydrophobic core, whereas larger fluctuations represent flexible regions such as the loops.
(B) Structures of the WT FSHR and the D408Y mutant colored according to the RMSF values, with rigid regions in red and flexible regions in blue. Flexibility seems to increase from helix 5 to helix 8 in the mutant receptor, since larger RMSF values were yield by the mutant than by the WT FSHR.

hinge region (FSHR$_{ED}$). That structure described in more detail the role of the glycoprotein hormones receptors ECD not only in ligand binding but also on receptor activation. Accordingly, this structure predicts that FSH is initially recruited by the previously described FSHR$_{HB}$ through high-affinity interactions between the gonadotropin and the concave surface of leucine-rich repeats (**Figure 1A**, gray arrows within the amino acid sequence of the ECD) 1–8. However, the interface between the FSH and the FSHR ECD is broader than that previously identified in the Fan and Hendrickson FSH-FSHR$_{HB}$ structure (49) due to the presence of secondary interaction sites (shown also in **Figure 1A**). According to this newer structure, binding of FSH to the FSHR hormone binding domain provokes conformational alterations in the L2β loop (residues V38β-Q48β) of FSH leading to interactions between amino acid residues in the L2β loop and LRRs 8 and 9, as well as to interactions of FSHR residues located in the hinge region with residues on FSH α- and β-subunits. Several residues on the FSHR determine specificity of the receptor for its ligand, including L55, E76, R101, K179, and I222, in which L55 and K179 are important to distinctly identify LH, human chorionic gonadotropin (hCG) and FSH due to their interaction with the FSHβ "seat belt," whereas the other residues dictate specificity preventing binding to TSH (7, 14). A more detailed map of interaction between residues from FSH and the FSH$_{ED}$ is shown in **Figure 5**. The FSHR ECD structure reported by Jiang and colleagues (7), identified the hinge region as an *integral* part of the ECD (**Figure 1B**), and confirmed previously reported biochemical data on the FSHR and TSHR (85, 90–93), underlying the role of this region in ligand-stimulated receptor activation. These and other studies (94) have also suggested that the ECD of the glycoprotein hormone receptors acts as a tethered inverse agonist. In this scenario, the ECD acts as an agonist upon ligand binding and activates the sequence 353FNPCEDIMGY362 located in the junction of the carboxyl-terminal end of the hinge region and the 7TMD helix 1, which function as an internal agonist unit (**Figure 1B**).

The agonist-stimulated activation mechanism of the FSHR includes a sulfated tyrosine residue at position 335 of the hinge region. Here, exposure of a pocket located in the interface of the α- and β-subunits of FSH formed upon binding of the ligand to the hormone binding domain, is the binding site for the sulfated tyrosine residue located immediately adjacent to the rigid hairpin loop (**Figure 1B**). The proposal is that this initial binding event is followed by lifting of the hairpin loop leading to relieving of the inhibitory effects of the loop on the 7TMD. Rotation of a fixed short helix formed by residues S273 to A279 (**Figure 1B**) additionally contributes to the conformational change of the hinge region that leads to receptor activation (7, 14). The fact that substitution of the S273 residue with a non-polar hydrophobic residue (isoleucine; S273I) leads to constitutive activation of the receptor, emphasizes on the importance of this helix movements on FSHR activation; this mechanism may also explain the effect of the S277I mutation on LHCGR constitutive activation (95). The disulfide bridges C275-C346 and C276-C356 play an additional role in FSHR activation through fastening the last β-strand (LRR 12) to the short helix forming a rigid body and tying this helix to the last few residues before the 7TMD helix 1 (internal

and biochemical analyses of FSH mutants provided an immediate validation of the dogma that both non-covalently linked α- and β-subunits (present in all glycoprotein hormones) are involved in specific binding to the receptor. Importantly, this structure also demonstrated that carbohydrates *are not* actually involved in the formation of the binding interface of the FSH–FSHR$_{HB}$ structure, but are rather sequestered to the periphery of the complex (88, 89). This observation would argue against the notion that pharmacodynamics of FSH biosimilars may vary depending on their carbohydrate composition. The second and subsequent crystal structure of the FSH-FSHR complex shed additional light on this topic while suggesting even more complicated structure-function correlates to consider.

The second crystal structure of FSH bound with the entire FSHR ECD reported by Jiang and colleagues (7) includes the

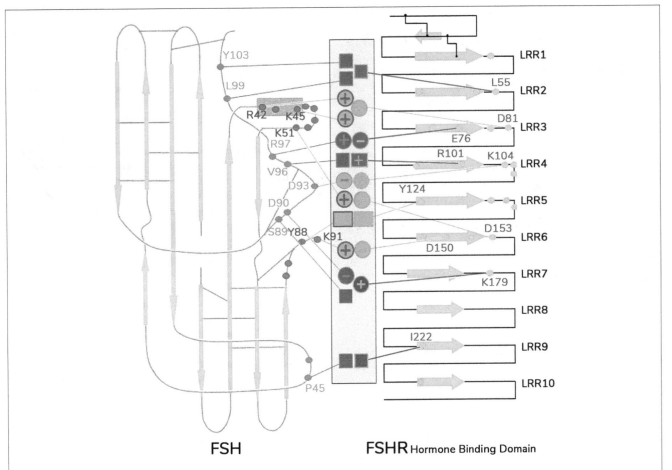

FSH

FSHR Hormone Binding Domain

FIGURE 5 | Schematic representation of detailed interaction of FSH and FSHR interface. Contacting residues from FSHR hormone binding domain are shown as yellow dots, those from FSHα as red dots, and FSHβ as blue dots. The middle area indicates the specific side-chain interactions between FSHR and its ligand. Interactions that contribute to common affinities among all the GPH–GPHR family members are shown as green-filled circles (for charge–charge interactions) or boxes (for non-charged atomic contacts), and they are connected by green lines toward the yellow dots in FSHR or red or blue dots in FSH α- or β-subunits, respectively. Interactions involved in specificity are shown as purple- or red-filled circles or boxes connected by lines of the same color to the dotted residues in the receptor and ligand. LRR, leucine-rich repeats.

agonist in **Figure 1B**). The movement of the hairpin loop occurring upon ligand binding presumably affects and influences the conformation of this and the remaining TMDs, thereby provoking receptor activation (see below). This structure has far-reaching impact. Given the similarity among the structures of glycoprotein hormones and glycoprotein hormone receptors, it is highly possible that all glycoprotein hormone receptors share the 2-step recognition/activation process described above. For example, mutants of glycoprotein hormone receptors created to remove this critical sulfated tyrosine, exhibit a marked loss of sensitivity to their corresponding ligands (86, 87, 96). Moreover, FSH with mutations in residues located below the sulfated tyrosine-binding pocket or at the potential exosite (αF74E and βL73E, respectively) promote signaling presumably by taking the hairpin loop up toward the top of the pocket (7).

FSHR (and TSHR as well) promiscuity for ligand specificity caused by particular mutations in the ECD (and the 7TMD as well, see below) (**Figure 1**) is an issue that has important

implications in the clinical setting. This is because of the structural similarities among the glycoprotein hormones and their receptors and the limited number of residues in the ligand and the LRRs at the hormone-binding domain that participate in ligand-receptor interactions. For example, a ligand structurally similar to a glycoprotein hormone receptor cognate ligand could interact with and activate the receptor. This could even occur with a low affinity and without triggering detectable receptor activation under basal conditions. In this regard, replacements of key residues that presumably participate in receptor-ligand interaction may hamper ligand discrimination of the receptor and result in recognition and interaction of the mutant receptor with other than its specific ligand. In this setting, the S128Y mutation at the FSHR (**Figure 1**) may provoke ovarian hyperstimulation syndrome [OHSS; which may be life-threatening in its severe form (97)] associated to pregnancy due to increased responsiveness of the FSHR to high levels of hCG present during the first trimester of pregnancy (98). In this mutation, replacement of serine with tyrosine allows the FSHR to hydrogen bond αR95 at the hCG molecule, leading to receptor activation.

Since the ELs are extracellular projections of the TMDs, it was anticipated that these loops also may be involved in ligand-receptor interaction and receptor activation, particularly EL1 and EL3, which is, indeed, the case. The role of the FSHR ELs in these processes has been described in detail in a recent review (4).

The 7TMD and Receptor Activation

Given that no structural data are currently available on gonadotropin receptors 7TMD, homology modeling with other GPCRs has been a very useful tool to explore the potential molecular mechanisms occurring at the 7TMD level that lead to the initial activation of FSHR by its ligand. Among a number of ligand-bound GPCR structures currently available, the following structures are important to understand the activation mechanism: a. A ligand-free form of opsin that is co-crystalized with the carboxyl-terminus of the α-subunit of $G_{\alpha t}$ (99); b. A β_2AR bound to agonist and stabilized in the active conformation by a nanobody mimicking the G protein (100); c. Agonist-bound β_2AR and adenosine A_{2A} receptor co-crystallized with heterotrimeric stimulatory G protein ($G\alpha_s$ — $\beta_1\gamma_2$) (101, 102); and d. The structures of four GPCRs bound to G_i obtained through cryo-electron microscopy (103–106). Previously described crystal structures, may be useful as a first approximation of ligand-induced activation of FSHR. However, since none of those receptors entertain a large extracellular domain for ligand binding, the common structural rearrangements noted may not translate well to the FSHR or other glycoprotein hormone receptors (107). Upon ligand binding, the extracellular portion of the 7TMD is initially affected by agonist-evoked local structural changes, including: a. A small distortion of TM helix 5; b. Relocation of TM helices 3 and 7; and c. Translation/rotation of TM helix 5 and helix 6. These movements occur concurrently with rearrangements in a cluster of conserved hydrophobic and aromatic residues (positions 3.40, 5.51, 6.44, and 6.48)[1], that constitute a transmission switch deeper in the core of the receptor leading to rearrangement at the TMD helix 3–helix 5 interface, and formation of new non-covalent contacts at the TMD helix 5–TMD helix 6 interface (109). Several residues in this transmission switch are highly conserved among Class A GPCRs, suggesting that they are a common feature of GPCR activation of effector proteins. These local changes are translated into large-scale helix movements occurring intracellularly at the cytoplasmic side of the plasma membrane (107), yielding rearrangements of TMD helix 5 at its cytoplasmic side (110) associated with a modification of theTMD helix 5–helix 6 interface, which result in the large-scale relocation of the cytoplasmic side of TMD helix 6 (111). Consequently, a cleft required for *hosting G protein α-subunits* opens. Further, recent studies on receptor-G_i complexes suggest that a smaller displacement of the TMD helix 6 might interfere

with binding of the receptor to G_s and allow to selectively bind G_i (103–106). Importantly, residues from the IL2 and the cytoplasmic end of TMD helix 3 (R3.50 of the conserved E/DRY/W sequence) participate in interaction with the G protein following activation (101, 112). As a result of receptor activation, the salt bridge between residues R3.50 and E6.30 in the inactive state is broken (99). These structural and biophysical studies indicate that agonist binding may not be solely sufficient to stabilize fully active states of the receptor and that binding of an effector protein on the cytosolic face of the receptor seems *necessary* to fully attain the active state of the receptor (113). Further, there may not be a single active state arguing that different ligands with or without allosteric modulators, can stabilize distinct conformations and give rise to diverse and distinct downstream responses (114, 115). It would follow then that CAM receptors might exist in conformations that facilitate recruitment of non-G protein effectors such as β-arrestins (116, 117), giving rise to biased signaling. Thus, from a clinical point of view understanding or determining their structure can guide development of therapeutically useful negative allosteric modulators. From a basic view, solving the structures of the constitutively active receptors will lead to additional insights about ligand-induced activation of FSHR, particularly with regard to engagement of downstream effectors.

Long-range conformational changes and rearrangements transmitted down stream the intracellular extensions of the TMD helices and associated with the ILs and C-tail of the receptor induce reorganization that allows accommodation and activation of multiple downstream effectors. The α-helices conforming the 7TMD may oscillate between multiple active conformations, which eventually determine the activation of several or distinct downstream signaling pathways and account for functional selectivity (see below). Given the structural and functional similarities among Class A GPCRs, it is highly possible that the FSHR (and other glycoprotein hormone receptors as well) may share some of recently described structural mechanisms of activation at the 7TMD exhibited by other members of this particular Class of GPCRs. Here it is important to note that in the case of rhodopsin the active conformation is not as variable as in other GPCRs with diffusible ligands, because upon light exposure rhodopsin exhibits (and, in fact, vision requires) a high switching fidelity and very fast activation dynamics than other GPCRs, which switch asynchronically during the ligand-stimulated activation process (118). In fact, a recent crystal structure of rhodopsin in complex with a mini-G_o protein (119) showed that the structure and active conformational state of rhodopsin bound to G_o is very similar to that previously observed for the rhodopsin-arrestin complex (120), implying that rhodopsin exposes the same sites to recognize its cognate G protein (G_t) and arrestin and that fewer stable conformations in the active state exist in this receptor compared to other GPCRs (119).

The specific intermolecular interactions and nature of the conformational changes subserving stabilization of the glycoprotein hormone receptors 7TMD in different (inactive or active) conformations are not yet fully understood at atomic resolution. Yet evidence derived from combined experimental

---

[1] Amino acid numbering according to the Ballesteros and Weinstein nomenclature, in which the first number denotes the helix (1–7) and the second the residue position relative to the most conserved position, which is assigned the number 50. [see Ballesteros and Weinstein (108)].

approaches (mutagenic, structural, and *in silico* strategies) as well as from *in vitro* recreation of naturally occurring inactivating and activating mutations (see below), have allowed identification of potential structural determinants and network interactions that predominate during the inactive and active conformations of these receptors (7, 121–126). Application of *in silico* and mutagenesis approaches, particularly on the LHCGR, have unveiled important information about TMD helices and particular amino acid residues involved in intra- and inter-helical non-covalent ionic interactions, network formation, and pathways that are associated with the different activation states of the gonadotropin receptors. In this regard, almost all conserved amino acid residues in the majority of the LHCGR helices participate in the formation of intramolecular networks in either inactive and/or active states. Moreover, highly conserved and non-conserved residues form ionic inter-helix network pathways that connect the extracellular and intracellular components of this receptor during different conformational states. Finally, salt bridging of R464 (R467 in the FSHR) at the ERW highly conserved motif located at the COOH-end of the TM3 (**Figure 1C**) with E463 (FSHR E466) and D564 (FSHR D567) (at the IL3-TMD helix 6 junction) represents a key network important for stabilization of the *inactive* conformation of the receptor (122, 123, 125, 127). This is the case for other GPCRs belonging to the rhodopsin/β-adrenergic-like family. As shown by recent crystal structures of GPCRs-coupled with G proteins, the majority of LHCGR CAMs would disrupt this essential TMD3-TMD6 inter-helical stabilizing bridge. That would enable flexibility for the opening of an intracellular crevice *between the IL2 and IL3 and TMD helix 3 and helix 6*, which in turn would allow exposure of key residues potentially involved in G_s and G_i activation, (99–106). Integrity of the TMD helix 3-helix 6 salt bridge as a requisite for keeping the inactive conformation of glycoprotein hormone receptors is further emphasized by experimental evidence. For example, D567G/N and D619G mutations lead to constitutive activation of the FSH and TSH receptors, respectively (128–133). In addition, *in silico* studies on a number of laboratory manufactured CAM FSHRs harboring mutations at residues 401, 580, 545, and 460 (**Figure 1**) are known to provoke constitutive activation of the LHCGR (127). It is also noteworthy that the majority of naturally occurring CAMs in the LHCG and TSH receptors are located at the TMD helix 6, which again underlines the importance of this particular helix on G protein coupling and signal transduction.

In contrast to the LHCGR or TSHR, gain-of-function mutations in the 7TMD of the FSHR leading to constitutive activation are relatively rare (**Figure 1**) despite the relatively high homology between their 7TMD [reviewed in (134)]. This observation suggests a higher stability of the FSHR 7TMD in the inactive state compared with those of other glycoprotein hormone receptors (135). Nevertheless, it is important to keep in mind that CAMs of the FSHR are actually difficult to detect in the clinic because they usually do not exhibit severe phenotypes (136). In fact, mutations leading to ligand-independent activation of LHCGR show low constitutive activity when introduced into the FSHR (127, 135), despite strong promiscuous activation by hCG and TSH (127). Promiscuous activation also has been observed in three out of six naturally occurring FSHR CAMs (134), suggesting a close link between constitutive activation of this receptor and ligand promiscuity, an association not always observed in the other related receptors (91, 130). Partial activation of the FSHR apparently facilitates relaxing the inhibitory constraints of the 7TMD, making the receptor prone to full activation by related ligands when present at high concentrations.

FSHR DOMAINS AND SIGNAL TRANSDUCTION

As described above, binding of agonist to the FSHR provokes conformational changes in the receptor molecule, that are transmitted through the 7TMD to the intracellular domains, where coupling to effectors, interaction with adapter proteins, and triggering of downstream intracellular signaling takes place. As in other GPCRs, the intracellular domains of the glycoprotein hormone receptors are extensions of the TMDs, that participate in downstream effector activation. Accordingly, conformational changes in the 7TMD helices lead to activation of G proteins and other interacting proteins involved in signaling, desensitization and internalization of the receptor (15, 56, 58, 122, 137–142) (**Figure 1C**). In addition to activation of the canonical G_s/adenylyl ciclase(cAMP/protein kinase A (PKA) pathway, the FSHR also activates signaling cascades involved in a variety of cellular processes, including proliferation and/or differentiation, functional selectivity and differential gene expression [reviewed in (143)]. Some of the motifs involved in these complex signaling networks are shown in **Figure 1**. For example interaction of the FSHR with the adaptor protein containing pleckstrin homology domain, phosphotyrosine binding domain, and leucine zipper motif (APPL), has been mapped to the IL-1, specifically to K393, L394, and F399 (144, 145). The adapter APPL1 may regulate signal specificity and trafficking through the interaction with PI3K and Akt, which is followed by FOXO1a phosphorylation, leading to abrogation of apoptosis (145); in addition, this adaptor is also involved in FSHR-mediated Ca^{2+} signaling and other functions (84, 146). Meanwhile, association of the FSHR with the 14-3-3τ protein has been mapped to the IL2, overlapping the above mentioned ERW motif (138, 147); 14-3-3 proteins are involved in several cell processes and play an important role in modulating signaling pathways through interacting with activated signaling proteins (148). Mutagenesis studies also have identified other residues in this loop, such as Leu477, that are important for maintaining the receptor in an inactive conformation (142), and it has been suggested that this particular loop may function as a conformational switch to evoke G protein activation, as reported for the LHCGR (58, 149, 150). Sequences in IL3 have been identified that are involved in signal transduction, including the reverse BB*XX*B motif in the juxtamembrane region of this loop (56, 151, 152). Replacement of R573 with cysteine does not affect PM expression or binding to agonist yet signaling mediated by G_s is severely impaired (59).

The C-tail exhibits a putative class B S/T cluster closely related with receptor phosphorylation by G protein-coupled receptor kinases (GRKs) and β-arrestin recruitment, which are scaffold intermediates involved not only in receptor desensitization, internalization, and recycling, but also in G_s-independent ERK1/2-mediated signaling (see below) (153–156).

The C-tail of the FSHR also exhibits an aspargine residue at position 680, which is the site for the expression of the most common functional variant (N680S) of the WT FSHR resulting from a single nucleotide polymorfism (SNP) in the *FSHR* and that exists in strong linkage disequilibrium with the amino acid residue in position 307 (T307A) at the ECD (157). Expression of the S680S FSHR variant *in vivo* has been associated with variations in the sensitivity of the FSHR to its cognate ligand (158, 159), whereas *in vitro* this variant exhibited attenuated intracellular signaling kinetics, enhanced β-arresting recruitment and ligand-stimulated internalization, and decreased CREB-dependent gene transcription and nuclear PKA activation (160, 161). The functional abnormalities of the S680S FSHR variant might be responsible for the altered response to exogenous FSH administration presented by women bearing the homozygous state as well as for the lower pregnancy rates observed in some particular populations (162).

Potentially important domains at the 7TMD and ILs involved in receptor-G protein association have been described in the preceding section.

FSHR DOMAINS INVOLVED IN INTERNALIZATION AND POST-ENDOCYTIC PROCESSING

G protein-coupled receptor interaction with agonist at the PM triggers downward trafficking of the receptor, which occurs through a series of well-known distinct processes. These include: a. phosphorylation and β-arrestin recruitment, which by interacting with clathrin and the clathrin adaptor AP2 promote receptor internalization into endosomes, and b. either targeting of the receptor to the lysosomes and/or proteasomes or recycling of the receptor back to the PM. Hence, the balance between trafficking from the site of synthesis (the ER) to the PM and the endocytosis-recycling/degradation pathway is what defines the final density of receptor protein available to agonist and required to evoke a biological response. Recently, FSHR was identified in very early endosomes during its post-endocytic sorting, rather than to early endosomes as in most GPCRs; apparently, sorting to very early endosomes represents an important mechanism subserving receptor recycling, where PKA-phosphorylated APPL1 present in this particular endosomal compartment plays an essential role (163–165). In addition to phosphorylation by PKA and PKC (both second messenger-dependent kinases), FSHR is phosphorylated by GRKs 2, 3, 5, and 6 (153, 155, 166, 167). Although both PKA and PKC participate in agonist-dependent and -independent desensitization (homologous and heterologous desensitization, respectively) of the FSHR, phosphorylation mediated by GRK results in more complex effects, including homologous desensitization, regulation of β-arrestin recruitment, internalization, and G protein-independent signaling (153). As described in the

previous section, a cluster of five serine and threonine residues has been identified in the C-tail of the FSHR as target for phosphorylation by GRKs (153). β-arrestins associated with the GRK2- or GRK5/6-phosphorylated, agonist-occupied FSHR, apparently extert distinct intracellular functions: the FSHR phosphorylated by GRK2 predominates in the β-arrestin-stimulated desensitization process, while phosphorylation by GRK5- and GRK6- is necessary for β-arrestin-mediated MAPK-ERK1/2 activation (153, 154, 168).

β-arrestin recruitment to GRK-phosphorylated FSHR is a well-recognized process leading to receptor internalization (153, 167, 169). In the case of the LHCGR this effect is rather mediated by the interaction with ADP ribosylation factor nucleotide-binding site opener (ARNO), which is an exchange factor for ADP ribosylation factor 6 (ARF6) that recruits β-arrestins when bound to GTP (170, 171). In contrast with the LHCGR (in which only 30% of the internalized receptor recycles back to the PM), most of the internalized FSHR is recycled back to the cell surface (166, 172). Palmitoylation plays and important role in determining the post-endocytic fate (degradation vs. recycling) of gonadotropin receptors (17, 18, 173–175). The importance of this S-acylation in internalization and post-endocytic processing of GPCRs varies depending on the particular receptor. In contrast to the LHCGR in which prevention of palmitoylation by site-directed mutagenesis increased the rate of agonist-stimulated internalization (174), abrogation of palmitoylation of the C-tail cysteine residues (cysteines 644, 646, and 672, **Figure 1C**) at the FSHR did not affect the dynamics of internalization of the hormone/FSHR complex (172). Nevertheless, in both unpalmitoylated receptors, recycling to the cell surface was impaired and the fraction of receptor/hormone complex submitted to degradation via the proteasome/lysosome pathway was increased (17, 174). Further, studies in HEK293 cells showed that in the non-palmitoylated FSHR degradation through proteasomes predominated over that mediated by lysosomes, as revealed by experiments in which proteosomal but not lysosomal degradation was inhibited (17). In fact, the FSHR is ubiquitinated in IL3 (**Figure 1C**) and proteosomal inhibitors increase cell surface residency of this receptor (17, 176). Thus in both gonadotropin receptors, S-acylation plays an important role in postendocytic processing.

In addition to palmitoylation, postendocytic trafficking also may be influenced by specific amino acid residues present in the C-tail of the FSHR. Similar to the LHCGR, truncations involving the last eight residues of the FSHR resulted in re-routing of a substantial amount of the internalized FSH-FSHR complex to the degradation pathway (166).

CONCLUSIONS

This review summarizes the information available on the relationship between structure and function of the FSHR. Although a substantial amount of information on this particular receptor structure-activity relationship has emerged during the last decade, there are still several issues that remain to be resolved, including elucidation of the entire crystal structure of the receptor including the 7TMD. This critical step will unambiguously and more precisely identify those residues and domains within the 7TMD and intracellular domains involved in receptor activation, FSHR-FSHR and FSHR/LHCGR association, and interaction with the array of proteins involved in intracellular signaling, and also in specific binding of allosteric modulators, the latter with important implications in the clinical arena.

Since there is no firm structural data on whether reported extragonadal FSHRs are variants of the canonical FSHR structure, particularly the FSHRs represented to be in bone, adipose tissue and malignant tumors (33, 177, 178), a more precise identification of such structural features might allow the design of highly specific therapeutic strategies, which block putative deleterious FSH effects on these particular tissues. In this vein, application of novel imaging techniques (179) may be useful to critically evaluate whether expression levels of FSHR in those extragonadal tissues are sufficient to incur these deleterious effects or whether their density changes as the menopausal status progresses. Without any doubt, crystals of gonadotropin receptors also will aid to clarify many aspects on extragonadal FSHRs function that may be translated in the near-term to human therapeutics.

Finally, another interesting issue concerns to the altered response of the S680S FSHR variant to the FSH stimulus. In this regard, two novel therapeutic FSH compounds produced by human cell lines have emerged; comparatively, these preparations differ somehow in glycosylation pattern and apparently exhibit a more favorable pharmacodynamic profile than the recombinant preparations synthesized by non-human cell lines (180–182). Those novel FSH preparations might be more advantageous than the widely used non-human cell-derived FSH compounds in women bearing the less favorable S680S FSHR variant. Nonetheless, more detailed data on the structural and biochemical features of these human cell-derived FSH preparations as well as on their binding dynamics at the FSHR and, more importantly, their effects on intracellular signaling, still are necessary before considering these new FSH formulations as a worthy option for these women.

AUTHOR CONTRIBUTIONS

AU-A, TZ, EJ-V, RG-S, and JD wrote the manuscript. AU-A and JD reviewed and edited the final version.

FUNDING

Research in the authors' laboratory, is supported by a CONACyT (Mexico) grant 240619 (to AU-A), and by internal support from the Coordinación de la Investigación Científica, UNAM, to the Red de Apoyo a la Investigación.

ACKNOWLEDGMENTS

The authors thank Ari Kleinberg B.Sc., from the Red de Apoyo a la Investigación-UNAM, for the artwork of **Figures 1** and **5**.

REFERENCES

1. Kleinau G, Neumann S, Gruters A, Krude H, Biebermann H. Novel insights on thyroid-stimulating hormone receptor signal transduction. *Endocr Rev.* (2013) 34:691–724. doi: 10.1210/er.2012-1072

2. Kreuchwig A, Kleinau G, Krause G. Research resource: novel structural insights bridge gaps in glycoprotein hormone receptor analyses. *Mol Endocrinol.* (2013) 27:1357–63. doi: 10.1210/me.2013-1115

3. Simoni M, Gromoll J, Nieschlag E. The follicle-stimulating hormone receptor: biochemistry, molecular biology, physiology, and pathophysiology. *Endocr Rev.* (1997) 18:739–73.

4. Ulloa-Aguirre A, Zarinan T. The follitropin receptor: matching structure and function. *Mol Pharmacol.* (2016) 90:596–608. doi: 10.1124/mol.116.104398

5. Fredriksson R, Lagerstrom MC, Lundin LG, Schioth HB. The G-protein-coupled receptors in the human genome form five main families. Phylogenetic analysis, paralogon groups, and fingerprints. *Mol Pharmacol.* (2003) 63:1256–72. doi: 10.1124/mol.63.6.1256

6. Kreuchwig A, Kleinau G, Kreuchwig F, Worth CL, Krause G. Research resource: update and extension of a glycoprotein hormone receptors web application. *Mol Endocrinol.* (2011) 25:707–12. doi: 10.1210/me.2010-0510

7. Jiang X, Liu H, Chen X, Chen PH, Fischer D, Sriraman V, et al. Structure of follicle-stimulating hormone in complex with the entire ectodomain of its receptor. *Proc Natl Acad Sci USA.* (2012) 109:12491–6. doi: 10.1073/pnas.1206643109

8. Krause G, Kreuchwig A, Kleinau G. Extended and structurally supported insights into extracellular hormone binding, signal transduction and organization of the thyrotropin receptor. *PLoS ONE* (2012) 7:e52920. doi: 10.1371/journal.pone.0052920

9. Mueller S, Jaeschke H, Gunther R, Paschke R. The hinge region: an important receptor component for GPHR function. *Trends Endocrinol Metab.* (2009) 21:111–22. doi: 10.1016/j.tem.2009.09.001

10. Bogerd J. Ligand-selective determinants in gonadotropin receptors. *Mol Cell Endocrinol.* (2007) 260–262:144–52. doi: 10.1016/j.mce.2006.01.019

11. Gromoll J, Ried T, Holtgreve-Grez H, Nieschlag E, Gudermann T. Localization of the human FSH receptor to chromosome 2 p21 using a genomic probe comprising exon 10. *J Mol Endocrinol.* (1994) 12:265–71.

12. Dias JA, Cohen BD, Lindau-Shepard B, Nechamen CA, Peterson AJ, Schmidt A. Molecular, structural, and cellular biology of follitropin and follitropin receptor. *Vitam Horm.* (2002) 64:249–322. doi: 10.1016/S0083-6729(02)64008-7

13. Thomas RM, Nechamen CA, Mazurkiewicz JE, Muda M, Palmer S, Dias JA. Follicle-stimulating hormone receptor forms oligomers and shows evidence of carboxyl-terminal proteolytic processing. *Endocrinology* (2007) 148:1987–95. doi: 10.1210/en.2006-1672

14. Jiang X, Dias JA, He X. Structural biology of glycoprotein hormones and their receptors: insights to signaling. *Mol Cell Endocrinol.* (2014) 382:424–51. doi: 10.1016/j.mce.2013.08.021

15. Kleinau G, Krause G. Thyrotropin and homologous glycoprotein hormone receptors: structural and functional aspects of extracellular signaling mechanisms. *Endocr Rev.* (2009) 30:133–51. doi: 10.1210/er.2008-0044

16. Duvernay MT, Zhou F, Wu G. A conserved motif for the transport of G protein-coupled receptors from the endoplasmic reticulum to the cell surface. *J Biol Chem.* (2004) 279:30741–50. doi: 10.1074/jbc.M313881200

17. Melo-Nava B, Casas-Gonzalez P, Perez-Solis MA, Castillo-Badillo J, Maravillas-Montero JL, Jardon-Valadez E, et al. Role of cysteine residues in the carboxyl-terminus of the follicle-stimulating hormone receptor in intracellular traffic and postendocytic processing. *Front Cell Dev Biol.* (2016) 4:76. doi: 10.3389/fcell.2016.00076

18. Uribe A, Zarinan T, Perez-Solis MA, Gutierrez-Sagal R, Jardon-Valadez E, Pineiro A, et al. Functional and Structural roles of conserved cysteine residues in the carboxyl-terminal domain of the follicle-stimulating hormone

receptor in human embryonic kidney 293 cells. *Biol Reprod.* (2008) 78:869–82. doi: 10.1095/biolreprod.107.063925

19. Richards JS, Pangas SA. The ovary: basic biology and clinical implications. *J Clin Invest.* (2010) 120:963–72. doi: 10.1172/JCI41350

20. Huhtaniemi I. A short evolutionary history of FSH-stimulated spermatogenesis. *Hormones (Athens)* (2015) 14:468–78. doi: 10.14310/horm.2002.1632

21. Walker WH, Cheng J. FSH and testosterone signaling in Sertoli cells. *Reproduction* (2005) 130:15–28. doi: 10.1530/rep.1.00358

22. Oduwole OO, Peltoketo H, Poliandri A, Vengadabady L, Chrusciel M, Doroszko M, et al. Constitutively active follicle-stimulating hormone receptor enables androgen-independent spermatogenesis. *J Clin Invest.* (2018) 128:1787–92. doi: 10.1172/JCI96794

23. Sun L, Peng Y, Sharrow AC, Iqbal J, Zhang Z, Papachristou DJ, et al. FSH directly regulates bone mass. *Cell* (2006) 125:247–60. doi: 10.1016/j.cell.2006.01.051

24. Sun L, Zhang Z, Zhu LL, Peng Y, Liu X, Li J, et al. Further evidence for direct pro-resorptive actions of FSH. *Biochem Biophys Res Commun.* (2010) 394:6–11. doi: 10.1016/j.bbrc.2010.02.113

25. Cannon JG, Kraj B, Sloan G. Follicle-stimulating hormone promotes RANK expression on human monocytes. *Cytokine* (2011) 53:141–4. doi: 10.1016/j.cyto.2010.11.011

26. Robinson LJ, Tourkova I, Wang Y, Sharrow AC, Landau MS, Yaroslavskiy BB, et al. FSH-receptor isoforms and FSH-dependent gene transcription in human monocytes and osteoclasts. *Biochem Biophys Res Commun.* (2010) 394:12–7. doi: 10.1016/j.bbrc.2010.02.112

27. Stilley JA, Christensen DE, Dahlem KB, Guan R, Santillan DA, England SK, et al. FSH receptor (FSHR). expression in human extragonadal reproductive tissues and the developing placenta, and the impact of its deletion on pregnancy in mice. *Biol Reprod.* (2014) 91:74. doi: 10.1095/biolreprod.114.118562

28. Stilley JA, Guan R, Duffy DM, Segaloff DL. Signaling through FSH receptors on human umbilical vein endothelial cells promotes angiogenesis. *J Clin Endocrinol Metab.* (2014) 99:E813–20. doi: 10.1210/jc.2013-3186

29. Planeix F, Siraj MA, Bidard FC, Robin B, Pichon C, Sastre-Garau X, et al. Endothelial follicle-stimulating hormone receptor expression in invasive breast cancer and vascular remodeling at tumor periphery. *J Exp Clin Cancer Res.* (2015) 34:12. doi: 10.1186/s13046-015-0128-7

30. Radu A, Pichon C, Camparo P, Antoine M, Allory Y, Couvelard A, et al. Expression of follicle-stimulating hormone receptor in tumor blood vessels. *N Engl J Med.* (2010) 363:1621–30. doi: 10.1056/NEJMoa1001283

31. Siraj A, Desestret V, Antoine M, Fromont G, Huerre M, Sanson M, et al. Expression of follicle-stimulating hormone receptor by the vascular endothelium in tumor metastases. *BMC Cancer* (2013) 13:246. doi: 10.1186/1471-2407-13-246

32. Song Y, Wang ES, Xing LL, Shi S, Qu F, Zhang D, et al. Follicle-stimulating hormone induces postmenopausal dyslipidemia through inhibiting hepatic cholesterol metabolism. *J Clin Endocrinol Metab.* (2016) 101:254–63. doi: 10.1210/jc.2015-2724

33. Feng Y, Zhu S, Antaris AL, Chen H, Xiao Y, Lu X, et al. Live imaging of follicle stimulating hormone receptors in gonads and bones using near infrared II fluorophore. *Chem Sci.* (2017) 8:3703–11. doi: 10.1039/c6sc04897h

34. Zaidi M, Blair HC, Iqbal J, Davies TF, Zhu LL, Zallone A, et al. New insights: elevated follicle-stimulating hormone and bone loss during the menopausal transition. *Curr Rheumatol Rep.* (2009) 11:191–5. doi: 10.1007/s11926-009-0026-0

35. Zaidi M, Blair HC, Iqbal J, Zhu LL, Kumar TR, Zallone A, et al. Proresorptive actions of FSH and bone loss. *Ann N Y Acad Sci.* (2007) 1116:376–82. doi: 10.1196/annals.1402.056

36. Zaidi S, Zhu LL, Mali R, Iqbal J, Yang G, Zaidi M, et al. Regulation of FSH receptor promoter activation in the osteoclast. *Biochem Biophys Res Commun.* (2007) 361:910–5. doi: 10.1016/j.bbrc.2007.07.081

37. Wang J, Zhang W, Yu C, Zhang X, Zhang H, Guan Q, et al. Follicle-stimulating hormone increases the risk of postmenopausal osteoporosis by stimulating osteoclast differentiation. *PLoS ONE* (2015) 10:e0134986. doi: 10.1371/journal.pone.0134986

38. Ji Y, Liu P, Yuen T, Haider S, He J, Romero R, et al. Epitope-specific monoclonal antibodies to FSHbeta increase bone mass. *Proc Natl Acad Sci USA.* (2018) 115:2192–97. doi: 10.1073/pnas.1718144115

39. Zaidi M, Lizneva D, Kim SM, Sun L, Iqbal J, New MI, et al. FSH, bone mass, body fat, and biological aging. *Endocrinology* (2018) 159:3503–14. doi: 10.1210/en.2018-00601

40. Ghinea N. Vascular endothelial FSH receptor, a target of interest for cancer therapy. *Endocrinology* (2018) 159:3268–74. doi: 10.1210/en.2018-00466

41. Stelmaszewska J, Chrusciel M, Doroszko M, Akerfelt M, Ponikwicka-Tyszko D, Nees M, et al. Revisiting the expression and function of follicle-stimulation hormone receptor in human umbilical vein endothelial cells. *Sci Rep.* (2016) 6:37095. doi: 10.1038/srep37095

42. Liu P, Ji Y, Yuen T, Rendina-Ruedy E, DeMambro VE, Dhawan S, et al. Blocking FSH induces thermogenic adipose tissue and reduces body fat. *Nature* (2017) 546:107–12. doi: 10.1038/nature22342

43. Cohen P, Spiegelman BM. Brown and beige fat: molecular parts of a thermogenic machine. *Diabetes* (2015) 64:2346–51. doi: 10.2337/db15-0318

44. Broadley SA, Hartl FU. The role of molecular chaperones in human misfolding diseases. *FEBS Lett.* (2009) 583:2647–53. doi: 10.1016/j.febslet.2009.04.029

45. Hou ZS, Ulloa-Aguirre A, Tao YX. Pharmacoperone drugs: targeting misfolded proteins causing lysosomal storage-, ion channels-, and G protein-coupled receptors-associated conformational disorders. *Expert Rev Clin Pharmacol.* (2018) 11:611–24. doi: 10.1080/17512433.2018.1480367

46. Ulloa-Aguirre A, Zarinan T, Gutierrez-Sagal R, Dias JA. Intracellular trafficking of gonadotropin receptors in health and disease. *Handb Exp Pharmacol.* (2018) 245:1–39. doi: 10.1007/164_2017_49

47. Helenius A, Aebi M. Roles of N-linked glycans in the endoplasmic reticulum. *Annu Rev Biochem.* (2004) 73:1019–49. doi: 10.1146/annurev.biochem.73.011303.073752

48. Helenius A, Aebi M. Intracellular functions of N-linked glycans. *Science* (2001) 291:2364–9. doi: 10.1126/science.291.5512.2364

49. Fan QR, Hendrickson WA. Structure of human follicle-stimulating hormone in complex with its receptor. *Nature* (2005) 433:269–77. doi: 10.1038/nature03206

50. Davis D, Liu X, Segaloff DL. Identification of the sites of N-linked glycosylation on the follicle-stimulating hormone (FSH). Receptor and assessment of their role in FSH receptor function *Mol Endocrinol.* (1995) 9:159–70. doi: 10.1210/mend.9.2.7776966

51. Aittomaki K, Lucena JL, Pakarinen P, Sistonen P, Tapanainen J, Gromoll J, et al. Mutation in the follicle-stimulating hormone receptor gene causes hereditary hypergonadotropic ovarian failure. *Cell* (1995) 82:959–68.

52. Huhtaniemi IT, Themmen AP. Mutations in human gonadotropin and gonadotropin-receptor genes. *Endocrine* (2005) 26:207–17. doi: 10.1385/ENDO:26:3:207

53. Nechamen CA, Dias JA. Human follicle stimulating hormone receptor trafficking and hormone binding sites in the amino terminus. *Mol Cell Endocrinol.* (2000) 166:101–10. doi: 10.1016/S0303-7207(00)00281-1

54. Nechamen CA, Dias JA. Point mutations in follitropin receptor result in ER retention. *Mol Cell Endocrinol.* (2003) 201:123–31. doi: 10.1016/S0303-7207(02)00424-0

55. Duvernay MT, Filipeanu CM, Wu G. The regulatory mechanisms of export trafficking of G protein-coupled receptors. *Cell Signal.* (2005) 17:1457–65. doi: 10.1016/j.cellsig.2005.05.020

56. Timossi C, Ortiz-Elizondo C, Pineda DB, Dias JA, Conn PM, Ulloa-Aguirre A. Functional significance of the BBXXB motif reversed present in the cytoplasmic domains of the human follicle-stimulating hormone receptor. *Mol Cell Endocrinol.* (2004) 223:17–26. doi: 10.1016/j.mce.2004.06.004

57. Zarinan T, Perez-Solis MA, Maya-Nunez G, Casas-Gonzalez P, Conn PM, Dias JA, et al. Dominant negative effects of human follicle-stimulating hormone receptor expression-deficient mutants on wild-type receptor cell surface expression. Rescue of oligomerization-dependent defective receptor expression by using cognate decoys *Mol Cell Endocrinol.* (2010) 321:112–22. doi: 10.1016/j.mce.2010.02.027

58. Schulz A, Schoneberg T, Paschke R, Schultz G, Gudermann T. Role of the third intracellular loop for the activation of gonadotropin receptors. *Mol Endocrinol.* (1999) 13:181–90.

59. Beau I, Touraine P, Meduri G, Gougeon A, Desroches A, Matuchansky C, et al. A novel phenotype related to partial loss of function mutations of the follicle stimulating hormone receptor. *J Clin Invest.* (1998) 102:1352–9.

60. Touraine P, Beau I, Gougeon A, Meduri G, Desroches A, Pichard C, et al. New natural inactivating mutations of the follicle-stimulating hormone receptor: correlations between receptor function and phenotype. *Mol Endocrinol.* (1999) 13:1844–54.

61. Bramble MS, Goldstein EH, Lipson A, Ngun T, Eskin A, Gosschalk JE, et al. A novel follicle-stimulating hormone receptor mutation causing primary ovarian failure: a fertility application of whole exome sequencing. *Hum Reprod.* (2016) 31:905–14. doi: 10.1093/humrep/dew025

62. Meduri G, Touraine P, Beau I, Lahuna O, Desroches A, Vacher-Lavenu MC, et al. Delayed puberty and primary amenorrhea associated with a novel mutation of the human follicle-stimulating hormone receptor: clinical, histological, and molecular studies. *J Clin Endocrinol Metab.* (2003) 88:3491–8. doi: 10.1210/jc.2003-030217

63. Ma J, Wang S, Zhao F, Xu J. Protein threading using context-specific alignment potential. *Bioinformatics* (2013) 29:i257–65. doi: 10.1093/bioinformatics/btt210

64. Thal DM, Vuckovic Z, Draper-Joyce CJ, Liang YL, Glukhova A, Christopoulos A, et al. Recent advances in the determination of G protein-coupled receptor structures. *Curr Opin Struct Biol.* (2018) 51:28–34. doi: 10.1016/j.sbi.2018.03.002

65. Almeida JG, Preto AJ, Koukos PI, Bonvin A, Moreira IS. Membrane proteins structures: a review on computational modeling tools. *Biochim Biophys Acta.* (2017) 1859:2021–39. doi: 10.1016/j.bbamem.2017.07.008

66. Ferre S, Casado V, Devi LA, Filizola M, Jockers R, Lohse MJ, et al. G protein-coupled receptor oligomerization revisited: functional and pharmacological perspectives. *Pharmacol Rev.* (2014) 66:413–34. doi: 10.1124/pr.113.008052

67. Rivero-Muller A, Jonas KC, Hanyaloglu AC, Huhtaniemi I. Di/oligomerization of GPCRs-mechanisms and functional significance. *Prog Mol Biol Transl Sci.* (2013) 117:163–85. doi: 10.1016/B978-0-12-386931-9.00007-6

68. Sleno R, Hebert TE. The dynamics of GPCR Oligomerization and their functional consequences. *Int Rev Cell Mol Biol.* (2018) 338:141–71. doi: 10.1016/bs.ircmb.2018.02.005

69. Guan R, Wu X, Feng X, Zhang M, Hebert TE, Segaloff DL. Structural determinants underlying constitutive dimerization of unoccupied human follitropin receptors. *Cell Signal.* (2010) 22:247–56. doi: 10.1016/j.cellsig.2009.09.023

70. Mazurkiewicz JE, Herrick-Davis K, Barroso M, Ulloa-Aguirre A, Lindau-Shepard B, Thomas RM, et al. Single-molecule analyses of fully functional fluorescent protein-tagged follitropin receptor reveal homodimerization and specific heterodimerization with lutropin receptor. *Biol Reprod.* (2015) 92:100. doi: 10.1095/biolreprod.114.125781

71. Balasubramanian S, Teissere JA, Raju DV, Hall RA. Hetero-oligomerization between GABAA and GABAB receptors regulates GABAB receptor trafficking. *J Biol Chem.* (2004) 279:18840–50. doi: 10.1074/jbc.M313470200M313470200

72. Bulenger S, Marullo S, Bouvier M. Emerging role of homo- and heterodimerization in G-protein-coupled receptor biosynthesis and maturation. *Trends Pharmacol Sci.* (2005) 26:131–7. doi: 10.1016/j.tips.2005.01.004

73. Hague C, Uberti MA, Chen Z, Hall RA, Minneman KP. Cell surface expression of alpha1D-adrenergic receptors is controlled by heterodimerization with alpha1B-adrenergic receptors. *J Biol Chem.* (2004) 279:15541–9. doi: 10.1074/jbc.M314014200

74. Margeta-Mitrovic M, Jan YN, Jan LY. A trafficking checkpoint controls GABA(B). receptor heterodimerization. *Neuron* (2000) 27:97–106. doi: 10.1016/S0896-6273(00)00012-X

75. Salahpour A, Angers S, Mercier JF, Lagace M, Marullo S, Bouvier M. Homodimerization of the beta2-adrenergic receptor as a prerequisite for cell surface targeting. *J Biol Chem.* (2004) 279:33390–7. doi: 10.1074/jbc.M403363200

76. Terrillon S, Bouvier M. Roles of G-protein-coupled receptor dimerization. *EMBO Rep.* (2004) 5:30–4. doi: 10.1038/sj.embor.7400052 7400052

77. White JH, Wise A, Main MJ, Green A, Fraser NJ, Disney GH, et al. Heterodimerization is required for the formation of a functional GABA(B). receptor *Nature* (1998) 396:679–82.

78. Guo W, Shi L, Javitch JA. The fourth transmembrane segment forms the interface of the dopamine D2 receptor homodimer. *J Biol Chem.* (2003) 278:4385–8. doi: 10.1074/jbc.C200679200C200679200

79. Hernanz-Falcon P, Rodriguez-Frade JM, Serrano A, Juan D, del Sol A, Soriano SF, et al. Identification of amino acid residues crucial for chemokine receptor dimerization. *Nat Immunol.* (2004) 5:216–23. doi: 10.1038/ni1027

80. Lopez-Gimenez JF, Canals M, Pediani JD, Milligan G. The alpha1b-adrenoceptor exists as a higher-order oligomer: effective oligomerization is required for receptor maturation, surface delivery, and function. *Mol Pharmacol.* (2007) 71:1015–29. doi: 10.1124/mol.106.033035

81. Jiang X, Fischer D, Chen X, McKenna SD, Liu H, Sriraman V, et al. Evidence for follicle-stimulating hormone receptor as a functional trimer. *J Biol Chem.* (2014) 289:14273–82. doi: 10.1074/jbc.M114.549592

82. Navarro G, Cordomi A, Casado-Anguera V, Moreno E, Cai NS, Cortes A, et al. Evidence for functional pre-coupled complexes of receptor heteromers and adenylyl cyclase. *Nat Commun.* (2018) 9:1242. doi: 10.1038/s41467-018-03522-3

83. Feng X, Zhang M, Guan R, Segaloff DL. Heterodimerization between the lutropin and follitropin receptors is associated with an attenuation of hormone-dependent signaling. *Endocrinology* (2013) 154:3925–30. doi: 10.1210/en.2013-1407

84. Jonas KC, Chen S, Virta M, Mora J, Franks S, Huhtaniemi I, et al. Temporal reprogramming of calcium signalling via crosstalk of gonadotrophin receptors that associate as functionally asymmetric heteromers. *Sci Rep.* (2018) 8:2239. doi: 10.1038/s41598-018-20722-5

85. Agrawal G, Dighe RR. Critical involvement of the hinge region of the follicle-stimulating hormone receptor in the activation of the receptor. *J Biol Chem.* (2009) 284:2636–47. doi: 10.1074/jbc.M808199200

86. Bruysters M, Verhoef-Post M, Themmen AP. Asp330 and Tyr331 in the C-terminal cysteine-rich region of the luteinizing hormone receptor are key residues in hormone-induced receptor activation. *J Biol Chem.* (2008) 283:25821–8. doi: 10.1074/jbc.M804395200

87. Costagliola S, Panneels V, Bonomi M, Koch J, Many MC, Smits G, et al. Tyrosine sulfation is required for agonist recognition by glycoprotein hormone receptors. *EMBO J.* (2002) 21:504–13. doi: 10.1093/emboj/21.4.504

88. Fan QR, Hendrickson WA. Structural biology of glycoprotein hormones and their receptors. *Endocrine* (2005) 26:179–88. doi: 10.1385/endo:26:3:179

89. Fan QR, Hendrickson WA. Assembly and structural characterization of an authentic complex between human follicle stimulating hormone and a hormone-binding ectodomain of its receptor. *Mol Cell Endocrinol.* (2007) 260–262:73–82. doi: 10.1016/j.mce.2005.12.055

90. Chen CR, Chazenbalk GD, McLachlan SM, Rapoport B. Evidence that the C terminus of the a subunit suppresses thyrotropin receptor constitutive activity. *Endocrinology* (2003) 144:3821–27. doi: 10.1210/En.2003-0430

91. Vassart G, Pardo L, Costagliola S. A molecular dissection of the glycoprotein hormone receptors. *Trends Biochem Sci.* (2004) 29:119–26. doi: 10.1016/j.tibs.2004.01.006

92. Vlaeminck-Guillem V, Ho SC, Rodien P, Vassart G, Costagliola S. Activation of the cAMP pathway by the TSH receptor involves switching of the ectodomain from a tethered inverse agonist to an agonist. *Mol Endocrinol.* (2002) 16:736–46. doi: 10.1210/mend.16.4.0816

93. Zhang M, Tong KP, Fremont V, Chen J, Narayan P, Puett D, et al. The extracellular domain suppresses constitutive activity of the transmembrane domain of the human TSH receptor: implications for hormone-receptor interaction and antagonist design. *Endocrinology* (2000) 141:3514–7. doi: 10.1210/endo.141.9.7790

94. Bruser A, Schulz A, Rothemund S, Ricken A, Calebiro D, Kleinau G, et al. The activation mechanism of glycoprotein hormone receptors with implications in the cause and therapy of endocrine diseases. *J Biol Chem.* (2016) 291:508–20. doi: 10.1074/jbc.M115.701102

95. Nakabayashi K, Kudo M, Kobilka B, Hsueh AJ. Activation of the luteinizing hormone receptor following substitution of Ser-277 with selective hydrophobic residues in the ectodomain hinge region. *J Biol Chem.* (2000) 275:30264–71. doi: 10.1074/jbc.M005568200

96. Bonomi M, Busnelli M, Persani L, Vassart G, Costagliola S. Structural differences in the hinge region of the glycoprotein hormone receptors: evidence from the sulfated tyrosine residues. *Mol Endocrinol.* (2006) 20:3351–63. doi: 10.1210/me.2005-0521

97. Kumar P, Sait SF, Sharma A, Kumar M. Ovarian hyperstimulation syndrome. *J Hum Reprod Sci.* (2011) 4:70–5. doi: 10.4103/0974-1208.86080

98. De Leener A, Montanelli L, Van Durme J, Chae H, Smits G, Vassart G, et al. Presence and absence of follicle-stimulating hormone receptor mutations provide some insights into spontaneous ovarian hyperstimulation syndrome physiopathology. *J Clin Endocrinol Metab.* (2006) 91:555–62. doi: 10.1210/jc.2005-1580

99. Scheerer P, Park JH, Hildebrand PW, Kim YJ, Krauss N, Choe HW, et al. Crystal structure of opsin in its G-protein-interacting conformation. *Nature* (2008) 455:497–502. doi: 10.1038/nature07330

100. Rasmussen SGF, Choi HJ, Fung JJ, Pardon E, Casarosa P, Chae PS, et al. Structure of a nanobody-stabilized active state of the beta(2). adrenoceptor. *Nature* (2011) 469:175–80. doi: 10.1038/Nature09648

101. Rasmussen SGF, DeVree BT, Zou YZ, Kruse AC, Chung KY, Kobilka TS, et al. Crystal structure of the beta(2). adrenergic receptor-Gs protein complex. *Nature* (2011) 477:549–U311. doi: 10.1038/Nature10361

102. Garcia-Nafria J, Lee Y, Bai X, Carpenter B, Tate CG. Cryo-EM structure of the adenosine A2A receptor coupled to an engineered heterotrimeric G protein. *Elife* (2018) 7:e35946. doi: 10.7554/eLife.35946

103. Draper-Joyce CJ, Khoshouei M, Thal DM, Liang YL, Nguyen ATN, Furness SGB, et al. Structure of the adenosine-bound human adenosine A1 receptor-Gi complex. *Nature* (2018) 558:559–63. doi: 10.1038/s41586-018-0236-6

104. Garcia-Nafria J, Nehme R, Edwards PC, Tate CG. Cryo-EM structure of the serotonin 5-HT1B receptor coupled to heterotrimeric Go. *Nature* (2018) 558:620–23. doi: 10.1038/s41586-018-0241-9

105. Kang Y, Kuybeda O, de Waal PW, Mukherjee S, Van Eps N, Dutka P, et al. Cryo-EM structure of human rhodopsin bound to an inhibitory G protein. *Nature* (2018) 558:553–58. doi: 10.1038/s41586-018-0215-y

106. Koehl A, Hu H, Maeda S, Zhang Y, Qu Q, Paggi JM, et al. Structure of the micro-opioid receptor-Gi protein complex. *Nature* (2018) 558:547–52. doi: 10.1038/s41586-018-0219-7

107. Venkatakrishnan AJ, Deupi X, Lebon G, Tate CG, Schertler GF, Babu MM. Molecular signatures of G-protein-coupled receptors. *Nature* (2013) 494:185–94. doi: 10.1038/nature11896

108. Ballesteros JA, Weinstein H. Integrated methods for the construction of three-dimensional models and computational probing of structure-function relations in G protein-coupled receptors.. *Methods Neurosci.* (1995) 25:366–428.

109. Deupi X, Standfuss J. Structural insights into agonist-induced activation of G-protein-coupled receptors. *Curr Opin Struct Biol.* (2011) 21:541–51. doi: 10.1016/j.sbi.2011.06.002

110. Sansuk K, Deupi X, Torrecillas IR, Jongejan A, Nijmeijer S, Bakker RA, et al. A structural insight into the reorientation of transmembrane domains 3 and 5 during family A G protein-coupled receptor activation. *Mol Pharmacol.* (2011) 79:262–9. doi: 10.1124/mol.110.066068

111. Standfuss J, Edwards PC, D'Antona A, Fransen M, Xie G, Oprian DD, et al. The structural basis of agonist-induced activation in constitutively active rhodopsin. *Nature* (2011) 471:656–60. doi: 10.1038/nature09795

112. Rasmussen SG, Choi HJ, Rosenbaum DM, Kobilka TS, Thian FS, Edwards PC, et al. Crystal structure of the human beta2 adrenergic G-protein-coupled receptor. *Nature* (2007) 450:383–7. doi: 10.1038/nature06325

113. Nygaard R, Zou YZ, Dror RO, Mildorf TJ, Arlow DH, Manglik A, et al. The dynamic process of beta(2)-adrenergic receptor activation. *Cell* (2013) 152:532–42. doi:. 10.1016/j.cell.2013.01.008

114. Kahsai AW, Xiao KH, Rajagopal S, Ahn S, Shukla AK, Sun JP, et al. Multiple ligand-specific conformations of the beta(2)-adrenergic receptor. *Nat Chem Biol.* (2011) 7:692–700. doi:. 10.1038/Nchembio.634

115. Reiter E, Ahn S, Shukla AK, Lefkowitz RJ. Molecular mechanism of beta-arrestin-biased agonism at seven-transmembrane receptors. *Annu Rev Pharmacol Toxicol.* (2012) 52:179–97. doi: 10.1146/annurev.pharmtox.010909.105800

116. Barak LS, Oakley RH, Laporte SA, Caron MG. Constitutive arrestin-mediated desensitization of a human vasopressin receptor mutant associated with nephrogenic diabetes insipidus. *Proc Natl Acad Sci USA.* (2001) 98:93–8. doi: 10.1073/pnas.011303698011303698[pii]

117. Vassart G, Costagliola S. G protein-coupled receptors: mutations and endocrine diseases. *Nat Rev Endocrinol.* (2011) 7:362–72. doi:. doi 10.1038/nrendo.2011.20

118. Lohse MJ, Maiellaro I, Calebiro D. Kinetics and mechanism of G protein-coupled receptor activation. *Curr Opin Cell Biol.* (2014) 27:87–93. doi: 10.1016/j.ceb.2013.11.009

119. Tsai CJ, Pamula F, Nehme R, Muhle J, Weinert T, Flock T, et al. Crystal structure of rhodopsin in complex with a mini-Go sheds light on the principles of G protein selectivity. *Sci Adv.* (2018) 4:eaat7052. doi: 10.1126/sciadv.aat7052

120. Kang Y, Zhou XE, Gao X, He Y, Liu W, Ishchenko A, et al. Crystal structure of rhodopsin bound to arrestin by femtosecond X-ray laser. *Nature* (2015) 523:561–7. doi: 10.1038/nature14656

121. Angelova K, Fanelli F, Puett D. A model for constitutive lutropin receptor activation based on molecular simulation and engineered mutations in transmembrane helices 6 and 7. *J Biol Chem.* (2002) 277:32202–13. doi: 10.1074/jbc.M203272200

122. Angelova K, Fanelli F, Puett D. Contributions of Intracellular Loops 2 and 3 of the lutropin receptor in Gs coupling. *Mol Endocrinol.* (2008) 22:126–38. doi: 10.1210/me.2007-0352

123. Angelova K, Felline A, Lee M, Patel M, Puett D, Fanelli F. Conserved amino acids participate in the structure networks deputed to intramolecular communication in the lutropin receptor. *Cell Mol Life Sci.* (2011) 68:1227–39. doi: 10.1007/s00018-010-0519-z

124. Angelova K, Narayan P, Simon JP, Puett D. Functional role of transmembrane helix 7 in the activation of the heptahelical lutropin receptor. *Mol Endocrinol.* (2000) 14:459–71. doi: 10.1210/mend.14.4.0439

125. Fanelli F, De Benedetti PG. Computational modeling approaches to structure-function analysis of G protein-coupled receptors. *Chem Rev.* (2005) 105:3297–351. doi: 10.1021/cr000095n

126. Fanelli F, Verhoef-Post M, Timmerman M, Zeilemaker A, Martens JW, Themmen AP. Insight into mutation-induced activation of the luteinizing hormone receptor: molecular simulations predict the functional behavior of engineered mutants at M398. *Mol Endocrinol.* (2004) 18:1499–508. doi: 10.1210/me.2003-0050

127. Zhang M, Tao YX, Ryan GL, Feng X, Fanelli F, Segaloff DL. Intrinsic differences in the response of the human lutropin receptor versus the human follitropin receptor to activating mutations. *J Biol Chem.* (2007) 282:25527–39. doi: 10.1074/jbc.M703500200

128. Gromoll J, Simoni M, Nieschlag E. An activating mutation of the follicle-stimulating hormone receptor autonomously sustains spermatogenesis in a hypophysectomized man. *J Clin Endocrinol Metab.* (1996) 81:1367–70.

129. Montanelli L, Delbaere A, Di Carlo C, Nappi C, Smits G, Vassart G, et al. A mutation in the follicle-stimulating hormone receptor as a cause of familial spontaneous ovarian hyperstimulation syndrome. *J Clin Endocrinol Metab.* (2004) 89:1255–8. doi: 10.1210/jc.2003-031910

130. Montanelli L, Van Durme JJ, Smits G, Bonomi M, Rodien P, Devor EJ, et al. Modulation of ligand selectivity associated with activation of the transmembrane region of the human follitropin receptor. *Mol Endocrinol.* (2004) 18:2061–73. doi: 10.1210/me.2004-0036

131. Parma J, Duprez L, Van Sande J, Cochaux P, Gervy C, Mockel J, et al. Somatic mutations in the thyrotropin receptor gene cause hyperfunctioning thyroid adenomas. *Nature* (1993) 365:649–51. doi: 10.1038/365649a0

132. Parma J, Van Sande J, Swillens S, Tonacchera M, Dumont J, Vassart G. Somatic mutations causing constitutive activity of the thyrotropin receptor are the major cause of hyperfunctioning thyroid adenomas: identification of additional mutations activating both the cyclic adenosine 3',5'-monophosphate and inositol phosphate-Ca2+ cascades. *Mol Endocrinol.* (1995) 9:725–33.

133. Smits G, Olatunbosun O, Delbaere A, Pierson R, Vassart G, Costagliola S. Ovarian hyperstimulation syndrome due to a mutation in the follicle-stimulating hormone receptor. *N Engl J Med.* (2003) 349:760–6. doi: 10.1056/NEJMoa030064

134. Ulloa-Aguirre A, Reiter E, Bousfield G, Dias JA, Huhtaniemi I. Constitutive activity in gonadotropin receptors. *Adv Pharmacol.* (2014) 70:37–80. doi: 10.1016/B978-0-12-417197-8.00002-X

135. Kudo M, Osuga Y, Kobilka BK, Hsueh AJ. Transmembrane regions V and VI of the human luteinizing hormone receptor are required for constitutive activation by a mutation in the third intracellular loop. *J Biol Chem.* (1996) 271:22470–8.

136. Casas-Gonzalez P, Scaglia HE, Perez-Solis MA, Durand G, Scaglia J, Zarinan T, et al. Normal testicular function without detectable follicle-stimulating hormone. A novel mutation in the follicle-stimulating hormone receptor gene leading to apparent constitutive activity and impaired agonist-induced desensitization and internalization. *Mol Cell Endocrinol.* (2012) 364:71–82. doi: 10.1016/j.mce.2012.08.011

137. DeMars G, Fanelli F, Puett D. The extreme C-terminal region of Galphas differentially couples to the luteinizing hormone and beta2-adrenergic receptors. *Mol Endocrinol.* (2011) 25:1416–30. doi: 10.1210/me.2011-0009

138. Dias JA, Mahale SD, Nechamen CA, Davydenko O, Thomas RM, Ulloa-Aguirre A. Emerging roles for the FSH receptor adapter protein APPL1 and overlap of a putative 14-3-3tau interaction domain with a canonical G-protein interaction site. *Mol Cell Endocrinol.* (2010) 329:17–25. doi: 10.1016/j.mce.2010.05.009

139. Dias JA, Nechamen CA, Atari R. Identifying protein interactors in gonadotropin action. *Endocrine* (2005) 26:241–7.

140. Feng X, Muller T, Mizrachi D, Fanelli F, Segaloff DL. An intracellular loop (IL2). residue confers different basal constitutive activities to the human lutropin receptor and human thyrotropin receptor through structural communication between IL2 and helix 6, via helix 3. *Endocrinology* (2008) 149:1705–17. doi: 10.1210/en.2007-1341

141. Thompson MD, Percy ME, McIntyre Burnham W, Cole DE. G protein-coupled receptors disrupted in human genetic disease. *Methods Mol Biol.* (2008) 448:109–37. doi: 10.1007/978-1-59745-205-2_7

142. Timossi C, Maldonado D, Vizcaino A, Lindau-Shepard B, Conn PM, Ulloa-Aguirre A. Structural determinants in the second intracellular loop of the human follicle-stimulating hormone receptor are involved in G(s). protein activation. *Mol Cell Endocrinol.* (2002) 189:157–68. doi: 10.1016/S0303-7207(01)00720-1

143. Ulloa-Aguirre A, Reiter E, Crepieux P. FSH receptor signaling: complexity of interactions and signal diversity. *Endocrinology* (2018) 159:3020–35. doi: 10.1210/en.2018-00452

144. Nechamen CA, Thomas RM, Cohen BD, Acevedo G, Poulikakos PI, Testa JR, et al. Human follicle-stimulating hormone (FSH). receptor interacts with the adaptor protein APPL1 in HEK 293 cells: potential involvement of the PI3K pathway in FSH signaling. *Biol Reprod.* (2004) 71:629–36. doi: 10.1095/biolreprod.103.025833

145. Nechamen CA, Thomas RM, Dias JA. APPL1, APPL2, Akt2 and FOXO1a interact with FSHR in a potential signaling complex. *Mol Cell Endocrinol.* (2007) 260-262:93–9. doi: 10.1016/j.mce.2006.08.014

146. Thomas RM, Nechamen CA, Mazurkiewicz JE, Ulloa-Aguirre A, Dias JA. The adapter protein APPL1 links FSH receptor to inositol 1,4,5-trisphosphate production and is implicated in intracellular Ca(2+) mobilization. *Endocrinology* (2011) 152:1691–701. doi: 10.1210/en.2010-1353

147. Cohen BD, Nechamen CA, Dias JA. Human follitropin receptor (FSHR). interacts with the adapter protein 14-3-3tau. *Mol Cell Endocrinol.* (2004) 220:1–7. doi: 10.1016/j.mce.2004.04.012

148. Tzivion G, Avruch J. 14-3-3 proteins: active cofactors in cellular regulation by serine/threonine phosphorylation. *J Biol Chem.* (2002) 277:3061–4. doi: 10.1074/jbc.R100059200

149. Dhanwada KR, Vijapurkar U, Ascoli M. Two mutations of the lutropin/choriogonadotropin receptor that impair signal transduction also interfere with receptor-mediated endocytosis. *Mol Endocrinol.* (1996) 10:544–54.

150. Ulloa-Aguirre A, Uribe A, Zarinan T, Bustos-Jaimes I, Perez-Solis MA, Dias JA. Role of the intracellular domains of the human FSH receptor in G(alphaS). protein coupling and receptor expression. *Mol Cell Endocrinol.* (2007) 260-262:153–62. doi: 10.1016/j.mce.2005.11.050

151. Grasso P, Deziel MR, Reichert LE Jr. Synthetic peptides corresponding to residues 551 to 555 and 650 to 653 of the rat testicular follicle-stimulating hormone (FSH). receptor are sufficient for post-receptor modulation of Sertoli cell responsiveness to FSH stimulation. *Regul Pept.* (1995) 60:177–83.

152. Grasso P, Leng N, Reichert LE Jr. A synthetic peptide corresponding to the third cytoplasmic loop (residues 533 to 555). of the testicular follicle-stimulating hormone receptor affects signal transduction in rat testis membranes and in intact cultured rat Sertoli cells. *Mol Cell Endocrinol.* (1995) 110:35–41.

153. Kara E, Crepieux P, Gauthier C, Martinat N, Piketty V, Guillou F, et al. A phosphorylation cluster of five serine and threonine residues in the C-terminus of the follicle-stimulating hormone receptor is important for desensitization but not for beta-arrestin-mediated ERK activation. *Mol Endocrinol.* (2006) 20:3014–26. doi: 10.1210/me.2006-0098

154. Marion S, Kara E, Crepieux P, Piketty V, Martinat N, Guillou F, et al. G protein-coupled receptor kinase 2 and beta-arrestins are recruited to FSH receptor in stimulated rat primary Sertoli cells. *J Endocrinol.* (2006) 190:341–50. doi: 10.1677/joe.1.06857

155. Troispoux C, Guillou F, Elalouf JM, Firsov D, Iacovelli L, De Blasi A, et al. Involvement of G protein-coupled receptor kinases and arrestins in desensitization to follicle-stimulating hormone action. *Mol Endocrinol.* (1999) 13:1599–614. doi: 10.1210/mend.13.9.0342

156. Wehbi V, Tranchant T, Durand G, Musnier A, Decourtye J, Piketty V, et al. Partially deglycosylated equine LH preferentially activates beta-arrestin-dependent signaling at the follicle-stimulating hormone receptor. *Mol Endocrinol.* (2010) 24:561–73. doi: 10.1210/me.2009-0347

157. Simoni M, Casarini L. Genetics of FSH action: a 2014-and-beyond view. *Eur J Endocrinol.* (2014) 170:R91–107. doi: 10.1530/EJE-13-0624

158. Behre HM, Greb RR, Mempel A, Sonntag B, Kiesel L, Kaltwasser P, et al. Significance of a common single nucleotide polymorphism in exon 10 of the follicle-stimulating hormone (FSH) receptor gene for the ovarian response to FSH: a pharmacogenetic approach to controlled ovarian hyperstimulation. *Pharmacogenet Genomics* (2005) 15:451–6. doi: 10.1097/01.fpc.0000167330.92786.5e

159. de Koning CH, Benjamins T, Harms P, Homburg R, van Montfrans JM, Gromoll J, et al. The distribution of FSH receptor isoforms is related to basal FSH levels in subfertile women with normal menstrual cycles. *Hum Reprod.* (2006) 21:443–6. doi: 10.1093/humrep/dei317

160. Tranchant T, Durand G, Piketty V, Gauthier C, Ulloa-Aguirre A, Crepieux P, et al. N680S snp of the human FSH receptor impacts on basal FSH and estradiol level in women and modifies PKA nuclear translocation and creb-dependent gene transcription *in vitro*. *Hum Reprod.* (2012) 27:i45.

161. Casarini L, Moriondo V, Marino M, Adversi F, Capodanno F, Grisolia C, et al. FSHR polymorphism p.N680S mediates different responses to FSH *in vitro*. *Mol Cell Endocrinol.* (2014) 393:83–91. doi: 10.1016/j.mce.2014.06.013

162. Garcia-Jimenez G, Zarinan T, Rodriguez-Valentin R, Mejia-Dominguez NR, Gutierrez-Sagal R, Hernandez-Montes G, et al. Frequency of the T307A, N680S, and−29G>A single-nucleotide polymorphisms in the follicle-stimulating hormone receptor in Mexican subjects of Hispanic ancestry. *Reprod Biol Endocrinol.* (2018) 16:100. doi: 10.1186/s12958-018-0420-4

163. Jean-Alphonse F, Bowersox S, Chen S, Beard G, Puthenveedu MA, Hanyaloglu AC. Spatially restricted G protein-coupled receptor activity via divergent endocytic compartments. *J Biol Chem.* (2014) 289:3960–77. doi: 10.1074/jbc.M113.526350

164. Sposini S, Hanyaloglu AC. Spatial encryption of G protein-coupled receptor signaling in endosomes; Mechanisms and applications. *Biochem Pharmacol.* (2017) 143:1–9. doi: 10.1016/j.bcp.2017.04.028

165. Sposini S, Jean-Alphonse FG, Ayoub MA, Oqua A, West C, Lavery S, et al. Integration of GPCR signaling and sorting from very early endosomes via opposing APPL1 mechanisms. *Cell Rep.* (2017) 21:2855–67. doi: 10.1016/j.celrep.2017.11.023

166. Krishnamurthy H, Kishi H, Shi M, Galet C, Bhaskaran RS, Hirakawa T, et al. Postendocytotic trafficking of the follicle-stimulating hormone (FSH)-FSH receptor complex. *Mol Endocrinol.* (2003) 17:2162–76. doi: 10.1210/me.2003-0118

167. Lazari MF, Liu X, Nakamura K, Benovic JL, Ascoli M. Role of G protein-coupled receptor kinases on the agonist-induced phosphorylation and internalization of the follitropin receptor. *Mol Endocrinol.* (1999) 13:866–78.

168. Reiter E, Lefkowitz RJ. GRKs and beta-arrestins: roles in receptor silencing, trafficking and signaling. *Trends Endocrinol Metab.* (2006) 17:159–65. doi: 10.1016/j.tem.2006.03.008

169. Piketty V, Kara E, Guillou F, Reiter E, Crepieux P. Follicle-stimulating hormone (FSH). activates extracellular signal-regulated kinase phosphorylation independently of beta-arrestin- and dynamin-mediated FSH receptor internalization. *Reprod Biol Endocrinol.* (2006) 4:33. doi: 10.1186/1477-7827-4-33

170. Mukherjee S, Gurevich VV, Preninger A, Hamm HE, Bader MF, Fazleabas AT, et al. Aspartic acid 564 in the third cytoplasmic loop of the luteinizing hormone/choriogonadotropin receptor is crucial for phosphorylation-independent interaction with arrestin2. *J Biol Chem.* (2002) 277:17916–27. doi: 10.1074/jbc.M110479200

171. Mukherjee S, Gurevich VV, Jones JC, Casanova JE, Frank SR, Maizels ET, et al. The ADP ribosylation factor nucleotide exchange factor ARNO promotes beta-arrestin release necessary for luteinizing hormone/choriogonadotropin receptor desensitization. *Proc Natl Acad Sci USA.* (2000) 97:5901–6. doi: 10.1073/pnas.100127097

172. Menon KM, Clouser CL, Nair AK. Gonadotropin receptors: role of post-translational modifications and post-transcriptional regulation. *Endocrine* (2005) 26:249–57. doi: 10.1385/ENDO:26:3:249

173. Kawate N, Peegel H, Menon KM. Role of palmitoylation of conserved cysteine residues of luteinizing hormone/human choriogonadotropin receptors in receptor down-regulation. *Mol Cell Endocrinol.* (1997) 127:211–9.

174. Munshi UM, Clouser CL, Peegel H, Menon KM. Evidence that palmitoylation of carboxyl terminus cysteine residues of the human luteinizing hormone receptor regulates postendocytic processing. *Mol Endocrinol.* (2005) 19:749–58. doi: 10.1210/me.2004-0335

175. Munshi UM, Peegel H, Menon KM. Palmitoylation of the luteinizing hormone/human chorionic gonadotropin receptor regulates receptor interaction with the arrestin-mediated internalization pathway. *Eur J Biochem.* (2001) 268:1631–9. doi: 10.1046/j.1432-1327.2001.02032.x

176. Cohen BD, Bariteau JT, Magenis LM, Dias JA. Regulation of follitropin receptor cell surface residency by the ubiquitin-proteasome pathway. *Endocrinology* (2003) 144:4393–402. doi: 10.1210/en.2002-0063

177. Hsueh AJ, He J. Gonadotropins and their receptors: coevolution, genetic variants, receptor imaging, and functional antagonists. *Biol Reprod.* (2018) 99:3–12. doi: 10.1093/biolre/ioy012

178. Kumar TR. Extragonadal Actions of FSH: a critical need for novel genetic models. *Endocrinology* (2018) 159:2–8. doi: 10.1210/en.2017-03118

179. Zhu S, Herraiz S, Yue J, Zhang M, Wan H, Yang Q, et al. 3D NIR-II molecular imaging distinguishes targeted organs with high-performance NIR-II bioconjugates. *Adv Mater.* (2018) 30:e1705799. doi: 10.1002/adma.201705799

180. Abd-Elaziz K, Duijkers I, Stockl L, Dietrich B, Klipping C, Eckert K, et al. A new fully human recombinant FSH (follitropin epsilon): two phase I randomized placebo and comparator-controlled pharmacokinetic and pharmacodynamic trials. *Hum Reprod.* (2017) 32:1639–47. doi: 10.1093/humrep/dex220

181. Olsson H, Sandstrom R, Grundemar L. Different pharmacokinetic and pharmacodynamic properties of recombinant follicle-stimulating hormone (rFSH). derived from a human cell line compared with rFSH from a non-human cell line. *J Clin Pharmacol.* (2014) 54:1299–307. doi: 10.1002/jcph.328

182. Koechling W, Plaksin D, Croston GE, Jeppesen JV, Macklon KT, Andersen CY. Comparative pharmacology of a new recombinant FSH expressed by a human cell line. *Endocr Connect.* (2017) 6:297–305. doi: 10.1530/EC-17-0067

19

FSHR Trans-Activation and Oligomerization

Kamila Szymańska[1], Joanna Kałafut[1], Alicja Przybyszewska[1], Beata Paziewska[1], Grzegorz Adamczuk[2], Michał Kiełbus[1] and Adolfo Rivero-Müller[1,3]*

[1] Department of Biochemistry and Molecular Biology, Medical University of Lublin, Lublin, Poland, [2] Independent Medical Biology Unit, Medical University of Lublin, Lublin, Poland, [3] Cell Biology, Biosciences, Faculty of Science and Engineering, Åbo Akademi University, Turku, Finland

*Correspondence:
Adolfo Rivero-Müller
a.rivero@umlub.pl; adoriv@utu.fi

Follicle stimulating hormone (FSH) plays a key role in human reproduction through, among others, induction of spermatogenesis in men and production of estrogen in women. The function FSH is performed upon binding to its cognate receptor—follicle-stimulating hormone receptor (FSHR) expressed on the surface of target cells (granulosa and Sertoli cells). FSHR belongs to the family of G protein-coupled receptors (GPCRs), a family of receptors distinguished by the presence of various signaling pathway activation as well as formation of cross-talking aggregates. Until recently, it was claimed that the FSHR occurred naturally as a monomer, however, the crystal structure as well as experimental evidence have shown that FSHR both self-associates and forms heterodimers with the luteinizing hormone/chorionic gonadotropin receptor—LHCGR. The tremendous gain of knowledge is also visible on the subject of receptor activation. It was once thought that activation occurs only as a result of ligand binding to a particular receptor, however there is mounting evidence of trans-activation as well as biased signaling between GPCRs. Herein, we describe the mechanisms of aforementioned phenomena as well as briefly describe important experiments that contributed to their better understanding.

Keywords: follicle-stimulating hormone (FSH), follicle-stimulating hormone receptor (FSHR), G protein-coupled receptor (GPCR), transactivation, biased signaling, oligomerization, homodimers, heterodimers

INTRODUCTION

Gonadotrophin hormones, which include luteinizing hormone (LH), follicle stimulating hormone (FSH) and human chorionic gonadotropin (hCG), perform a number of functions pivotal for the process of sexual development and reproduction as well as for the fetal development in the case of the latter hormone. Alongside the thyroid-stimulating hormone (TSH) they comprise a glycoprotein hormone family. LH, FSH, and TSH are synthesized and secreted by the cells of the anterior pituitary gland (gonadotrophs), while hCG is produced by placental syncytiotrophoblasts.

The action of these hormones is achieved by the presence of receptors belonging to the class A of G protein-coupled receptors (GPCRs)—FSH constitutes ligand for FSHR, TSH for TSHR, whereas LH and hCG for their common LHCGR (1). GPCRs constitute the largest protein superfamily and the most various group of all membrane receptors in human genome, and they transmit a broad spectrum of extracellular signals in cell physiology and homeostasis (2, 3). Receptors belonging to the GPCRs are distinguished by the presence of transmembrane domain built of seven α-helices and coupling with G proteins responsible for the signal transduction following the activation of receptor with corresponding ligand. Due to their structure, one could define three areas of the protein: the extracellular domain (*N*-terminus and three extracellular loops), transmembrane domain, and the intracellular domain (three intracellular loops as well as the *C*-terminus) (4). Glycoprotein receptors differ from other class A GPCRs due to the presence of large *N*-terminal domain (exodomain) within which the ligand-binding site is located (5, 6). Their exodomain is composed of nine subdomains containing leucine-rich repeats (LRR) as well as cysteine-rich subdomains located at the *C*- and *N*-terminus of this domain, respectively (7).

Binding of LH/hCG, TSH or FSH to their cognate receptors results in activation of intracellular signaling pathways which in turn leads to the stimulation of cell growth, differentiation, and proliferation. In the case of FSHR and LHCGR, the cyclic AMP (cAMP) pathway plays a major role in intracellular signaling and it involves the coupling of receptor with $G_{\alpha s}$ protein that is responsible for activation of adenylyl cyclase and thereby an increased level of cAMP. Aside from the cAMP pathway, other signaling pathways can be distinguished herein, including the extracellular regulated kinases (ERKs), phosphatidylinositol-3 kinase (PI3K), protein kinase B (PKB), p38 mitogen-activated protein kinases (MAPKs), and protein kinase C (PKC) pathways (8, 9). Although not all of them are solely G protein-dependent, such as the ERK pathway which can also be activated via β-arrestins (10).

The major expression sites of FSHR, posing the subject of this review article, constitute Sertoli cells in the testis and granulosa cells in the ovary (11). Extragonadal FSHR expression has been detected in a variety of other cell types and tissues including osteoclasts (12, 13), human umbilical vein endothelial cells (14), monocytes (15, 16), female reproductive tract (17), and liver (18), although the functional and physiological significance of this is debatable (19). FSH stimulates estrogen production by granulosa cells, the growth and maturation of ovarian follicles as well as it regulates the ovulatory cycle, whereas in males it induces the secretion of androgen-binding protein, stimulates Sertoli cells and thereby the spermatogenesis process (5).

In the last one and a half decades, GPCRs have been found to form functional oligomers composed of two or more receptors (20). Furthermore, these protomers are built of either one type or different types of GPCRs, thus they can form homo- and/or heterodimers. The significance of GPCR oligomerization for proper cellular functioning consists in regulation of intracellular signaling via diversification and/or modulation of the signal, as well as during biosynthesis and desensitization. Presumably, monomers and oligomers remain in equilibrium, thus enabling the control of ligand action and intracellular signaling in response to ligand binding (21).

GPCRs OLIGOMERIZATION

Oligomerization is a term used to describe the GPCR complexes composed of two (dimers), three (trimers) or higher number of protomers. Heretofore, a number of reports have been published about the formation of oligomers by receptors belonging to different classes of the GPCR family. Among the oligomers, we can distinguish homomers created by receptors of the same type, as well as heteromers composed of various closely related types of GPCRs (21). GPCRs must fulfill certain conditions to be classified as heteromers such as colocalization and physical interaction between protomers (**Figure 1A**). Additionally, they should be distinguished by acquisition of new properties, absence of monomers, or the loss of the characteristics typical for single protomers (22).

The first mention of presumable dimerization by GPCRs dates from the 1980s and it comes from the work of Birdsall (23). This conclusion was derived from experimental observations carried out by another research group several years earlier, where decreased binding affinity of β2 adrenergic receptor (β2AR) in the presence of GTP was noticed. Further treatment with methacholine, being the agonist for muscarinic cholinergic receptor, restored the binding affinity of β2AR, suggesting that the ligand binding by one receptor may affect the binding affinity of other receptor (24).

The first tangible evidence confirming the existence of oligomers among members of GPCRs family concerned mainly the C class of GPCRs, as several of these receptors are *forced oligomers*—they need to form oligomers to function (25). Co-immunoprecipitation studies performed by Romano et al. showed that metabotropic glutamate receptors (mGluRs) form dimers through the presence of one or more intermolecular disulphide bridges within the extracellular domain (26, 27). Yet, later they discovered that covalent dimerization is not a prerequisite for ligand binding but mGluRs form a non-covalent dimers in the absence of disulphide bridges (28). Simultaneously, the group led by Julia H. White studied the metabotropic γ-aminobutyric acid receptor, which was found to heterodimerize by two polypeptide chains within the carboxyl terminus, and its heterodimerization is required for its proper membrane expression as well as ligand binding affinity (29). Methodological developments have made possible to study oligomerization of GPCRs in more detail (see section *Methods to investigate the oligomerization of FSHR* for a better description of methods). For example, bioluminescence resonance energy transfer (BRET) was used by the group of Ali Salahpour for studying the homodimerization of β2AR. The researchers created β2AR mutants either carrying an endoplasmic reticulum (ER)-retention signal or lacking the ER-export motif as well as mutants with disturbed putative dimerization motif. All of the aforementioned mutant receptors formed dimers with the WT receptors, thus they inhibited the transport of WT β2AR to the cell membrane (30).

The abovementioned examples as well as many other dimer-forming C class of GPCRs provided evidence that made possible to ascertain that receptor dimerization is of vital importance for receptor functionality. Moreover, they have provided evidence for the existence of both homomerization and heteromerization at multiple levels in their live cycles. Homomerization of β2AR constitute an example of dimerization at the protein synthesis level. Alteration of one protomer results in inhibition of dimer trafficking, thus it prevents the expression of abnormal receptor on the cell membrane. Hence, dimerization seems to

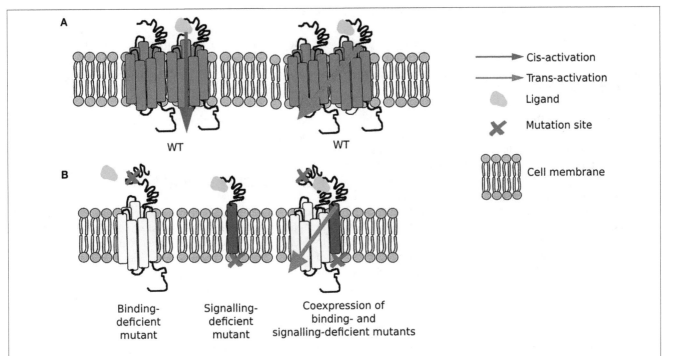

FIGURE 1 | Schematic representation of possible options for GPCR activation **(A)** The function of the wild-type (WT) receptor is possible due to either cis-activation or trans-activation. **(B)** Two mutant receptors, a binding-deficient and a signaling-deficient are unable to function separately. Nonetheless, when they are co-expressed, they interact together and form a functional complex as a result of transactivation.

occasionally be a quality control mechanism during biosynthesis (31). Di/oligomerization may also occur during the next stages of receptor biosynthesis, such as protein maturation at Golgi apparatus as well as following ligand binding and activation of mature receptor on the plasma membrane (32).

Oligomer formation involves different regions of GPCRs with the special contribution of transmembrane domains and extracellular domains among receptors with large exodomains (31). Di- or oligomerization divided opinions: those who claimed there were no di/oligomers (seen as biochemical artifacts), those saying that di/oligomers existed but had no effect, and those that professed that only di/oligomers were functional. As often in biological systems, there was no single answer, instead more than 15 years of active research provided evidence that while some GPCRs work as monomers (*cis*-activation), others work in congregates, and others do both. What was less expected was the number of combinations these receptors can create, in particular at hetero-dimers/hetero-oligomers rendezvous. These aggregates often result in *allosteric modulation*—where the activation of one receptor can modify the affinity or responses of the second receptor to its ligand; or in the activation of (an) unliganded receptor(s) by the activation of another (or several) neighboring receptor(s)—this latter sequential signal activation is often called *receptor trans-activation*.

As many other GPCRs, the glycoprotein hormone receptors (LHCGR, TSHR and FSHR) have also been found to self-associate as well as to form heterodimers with other GPCRs (32–37). Moreover, the glycoprotein hormone receptors are also able

to trans-activate, often in what seems to be another example of the regulatory mechanism for intracellular signaling via signal selection (38).

GPCRs TRANS-ACTIVATION

The first report on GPCR trans-activation was published by Daub et al. in (39), where they found that the epidermal growth factor receptor (EGFR), not a GPCR, became tyrosine-phosphorylated when rat fibroblasts were stimulated with GPCR agonists such as thrombin, endothelin-1 and lysoposphatic acid. These results provided evidence that the activation of a GPCR may result in the activation of another receptor, not necessarily another member of GPCR family (39).

It is worth mentioning that initially only *cis*-activation of GPCRs was postulated, meaning the activation of a single receptor (monomer) upon ligand binding (38). The phenomenon of trans-activation on the other hand, involves the interaction of two receptors either of the same type or different type. The earliest reports on GPCR trans-activation found that the ligand to one GPCR, e.g., muscarinic receptor, could alter, by binding to its own receptor, the affinity of a neighboring receptor e.g., β2AR for its own ligand (24). With the advent of molecular biology, the search for interacting GPCRs began, with unexpectedly large numbers of receptors found in dimers or higher order oligomers (20). The next problems to solve were to understand how these interactions affect the receptors, how to map the interacting domains between receptors, and whether oligomerization equals trans-activation (38).

Trans-activation of GPCRs has then been further elucidated by many elegant experiments using chimeric or mutant receptors, where only the presence of two complementary receptors would trigger downstream signaling (40). Large part of the interactions between heterodimeric receptors have been mapped to their transmembrane helices and C-terminal tails (29, 31).

FSHR Trans-activation

Unlike other class A GPCRs, the glycoprotein hormone receptors (TSHR, LHCGR, and FSHR) have a very large extracellular N-terminal that is responsible for binding their respective hormones (41, 42). Such large extracellular binding arm could potentially reach another uncoupled receptor in a close proximity. In an attempt to test its feasibility, the group of Tae Ji generated a series of chimeric LHCGRs (37), and later on FSHRs (36), where the large N-terminal was fused to a membrane protein while a binding-deficient receptor was used as acceptor to transmit downstream signaling. The first set of mutants involved changes in the LRR of the LHCGR (or LHR as in some cases the mouse or rat LHR was used) as non-binding mutants, yet these still possess the intact transmembrane and intracellular domains to convey signaling. The first LHR signal-deficient mutant was created by substitution of lysine to arginine at position 605 of the polypeptide chain (initially referred as K578R due to old nomenclature). The co-expression of these two mutants in HEK293 cells resulted in binding of hCG, by the signal-deficient mutant, with the same affinity as in the case of the LHR WT, and a concomitant cAMP generation of about 30% of that of WT LHR via trans-activation of the binding-deficient mutant (37, 43).

Two years later, the same group of researchers created several FSHR constructs—some binding-deficient and the other signal-deficient. For the latter, the exodomain of FSHR (exoFSHR) was fused with either the glycosyl phosphatidylinositol (exoGPI) or the transmembrane domain of CD8 receptor (exoCD) (**Figure 1B**). Afterwards, stable lines expressing the signal-deficient FSHR mutants were transiently transfected with one of the plasmids encoding the exo-FSHR. The results revealed that a binding-deficient receptor could be trans-activated by signaling-deficient receptors. Unexpectedly, exoFSHR-GPI was able to activate the binding-deficient mutants FSHR[P24A], FSHR[D26A], and FSHR[F36A] only via the cAMP pathway, whereas trans-activation of FSHR[L27A] resulted in no cAMP but only activation of the IP signaling pathway. This form of trans-activation, subsequently named *intermolecular cooperation* to differentiate from the TMD-TMD trans-activation, maintains its specificity as the exo-FSHR could not trans-activate the LHR (36). Similar results were obtained by the group led by Jeoung (38).

Intermolecular cooperation was further tested in mice, using the *LHR* knockout mice (LuRKO), to avoid cofounding effects by the presence of the WT LHR, and signal-deficient and binding-deficient mutant LHRs. The expression of the two mutants was able to partly rescue LHR signaling, and generate measurable levels of testosterone, which was enough to rescue the fertility of male mice (40). Although, these experiments were performed using the LHR, one could speculate, due to their structural similarities and previous results *in vitro*, that the FSHR would

be able to do the same. Evidence supporting intermolecular cooperation continuous to accumulate over the years (44, 45).

One lesson we can learn from intermolecular cooperation is that a ligand-exodomain is sometimes able to activate single pathways on the binding-deficient receptor, pointing out that GPCRs have different *switches* for triggering different pathways. This is a major focus in pharmacology where the search for compounds that trigger bias signaling is of clinical importance.

FSHR BIASED SIGNALING

Another interesting issue related to trans-activation constitutes the phenomenon of *biased signaling*. Nevertheless, in order to be able to expound the biased signaling in the context of the FSHR, it is necessary to first clarify this term and take into account the entire GPCR family. GPCRs adopt multiple conformational states, both active and inactive. Each conformation is associated with different signaling pathway, and thus various downstream effects (46). Therefore, the presence of one particular conformational state can lead to the recruitment of G proteins and/or β-arrestins and thus lead to the activation of different signaling pathways (**Figure 2**). Furthermore, biased signaling may also be considered for the strength to which the signaling pathways are activated. Biased agonism occurs when binding of certain ligands to a GPCR results in transduction of different intracellular signaling to varying extents. Although most of the studies on GPCR biased signaling have been carried out on the β2AR and angiotensin receptors, it is speculated that this phenomenon concerns the vast majority of GPCR family (46, 47).

In the case of FSHR, we can distinguish three main types of biased signaling. The first type may occur due to the attachment of small chemical ligands to the FSHR transmembrane domain resulting in a stabilization of conformation and thus leading to biased signaling. This category of biased signaling arises greatest interest in the scientific community due to its therapeutic potential. The second type constitutes a consequence of modifications in the receptor structure due to the presence of mutation or polymorphism. In turn, the last type, also referred as *conditional effectiveness*, is caused by the presence of interacting proteins in the same environment as the FSHR (48). All these are of physiological and clinical importance as we will discuss below.

Clinical treatment using hormones is associated with the presence of a wide range of side effects resulting from the activation of multiple signaling pathways. Therefore, the possibility of influencing single signaling pathways constitutes another useful tool during research aimed at eliminating the side effects of hormone therapy (36).

With the above in mind, a high throughput screen for FSHR modulators that induce biased signaling was carried out by the group led by James A. Dias in collaboration with Addex Pharmaceuticals. They identified a small chemical molecule referred as ADX61623 which behaves as a negative allosteric modulator (NAM) of FSHR. When FSH and ADX61623 were simultaneously bound to the FSHR of rat granulosa primary cells, no cAMP nor progesterone production but

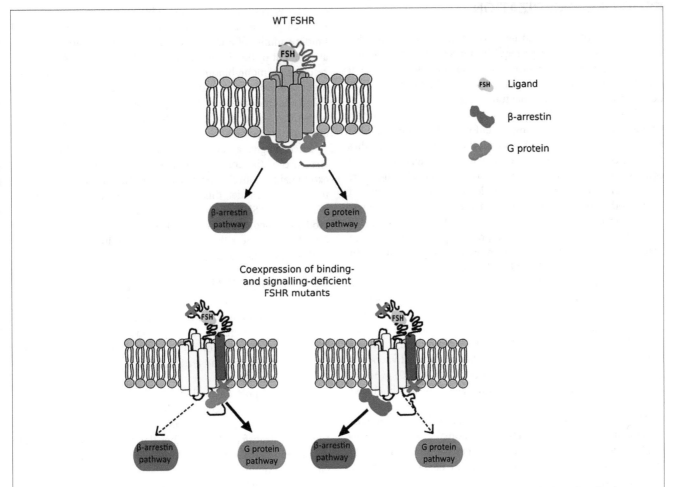

FIGURE 2 | Scheme illustrating the FSHR biased signaling. The upper part of the figure presents the G protein-dependent and β-arrestin-dependent signal transduction of the wild-type FSHR. The lower part of the figure shows the bias toward either the G protein-dependent pathway **(left)** or the β-arrestin pathway **(right)** when a binding-deficient and a signal-deficient FSHR are co-expressed.

concurrent estrogen production occurred. Nonetheless, *in vivo* studies carried out on female rats did not find any effect in follicular development (49). Three years later, the same research group described two new NAMs, structurally similar to ADX61623, termed ADX68692 and ADX68693. Whilst ADX68692 effectively inhibited cAMP, progesterone production and oestradiol synthesis in rat granulosa cells, as well as follicular growth in female rats, ADX68693 blocked cAMP and progesterone production but it was ineffectual in the case of oestradiol and *in vivo* experiments (50, 51).

In addition to studies focused on NAMs and their potential use in contraception, attention was also devoted to development of a positive allosteric modulators (PAMs) aimed for the treatment of infertility. Sriraman et al. discovered the efficacy of a thiazolidinone derivative as a PAM of FSHR. The treatment of rat granulosa cell line with aforementioned compound resulted in activation of ERK/Akt pathways and increased production of oestradiol. The latter was also present in the case of human granulosa cell line treated with this compound. Furthermore,

stimulation of cultured preantral follicles with the thiazolidinone derivative triggered their maturation, in line with its FSH-like properties. Although, this compound has high genotoxicity and unfavorable pharmacokinetics and oral availability (52).

FSHR biased signaling was first identified in clinical samples by Aittomaki et al. in 1995 as the cause of hereditary hypergonadotropic ovarian failure in women and subfertility in men. A mutation at position 189, alanine to valine A189V, caused complete suppression of cAMP/PKA pathway, whereas it induced the ERK/MAPK pathway (53). Detailed *in vitro* experiments found that FSHR-A189V-induced ERK phosphorylation via β-arrestins (54), and that this was the result of the number of membrane-localized receptors—since an increase of receptor number in the presence of phosphodiesterase inhibitors resulted in elevated cAMP generation via G proteins. Thus, this suggests that the density of FSHRs affects the biased signaling where activation of G proteins requires a higher density of the FSHRs than those required by β-arrestins (55).

FSHR OLIGOMERIZATION

In the case of rhodopsin-like receptors, class A GPCRs, oligomerization is not a prerequisite for signaling occurrence, but it constitutes another form of its regulatory mechanism that can affect membrane expression of the receptor, ligand binding, desensitization as well as signal transduction (21).

FSHR oligomerization was first observed on the surface of Chinese hamster ovary using a confocal microscope in 1994 (56). However, for further biochemical and biophysical studies it was necessary to wait for the development of techniques and equipment. Nevertheless, before the presence of FSHR oligomers was confirmed, a number of studies have been carried out on the other two glycoprotein hormone receptors. Oligomers formed by the LHCGR were first reported in studies carried out by Osuga et al. (54) They co-expressed the binding-deficient LHCGR and either the chimeric receptor composed of FSHR extracellular region and LHCGR transmembrane domain or N-terminally truncated LHCGR, thereby providing information on the interactions between the two receptors (54). Shortly thereafter, the presence of TSHR dimers and oligomers was observed in thyroid tissue using FRET (57). Tao et al. revealed that LHCGR self-associates and forms both dimers and oligomers (58). Other research groups have shown that activation of LHCGR with either of its ligands causes clustering (59), whereas in the case of TSHR, stimulation with agonist results in cluster dissociation (60).

The crystal structure of FSHR revealed a dimeric complex composed of FSH-bound FSHR exodomain, or hormone-binding domain, (FSH/FSHR$_{HB}$), suggesting that this dimer is, at least one of, the functional form of FSHR. The atomic organization also showed that FSHR oligomers are formed via hydrophobic interactions between LRR 2–4 (42). Next was to find FSHR oligomers in cells, which was firstly reported by the group of Richard M. Thomas, involving complementary coimmunoprecipitation of Myc- and FLAG-tagged FSHRs. This revealed the presence of FSHR oligomers in the ER, suggesting that the formation of FSHR oligomers takes place at the early stages of the biosynthesis of this receptor. Unlike the LHCGR and TSHR, the FSHR oligomers seem to be barely affected by ligand stimulation. An additional peculiarity of the FSHR, as compared to other glycoprotein receptors, is that its C-terminal is proteolytically processed just as oligomerization during protein biosynthesis—which was a limitation to tag this receptor using fluorescent proteins at its C-terminus (61). The constitutive formation of FSHR oligomers during the protein biosynthesis was confirmed by the group led by Rongbin Guan. They have also showed that the exodomain and the serpentine region are involved in the oligomerization (62). The issue of inserting a tag or florescent protein fusion to the C-terminus of FSHR was solved by Mazurkiewicz et al. by creating a construct in which the C-terminus of FSHR was replaced by that of the LHR, to which the fluorescent protein (FP) was subsequently joined to form the FSHR-LHRcT-FP chimera (63).

Another indication of FSHR homomerization, and one that suggests functional consequences, constitutes the phenomenon of negative cooperativity reported by a number of independent research groups. This allosteric mechanism involves decreased binding affinity of one homodimer-forming receptor due to the attachment of the ligand to the second protomer (64, 65). As a result of hormone-binding by FSHR, conformational changes in the receptor occur (65). As mentioned above, the existence of the FSHR oligomerization is also fully supported by the phenomenon of its trans-activation and intramolecular cooperation described, among others, by Ji et al. (36).

Interestingly, a few years after revealing the first crystal structure of the complex built of FSH and part of the FSHR exodomain, a novel crystal structure was unveiled. In contrast to the earlier model, this one includes the entire exodomain of FSHR (FSH-FSHR$_{ED}$ complex) as well as a hinge region. This model revealed the presence of trimers in an asymmetrical unit (66) that can bind either one molecule of fully glycosylated FSH or three molecules of deglycosylated FSH (67).

FSHR/LHCGR Heteromerization

In addition to the self-association of FSHR, this receptor also heteromerizes (**Figure 3**). While in testes the FSHR and LHCGR are expressed in different cells types, in the ovary both receptors are expressed at least in one cell type—granulosa cells. Therefore, the heteromerization and cross-talk between these two receptors is of particular interest.

The first report on the heteromerization between the FSHR and LHCGR was made as a result of an experiment carried out by Feng et al. (65) in 2013. In that study, HEK293 cells were transiently transfected with either the hFSHR-Renilla luciferase (RLuc) and LHCGR-GFP pair or the LHCGR-RLuc and hFSHR-GFP pair. Importantly, the expression of the RLuc constructs was constant, whereas the expression the GFP^2 constructs was incremented. Following co-transfection of HEK293 cells, BRET was performed showing that the FSHR and LHCGR form heteromers on the cell membrane. Interestingly, dimerization of LHCGR with FSHR resulted in the attenuation of the cAMP production upon stimulation with either hCG or LH, whereas FSH stimulation led to the attenuation of cAMP production (**Figure 4**). Therefore, the results of this study show that heteromerization between these two receptors occurs and that it leads to the attenuation of hormone-dependent signaling. This is physiologically relevant since these two receptors play essential roles in signal regulation in mature granulosa cells in ovaries (68).

The work of Mazurkiewicz et al. provided another evidence of FSHR/LHCGR heteromerization. HEK293 cells co-transfected with a pair of constructs—hFSHR-rLHR-cT-mCherry and LHR-YFP, revealed the presence of FSHR/LHCGR heteromers on the plasma membrane by FRET, thereby confirming previous reports (63).

More detailed reports on FSHR/LHCGR heteromerization suggest that LHCGR couples with the G$_{\alpha q/11}$ protein that activates phospholipase C. That in turn lead to increased concentration of intracellular diacyl glycerol and inositol phosphates triggering the release of Ca^{2+}. Nonetheless, the G$_{\alpha q/11}$-Ca^{2+} signaling is induced only under conditions of high LHCGR membrane expression and high hormone

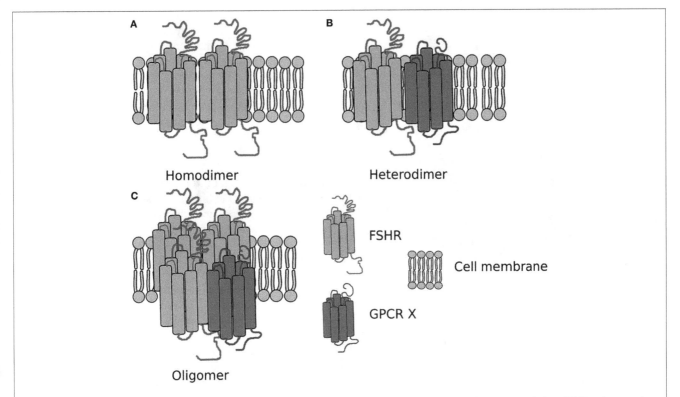

FIGURE 3 | Scheme showing the FSHR complexes. (A) Homodimer composed of two FSHR protomers. (B) Heterodimer composed of one FSHR protomer and one different GPCR X protomer. (C) Oligomer composed of FSHR protomers and one different GPCR protomer (in ratio 3:1).

concentrations. HEK293 transiently transfected with either HA-FSHR or FLAG-LHCGR or both plasmids simultaneously, established that only co-expression of both receptors simultaneously induced a sustained LH-induced Ca^{2+} release, showing that the non-liganded FSHR is able to disrupt the $G_{\alpha q/11}$-dependent Ca^{2+} signaling of engaged LHCGR. Primary human granulosa cell line expressing both receptors resulted in similar results to those derived from the experiment with HEK293 cells. The LHCGR/FSHR crosstalk is able to alter LHCGR signaling, presumably constituting a regulatory mechanism of the functions of granulosa cells (69).

The phenomenon of FSHR/LHCGR heteromerization seems to play an important role in terms of antral follicular development. A recently suggested model infers that low expression of LHCGR is yet noticeable during the FSH/FSHR-dependent early antral stages (Figure 4). At the time, both receptors form heteromers, and binding of FSH to its cognate receptor results in the trans-activation of LHCGR in an environment of very low LH. Low LH is likely required for keeping LHCGR-expressing theca cells under low steroidogenesis while proper follicular selection occurs. Therefore, FSHR/LHCGR crosstalk in granulosa cells may explain their steroidogenic activity at this stage of folliculogenesis, an activity otherwise associated to LH-activation in large antral stages (70). Clinical and *in vivo* studies will help to elucidate some of the remaining unsolved conundrums in folliculogenesis and its relation with FSHR/LHCGR interactions.

Methods to Investigate the Oligomerization of FSHR

Oligomerization and trans-activation of GPCRs have taken long to be widely accepted, due to (partly) the need for novel techniques and equipment such as super-resolution microscopy, to visualize these molecules with enough definition. One of the first and most common methods used to study GPCR oligomerization was co-immunoprecipitation (co-IP) (64). This is a technique that allows the precipitation of protein complexes using specific binding antibodies, followed by visualization with SDS-PAGE and Western Blotting. The advantages of co-IP include relatively low costs and its simplicity. The key issue for the widespread use of co-IP for detection of GPCRs homo- and heterodimers was the cloning of epitope-tags on GPCRs (71). However, co-IP requires many controls to rule out non-specific aggregation, non-specific antibody binding and appropriate lysis protocols. An additional limitation of this method is the lack of specific antibodies recognizing endogenous GPCRs (64, 72, 73). Co-IP has been used to detect many oligomeric complexes, including Myc- and FLAG-tagged FSHRs. Discovering that FSHR forms oligomers at the early stages of biosynthesis as mentioned above (61).

Another biochemical method allowing the electrophoretic separation of intact protein complexes is Blue Native Electrophoresis (BN-PAGE). This method is characterized by the use of non-denaturing detergents that do not affect

212

Reproductive Medicine: Role of Follicle Stimulating Hormone

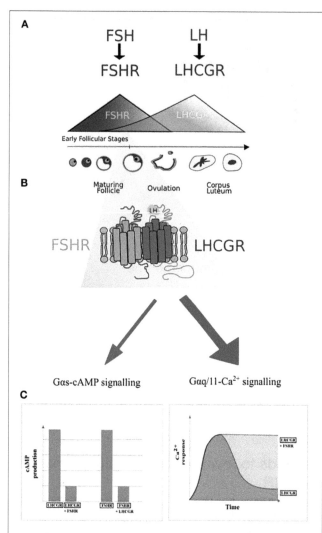

FIGURE 4 | Schematic representation of FSHR and LHCGR expression in the ovarian granulosa cells during the menstrual cycle. **(A)** The domination of FSHR expression is noticeable during the first half of the cycle, while the second half of the cycle is dominated by the LHCGR expression. However, small expression of the LHCGR receptor is present during the early follicular stages. **(B)** During the simultaneous expression of LHCGR and FSHR both receptors form heterodimers. **(C)** Co-expression of liganded LHCGR and non-liganded FSHR results in either decreased cAMP production or prolonged Ca^{2+} release in LHCGR.

another at a distance no >100 Å. An additional condition for the occurrence of this phenomenon is the overlap of the emission spectrum of the donor molecule and the excitation spectrum of the acceptor molecule. The most frequent donor-acceptor pair is GFP and one of its variant with different spectral characteristics (78, 79). Using FRET it is possible to detect both ligand-induced signal transduction of GPCR (80), activation of GPCR in response to ligands (81) and GPCR oligomerization (82). In FRET studies two different GFP variants, meeting the energy transfer conditions, are linked to the same or different type of GPCRs or GPCR and their corresponding ligands. Detection of the ratio of donor:acceptor protein emission spectrum indicates the interaction between the proteins tested. Nonetheless, the fluorescent proteins used in this method are relatively large, which can affect the interaction or function of the proteins (83). In addition, accuracy of measurements can be affected by bleed-through, background signals, cross-talk and photobleaching (83, 84). This method has been used repeatedly for studies on oligomerization of the full-length native FSHR. The use of specific monoclonal antibodies or Fab fragments that have been tagged with various fluorophores has shown that FSHRs are present as oligomers on the plasma membrane (61).

Some of the limitations of FRET have been solved by Time Resolved FRET (TR-FRET), which is based on the use of a fluorescent donor containing lanthanides. Terbium and europium are characterized by long-lasting fluorescent light emission. This results in a significant reduction in noise, and thus a higher signal-to-noise ratio. These elements are trapped in stable cryptates that absorb light and transfer energy to the lanthanide (85, 86). Receptors can be tagged non-covalently using antibodies or covalently using tag proteins such as SNAP, CLIP or Halotag. If the labeled receptors form dimers, the tags are located close to each other and a TR-FRET signal is generated (87).

Bioluminescence resonance energy transfer (BRET) is the transfer of energy from a luminescent donor to a fluorescent protein as an acceptor. Depending on the type of substrate, the luciferase and the fluorescent protein, the BRET method can be divided into: BRET1, BRET2, BRET3, eBRET, and QD-BRET (88). In first generation of BRET (BRET1), the energy transfer pairing was the most popular bioluminescent protein—RLuc and enhanced yellow fluorescent protein (eYFP). The substrate of RLuc is coelenterazine (71, 89). Nevertheless, the BRET1 system is distinguished by the presence of a high background due to the bleed-through of donor emission peak at the acceptor emission wavelength. Therefore, the second generation of BRET (BRET2) was developed with a better separation of the acceptor and donor spectra in comparison to BRET1. This was achieved by the use of different substrate, referred as DeepBlueC, which is an analog of coelenterazine that is characterized by lower emission interference with the acceptor, better biophysical properties, cell permeability as well as reduced toxicity. DeepBlueC is used with modified GPF2 instead of eYFP. Nonetheless, DeepBlueC has some disadvantages that include its short lifetime and low light emission. In the third generation of BRET (BRET3) the firefly luciferase is used as a donor, while various types of fluorescent proteins that are excited by the wavelength emitted by luciferase

the quaternary structure of proteins, unlike SDS. In addition, Coomassie Blue dye gives the proteins a negative charge and prevents non-specific protein aggregation during electrophoresis. Visualization of the examined types of GPCR is possible by means of immunoblotting (74, 75). The use of this method allows simple determination of the proportion of different oligomeric types of GPCR (76).

Förster resonance energy transfer (FRET) is a method for studying the interaction between proteins in a living cell. The phenomenon of resonance energy transfer between donor and acceptor was pioneered by Förster (77). Non-radiative energy transfer occurs between one excited fluorescent protein and

(565 nm) are used as acceptors. Other types of BRET constitute extended BRET (eBRET) that enables to monitor experiments in real-time using coelentrazine as well as QD-BRET based on the use of quantum dots (90, 91). Compared with FRET, the advantage in favor of this method is that there is no need to use a light source to excite the donor and thus no-photobleaching. However, BRET is characterized by low sensitivity and to be unable to determine the location of the signal in a cell (71). BRET is a method enabling the study of oligomerization (92) and GPCR interactions with other proteins as well as receptor signaling and activation (90).

Determining the structure GPCR is performed by X-Ray crystallography. This method can contribute to the increase of our knowledge about the ligand-receptor and receptor-effector protein interactions, as well as GPCR oligomerization. However, care should be taken as some of these interfaces might be artificial and potentially may not represent a functional biological assembly (91).

Beside the methods to detect protein-protein interaction, the raise of biosensors and assays to analyze secondary metabolites and signaling players have been vital to determine the functionality of oligomers and complementing receptors (91, 93–95).

CONCLUSIONS

The last several years of research centered around the FSHR shed new light on the processes of its biosynthesis, maturation, membrane expression, activation and intracellular signaling. In this review we have discussed the evidence on the existence of trans-activation, oligomerization and biased signaling of the FSHR. Oligomerization studies revealed that the FSHR is present not only as a monomer, but it also forms higher-order complexes such as homo- and heteromers (with the LHCGR). Homomerization occurring during the protein biosynthesis constitutes the quality control checkpoint at the ER level. The discovery of FSHR oligomers resulted in further dissecting the interaction between receptors, which led to the conclusion that the FSHR can be activated not only via cis- but also trans-activation. Furthermore, trans-activation studies have also provided evidence for the existence of biased FSHR signaling at various levels. All aforementioned phenomena constitute FSHR

regulatory mechanisms of intracellular signaling control through the determination, modification and fine-tuning of the signal.

Better insight in the molecular mechanisms and functioning of the FSHR may contribute to the development of new drugs to trigger single signaling pathways. Furthermore, it is worth noting that the importance of FSHR/LHCGR heteromerization is mainly due to their co-expression on the surface of granulosa cells and the participation of both receptors in the ovulation process. The expression of FSHR and LHCGR on the plasma membrane as well as the level of gonadotropins fluctuate during the menstrual cycle—the FSH/FSHR prevails during the first phase of the cycle, whereas the second phase is dominated by the LH/LHCGR. The expression of FSHR is induced at the beginning of the menstrual cycle and then decreases with the maturation of the ovarian follicle. Afterwards, the expression of *LHCGR* is induced due to the FSH-stimulation, via the FSHR, plus other factors. Following this, the LHCGR expression decreases upon desensitization by LH surge (**Figure 4**) (96). It is believed that the crosstalk between both receptors is responsible for switching the dominance between the FSHR and LHCGR expression during the cycle as a result of affecting the LHCGR and LH signaling (69). Therefore, disturbed interactions between FSHR and LHCGR may cause the development of several diseases. Presumably, crosstalk disturbances may lead to the overexpression of LHCGR and thus to the development of polycystic ovary syndrome (97, 98).

AUTHOR CONTRIBUTIONS

KS and AR-M outlined the manuscript. KS, JK, AP, BP, and MK collected the information and co-wrote the manuscript. GA and KS made the graphical work. AR-M coordinated the work and supervised the accuracy of the information. All authors critically read and approved the manuscript.

FUNDING

Our work as well as salaries, open access fees, are supported by the Polish National Science Centre (NCN): (1) DEC-2015/17/B/NZ1/01777; (2) DEC-2017/01/X/NZ1/00107, and (3) DEC-2017/25/B/NZ4/02364.

REFERENCES

1. Jiang X, Dias JA, He X. Structural biology of glycoprotein hormones and their receptors: insights to signaling. *Mol Cell Endocrinol.* (2014) 382:424–51. doi: 10.1016/j.mce.2013.08.021
2. Zhang Y, Devries ME, Skolnick J. Structure modeling of all identified G protein-coupled receptors in the human genome. *PLoS Comput Biol.* (2006) 2:e13. doi: 10.1371/journal.pcbi.0020013
3. Jonas KC, Rivero-Müller A, Huhtaniemi IT, Hanyaloglu AC. G protein-coupled receptor transactivation. From molecules to mice. *Methods Cell Biol.* (2013) 117:433–50. doi: 10.1016/B978-0-12-408143-7.00023-2
4. Menon KMJ, Menon B. Structure, function and regulation of gonadotropin receptors - a perspective. *Mol Cell Endocrinol.* (2012) 356:88–97. doi: 10.1016/j.mce.2012.01.021
5. Ulloa-Aguirre A, Timossi C. Structure-function relationship of follicle-stimulating hormone and its receptor. *Hum Reprod Update* (1998) 4:260–83. doi: 10.1093/humupd/4.3.260
6. Themmen APN, Huhtaniemi IT. Mutations of gonadotropins and gonadotropin receptors: elucidating the physiology and pathophysiology of pituitary-gonadal function. *Endocr Rev.* (2000) 21:551–83. doi: 10.1210/edrv.21.5.0409
7. Vischer HF, Granneman JCM, Bogerd J. Opposite contribution of two ligand-selective determinants in the N-terminal hormone-binding exodomain of human gonadotropin receptors. *Mol Endocrinol.* (2003) 17:1972–81. doi: 10.1210/me.2003-0172
8. Ulloa-Aguirre A, Reiter E, Bousfield G, Dias JA, Huhtaniemi I. Chapter two – constitutive activity in gonadotropin receptors. *Adv Pharmacol.* (2014) 70:37–80. doi: 10.1016/B978-0-12-417197-8.00002-X

9. Hunzicker-Dunn M, Maizels ET. FSH signaling pathways in immature granulosa cells that regulate target gene expression: branching out from protein kinase A. *Cell Signal.* (2006) 18:1351–9. doi: 10.1016/j.cellsig.2006.02.011

10. Kara E, Cre P, Gauthier C, Martinat N, Piketty V, Guillou F, et al. A phosphorylation cluster of five serine and threonine residues in the C-terminus of the follicle-stimulating hormone receptor is important for desensitization but not for β -arrestin-mediated ERK activation. *Mol Endocrinol.* (2011) 20:3014–26. doi: 10.1210/me.2006-0098

11. Simoni M, Gromoll J, Nieschlag E. The follicle-stimulating hormone receptor : biochemistry, molecular biology, physiology, and pathophysiology. *Endocr Rev.* (1997) 18:739–73.

12. Sun L, Peng Y, Sharrow AC, Iqbal J, Zhang Z, Papachristou DJ, et al. FSH directly regulates bone mass. *Cell* (2006) 125:247–60. doi: 10.1016/j.cell.2006.01.051

13. Sun L, Zhang Z, Zhu LL, Peng Y, Liu X, Li J, et al. Further evidence for direct pro-resorptive actions of FSH. *Biochem Biophys Res Commun.* (2010) 394:6–11. doi: 10.1016/j.bbrc.2010.02.113

14. Stilley JA, Guan R, Duffy DM, Segaloff DL. Signaling through FSH receptors on human umbilical vein endothelial cells promotes angiogenesis. *J Clin Endocrinol Metab.* (2014) 99:E813–20. doi: 10.1210/jc.2013-3186

15. Cannon JG, Kraj B, Sloan G. Follicle-stimulating hormone promotes RANK expression on human monocytes. *Cytokine* (2011) 53:141–4. doi: 10.1016/j.cyto.2010.11.011

16. Robinson LJ, Tourkova I, Wang Y, Sharrow AC, Michael S, Yaroslavskiy BB, et al. FSH-receptor isoforms and FSH-dependent gene transcription in human monocytes and osteoclasts. *Biochem Biophys Res Commun.* (2010) 394:12–7. doi: 10.1016/j.bbrc.2010.02.112

17. Stilley JAW, Christensen DE, Dahlem KB, Guan R, Santillan DA, England SK, et al. FSH receptor (FSHR) expression in human extragonadal reproductive tissues and the developing placenta, and the impact of its deletion on pregnancy in mice. *Biol Reprod.* (2014) 91:1–15. doi: 10.1095/biolreprod.114.118562

18. Song Y, Wang ES, Xing LL, Shi S, Qu F, Zhang D, et al. Follicle-stimulating hormone induces postmenopausal dyslipidemia through inhibiting hepatic cholesterol metabolism. *J Clin Endocrinol Metab.* (2016) 101:254–63. doi: 10.1210/jc.2015-2724

19. Stelmaszewska J, Chrusciel M, Doroszko M, Akerfelt M, Ponikwicka-Tyszko D, Nees M, et al. Revisiting the expression and function of follicle-stimulation hormone receptor in human umbilical vein endothelial cells. *Sci Rep.* (2016) 6:1–12. doi: 10.1038/srep37095

20. Rivero-Müller A, Jonas KC, Hanyaloglu AC, Huhtaniemi I. Di/Oligomerization of GPCRs - mechanisms and functional significance. *Prog Mol Biol Transl Sci.* (2013) 117:163–85. doi: 10.1016/B978-0-12-386931-9.00007-6

21. Kleinau G, Müller A, Biebermann H. Oligomerization of GPCRs involved in endocrine regulation. *J Mol Endocrinol.* (2016) 57:R59–80. doi: 10.1530/JME-16-0049

22. Gomes I, Ayoub MA, Fujita W, Jaeger WC, Pfleger KD, Devi LA. G protein-coupled receptor heteromers. *Annu Rev Pharmacol Toxicol.* (2016) 56:403–25. doi: 10.1146/annurev-pharmtox-011613-135952

23. Birdsall NJM. Can different receptors interact directly with each other? *Trends Neurosci.* (1982) 5:137–8. doi: 10.1016/0166-2236(82)90081-9

24. Watanabe AM, Mcconnaughey MM, Strawbridge RA, Fleming JW, Besch HR. Muscarinic cholinergic receptor modulation of beta-adrenergic receptor affinity for catecholamines. *J Biol Chem.* (1978) 253:4833–6.

25. Dalrymple MB, Pfleger KDG, Eidne KA. G protein-coupled receptor dimers: functional consequences, disease states and drug targets. *Pharmacol Ther.* (2008) 118:359–71. doi: 10.1016/j.pharmthera.2008.03.004

26. Romano C, Yang WL, O'Malley KL. Metabotropic glutamate receptor 5 is a disulfide-linked dimer. *J Biol Chem.* (1996) 271:28612–6.

27. Marshall FH, Jones KA, Kaupmann K, Bettler B. GABA(B) receptors - the first 7TM heterodimers. *Trends Pharmacol Sci.* (1999) 20:396–9. doi: 10.1016/S0165-6147(99)01383-8

28. Romano C, Miller JK, Hyrc K, Dikranian S, Mennerick S, Takeuchi Y, et al. Covalent and noncovalent interactions mediate metabotropic glutamate receptor mGlu5 dimerization. *Mol Pharmacol.* (2001) 59:46–53. doi: 10.1124/mol.59.1.46

29. White JH, Wise A, Main MJ, Green A, Fraser NJ, Disney GH, et al. Heterodimerization is required for the formation of a functional GABA(B) receptor. *Nature* (1998) 396:679–82. doi: 10.1038/25354

30. Salahpour A, Angers S, Mercier JF, Lagacé M, Marullo S, Bouvier M. Homodimerization of the β2-adrenergic receptor as a prerequisite for cell surface targeting. *J Biol Chem.* (2004) 279:33390–7. doi: 10.1074/jbc.M403363200

31. Bulenger S, Marullo S, Bouvier M. Emerging role of homo- and heterodimerization in G-protein-coupled receptor biosynthesis and maturation. *Trends Pharmacol Sci.* (2005) 26:131–7. doi: 10.1016/j.tips.2005.01.004

32. Ulloa-Aguirre A, Zarinan T. The follitropin receptor: matching structure and function. *Mol Pharmacol.* (2016) 90:596–608. doi: 10.1124/mol.116.104398

33. Chen J, Ishii M, Wang L, Ishii K, Coughlin SR. Thrombin receptor activation. Confirmation of the intramolecular tethered liganding hypothesis and discovery of an alternative intermolecular liganding mode. *J Biol Chem.* (1994) 269:16041–5.

34. O'Brien PJ, Prevost N, Molino M, Hollinger MK, Woolkalis MJ, Woulfe DS, et al. Thrombin responses in human endothelial cells. Contributions from receptors other than PAR1 include the transactivation of PAR2 by thrombin-cleaved PAR1. *J Biol Chem.* (2000) 275:13502–9. doi: 10.1074/jbc.275.18.13502

35. Han Y, Moreira IS, Urizar E, Weinstein H, Jonathan A. Allosteric communication between protomers of dopamine Class A GPCR dimers modulates activation. *Nat Chem Biol.* (2009) 5:688–95. doi: 10.1038/nchembio.199

36. Ji I, Lee C, Jeoung M, Koo Y, Sievert GA, Ji TH. Trans -activation of mutant follicle-stimulating hormone receptors selectively generates only one of two hormone signals. *Mol Endocrinol.* (2004) 18:968–78. doi: 10.1210/me.2003-0443

37. Ji I. Cis- and trans-activation of hormone receptors: the LH receptor. *Mol Endocrinol.* (2002) 16:1299–308. doi: 10.1210/mend.16.6.0852

38. Jeoung M, Lee C, Ji I, Ji TH. Trans-activation, Cis-activation and signal selection of gonadotropin receptors. *Mol Cell Endocrinol.* (2007) 260–262:137–43. doi: 10.1016/j.mce.2005.09.015

39. Daub H, Weiss FU, Wallasch C, Ullrich A. Role of transactivation of the EGF receptor in signalling by G-protein-coupled receptors. *Nature* (1996) 379:557–60. doi: 10.1038/379557a0

40. Rivero-Müller A, Chou YY, Ji I, Lajic S, Hanyaloglu AC, Jonas K, et al. Rescue of defective G protein-coupled receptor function *in vivo* by intermolecular cooperation. *Proc Natl Acad Sci USA.* (2010) 107:2319–24. doi: 10.1073/pnas.0906695106

41. Smits G, Campillo M, Govaerts C, Janssens V, Richter C, Vassart G, et al. Glycoprotein hormone receptors: determinants in leucine-rich repeats responsible for ligand specificity. *EMBO J.* (2003) 22:2692–703. doi: 10.1093/emboj/cdg260

42. Fan QR, Hendrickson WA. Structure of human follicle-stimulating hormone in complex with its receptor. *Nature* (2005) 433:269–77. doi: 10.1038/nature03206

43. Lee C, Ji I, Ryu K, Song Y, Michael Conn P, Ji TH. Two defective heterozygous luteinizing hormone receptors can rescue hormone action. *J Biol Chem.* (2002) 277:15795–800. doi: 10.1074/jbc.M111818200

44. Jonas KC, Fanelli F, Huhtaniemi IT, Hanyaloglu AC. Single molecule analysis of functionally asymmetric G protein-coupled receptor (GPCR) oligomers reveals diverse spatial and structural assemblies. *J Biol Chem.* (2015) 290:3875–92. doi: 10.1074/jbc.M114.622498

45. Jonas KC, Huhtaniemi I, Hanyaloglu AC. Single-molecule resolution of G proteincoupled receptor (GPCR) complexes. *Methods Cell Biol.* (2016) 132:55–72. doi: 10.1016/bs.mcb.2015.11.005

46. Bologna Z, Teoh J, Bayoumi AS, Tang Y, Kim I. Biased G protein-coupled receptor signaling: new player in modulating physiology and pathology. *Biomol Ther.* (2017) 25:12–25. doi: 10.4062/biomolther.2016.165

47. Liu J, Horst R, Katritch V, Stevens R, Wuthrich K. Biased signalling pathways in beta2-adrenergic receptor characterized by 19F-NMR. *Science* (2013) 335:1106–10. doi: 10.1126/science.1215802

48. Landomiel F, Gallay N, Jégot G, Tranchant T, Durand G, Bourquard T, et al. Biased signalling in follicle stimulating hormone action. *Mol Cell Endocrinol.* (2014) 382:452–9. doi: 10.1016/j.mce.2013.09.035

49. Dias JA, Bonnet B, Weaver BA, Watts J, Kluetzman K, Thomas RM, et al. A negative allosteric modulator demonstrates biased antagonism of the follicle stimulating hormone receptor. *Moll Cell Endocrinol.* (2011) 333:143–50. doi: 10.1016/j.mce.2010.12.023

50. Dias JA, Campo B, Weaver BA, Watts J, Kluetzman K, Thomas RM, et al. Inhibition of follicle-stimulating hormone-induced preovulatory follicles in rats treated with a nonsteroidal negative allosteric modulator of follicle-stimulating hormone receptor[1]. *Biol Reprod.* (2014) 90:1–11. doi: 10.1095/biolreprod.113.109397

51. Ayoub MA, Yvinec R, Jégot G, Dias JA, Poli SM, Poupon A, et al. Profiling of FSHR negative allosteric modulators on LH/CGR reveals biased antagonism with implications in steroidogenesis. *Mol Cell Endocrinol.* (2016) 436:10–22. doi: 10.1016/j.mce.2016.07.013

52. Sriraman V, Denis D, De Matos D, Yu H, Palmer S, Nataraja S. Investigation of a thiazolidinone derivative as an allosteric modulator of follicle stimulating hormone receptor: evidence for its ability to support follicular development and ovulation. *Biochem Pharmacol.* (2014) 89:266–75. doi: 10.1016/j.bcp.2014.02.023

53. Aittomäki K, Lucena JL, Pakarinen P, Sistonen P, Tapanainen J, Gromoll J, et al. Mutation in the follicle-stimulating hormone receptor gene causes hereditary hypergonadotropic ovarian failure. *Cell* (1995) 82:959–68.

54. Osuga Y, Hayashi M, Kudo M, Conti M, Kobilka B, Hsueh AJW. Co-expression of defective luteinizing hormone receptor fragments partially reconstitutes ligand-induced signal generation. *J Biol Chem.* (1997) 272:25006–12. doi: 10.1074/jbc.272.40.25006

55. Rannikko A, Pakarinen P, Manna PR, Beau I, Misrahi M, Huhtaniemi I. Functional characterization of the human FSH receptor with an inactivating Ala189Val mutation. *Mol Hum Reprod.* (2002) 8:311–7. doi: 10.1093/molehr/8.4.311

56. Liu X, DePasquale JA, Griswold MD, Dias JA. Accessibility of rat and human follitropin primary sequence (R265-S296) *in situ*. *Endocrinology* (1994) 135:682–91. doi: 10.1210/endo.135.2.8033817

57. Latif R, Graves P, Davies TF. Oligomerization of the human thyrotropin receptor: fluorescent protein-tagged hTSHR reveals post-translational complexes. *J Biol Chem.* (2001) 276:45217–24. doi: 10.1074/jbc.M103727200

58. Tao YX, Johnson NB, Segaloff DL. Constitutive and agonist-dependent self-association of the cell surface human lutropin receptor. *J Biol Chem.* (2004) 279:5904–14. doi: 10.1074/jbc.M311162200

59. Horvat RD, Nelson S, Clay CM, Barisas BG, Roess DA. Intrinsically fluorescent luteinizing hormone receptor demonstrates hormone-driven aggregation. *Biochem Biophys Res Commun.* (1999) 255:382–5. doi: 10.1006/bbrc.1999.0185

60. Latif R, Graves P, Davies TF. Ligand-dependent inhibition of oligomerization at the human thyrotropin receptor. *J Biol Chem.* (2002) 277:45059–67. doi: 10.1074/jbc.M206693200

61. Thomas RM, Nechamen CA, Mazurkiewicz JE, Muda M, Palmer S, Dias JA. Follice-stimulating hormone receptor forms oligomers and shows evidence of carboxyl-terminal proteolytic processing. *Endocrinology* (2007) 148:1987–95. doi: 10.1210/en.2006-1672

62. Guan R, Wu X, Feng X, Zhang M, Hébert TE, Segaloff DL. Structural determinants underlying constitutive dimerization of unoccupied human follitropin receptors. *Cell Signal.* (2010) 22:247–56. doi: 10.1016/j.cellsig.2009.09.023

63. Mazurkiewicz JE, Herrick-Davis K, Barroso M, Ulloa-Aguirre A, Lindau-Shepard B, Thomas RM, et al. Single-molecule analyses of fully functional fluorescent protein-tagged follitropin receptor reveal homodimerization and specific heterodimerization with lutropin receptor. *Biol Reprod.* (2015) 92:1–12. doi: 10.1095/biolreprod.114.125781

64. Bonomi M, Persani L. Modern methods to investigate the oligomerization of glycoprotein hormone receptors (TSHR, LHR, FSHR). *Methods Enzymol.* (2013) 521:367–83. doi: 10.1016/B978-0-12-391862-8.00020-X

65. Urizar E, Montanelli L, Loy T, Bonomi M, Swillens S, Gales C, et al. Glycoprotein hormone receptors: link between receptor homodimerization and negative cooperativity. *EMBO J.* (2005) 24:1954–64. doi: 10.1038/sj.emboj.7600686

66. Jiang X, Liu H, Chen X, Chen PH, Fischer D, Sriraman V, et al. Structure of follicle-stimulating hormone in complex with the entire ectodomain of its receptor. *Proc Natl Acad Sci USA.* (2012) 109:12491–6. doi: 10.1073/pnas.1206643109

67. Jiang X, Fischer D, Chen X, McKenna SD, Liu H, Sriraman V, et al. Evidence for follicle-stimulating hormone receptor as a functional trimer. *J Biol Chem.* (2014) 289:14273–82. doi: 10.1074/jbc.M114.549592

68. Feng X, Zhang M, Guan R, Segaloff DL. Heterodimerization between the lutropin and follitropin receptors is associated with an attenuation of hormone-dependent signaling. *Endocrinology* (2013) 154:3925–30. doi: 10.1210/en.2013-1407

69. Jonas KC, Chen S, Virta M, Mora J, Franks S, Huhtaniemi I, et al. Temporal reprogramming of calcium signalling via crosstalk of gonadotrophin receptors that associate as functionally asymmetric heteromers. *Sci Rep.* (2018) 8:1–11. doi: 10.1038/s41598-018-20722-5

70. Casarini L, Santi D, Simoni M, Potì F. 'Spare' luteinizing hormone receptors : facts and fiction. *Trends Endocrinol Metab.* (2018) 29:208–17. doi: 10.1016/j.tem.2018.01.007

71. Milligan G, Bouvier M. Methods to monitor the quaternary structure of G protein-coupled receptors. *FEBS J.* (2005) 272:2914–25. doi: 10.1111/j.1742-4658.2005.04731.x

72. Bryen A. Jordan LAD. G-protein-coupled receptor heterodimerization modulates receptor function. *Nature* (1999) 399:697–700. doi: 10.1038/21441

73. Salim K, Fenton T, Bacha J, Urien-Rodriguez H, Bonnert T, Skynner HA, et al. Oligomerization of G-protein-coupled receptors shown by selective co-immunoprecipitation. *J Biol Chem.* (2002) 277:15482–5. doi: 10.1074/jbc.M201539200

74. Fiala GJ, Schamel WWA, Blumenthal B. Blue Native Polyacrylamide Gel Electrophoresis (BN-PAGE) for analysis of multiprotein complexes from cellular lysates. *J Vis Exp.* (2011) 48:2164. doi: 10.3791/2164

75. Swamy M, Siegers GM, Minguet S, Wollscheid B, Schamel WWA. Blue native polyacrylamide gel electrophoresis (BN-PAGE) for the identification and analysis of multiprotein complexes. *Sci STKE* (2006) 2006:Pl4. doi: 10.1126/stke.3452006pl4

76. Xu T-R, Ward RJ, Pediani JD, Milligan G. The orexin OX$_1$ receptor exists predominantly as a homodimer in the basal state: potential regulation of receptor organization by both agonist and antagonist ligands. *Biochem J.* (2011) 439:171–83. doi: 10.1042/BJ20110230

77. Forster T. Zwischenmolekulare Energiewanderung und Fluoreszenz. *Ann der Phys.* (1948) 6:55–75. doi: 10.1002/andp.19484370105

78. Jares-Erijman EA, Jovin TM. FRET imaging. *Nat Biotechnol.* (2003) 21:1387–95. doi: 10.1038/nbt896

79. Vogel SS, Thaler C, Koushik SV. Fanciful FRET. *Sci STKE* (2006) 2006:re2. doi: 10.1126/stke.3312006re2

80. Chachisvilis M, Zhang YL, Frangos JA. G protein-coupled receptors sense fluid shear stress in endothelial cells. *Proc Natl Acad Sci USA.* (2006) 103:15463–8. doi: 10.1073/pnas.0607224103

81. Carlson HJ, Campbell RE. Genetically encoded FRET-based biosensors for multiparameter fluorescence imaging. *Curr Opin Biotechnol.* (2009) 20:19–27. doi: 10.1016/j.copbio.2009.01.003

82. Lopez-Gimenez JF, Canals M, Pediani JD, Milligan G. The alpha 1b-adrenoceptor exists as a higher-order oligomer: effective oligomerization is required for receptor maturation, surface delivery, and function. *Mol Pharmacol.* (2007) 71:1015–29. doi: 10.1124/mol.106.033035

83. Piston DW, Kremers GJ. Fluorescent protein FRET: the good, the bad and the ugly. *Trends Biochem Sci.* (2007) 32:407–14. doi: 10.1016/j.tibs.2007.08.003

84. Kirber MT, Chen K, Keaney JF. YFP photoconversion revisited: confirmation of the CFP-like species. *Nat Methods* (2007) 4:767–8. doi: 10.1038/nmeth1007-767

85. Selvin PR. Principles and biophysical applications of lanthanide-based probes. *Annu Rev Biophys Biomol Struct.* (2002) 31:275–302. doi: 10.1146/annurev.biophys.31.101101.140927

86. Cottet M, Faklaris O, Maurel D, Scholler P, Doumazane E, Trinquet E, et al. BRET and time-resolved FRET strategy to study GPCR oligomerization: from cell lines toward native tissues. *Front Endocrinol.* (2012) 3:1–14. doi: 10.3389/fendo.2012.00092

87. Albizu L, Cottet M, Kralikova M, Stoev S, Seyer R, Brabet I, et al. Time-resolved FRET between GPCR ligands reveals oligomers in native tissues. *Nat Chem Biol.* (2010) 6:587–94. doi: 10.1038/nchembio.396

88. Bacart J, Corbel C, Jockers R, Bach S, Couturier C. The BRET technology and its application to screening assays. *Biotechnol J.* (2008) 3:311–24. doi: 10.1002/biot.200700222

89. Borroto-Escuela DO, Flajolet M, Agnati LF, Greengard P, Fuxe K. Bioluminiscence Resonance Energy Transfer (Bret) methods to study G protein-coupled receptor - receptor tyrosine kinase heteroreceptor complexes. *Methods Cell Biol.* (2013) 117:141–64. doi: 10.1016/B978-0-12-408143-7.00008-6

90. Kaczor A, Makarska-Bialokoz M, Selent J, Fuente R, Marti-Solano M, Castro M. Application of BRET for studying G protein-coupled receptors. *Mini Rev Med Chem.* (2014) 14:411–25. doi: 10.2174/1389557514666140428113708

91. Guo H, An S, Ward R, Yang Y, Liu Y, Guo XX, et al. Methods used to study the oligomeric structure of G-protein-coupled receptors. *Biosci Rep.* (2017) 37:BSR20160547. doi: 10.1042/BSR20160547

92. Achour L, Kamal M, Jockers R, Marullo S. Using quantitative BRET to assess G protein-coupled receptor homo- and heterodimerization. *Methods Mol Biol.* (2011) 756:183–200. doi: 10.1007/978-1-61779-160-4_9

93. Paramonov VM, Mamaeva V, Sahlgren C, Rivero-Müller A. Genetically-encoded tools for cAMP probing and modulation in living systems. *Front Pharmacol.* (2015) 6:196. doi: 10.3389/fphar.2015.00196

94. Clister T, Mehta S, Zhang J. Single-cell analysis of G-protein signal transduction. *J Biol Chem.* (2015) 290:6681–8. doi: 10.1074/jbc.R114.616391

95. Trehan A, Rotgers E, Coffey ET, Huhtaniemi I, Rivero-Müller A. CANDLES, an assay for monitoring GPCR induced cAMP generation in cell cultures. *Cell Commun Signal.* (2014) 12:70. doi: 10.1186/s12964-014-0070-x

96. Kishi H, Kitahara Y, Imai F, Nakao K, Suwa H. Expression of the gonadotropin receptors during follicular development. *Reprod Med Biol.* (2018) 17:11–9. doi: 10.1002/rmb2.12075

97. Risma KA, Clay CM, Nett TM, Wagner T, Yun J, Nilson JH. Targeted overexpression of luteinizing hormone in transgenic mice leads to infertility, polycystic ovaries, and ovarian tumors. *Proc Natl Acad Sci USA.* (1995) 92:1322–6. doi: 10.1073/pnas.92.5.1322

98. Willis DS. Premature response to luteinizing hormone of granulosa cells from anovulatory women with polycystic ovary syndrome: relevance to mechanism of anovulation. *J Clin Endocrinol Metab.* (1998) 83:3984–91. doi: 10.1210/jc.83.11.3984

20

Molecular Mechanisms of Action of FSH

Livio Casarini [1,2]* and Pascale Crépieux [3]

[1] Unit of Endocrinology, Department Biomedical, Metabolic and Neural Sciences, University of Modena and Reggio Emilia, Modena, Italy, [2] Center for Genomic Research, University of Modena and Reggio Emilia, Modena, Italy, [3] PRC, UMR INRA0085, CNRS 7247, Centre INRA Val de Loire, Nouzilly, France

*Correspondence:
Livio Casarini
livio.casarini@unimore.it

The glycoprotein follicle-stimulating hormone (FSH) acts on gonadal target cells, hence regulating gametogenesis. The transduction of the hormone-induced signal is mediated by the FSH-specific G protein-coupled receptor (FSHR), of which the action relies on the interaction with a number of intracellular effectors. The stimulatory Gαs protein is a long-time known transducer of FSH signaling, mainly leading to intracellular cAMP increase and protein kinase A (PKA) activation, the latter acting as a master regulator of cell metabolism and sex steroid production. While *in vivo* data clearly demonstrate the relevance of PKA activation in mediating gametogenesis by triggering proliferative signals, some *in vitro* data suggest that pro-apoptotic pathways may be awakened as a "dark side" of cAMP/PKA-dependent steroidogenesis, in certain conditions. P38 mitogen-activated protein kinases (MAPK) are players of death signals in steroidogenic cells, involving downstream p53 and caspases. Although it could be hypothesized that pro-apoptotic signals, if relevant, may be required for regulating *atresia* of *non*-dominant ovarian follicles, they should be transient and counterbalanced by mitogenic signals upon FSHR interaction with opposing transducers, such as Gαi proteins and β-arrestins. These molecules modulate the steroidogenic pathway *via* extracellular-regulated kinases (ERK1/2), phosphatidylinositol-4,5-bisphosphate 3-kinases (PI3K)/protein kinase B (AKT), calcium signaling and other intracellular signaling effectors, resulting in a complex and dynamic signaling network characterizing sex- and stage-specific gamete maturation. Even if the FSH-mediated signaling network is not yet entirely deciphered, its full comprehension is of high physiological and clinical relevance due to the crucial role covered by the hormone in regulating human development and reproduction.

Keywords: FSH, FSHR, signaling, PKA, arrestin

INTRODUCTION

Follicle-stimulating hormone (FSH) is a glycoprotein playing a central role in mammalian reproduction and development. In the ovary, FSH regulates folliculogenesis, oocyte selection, and the synthesis of sex steroid hormones, thus preparing the reproductive tract for fertilization, implantation, and pregnancy (1). In the male, this gonadotropin mediates testicular development and spermatogenesis (2). The hormone is secreted by the gonadotrope cells of the pituitary, upon pulsatile regulation by the hypothalamic gonadotropin-releasing hormone (GnRH) (3), and acts on the surface of target cells located in the gonads of both males and females, where hormone-induced cell proliferation- and apoptosis-linked signals are triggered. FSH displays an α subunit, common to other gonadotropins and to thyrotropin, and a β subunit specifically binding to its G protein-coupled receptor (GPCR), namely FSHR (4). *In silico* and crystallographic structural analyzes found also interaction between the α subunit and FSHR, demonstrating that receptor binding is not exclusive of the β subunit (5). Hormone binding implies conformational changes of the receptor (6) that transduce the signal *via* direct protein interactions at the plasma membrane, resulting in a cascade of biochemical reactions that constitute an intertwined complex signaling network (7). In this review, signaling pathways activated in gonadal cells upon FSH binding to its membrane receptor are discussed in detail, providing a comprehensive view on the downstream life and death signals regulating reproductive functions.

FSHR INTERACTION WITH MEMBRANE RECEPTORS

The FSHR has been shown to functionally and/or physically interact with other membrane receptors (8, 9), hence intensifying the diversity of FSH action (10). For example, the FSHR may exist as a unit of di/trimeric homomers (5). Interestingly, heterodimerization of the FSHR with the luteinizing hormone (LH) receptor (LHCGR) (11) may play a key role in regulating the ovarian growth and selection (12), by virtue of the physical interaction between these two receptors. Interestingly, intracellular signals delivered by LH at the LHCGR may be modulated by the presence of FSHR on the cell surface, and *vice versa*, through the formation of receptor heteromers. For example, unliganded co-expressed FSHR amplifies Gαq- mediated signaling initiated at the LHCGR (13), whereas the LHCGR may inhibit FSHR-dependent cAMP production (11). In addition, other classes of receptors, such as tyrosine kinase receptors, may also contribute to the modulation of FSH activity. The insulin-like growth factor-1 receptor (IGF-1R) is one of those, as it appears necessary for FSH-induced granulosa cell differentiation *via* a signaling cascade involving the thymoma viral oncogene homolog 3 (AKT3) (14). Similarly, action of the epidermal growth factor receptor (EGFR) during granulosa cell differentiation is required for activation of ERK1/2 (15). Interestingly, the interaction between FSHR and EGFR signaling networks was analyzed using an automated, logic- based approach, suggesting that the ERK1/2-pathway may be activated by EGFR-dependent signals *via* p38 mitogen- activated protein kinases (MAPK) (16). Moreover, this study confirmed that EGFR is trans-activated through FSHR-mediated pathways involving the proto-oncogene tyrosine-protein kinase *SRC*. On the other hand, EGFR signaling network overlaps, at least in part, that of FSHR, contributing to modulation of the ERK1/2, the phosphatidylinositol-4,5-bisphosphate 3- kinases (PI3K)/protein kinase B (AKT), and the Janus kinase (JAK)/signal transducer and activator of transcription protein (STAT) pathways (16).

INTRACELLULAR FSHR SIGNAL TRANSDUCING PARTNERS

Typically, G proteins are directly activated by the FSHR, by splitting of the βγ dimer from the α subunit (17), that act as regulators of intracellular enzymes, such as G protein-coupled receptor kinases (GRKs), or adenylyl cyclase, respectively, among many others (18). Moreover, βγ dimer was demonstrated to be able of modulating intracellular signaling cascades (19, 20).

G protein activation is followed by FSHR phosphorylation at the intracellular level, operated by GRKs and resulting in receptor association with β-arrestins (21, 22). β-arrestins are scaffold proteins (23) that mediate GPCR desensitization, recycling, and G protein-independent signaling (24). Another direct FSHR-interacting partner is adaptor protein, phosphotyrosine interacting with PH domain and leucine zipper 1 (APPL1), that is linked to the activation of the PI3K/AKT anti-apoptotic pathway and calcium ion mobilization (25). By these means, APPL1 might regulate the selection of the dominant follicle by mediating the anti-apoptotic effects exerted by FSH *via* inhibitory phosphorylation of forkhead homolog in rhabdomyosarcoma (FOXO1a) (26). Interestingly, APPL1 is involved in cAMP signaling exerted by GPCR activity in very early endosomal compartments, hence contributing to the spatial encoding of intracellular signaling, as shown for the LHR (27). Similarly, GAIP-interacting protein C terminus (GIPC), a PDZ protein, redirects the FSHR to pre-early endosomes, hence promoting sustained, intracellular MAPK (28). Another protein directly interacting with FSHR is the 14-3-3τ adapter protein (29), which may contact the canonical G protein-receptor interaction site located at the intracellular level and mediates the activation of the AKT-pathway (30).

In the gonads, FSH-mediated signaling results in the transcription of target genes, which include *LHCGR* and other genes encoding membrane receptors, protein kinases, growth factors, enzymes regulating steroid synthesis, genes involved in the regulation of cell cycle, proliferation and differentiation, apoptosis, and circadian rhythm (31–33). Despite the wide diversity of FSH target genes, effects of gonadal stimulation by the hormone was defined as both proliferative and anti- apoptotic due to the positive impact on gametogenesis (34, 35) and on growth of certain cancer cells (36). Nevertheless, pro-apoptotic functions emerged as a condition related to FSH-mediated steroid production (37, 38). In this review, molecular mechanisms of FSH action and their relationships with downstream steroidogenic, life, and death signals regulating reproduction (**Figure 1**) are discussed.

ACTIVATION OF THE CAMP/PKA STEROIDOGENIC PATHWAY

While FSH is mainly known to support the maturation of gametes *via* Sertoli cell nurturing functions in the male, the hormone has steroidogenic activity in ovarian granulosa cells (4). This action is exerted *via* the protein kinase A (PKA) pathway, whose activation depends on ATP conversion into the second

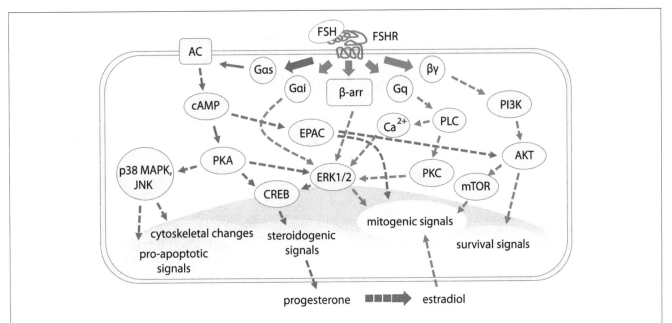

FIGURE 1 | Cross-talk between FSH-dependent steroidogenic, life, and death signals in granulosa cells. G protein subunits and β-arrestins mediate the activation of multiple signaling pathways modulating different events downstream. Gαs protein/cAMP-related signaling are represented by orange arrows while signaling cascades depending on other FSHR intracellular interactors are indicated by blue arrows. Steroidogenic events are mainly mediated through cAMP/PKA-pathway, which is linked to p38 MAPK signaling, while ERK1/2 and AKT are key players for mitogenic and survival signals activation. Some pathways were omitted.

messenger cAMP by adenylyl cyclases, primary targets of the Gαs protein subunit. The interaction between cAMP and PKA was described several decades ago (39). Intracellular cAMP increase is under the negative control of phosphodiesterase (PDE) enzymes, which metabolize the second messenger into 5′AMP (40). As mentioned above, cAMP signaling is spatially and temporally compartmentalized within the cell (41). Versatility in cAMP-dependent signaling depends on the expression of factors such as the isoform of adenylyl cyclase (42), PDE (43), β-arrestins (44), and A kinase anchoring proteins (AKAP) (45) that target the subcellular distribution of PKA.

In Sertoli cells, cAMP binding to PKA results in the release of PKA catalytic subunits (46) and indirectly mediates the phosphorylation of the extracellular signal-regulated kinase 1/2 (ERK1/2) MAPK, in order to promote cell proliferation (47). In granulosa cells, the mechanism whereby ERK is activated likely consists in the removal of a tonic inhibition exerted by a phosphotyrosine phosphatase on MEK1 (48), recently identified as DUSP6 (49). An alternative mechanism consists in the activation of ERK1/2 by β-arrestins, with a different kinetics than G proteins (**Figure 2**), since it is delayed and sustained (50). It was demonstrated that pERK1/2 is involved in both cAMP-dependent (51) and -independent (52) steroidogenesis. In the first case, depletion of ERK1/2 phosphorylation by specific MEK inhibition resulted in attenuated early (10–15 min) phosphorylation of the cAMP response element-binding protein (CREB) (51), a nuclear transcription factor up-regulating steroidogenic enzymes in gonadal cells (53). In this case, pERK1/2 inhibition negatively impacts on progesterone synthesis, indicating that cAMP-dependent ERK1/2

phosphorylation plays a stimulatory role in the rapidly delivered FSH-dependent steroidogenic signal. Interestingly, molecular mechanisms regulating steroidogenic stimuli in the Leydig cell may be different to those occurring in FSH-responsive cells. In Leydig cells, steroid hormones may be produced *via* ERK1/2- and CREB-dependent signaling in the absence of cAMP recruitment, *via* an EGFR-regulated mechanism (52). In granulosa cells, selective blockade of MAPK activation results in the inhibition of FSH-dependent StAR and progesterone synthesis while androgens to estrogen conversion by the enzyme aromatase is enhanced (54), demonstrating a differential regulation of FSH-induced sex steroid synthesis in target cells. Similar results were found by treating theca cells with LH, that induced differential, ERK1/2-dependent regulation of progesterone and androgen production (55). However, the role of ERK1/2 in mediating steroidogenesis is a still debated matter, since it was reported to be inhibitory (56) while other studies demonstrated the positive impact of the MAPK activation on the synthesis of sex steroids (57).

ROLES OF cAMP-DEPENDENT PKA ACTIVATION

Whereas, ERK is an indirect cytosolic target of PKA that can affect CREB phosphorylation (51), the latter may be directly activated upon translocation of PKA catalytic subunit in the nucleus (48), hence inducing the transcription of CREB target genes characterized by cAMP-response elements (CRE) within their promoter region (53). Nuclear PKA was also shown

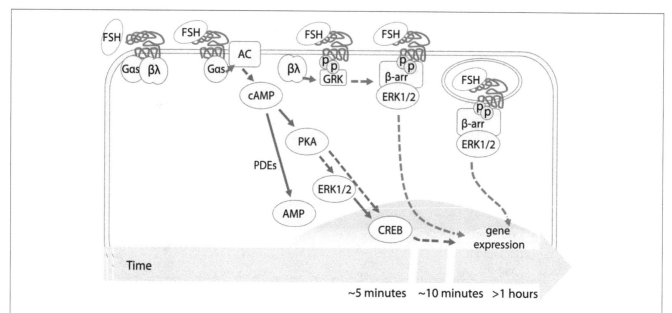

FIGURE 2 | Temporal succession of FSH-dependent events across the cAMP/PKA-pathway. cAMP-related signaling involves PKA, ERK1/2, and CREB activation. FSHR phosphorylation by GRKs occurs before β-arrestin recruitment and subsequent receptor internalization.

to phosphorylate histone H3, thus mediating FSH mitogenic activity in granulosa cells (58, 59). These interesting observations suggest that PKA could be endowed with a more general role in gene transcription, by promoting chromatin remodeling through histone H3 post-translational modifications. In addition, recent genome-wide experiments have highlighted that FSH-responsive genes contain far less CRE than expected in their promoters, that are notably enriched in GATA-binding sites (32).

The wide range of PKA-dependent signaling pathways suggests that the kinase is a master regulator of several FSH-dependent cell functions, especially those related to steroidogenesis and cell differentiation. However, intracellular signaling cascades regulated by PKA do not completely overlap those depending on FSH. For example, FSH induces p38 MAPK activation while PKA *per se* does not (60).

FSH-induced cAMP production does not only lead to activation of PKA but also of the exchange protein directly activated by cAMP (EPAC) activation. EPAC is a relatively newly discovered cAMP target mediating the activation of the small GTPases RAS and RAP and resulting in the regulation of several cell functions, such as mitogen-activated protein kinase activation, cytoskeletal changes, and calcium homeostasis (61). EPAC was suggested to be a modulator of EGFR expression (62) and granulosa cell differentiation (15) in the ovary, as well as AKT phosphorylation in Sertoli cells (63). However, the role of EPAC in the FSH-mediated signaling cascade is not yet completely elucidated.

REGULATION OF PROLIFERATIVE AND PRO-APOPTOTIC SIGNALS

In gonadal cells, part of the steroidogenic process and the proteasome are compartmentalized into different organelles,

avoiding cell collapse before adequate amount of sex steroid hormones are produced (64). This function is likely enabled to limit the number of follicles that can achieve ovulation and to maintain intact the synthesis of sex steroids during the initial steps of apoptosis. These issues reflect the connection between intracellular signaling cascades regulating steroidogenic signals and pro-apoptotic stimuli, whose dominance is stage-specific, depends on several paracrine factors and is regulated *via* a complex intracellular network involving cAMP and activating the pro-apoptotic protein p53 (65). In this context, the link between cAMP/PKA and p38 MAPK activation may provide a molecular mechanism of apoptosis in steroidogenic cells. The role of p38, as well as Jun N-terminal kinase (JNK), is associated to apoptotic events in pre-ovulatory granulosa cells of primates (66), suggesting that these enzymes could be involved in the selection of the dominant follicle. This role would be counteracted by pERK1/2 activation in the dominant follicle (57), confirming the anti-apoptotic and proliferative functions mediated by this MAP kinase. Indeed, ovarian granulosa cell death is associated with reduced ERK1/2 activity, that is linked to phosphorylation of BCL-2 associated agonist of cell death (BAD) protein leading to a loss of its pro-apoptotic activity (67, 68).

PRO- AND ANTI-APOPTOTIC PATHWAYS ARE ACTIVATED SIMULTANEOUSLY

In steroidogenic cells, apoptosis is preceded by cell rounding, a cAMP-dependent conformational changes involving actin filaments breakdown (69, 70) that can be prevented by selective blockade of PKA, and also depends on p38 MAPK (71). Both PKA and p38 MAPK may be activated by FSH in a dose-dependent manner, resulting in cytoskeletal rearrangements and shape changes. These data suggest that the gonadotropin retains both pro- and anti-apoptotic potential, exerted *via* p38 MAPK and ERK1/2, respectively, and this dual action of FSH provides an interesting point of view on gonadotropin functioning. On the one side, the hormone induces the synthesis of steroid hormones *via* the cAMP/PKA-pathway, as a requisite for gamete growth and reproduction (72). However, the steroidogenic signaling cascade is cross-linked to pro-apoptotic signals occurring through p38 MAPK, activated simultaneously and necessary for regulating steroid synthesis (73, 74). This cross-talk was described even in the mouse adrenal Y1 cell line, where p38 MAPK activation negatively impacts on CREB phosphorylation and StAR activity, inhibiting FSH-induced steroid synthesis (75). On the other side, survival signals are provided through the PKA/ERK1/2 signaling package, counterbalancing the pro-apoptotic effect and, to a certain extent, even inhibiting steroidogenesis (56). While further efforts should be performed to fully solve this question, some hints suggest that the FSH-dependent molecular mechanism underlying cell fate may depend on the potency and persistence of cAMP at the intracellular levels. Indeed, proliferative signals could be predominant at relatively low FSHR expression levels (38), due to preferential activation of ERK1/2 signaling through β-arrestins (38, 76). Relatively high and persistent intracellular cAMP levels due to β-arrestin depletion or FSHR over-expression result in caspase 3 cleavage and apoptosis (38) and this mechanism could contribute to regulating the selection of the dominant ovarian follicles (12). In granulosa cells, *FSHR* over-expression is linked to upregulation of pro-apoptotic genes and increased cell death, compared to cells expressing relatively low *FSHR* levels (77). Thus, it is possible that proliferative signals exerted *via* ERK1/2-pathway could be not sufficient to counteract the pro-apoptotic stimulus during the early/mid-antral follicular phase, when FSHR expression achieves maximal levels (78). In the ovary, this situation should be dynamic and transient, as well as the *FSHR* over-expression (78), follicle-specific and stage-dependent, in order to coordinate the maturation of one single follicle achieving ovulation while the others become *atretic*. This regulatory mechanism may be juxtaposed to what was previously described in Sertoli cell, that is assumed to be the male counterpart of granulosa cell. In 5-day rat Sertoli cells, the ERK1/2-pathway is stimulated by FSH upon dual coupling of FSHR to both stimulatory Gαs and inhibitory Gαi proteins, resulting in cyclin D1 activation and cell proliferation (47). As cells proceed throughout the differentiation program, FSH treatment is linked to consistent ERK1/2 inhibition and decreased cell proliferation, while gradually stabilizing PTEN (79). Thus, the ERK1/2 signaling pathway is a key regulator of FSH-induced life and death signals.

PKC AND CALCIUM ION SIGNALING

Increasing evidence indicates that one of the actions exerted by FSH consists in the activation of the protein kinase C (PKC) pathway that is involved in expansion of the cumulus, meiotic maturation of oocytes, and modulation of progesterone production in the ovary (80). Cross-talk between cAMP/PKA

and PKC pathways was also described in Sertoli cells (81), where the FSH-dependent activation of these kinases is connected to calcium ion (Ca^{2+}) signaling (82), resulting from intracellular release as well as from rapid influx from T-type Ca^{2+} channels (83, 84) or through a Gαh transglutaminase/PLCδ interaction (85). *In vitro* experiments in transiently FSHR over-expressing human embryonic kidney (HEK) and virally transduced human granulosa (KGN) cells demonstrated that intracellular Ca^{2+} increase may occur *via* a molecular mechanism dependent on the interaction between APPL-1 and FSHR, and involving inositol 1,4,5-trisphosphate (IP_3) (25). Interestingly, IP_3 production dampens the expression of the aromatase enzyme, at least under FSHR over-expression (86), suggesting an inhibitory role of the APPL-1/IP_3/Ca^{2+} signaling module on sex steroid synthesis. While further studies are required to confirm these results in the presence of physiological FSHR expression levels, these data show that APPL-1-mediated Ca^{2+} signaling does not necessarily depend on cAMP, as previously demonstrated (87). Moreover, human PKC belongs to a superfamily of about 15 isoenzymes activated upon Gq protein-mediated production of diacylglycerol (DAG) and/or Ca^{2+} by phospholipases at the intracellular level (88). In the mouse ovary, expression of PKC isoforms is dynamic and changes according to the developmental stage, from pre-puberty to the adulthood, suggesting that different isoenzymes may control specific ovarian functions, such as follicular maturation, ovulation, and luteinization (89).

It is known that PKC counteracts the PKA-mediated steroidogenesis through cAMP inhibition in granulosa (90, 91), and this function was further confirmed in both mammalian (92) and avian models (93). Moreover, PKC attenuates the Gαs protein-dependent signaling (94, 95), as well as proteoglycan synthesis in Sertoli cells (96). Interestingly, several reports demonstrated an up-regulatory role of PKC in Leydig cell steroidogenesis (97). Indeed, the enzyme is involved in the positive modulation of cAMP, pCREB and StAR activation, increasing the rate of steroid synthesis in the mouse Leydig MA-10 cell line (98, 99), and in mouse primary Leydig cells (100). In this case, PKC activation would not depend on FSH, due to the lack of FSHR expression in Leydig cells. On the contrary, PKC up-regulation in ovarian theca cells may be LH-dependent and negatively impacts on androstenedione synthesis *in vitro* (101), suggesting the existence of a sex-specific function of the kinase in regulating the synthesis of sex steroids in androgenic cells.

THE pAKT ANTI-APOPTOTIC PATHWAY

FSH binding to its receptor mediates the activation of PI3K, that are enzymes involved in the regulation of cell survival, growth and differentiation (102). In Sertoli cells, FSH increases phosphatase and tensin homolog deleted in chromosome 10 (PTEN) synthesis within minutes, independently of mRNA transcription (79), but rather mediated by FSH-mediated destabilization of several anti-PTEN miRNAs (103). PTEN stabilization in mature rat counteracts PI3K activity, when cell proliferation ceases prior puberty. AKT activation *via* PI3K may occur through both PKA-dependent (104) and independent mechanisms (63), reflecting the relevance of this kinase in modulating proliferative and anti-apoptotic signals in steroidogenic cells. Indeed, in granulosa cells, an interplay between AKT- and cAMP/PKA-pathway up-regulating steroidogenesis was demonstrated (105). Moreover, FSH-dependent activation of the AKT/mammalian target of rapamycin (mTOR) signaling module (106), a positive regulator of cell cycle progression and cell proliferation (107), was also described (108–110). AKT phosphorylation was observed in mouse granulosa cells, where the kinase induces the inactivation of FOXO1 and expression of cyclin D2, resulting in cell proliferation and differentiation in response to FSH (111). In fact, recent genome-wide studies have revealed that most FSH-responsive genes in granulosa cells are FOXO target genes (33). New insights onto FSH-mediated protection from atresia came from the discovery that FOXO nuclear exclusion (inhibition) upon activation of the PIK3/AKT/mTOR signaling pathway prevents granulosa cell autophagy (112, 113). The relevance of pAKT activation for reproduction was highlighted by in vitro experiments where mouse preantral follicular granulosa cells were co-cultured with oocytes (114). The presence of granulosa cells inhibited oocyte apoptosis via PI3K/AKT, promoting gamete growth. Especially, AKT was described to regulate meiotic resumption in several animal models (115–117). Finally, the AKT pathway is a preferential target of LH (118) and its activation is even enhanced in the presence of FSH (119, 120), suggesting that anti-apoptotic and proliferative stimuli would be required during the late antral follicular phase to prepare the late stages of oocyte maturation and achieve ovulation. Taken together, the PI3K/AKT-pathway may act in concert with mTOR (108) regulating survival signal in the ovary. These signals are fundamental for primordial to Graafian follicles survival, as well as for oocyte maturation and growth. In this context, it is reasonable that the PI3K/AKT anti-apoptotic activity mediated through FSHR is fundamental to counteract cAMP/PKA pro-apoptotic stimuli and rescue the follicle from atresia (121). In fact, dysregulation of this signaling cascade may impair female gametogenesis and it was described as a cause of infertility (122). Interesting data explaining how signals delivered through the cAMP/PKA- and PI3K/AKT-pathway are counterbalanced come from the analysis of FSH treatment of Sertoli cells. In this model, FSH has a dual, stage-dependent action. While the hormone stimulates the proliferation of immature cells through activation of PI3K/AKT-, mTOR- and ERK1/2-pathways, it preferentially stimulates cAMP production in mature Sertoli cells, resulting in PI3K/AKT inhibition and arrest of cell proliferation (110, 123).

While this effect is maybe due to the change of Sertoli cell competence, where PI3K/AKT-pathway activation becomes dependent on paracrine factors during the late stages of the maturation (124), it provides an example of dual regulation of life and death signals exerted by FSH.

CONCLUSIONS

FSH mediates multiple signaling pathways by binding to its unique GPCR (125). At the intracellular level, FSH is capable of promoting cell growth and survival opposed to steroidogenic signals cross-linked to apoptosis, resulting in a fine-tuned regulation of the gametogenesis and, in general, of reproduction. In the male gonads, FSH induces proliferation of Sertoli cells via AKT- and ERK1/2-pathways and the role of these signaling cascades, which are proliferative and anti-apoptotic, is reflected during folliculogenesis, oocyte maturation, and growth in the ovary. The synthesis of steroid hormones mainly mediated by cAMP/PKA-pathway activation is a primary endpoint in FSH functioning in the granulosa cell during the antral stage of folliculogenesis. Estrogens are the final products required for proper development of the dominant follicle, at the cost of scarifying others which become atretic. It is well known that follicular atresia is due to lowering of FSH support. However, in vitro data support unexpected, stage-specific pro-apoptotic signals delivered by the hormone that may play a role in vivo and this issue merits further investigations.

AUTHOR CONTRIBUTIONS

All authors listed have made a substantial, direct and intellectual contribution to the work, and approved it for publication.

ACKNOWLEDGMENTS

Authors are grateful to the Italian Ministry of University and Research for supporting the Department of Biomedical, Metabolic, and Neural Sciences (University of Modena and Reggio Emilia, Italy) in the context of the Departments of Excellence Programme. We are also indebted to the Institut National de la Recherche Agronomique PHASE Department, to the Centre National de la Recherche Scientifique, the French National Research Agency under the program Investissements d'avenir Grant Agreement LabEx MabImprove: ANR-10-LABX-53, and to the GPCRAb (ARD2020 BIOMEDICAMENTS, contract #32000593) grants from Région Center.

REFERENCES

1. Messinis IE, Messini CI, Dafopoulos K. Novel aspects of the endocrinology of the menstrual cycle. *Reproduct BioMed.* (2014) 28:714–22. doi: 10.1016/j.rbmo.2014.02.003
2. Huhtaniemi I. A short evolutionary history of FSH-stimulated spermatogenesis. *Hormones.* (2015) 14:468–78. doi: 10.14310/horm.2002.1632
3. Stamatiades GA, Kaiser UB. Gonadotropin regulation by pulsatile GnRH: signaling and gene expression. *Mol Cell Endocrinol.* (2018) 463:131–41. doi: 10.1016/j.mce.2017.10.015
4. Simoni M, Gromoll J, Nieschlag E. The follicle-stimulating hormone receptor: biochemistry, molecular biology, physiology, and pathophysiology. *Endocr Rev.* (1997) 18:739–73. doi: 10.1210/edrv.18.6.0320

5. Jiang X, Fischer D, Chen X, McKenna SD, Liu H, Sriraman V, et al. Evidence for follicle-stimulating hormone receptor as a functional trimer. *J Biol Chem.* (2014) 289:14273–82. doi: 10.1074/jbc.M114.549592

6. Jiang X, Liu H, Chen X, Chen P-H, Fischer D, Sriraman V, et al. Structure of follicle-stimulating hormone in complex with the entire ectodomain of its receptor. *Proc Natl Acad Sci.* (2012) 109:12491–6. doi: 10.1073/pnas.1206643109

7. Gloaguen P, Crépieux P, Heitzler D, Poupon A, Reiter E. Mapping the follicle-stimulating hormone-induced signaling networks. *Front Endocrinol.* (2011) 2:45. doi: 10.3389/fendo.2011.00045

8. Jonas KC, Rivero-Müller A, Huhtaniemi IT, Hanyaloglu AC. G protein-coupled receptor transactivation. *Methods Cell Biol.* (2013) 117:433–50. doi: 10.1016/B978-0-12-408143-7.00023-2

9. Rivero-Muller A, Chou Y-Y, Ji I, Lajic S, Hanyaloglu AC, Jonas K, et al. Rescue of defective G protein-coupled receptor function *in vivo* by intermolecular cooperation. *Proc Natl Acad Sci.* (2010) 107:2319–24. doi: 10.1073/pnas.0906695106

10. Ulloa-Aguirre A, Reiter E, Crépieux P. FSH receptor signaling: complexity of interactions and signal diversity. *Endocrinology.* (2018) 159:3020–35. doi: 10.1210/en.2018-00452

11. Feng X, Zhang M, Guan R, Segaloff DL. Heterodimerization between the lutropin and follitropin receptors is associated with an attenuation of hormone-dependent signaling. *Endocrinology.* (2013) 154:3925–30. doi: 10.1210/en.2013-1407

12. Casarini L, Santi D, Simoni M, Potì F. 'Spare' luteinizing hormone receptors: facts and fiction. *Trends Endocrinol Metabol.* (2018) 29:208–17. doi: 10.1016/j.tem.2018.01.007

13. Jonas KC, Chen S, Virta M, Mora J, Franks S, Huhtaniemi I, et al. Temporal reprogramming of calcium signalling via crosstalk of gonadotrophin receptors that associate as functionally asymmetric heteromers. *Sci Rep.* (2018) 8:2239. doi: 10.1038/s41598-018-20722-5

14. Baumgarten SC, Convissar SM, Fierro MA, Winston NJ, Scoccia B, Stocco C. IGF1R signaling is necessary for FSH-induced activation of AKT and differentiation of human cumulus granulosa cells. *J Clin Endocrinol Metabol.* (2014) 99:2995–3004. doi: 10.1210/jc.2014-1139

15. Wayne CM, Fan H-Y, Cheng X, Richards JS. Follicle-stimulating hormone induces multiple signaling cascades: evidence that activation of Rous sarcoma oncogene, RAS, and the epidermal growth factor receptor are critical for granulosa cell differentiation. *Mol Endocrinol.* (2007) 21:1940–57. doi: 10.1210/me.2007-0020

16. Rougny A, Gloaguen P, Langonné N, Reiter E, Crépieux P, Poupon A, et al. A logic-based method to build signaling networks and propose experimental plans. *Sci Rep.* (2018) 8:7830. doi: 10.1038/s41598-018-26006-2

17. Kahn RA, Gilman AG. ADP-ribosylation of Gs promotes the dissociation of its alpha and beta subunits. *J Biol Chem.* (1984) 259:6235–40.

18. De Pascali F, Tréfier A, Landomiel F, Bozon V, Bruneau G, Yvinec R, et al. "Follicle-stimulating hormone receptor: advances and remaining challenges." *Int Rev Cell Mol Biol.* (2018) 338:1–58. doi: 10.1016/bs.ircmb.2018.02.001

19. Federman AD, Conklin BR, Schrader KA, Reed RR, Bourne HR. Hormonal stimulation of adenylyl cyclase through Gi-protein beta gamma subunits. *Nature.* (1992) 356:159–61. doi: 10.1038/356159a0

20. Koch WJ, Hawes BE, Inglese J, Luttrell LM, Lefkowitz RJ. Cellular expression of the carboxyl terminus of a G protein-coupled receptor kinase attenuates G beta gamma-mediated signaling. *J Biol Chem.* (1994) 269:6193–7.

21. Troispoux C, Guillou F, Elalouf JM, Firsov D, Iacovelli L, De Blasi A, et al. Involvement of G protein-coupled receptor kinases and arrestins in desensitization to follicle-stimulating hormone action. *Mol Endocrinol.* (1999) 13:1599–614. doi: 10.1210/mend.13.9.0342

22. Krishnamurthy H, Galet C, Ascoli M. The association of arrestin-3 with the follitropin receptor depends on receptor activation and phosphorylation. *Mol Cell Endocrinol.* (2003) 204:127–40. doi: 10.1016/S0303-7207(03)00088-1

23. Crépieux P, Poupon A, Langonné-Gallay N, Reiter E, Delgado J, Schaefer MH, et al. A comprehensive view of the β-arrestinome. *Front Endocrinol.* (2017) 8:32. doi: 10.3389/fendo.2017.00032

24. De Pascali F, Reiter E. β-arrestins and biased signalling in gonadotropin receptors. *Miner Ginecol.* (2018) 70:525–38. doi: 10.23736/S0026-4784.18.04272-7

25. Thomas RM, Nechamen CA, Mazurkiewicz JE, Ulloa-Aguirre A, Dias JA. The adapter protein APPL1 links FSH receptor to inositol 1,4,5-trisphosphate production and is implicated in intracellular Ca^{2+} mobilization. *Endocrinology.* (2011) 152:1691–701. doi: 10.1210/en.2010-1353

26. Nechamen CA, Thomas RM, Cohen BD, Acevedo G, Poulikakos PI, Testa JR, et al. Human follicle-stimulating hormone (FSH) receptor interacts with the adaptor protein APPL1 in HEK 293 cells: potential involvement of the PI3K pathway in FSH signaling. *Biol Reproduc.* (2004) 71:629–36. doi: 10.1095/biolreprod.103.025833

27. Sposini S, Jean-Alphonse FG, Ayoub MA, Oqua A, West C, Lavery S, et al. Integration of GPCR signaling and sorting from very early endosomes via opposing APPL1 mechanisms. *Cell Rep.* (2017) 21:2855–67. doi: 10.1016/j.celrep.2017.11.023

28. Jean-Alphonse F, Bowersox S, Chen S, Beard G, Puthenveedu MA, Hanyaloglu AC. Spatially restricted G protein-coupled receptor activity via divergent endocytic compartments. *J Biol Chem.* (2014) 289:3960–77. doi: 10.1074/jbc.M113.526350

29. Cohen BD, Nechamen CA, Dias JA. Human follitropin receptor (FSHR) interacts with the adapter protein 14-3-3τ. *Mol Cell Endocrinol.* (2004) 220:1–7. doi: 10.1016/j.mce.2004.04.012

30. Dias JA, Mahale SD, Nechamen CA, Davydenko O, Thomas RM, Ulloa-Aguirre A. Emerging roles for the FSH receptor adapter protein APPL1 and overlap of a putative 14-3-3τ interaction domain with a canonical G-protein interaction site. *Mol Cell Endocrinol.* (2010) 329:17–25. doi: 10.1016/j.mce.2010.05.009

31. Friedmann S, Sarit F, Dantes A, Ada D, Amsterdam A, Abraham A. Ovarian transcriptomes as a tool for a global approach of genes modulated by gonadotropic hormones in human ovarian granulosa cells. *Endocrine.* (2005) 26:259–65. doi: 10.1385/ENDO:26:3:259

32. Perlman S, Bouquin T, van den Hazel B, Jensen TH, Schambye HT, Knudsen S, et al. Transcriptome analysis of FSH and FSH variant stimulation in granulosa cells from IVM patients reveals novel regulated genes. *MHR Basic Sci Reproduc Med.* (2006) 12:135–44. doi: 10.1093/molehr/gah247

33. Herndon MK, Law NC, Donaubauer EM, Kyriss B, Hunzicker-Dunn M. Forkhead box O member FOXO1 regulates the majority of follicle-stimulating hormone responsive genes in ovarian granulosa cells. *Mol Cell Endocrinol.* (2016) 434:116–26. doi: 10.1016/j.mce.2016.06.020

34. Plant TM, Marshall GR. The functional significance of FSH in spermatogenesis and the control of its secretion in male primates. *Endocr Rev.* (2001) 22:764–86. doi: 10.1210/edrv.22.6.0446

35. Hillier SG. Gonadotropic control of ovarian follicular growth and development. *Mol Cell Endocrinol.* (2001) 179:39–46. doi: 10.1016/S0303-7207(01)00469-5

36. Choi J-H, Wong AST, Huang H-F, Leung PCK. Gonadotropins and ovarian cancer. *Endocr Rev.* (2007) 28:440–61. doi: 10.1210/er.2006-0036

37. Amsterdam A, Sasson R, Keren-Tal I, Aharoni D, Dantes A, Rimon E, et al. Alternative pathways of ovarian apoptosis: death for life. *Biochem Pharmacol.* (2003) 66:1355–62. doi: 10.1016/S0006-2952(03)00485-4

38. Casarini L, Reiter E, Simoni M. β-arrestins regulate gonadotropin receptor-mediated cell proliferation and apoptosis by controlling different FSHR or LHCGR intracellular signaling in the hGL5 cell line. *Mol Cell Endocrinol.* (2016) 437:11–21. doi: 10.1016/j.mce.2016.08.005

39. Gilman AG. A protein binding assay for adenosine 3':5'-cyclic monophosphate. *Proc Natl Acad Sci USA.* (1970) 67:305–12.

40. Conti M, Andersen CB, Richard F, Mehats C, Chun SY, Horner K, et al. Role of cyclic nucleotide signaling in oocyte maturation. *Mol Cell Endocrinol.* (2002) 187:153–9. doi: 10.1016/S0303-7207(01)00686-4

41. Sposini S, Hanyaloglu AC. Evolving view of membrane trafficking and signaling systems for G protein-coupled receptors. *Prog Mol Subcell Biol.* (2018) 57:273–99. doi: 10.1007/978-3-319-96704-2_10

42. Johnstone TB, Agarwal SR, Harvey RD, Ostrom RS. cAMP signaling compartmentation: adenylyl cyclases as anchors of dynamic signaling complexes. *Mol Pharmacol.* (2018) 93:270–6. doi: 10.1124/mol.117.110825

43. Conti M, Kasson BG, Hsueh AJ. Hormonal regulation of 3′,5′-adenosine monophosphate phosphodiesterases in cultured rat granulosa cells. *Endocrinology*. (1984) 114:2361–8. doi: 10.1210/endo-114-6-2361

44. Tréfier A, Musnier A, Landomiel F, Bourquard T, Boulo T, Ayoub MA, et al. G protein–dependent signaling triggers a β-arrestin–scaffolded p70S6K/rpS6 module that controls 5′TOP mRNA translation. *FASEB J*. (2018) 32:1154–69. doi: 10.1096/fj.201700763R

45. Carr DW, DeManno DA, Atwood A, Hunzicker-Dunn M, Scott JD. Follicle-stimulating hormone regulation of A-kinase anchoring proteins in granulosa cells. *J Biol Chem*. (1993) 268:20729–32.

46. Landmark BF, Fauske B, Eskild W, Skalhegg B, Lohmann SM, Hansson V, et al. Identification, characterization, and hormonal regulation of 3′,5′-cyclic adenosine monophosphate dependent protein kinases in rat sertoli cells*. *Endocrinology*. (1991) 129:2345–54. doi: 10.1210/endo-129-5-2345

47. Crépieux P, Marion S, Martinat N, Fafeur V, Vern YL, Kerboeuf D, et al. The ERK-dependent signalling is stage-specifically modulated by FSH, during primary Sertoli cell maturation. *Oncogene*. (2001) 20:4696–709. doi: 10.1038/sj.onc.1204632

48. Cottom J, Salvador LM, Maizels ET, Reierstad S, Park Y, Carr DW, et al. Follicle-stimulating hormone activates extracellular signal-regulated kinase but not extracellular signal-regulated kinase kinase through a 100-kDa phosphotyrosine phosphatase. *J Biol Chem*. (2003) 278:7167–79. doi: 10.1074/jbc.M203901200

49. Law NC, Donaubauer EM, Zeleznik AJ, Hunzicker-Dunn M. How protein kinase A activates canonical tyrosine kinase signaling pathways to promote granulosa cell differentiation. *Endocrinology*. (2017) 158:2043–51. doi: 10.1210/en.2017-00163

50. Kara E, Crépieux P, Gauthier C, Martinat N, Piketty V, Guillou F, et al. A phosphorylation cluster of five serine and threonine residues in the C-terminus of the follicle-stimulating hormone receptor is important for desensitization but not for beta-arrestin-mediated ERK activation. *Mol Endocrinol*. (2006) 20:3014–26. doi: 10.1210/me.2006-0098

51. Casarini L, Moriondo V, Marino M, Adversi F, Capodanno F, Grisolia C, et al. FSHR polymorphism p.N680S mediates different responses to FSH *in vitro*. *Mol Cell Endocrinol*. (2014) 393:83–91. doi: 10.1016/j.mce.2014.06.013

52. Manna PR, Chandrala SP, Jo Y, Stocco DM. cAMP-independent signaling regulates steroidogenesis in mouse Leydig cells in the absence of StAR phosphorylation. *J Mol Endocrinol*. (2006) 37:81–95. doi: 10.1677/jme.1.02065

53. Montminy MR, Bilezikjian LM. Binding of a nuclear protein to the cyclic-AMP response element of the somatostatin gene. *Nature*. (1987) 328:175–8. doi: 10.1038/328175a0

54. Moore RK, Otsuka F, Shimasaki S. Role of ERK1/2 in the differential synthesis of progesterone and estradiol by granulosa cells. *Biochem Biophys Res Commun*. (2001) 289:796–800. doi: 10.1006/bbrc.2001.6052

55. Tajima K, Yoshii K, Fukuda S, Orisaka M, Miyamoto K, Amsterdam A, et al. Luteinizing hormone-induced extracellular-signal regulated kinase activation differently modulates progesterone and androstenedione production in bovine theca cells. *Endocrinology*. (2005) 146:2903–10. doi: 10.1210/en.2005-0093

56. Amsterdam A, Hanoch T, Dantes A, Tajima K, Strauss JF, Seger R. Mechanisms of gonadotropin desensitization. *Mol Cell Endocrinol*. (2002) 187:69–74. doi: 10.1016/S0303-7207(01)00701-8

57. Peter AT, Dhanasekaran N. Apoptosis of granulosa cells: a review on the role of MAPK-signalling modules. *Reproduc Domestic Anim*. (2003) 38:209–13. doi: 10.1046/j.1439-0531.2003.00438.x

58. Salvador LM, Park Y, Cottom J, Maizels ET, Jones JC, Schillace RV, et al. Follicle-stimulating hormone stimulates protein kinase A-mediated histone H3 phosphorylation and acetylation leading to select gene activation in ovarian granulosa cells. *J Biol Chem*. (2001) 276:40146–55. doi: 10.1074/jbc.M106710200

59. DeManno DA, Cottom JE, Kline MP, Peters CA, Maizels ET, Hunzicker-Dunn M. Follicle-stimulating hormone promotes histone H3 phosphorylation on serine-10. *Mol Endocrinol*. (1999) 13:91–105. doi: 10.1210/mend.13.1.0222

60. Puri P, Little-Ihrig L, Chandran U, Law NC, Hunzicker-Dunn M, Zeleznik AJ. Protein kinase A: a master kinase of granulosa cell differentiation. *Sci Rep*. (2016) 6:28132. doi: 10.1038/srep28132

61. Schmidt M, Dekker FJ, Maarsingh H. Exchange protein directly activated by cAMP (epac): a multidomain cAMP mediator in the regulation of diverse biological functions. *Pharmacol Rev*. (2013) 65:670–709. doi: 10.1124/pr.110.003707

62. Choi J-H, Chen C-L, Poon SL, Wang H-S, Leung PCK. Gonadotropin-stimulated epidermal growth factor receptor expression in human ovarian surface epithelial cells: involvement of cyclic AMP-dependent exchange protein activated by cAMP pathway. *Endocr Relat Cancer*. (2009) 16:179–88. doi: 10.1677/ERC-07-0238

63. Meroni SB, Riera MF, Pellizzari EH, Cigorraga SB. Regulation of rat Sertoli cell function by FSH: possible role of phosphatidylinositol 3-kinase/protein kinase B pathway. *J Endocrinol*. (2002) 174:195–204. doi: 10.1677/joe.0.1740195

64. Amsterdam A, Dantes A, Selvaraj N, Aharoni D. Apoptosis in steroidogenic cells: structure-function analysis. *Steroids*. (1997) 62:207–11. doi: 10.1016/S0039-128X(96)00182-1

65. Amsterdam A, Gold RS, Hosokawa K, Yoshida Y, Sasson R, Jung Y, et al. Crosstalk among multiple signaling pathways controlling ovarian cell death. *Trends Endocrinol Metabol*. (1999) 10:255–62. doi: 10.1016/S1043-2760(99)00164-2

66. Uma J, Muraly P, Verma-Kumar S, Medhamurthy R. Determination of onset of apoptosis in granulosa cells of the preovulatory follicles in the bonnet monkey (*Macaca radiata*): correlation with mitogen-activated protein kinase activities. *Biol Reproduc*. (2003) 69:1379–87. doi: 10.1095/biolreprod.103.017897

67. Shiota M, Sugai N, Tamura M, Yamaguchi R, Fukushima N, Miyano T, et al. Correlation of mitogen-activated protein kinase activities with cell survival and apoptosis in porcine granulosa cells. *Zool Sci*. (2003) 20:193–201. doi: 10.2108/zsj.20.193

68. Gebauer G, Peter AT, Onesime D, Dhanasekaran N. Apoptosis of ovarian granulosa cells: correlation with the reduced activity of ERK-signaling module. *J Cell Biochem*. (1999) 75:547–54. doi: 10.1002/(SICI)1097-4644(19991215)75:43.3.CO;2-X

69. Schiffer Z, Keren-Tal I, Deutsch M, Dantes A, Aharoni D, Weinerb A, et al. Fourier analysis of differential light scattering for the quantitation of FSH response associated with structural changes in immortalized granulosa cells. *Mol Cell Endocrinol*. (1996) 118:145–53. doi: 10.1016/0303-7207(96)03774-4

70. Amsterdam A, Dantes A, Liscovitch M. Role of phospholipase-D and phosphatidic acid in mediating gonadotropin-releasing hormone-induced inhibition of preantral granulosa cell differentiation. *Endocrinology*. (1994) 135:1205–11. doi: 10.1210/endo.135.3.8070364

71. Maizels ET, Cottom J, Jones JC, Hunzicker-Dunn M. Follicle stimulating hormone (FSH) activates the p38 mitogen-activated protein kinase pathway, inducing small heat shock protein phosphorylation and cell rounding in immature rat ovarian granulosa cells. *Endocrinology*. (1998) 139:3353–6. doi: 10.1210/endo.139.7.6188

72. Di Giacomo M, Camaioni A, Klinger FG, Bonfiglio R, Salustri A. Cyclic AMP-elevating Agents promote cumulus cell survival and hyaluronan matrix stability, thereby prolonging the time of mouse oocyte fertilizability. *J Biol Chem*. (2016) 291:3821–36. doi: 10.1074/jbc.M115.680983

73. Yu F-Q, Han C-S, Yang W, Jin X, Hu Z-Y, Liu Y-X. Activation of the p38 MAPK pathway by follicle-stimulating hormone regulates steroidogenesis in granulosa cells differentially. *J Endocrinol*. (2005) 186:85–96. doi: 10.1677/joe.1.05955

74. Inagaki K, Otsuka F, Miyoshi T, Yamashita M, Takahashi M, Goto J, et al. p38-mitogen-activated protein kinase stimulated steroidogenesis in granulosa cell-oocyte cocultures: role of bone morphogenetic proteins 2 and 4. *Endocrinology*. (2009) 150:1921–30. doi: 10.1210/en.2008-0851

75. Li J, Zhou Q, Ma Z, Wang M, Shen W-J, Azhar S, et al. Feedback inhibition of CREB signaling by p38 MAPK contributes to the negative regulation of steroidogenesis. *Reproduc Biol Endocrinol*. (2017) 15:19. doi: 10.1186/s12958-017-0239-4

76. Tranchant T, Durand G, Gauthier C, Crépieux P, Ulloa-Aguirre A, Royère D, et al. Preferential β-arrestin signalling at low receptor density revealed by functional characterization of the human FSH receptor A189 V mutation?. *Mol Cell Endocrinol*. (2011) 331:109–18. doi: 10.1016/j.mce.2010.08.016

77. Sasson R, Dantes A, Tajima K, Amsterdam A. Novel genes modulated by FSH in normal and immortalized FSH-responsive cells: new

insights into the mechanism of FSH action. *FASEB J.* (2003) 17:1256–66. doi: 10.1096/fj.02-0740com

78. Jeppesen JV, Kristensen SG, Nielsen ME, Humaidan P, Dal Canto M, Fadini R, et al. LH-receptor gene expression in human granulosa and cumulus cells from antral and preovulatory follicles. *J Clin Endocrinol Metabol.* (2012) 97:E1524–31. doi: 10.1210/jc.2012-1427

79. Dupont J, Musnier A, Decourtye J, Boulo T, Lécureuil C, Guillou H, et al. FSH-stimulated PTEN activity accounts for the lack of FSH mitogenic effect in prepubertal rat Sertoli cells. *Mol Cell Endocrinol.* (2010) 315:271–6. doi: 10.1016/j.mce.2009.09.016

80. Yamashita Y, Okamoto M, Ikeda M, Okamoto A, Sakai M, Gunji Y, et al. Protein kinase C (PKC) increases TACE/ADAM17 enzyme activity in porcine ovarian somatic cells, which is essential for granulosa cell luteinization and oocyte maturation. *Endocrinology.* (2014) 155:1080–90. doi: 10.1210/en.2013-1655

81. Gorczynska E, Spaliviero J, Handelsman DJ. The relationship between 3′,5′-cyclic adenosine monophosphate and calcium in mediating follicle-stimulating hormone signal transduction in Sertoli cells. *Endocrinology.* (1994) 134:293–300. doi: 10.1210/endo.134.1.8275946

82. Meroni S, Cánepa D, Pellizzari E, Schteingart H, Cigorraga S. Regulation of gamma-glutamyl transpeptidase activity by Ca(2+)- and protein kinase C-dependent pathways in Sertoli cells. *Int J Androl.* (1997) 20:189–94. doi: 10.1046/j.1365-2605.1997.00053.x

83. Flores JA, Veldhuis JD, Leong DA. Follicle-stimulating hormone evokes an increase in intracellular free calcium ion concentrations in single ovarian (granulosa) cells. *Endocrinology.* (1990) 127:3172–9. doi: 10.1210/endo-127-6-3172

84. Loss ES, Jacobus AP, Wassermann GF. Rapid signaling responses in Sertoli cell membranes induced by follicle stimulating hormone and testosterone: calcium inflow and electrophysiological changes. *Life Sci.* (2011) 89:577–83. doi: 10.1016/j.lfs.2011.05.017

85. Lin Y-F, Tseng M-J, Hsu H-L, Wu Y-W, Lee Y-H, Tsai Y-H. A novel follicle-stimulating hormone-induced G alpha h/phospholipase C-delta1 signaling pathway mediating rat sertoli cell Ca2+-influx. *Mol Endocrinol.* (2006) 20:2514–27. doi: 10.1210/me.2005-0347

86. Donadeu FX, Ascoli M. The differential effects of the gonadotropin receptors on aromatase expression in primary cultures of immature rat granulosa cells are highly dependent on the density of receptors expressed and the activation of the inositol phosphate cascade. *Endocrinology.* (2005) 146:3907–16. doi: 10.1210/en.2005-0403

87. Flores JA, Leong DA, Veldhuis JD. Is the calcium signal induced by follicle-stimulating hormone in swine granulosa cells mediated by adenosine cyclic 3′,5′-monophosphate-dependent protein kinase? *Endocrinology.* (1992) 130:1862–6. doi: 10.1210/endo.130.4.1547716

88. Mellor H, Parker PJ. The extended protein kinase C superfamily. *Biochem J.* (1998) 332(Pt 2):281–92. doi: 10.1042/bj3320281

89. Tepekoy F, Ustunel I, Akkoyunlu G. Protein kinase C isoforms α, δ and ε are differentially expressed in mouse ovaries at different stages of postnatal development. *J Ovarian Res.* (2014) 7:117. doi: 10.1186/s13048-014-0117-z

90. Manna PR, Pakarainen P, Rannikko AS, Huhtaniemi IT. Mechanisms of desensitization of follicle-stimulating hormone (FSH) action in a murine granulosa cell line stably transfected with the human FSH receptor complementary deoxyribonucleic acid. *Mol Cell Endocrinol.* (1998) 146:163–76. doi: 10.1016/S0303-7207(98)00156-7

91. González Reyes J, Santana P, González Robaina I, Cabrera Oliva J, Estévez F, Hernández I, et al. Effect of the protein phosphatase inhibitor okadaic acid on FSH-induced granulosa cell steroidogenesis. *J Endocrinol.* (1997) 152:131–9. doi: 10.1677/joe.0.1520131

92. Nemer A, Azab AN, Rimon G, Lamprecht S, Ben-Menahem D. Different roles of cAMP/PKA and PKC signaling in regulating progesterone and PGE2 levels in immortalized rat granulosa cell cultures. *Gen Comp Endocrinol.* (2018) 269:88–95. doi: 10.1016/j.ygcen.2018.08.019

93. Jamaluddin M, Molnár M, Marrone BL, Hertelendy F. Signal transduction in avian granulosa cells: effects of protein kinase C inhibitors. *Gen Comp Endocrinol.* (1994) 93:471–9. doi: 10.1006/gcen.1994.1051

94. Eskola V, Ryhänen P, Savisalo M, Rannikko A, Kananen K, Sprengel R, et al. Stable transfection of the rat follicle-stimulating hormone receptor

complementary DNA into an immortalized murine Sertoli cell line. *Mol Cell Endocrinol.* (1998) 139:143–52. doi: 10.1016/S0303-7207(98)00063-X

95. Eikvar L, Taskén KA, Eskild W, Hansson V. Protein kinase C activation and positive and negative agonist regulation of 3′,5′-cyclic adenosine monophosphate levels in cultured rat Sertoli cells. *Acta Endocrinol.* (1993) 128:568–72. doi: 10.1530/acta.0.1280568

96. Fagnen G, Phamantu NT, Bocquet J, Bonnamy PJ. Activation of protein kinase C increases proteoglycan synthesis in immature rat Sertoli cells. *Biochim Biophys Acta.* (1999) 1472:250–61. doi: 10.1016/S0304-4165(99)00128-2

97. Cooke BA, Choi MC, Dirami G, Lopez-Ruiz MP, West AP. Control of steroidogenesis in Leydig cells. *J Steroid Biochem Mol Biol.* (1992) 43:445–9. doi: 10.1016/0960-0760(92)90083-U

98. Manna PR, Soh J-W, Stocco DM. The involvement of specific PKC isoenzymes in phorbol ester-mediated regulation of steroidogenic acute regulatory protein expression and steroid synthesis in mouse leydig cells. *Endocrinology.* (2011) 152:313–25. doi: 10.1210/en.2010-0874

99. Manna PR, Huhtaniemi IT, Stocco DM. Mechanisms of protein kinase C signaling in the modulation of 3′,5′-cyclic adenosine monophosphate-mediated steroidogenesis in mouse gonadal cells. *Endocrinology.* (2009) 150:3308–17. doi: 10.1210/en.2008-1668

100. Costa RR, Reis RI dos, Aguiar JF, Varanda WA. Luteinizing hormone (LH) acts through PKA and PKC to modulate T-type calcium currents and intracellular calcium transients in mice Leydig cells. *Cell Calcium.* (2011) 49:191–9. doi: 10.1016/j.ceca.2011.02.003

101. Zachow RJ, Terranova PF. Involvement of protein kinase C and protein tyrosine kinase pathways in tumor necrosis factor-alpha-induced clustering of ovarian theca-interstitial cells. *Mol Cell Endocrinol.* (1993) 97:37–49. doi: 10.1016/0303-7207(93)90209-3

102. Leevers SJ, Vanhaesebroeck B, Waterfield MD. Signalling through phosphoinositide 3-kinases: the lipids take centre stage. *Curr Opin Cell Biol.* (1999) 11:219–25. doi: 10.1016/S0955-0674(99)80029-5

103. Nicholls PK, Harrison CA, Walton KL, McLachlan RI, O'Donnell L, Stanton PG. Hormonal regulation of sertoli cell micro-RNAs at spermiation. *Endocrinology.* (2011) 152:1670–83. doi: 10.1210/en.2010-1341

104. Hunzicker-Dunn ME, Lopez-Biladeau B, Law NC, Fiedler SE, Carr DW, Maizels ET. PKA and GAB2 play central roles in the FSH signaling pathway to PI3K and AKT in ovarian granulosa cells. *Proc Natl Acad Sci.* (2012) 109:E2979–88. doi: 10.1073/pnas.1205661109

105. Chen Y-J, Hsiao P-W, Lee M-T, Mason JI, Ke F-C, Hwang J-J. Interplay of PI3K and cAMP/PKA signaling, and rapamycin-hypersensitivity in TGFbeta1 enhancement of FSH-stimulated steroidogenesis in rat ovarian granulosa cells. *J Endocrinol.* (2007) 192:405–19. doi: 10.1677/JOE-06-0076

106. Rehnitz J, Alcoba DD, Brum IS, Hinderhofer K, Youness B, Strowitzki T, et al. FMR1 and AKT/mTOR signalling pathways: potential functional interactions controlling folliculogenesis in human granulosa cells. *Reproduc BioMed.* (2017) 35:485–93. doi: 10.1016/j.rbmo.2017.07.016

107. King D, Yeomanson D, Bryant HE. PI3King the lock: targeting the PI3K/Akt/mTOR pathway as a novel therapeutic strategy in neuroblastoma. *J Pediatr Hematol/Oncol.* (2015) 37:245–51. doi: 10.1097/MPH.0000000000000329

108. Alam H, Maizels ET, Park Y, Ghaey S, Feiger ZJ, Chandel NS, et al. Follicle-stimulating hormone activation of hypoxia-inducible factor-1 by the phosphatidylinositol 3-kinase/AKT/Ras homolog enriched in brain (Rheb)/mammalian target of rapamycin (mTOR) pathway is necessary for induction of select protein markers of follicular differentiation. *J Biol Chem.* (2004) 279:19431–40. doi: 10.1074/jbc.M401235200

109. Lécureuil C, Tesseraud S, Kara E, Martinat N, Sow A, Fontaine I, et al. Follicle-stimulating hormone activates p70 ribosomal protein S6 kinase by protein kinase A-mediated dephosphorylation of Thr 421/Ser 424 in primary Sertoli cells. *Mol Endocrinol.* (2005) 19:1812–20. doi: 10.1210/me.2004-0289

110. Musnier A, Heitzler D, Boulo T, Tesseraud S, Durand G, Lécureuil C, et al. Developmental regulation of p70 S6 kinase by a G protein-coupled receptor dynamically modelized in primary cells. *Cell Mol Life Sci.* (2009) 66:3487–503. doi: 10.1007/s00018-009-0134-z

111. Park Y, Maizels ET, Feiger ZJ, Alam H, Peters CA, Woodruff TK, et al. Induction of cyclin D2 in rat granulosa cells requires FSH-dependent relief

from FOXO1 repression coupled with positive signals from Smad. *J Biol Chem.* (2005) 280:9135–48. doi: 10.1074/jbc.M409486200

112. Shen M, Jiang Y, Guan Z, Cao Y, Sun S-C, Liu H. FSH protects mouse granulosa cells from oxidative damage by repressing mitophagy. *Sci Rep.* (2016) 6:38090. doi: 10.1038/srep38090

113. Shen M, Jiang Y, Guan Z, Cao Y, Li L, Liu H, et al. Protective mechanism of FSH against oxidative damage in mouse ovarian granulosa cells by repressing autophagy. *Autophagy.* (2017) 13:1364–85. doi: 10.1080/15548627.2017.1327941

114. Li Z, Zhang P, Zhang Z, Pan B, Chao H, Li L, et al. A co-culture system with preantral follicular granulosa cells *in vitro* induces meiotic maturation of immature oocytes. *Histochem Cell Biol.* (2011) 135:513–22. doi: 10.1007/s00418-011-0812-4

115. Kalous J, Kubelka M, Šolc P, Šušor A, Motlík J. AKT (protein kinase B) is implicated in meiotic maturation of porcine oocytes. *Reproduction.* (2009) 138:645–54. doi: 10.1530/REP-08-0461

116. Han SJ, Vaccari S, Nedachi T, Andersen CB, Kovacina KS, Roth RA, et al. Protein kinase B/Akt phosphorylation of PDE3A and its role in mammalian oocyte maturation. *EMBO J.* (2006) 25:5716–25. doi: 10.1038/sj.emboj.7601431

117. Kishimoto T. A primer on meiotic resumption in starfish oocytes: the proposed signaling pathway triggered by maturation-inducing hormone. *Mol Reproduc Dev.* (2011) 78:704–7. doi: 10.1002/mrd.21343

118. Casarini L, Lispi M, Longobardi S, Milosa F, La Marca A, Tagliasacchi D, et al. LH and hCG action on the same receptor results in quantitatively and qualitatively different intracellular signalling. *PLoS ONE.* (2012) 7:e46682. doi: 10.1371/journal.pone.0046682

119. Casarini L, Santi D, Brigante G, Simoni M. Two hormones for one receptor: evolution, biochemistry, actions and pathophysiology of LH and hCG. *Endocr Rev.* (2018) 2018:65. doi: 10.1210/er.2018-00065

120. Casarini L, Riccetti L, De Pascali F, Nicoli A, Tagliavini S, Trenti T, et al. Follicle-stimulating hormone potentiates the steroidogenic activity of chorionic gonadotropin and the anti-apoptotic activity of luteinizing hormone in human granulosa-lutein cells *in vitro*. *Mol Cell Endocrinol.* (2016) 422:103–14. doi: 10.1016/j.mce.2015.12.008

121. Riccetti L, Sperduti S, Lazzaretti C, Casarini L, Simoni M. The cAMP/PKA pathway: steroidogenesis of the antral follicular stage. *Miner Ginecol.* (2018) 2018:4282. doi: 10.23736/S0026-4784.18.04282-X

122. Makker A, Goel MM, Mahdi AA. PI3K/PTEN/Akt and TSC/mTOR signaling pathways, ovarian dysfunction, and infertility: an update. *J Mol Endocrinol.* (2014) 53:R103–18. doi: 10.1530/JME-14-0220

123. Nascimento AR, Macheroni C, Lucas TFG, Porto CS, Lazari MFM. Crosstalk between FSH and relaxin at the end of the proliferative stage of rat Sertoli cells. *Reproduction.* (2016) 152:613–28. doi: 10.1530/REP-16-0330

124. Meroni SB, Riera MF, Pellizzari EH, Galardo MN, Cigorraga SB. FSH activates phosphatidylinositol 3-kinase/protein kinase B signaling pathway in 20-day-old Sertoli cells independently of IGF-I. *J Endocrinol.* (2004) 180:257–65. doi: 10.1677/joe.0.1800257

125. Hunzicker-Dunn M, Maizels E. FSH signaling pathways in immature granulosa cells that regulate target gene expression: branching out from protein kinase A. *Cell Signal.* (2006) 18:1351–9. doi: 10.1016/j.cellsig.2006.02.011

Permissions

The contributors of this book come from diverse backgrounds, making this book a truly international effort. This book will bring forth new frontiers with its revolutionizing research information and detailed analysis of the nascent developments around the world.

We would like to thank all the contributing authors for lending their expertise to make the book truly unique. They have played a crucial role in the development of this book. Without their invaluable contributions this book wouldn't have been possible. They have made vital efforts to compile up to date information on the varied aspects of this subject to make this book a valuable addition to the collection of many professionals and students.

This book was conceptualized with the vision of imparting up-to-date information and advanced data in this field. To ensure the same, a matchless editorial board was set up. Every individual on the board went through rigorous rounds of assessment to prove their worth. After which they invested a large part of their time researching and compiling the most relevant data for our readers.

The editorial board has been involved in producing this book since its inception. They have spent rigorous hours researching and exploring the diverse topics which have resulted in the successful publishing of this book. They have passed on their knowledge of decades through this book. To expedite this challenging task, the publisher supported the team at every step. A small team of assistant editors was also appointed to further simplify the editing procedure and attain best results for the readers.

Apart from the editorial board, the designing team has also invested a significant amount of their time in understanding the subject and creating the most relevant covers. They scrutinized every image to scout for the most suitable representation of the subject and create an appropriate cover for the book.

The publishing team has been an ardent support to the editorial, designing and production team. Their endless efforts to recruit the best for this project, has resulted in the accomplishment of this book. They are a veteran in the field of academics and their pool of knowledge is as vast as their experience in printing. Their expertise and guidance has proved useful at every step. Their uncompromising quality standards have made this book an exceptional effort. Their encouragement from time to time has been an inspiration for everyone.

The publisher and the editorial board hope that this book will prove to be a valuable piece of knowledge for researchers, students, practitioners and scholars across the globe.

List of Contributors

Hermann M. Behre
Center for Reproductive Medicine and Andrology, University Hospital Halle, Martin Luther University Halle-Wittenberg, Halle, Germany

Elodie Kara, Laurence Dupuy, Sophie Casteret and Marie-Christine Maurel
Igyxos SA, Nouzilly, France

Céline Bouillon
Igyxos SA, Nouzilly, France
Service de Médecine et Biologie de la Reproduction, CHRU de Tours, Tours, France
Biologie Intégrative de l'Ovaire, INRA, UMR85, Physiologie de la Reproduction et des Comportements Nouzilly, France
CNRS, UMR7247, Nouzilly, France
Université François Rabelais, Tours, France
IFCE, Nouzilly, France

Monica Muratori
Department of Experimental and Clinical Biomedical Sciences "Mario Serio", University of Florence, Florence, Italy

Elisabetta Baldi
Department Experimental and Clinical Medicine, University of Florence, Florence, Italy

Joop S. E. Laven
Division of Reproductive Endocrinology and Infertility, Department of Obstetrics and Gynaecology, Erasmus University Medical Center, Rotterdam, Netherlands

Daria Lizneva, Alina Rahimova, Se-Min Kim, Ihor Atabiekov, Seher Javaid, Bateel Alamoush, Charit Taneja, Ayesha Khan, Li Sun, Tony Yuen and Mone Zaidi
The Mount Sinai Bone Program, Department of Medicine, Icahn School of Medicine at Mount Sinai, New York, NY, United States

Ricardo Azziz
Academic Health and Hospital Affairs, State University of New York, Albany, NY, United States

Stella Campo, Luz Andreone and Verónica Ambao
Centro de Investigaciones Endocrinológicas "Dr. César Bergadá" (CEDIE), Buenos Aires, Argentina, Instituto

Ricardo S. Calandra and Susana B. Rulli
Medicina Experimental (IBYME-CONICET), Buenos Aires, Argentina

Alessandro Conforti, Francesca Bagnulo, Stefania Peluso, Luigi Carbone and Giuseppe De Placido
Department of Neuroscience, Reproductive Science and Odontostomatology, University of Naples Federico II, Naples, Italy

Alberto Vaiarelli, Danilo Cimadomo and Filippo Maria Ubaldi
G.E.N.E.R.A. Centre for Reproductive Medicine, Clinica Valle Giulia, Rome, Italy

Francesca Di Rella
Medical Oncology, Department of Senology, National Cancer Institute, IRCCS Fondazione G. Pascale, Naples, Italy

Ilpo Huhtaniemi
Department of Surgery and Cancer, Institute of Reproductive and Developmental Biology, Imperial College London, London, United Kingdom
Department of Physiology, University of Turku, Turku, Finland

Carlo Alvigg
Department of Neuroscience, Reproductive Science and Odontostomatology, University of Naples Federico II, Naples, Italy
Istituto per l'Endocrinologia e l'Oncologia Sperimentale (IEOS) Consiglio Nazionale delle Ricerche, Naples, Italy

Ross C. Anderson
Centre for Neuroendocrinology, Department of Physiology, Faculty of Health Sciences, University of Pretoria, Pretoria, South Africa

Claire L. Newton
Centre for Neuroendocrinology, Department of Immunology, Faculty of Health Sciences, University of Pretoria, Pretoria, South Africa

Robert P. Millar
Centre for Neuroendocrinology, Department of Immunology, Faculty of Health Sciences, University of Pretoria, Pretoria, South Africa
Department of Integrative Biomedical Sciences, Faculty of Health Sciences, University of Cape Town, Cape Town, South Africa

Bruno Lunenfeld
Faculty of Life Sciences, Bar-Ilan University, Ramat Gan, Israel

Wilma Bilger
Medical Affairs Fertility, Endocrinology and General Medicine, Merck Serono GmbH, Darmstadt, Germany

Salvatore Longobardi
Global Medical Affairs Fertility, Merck Healthcare KGaA, Darmstadt, Germany

Veronica Alam
Global Clinical Development, EMD Serono, Rockland, MA, United States
A Business of Merck KGaA, Darmstadt, Germany

Thomas D'Hooghe
Global Medical Affairs Fertility, Merck Healthcare KGaA, Darmstadt, Germany
Organ Systems, Group Biomedical Sciences, Department of Development and Regeneration, KU Leuven (University of Leuven), Leuven, Belgium
Department of Obstetrics and Gynecology, Yale University, New Haven, CT, United States

Sesh K. Sunkara
Assisted Conception Unit, King's College London, Guy's Hospital, London, United Kingdom

Carolyn Sadler
Division of Reproductive Sciences, Department of Obstetrics and Gynecology, University of Colorado Anschutz Medical Campus, Aurora, IL, United States

Rosemary McDonald
Division of Reproductive Sciences, Department of Obstetrics and Gynecology, University of Colorado Anschutz Medical Campus, Aurora, IL, United States
Integrated Physiology Graduate Program, University of Colorado Anschutz Medical Campus, Aurora, IL, United States

T. Rajendra Kumar
Division of Reproductive Sciences, Department of Obstetrics and Gynecology, University of Colorado Anschutz Medical Campus, Aurora, IL, United States,
Integrated Physiology Graduate Program, University of Colorado Anschutz Medical Campus, Aurora, IL, United States
Division of Reproductive Endocrinology and Infertility, Department of Obstetrics and Gynecology, University of Colorado Anschutz Medical Campus, Aurora, IL, United States
Department of Obstetrics and Gynecology, University of Colorado Anschutz Medical Campus, Aurora, CO, United States

James A. Dias
Department of Biomedical Sciences, School of Public Health, University at Albany, Albany, NY, United States

Niamh Sayers and Aylin C. Hanyaloglu
Department Surgery and Cancer, Institute of Reproductive and Developmental Biology, Imperial College London

Frank J. Broekmans
University Medical Center Utrecht, Utrecht, Netherlands

Maria Schubert
Department of Clinical and Surgical Andrology, Centre of Reproductive Medicine and Andrology, University Hospital Münster, Münster, Germany

Lina Pérez Lanuza and Jörg Gormoll
Medicine and Andrology, University Hospital Münster, Münster, Germany

Olayiwola O. Oduwole
Department of Surgery and Cancer, Institute of Reproductive and Developmental Biology, Imperial College London, London, United Kingdom

Hellevi Peltoketo
Cancer and Translational Medicine Research Unit, Laboratory of Cancer Genetics and Tumor Biology, Biocenter Oulu University of Oulu, Oulu, Finland

George R. Bousfield and Jeffrey V. May
Department of Biological Sciences, Wichita State University, Wichita, KS, United States

John S. Davis
Department of Obstetrics and Gynecology, University of Nebraska Medical Center, Omaha, NE, United States
Departments of Biochemistry and Molecular Biology, University of Nebraska Medical Center, Omaha, NE, United States
Nebraska-Western Iowa Health Care System, Omaha, NE, United States

Laura Riccetti, Samantha Sperduti and Silvia Limoncella
Unit of Endocrinology, Department of Biomedical, Metabolic and Neural Sciences, University of Modena and Reggio Emilia

Clara Lazzaretti and Elia Paradiso
Unit of Endocrinology, Department of Biomedical, Metabolic and Neural Sciences, University of Modena and Reggio Emilia
International PhD School in Clinical and Experimental Medicine, University of Modena and Reggio Emilia

Danièle Klett , Francesco De Pascali and Eric Reiter
PRC, INRA, CNRS, IFCE, Université de Tours, Nouzilly, France

Francesco Potì
Unit of Neurosciences, Department of Medicine and Surgery, University of Parma, Parma, Italy

Eugenio Galano, Angelo Palmese and Abhijeet Satwekar
Analytical Development Biotech Products, Merck Serono S.p.A. (an affiliate of Merck KGaA, Darmstadt, Germany), Rome, Italy

Jessica Daolio, Alessia Nicoli, Maria Teresa Villani and Lorenzo Aguzzoli
Azienda Unità Sanitaria Locale—IRCCS di Reggio Emilia, Department of Obstetrics and Gynaecology, Fertility Center, ASMN, Reggio Emilia, Italy

Adolfo Rivero-Müller
Department of Biochemistry and Molecular Biology, Medical University of Lublin, Lublin, Poland
Cell Biology, Biosciences, Faculty of Science and Engineering, Åbo Akademi University, Turku, Finland

Manuela Simoni
Unit of Endocrinology, Department of Biomedical, Metabolic and Neural Sciences, University of Modena and Reggio Emilia
PRC, INRA, CNRS, IFCE, Université de Tours, Nouzilly, France
Center for Genomic Research, University of Modena and Reggio Emilia, Modena, Italy
Unit of Endocrinology, Department of Medical Specialties, Azienda Ospedaliero-Universitaria, Modena, Italy Recombi

Flavie Landomiel, Pauline Raynaud, Frédéric Jean-Alphonse, Romain Yvinec, Lucie P. Pellissier, Véronique Bozon, Gilles Bruneau, Pascale Crépieux and Anne Poupon
PRC, INRA, CNRS, IFCE, Université de Tours, Nouzilly, France

Simonetta Tagliavini and Tommaso Trenti
Department of Laboratory Medicine and Pathological Anatomy, Azienda USL, NOCSAE, Modena, Italy

Alfredo Ulloa-Aguirre, Teresa Zariñán and Rubén Gutiérrez-Sagal
Red de Apoyo a la Investigación, Universidad Nacional Autónoma de México and Instituto Nacional de Ciencias Médicas y Nutrición Salvador Zubirán, Mexico City, Mexico

Eduardo Jardón-Valadez
Departamento de Ciencias Ambientales, Universidad Autónoma Metropolitana Unidad Lerma, Lerma, Mexico

Kamila Szymańska, Joanna Kałafut, Alicja Przybyszewska, Beata Paziewska and Michał Kiełbus
Department of Biochemistry and Molecular Biology, Medical University of Lublin, Lublin, Poland

Grzegorz Adamczuk
Independent Medical Biology Unit, Medical University of Lublin, Lublin, Poland

Livio Casarini
Unit of Endocrinology, Department of Biomedical, Metabolic and Neural Sciences, University of Modena and Reggio Emilia Center for Genomic Research, University of Modena and Reggio Emilia, Modena, Italy

Index

Printed in the USA
CPSIA information can be obtained
at www.ICGtesting.com
JSHW051359091023
49903JS00006B/207